Forensic Pathology

Rebekah Jacques
Editor

Forensic Pathology

Death Investigation Bioethics and Other Medicolegal Principles

Springer

Editor
Rebekah Jacques
London Health Sciences Centre
University Hospital
London, ON, Canada

ISBN 978-3-031-42037-5 ISBN 978-3-031-42038-2 (eBook)
https://doi.org/10.1007/978-3-031-42038-2

This Springer imprint is published by the registered company Springer Nature Switzerland AG
The registered company address is: Gewerbestrasse 11, 6330 Cham, Switzerland

Paper in this product is recyclable.

To murdered and missing Indigenous women and girls; their families and communities

Foreword

Although it surprises many people, forensic pathology in Canada is one of the smallest and newest subspecialties of Medicine. It was only in 2008 that the first Canadian forensic pathology postgraduate training program was accredited by the Royal College of Physicians and Surgeons of Canada at the University of Toronto. However, in the years that followed there has been a progressive development of forensic pathology in Canada. One milestone in this development has been the emergence of a strong new generation of forensic pathologists in Canada, who are making significant contributions to our field. One such contribution is this impressive volume on forensic pathology by Dr. Rebekah Jacques, who is one of the early graduates of our forensic pathology training program in Toronto. This book is only the third book ever written on the topic in Canada and its addition to the literature represents a truly modern synthesis of the subject matter. The observant reader will notice topics that are not typically included in introductory forensic texts, such as biomedical ethics, grief, and the role of molecular diagnostics in autopsies.

This book also underscores the pivotal centerpiece of forensic pathology: the autopsy. In the Twenty-first century, the autopsy is a tool that not only provides the truth about how people die, but it is also an important mechanism to sustain human rights and contribute to public health. The perspective in this book demonstrates how those important contributions of forensic pathology can be realized in the modern world. Furthermore, the description of classical topics, such as injury interpretation, and the interpretation of toxicological data is also provided.

Dr. Jacques and her colleagues have succeeded in producing a useful addition to medical and scientific literature. It is also wonderful to see that Canadian forensic pathologists and other forensic scientists have collaborated on such an important and impressive book. Dr. Jacques, who is one of the first Indigenous forensic pathologists in Canada, is clearly an emerging leader in our field in Canada, much to the benefit of society more broadly. This is even more important as Canada develops it approach to the forensic aspects of Indian Residential Schools.

It is my hope that many young people will read this book and become inspired to start their own journey in the world of forensic medicine and science!

Department of Laboratory Medicine and Pathobiology
University of Toronto,
Toronto, ON, Canada
Michael S. Pollanen

Preface

I first became interested in forensic pathology as a possible career by reading a book that discussed forensic pathology at the local library in my small hometown in northern Ontario, Canada. Forensic pathology was intriguing because this field of medicine deals with a broad spectrum of knowledge that can be collected at autopsy. This knowledge can be used to contribute to the understanding of what happened to a deceased person by establishing the cause and manner of death. In addition, this knowledge can be used to make an identification of a dead body so that repatriation to families can occur.

Today, there are many outstanding forensic pathology textbooks that bring the reader through the procedures that are required in the examination of a dead body. Such texts do not have a comprehensive analysis of the "softer" topics in forensic pathology, which are sometimes "harder" to master when compared to the procedural skills of the autopsy. These "softer" skills include speaking to next of kin, death investigation bioethics, and testifying as an expert witness. These topics have dedicated spaces and chapters in Part I of this textbook and reflect the experience in Ontario, Canada. Chapters in Part II covers topics that are included in many forensic pathology textbooks but also includes a chapter on the Negative Medicolegal Autopsy, which brings together various aspects and pathology frameworks that are covered in part by other textbooks and journal articles but have not previously been collated in one chapter. Part III covers the deaths from special populations that may enter medicolegal death investigation systems and the unique challenges associated with these deaths. This section has a designated chapter on geriatric populations, which includes a discussion on the emerging concern of fatal maltreatment of older adults. Guest authors have been invited to author topics to provide diversity of perspectives and expertise.

Although this book is written for trainees, pathologists, and non-pathologists that work in death investigation, it is hoped that a copy of this text will also fall into the hands of a novice and inspire a career in forensic pathology.

London, Canada Rebekah Jacques

Acknowledgments

I would like to acknowledge the assistance of the following for their contribution to this undertaking:

I am grateful to have been able to edit this work on the Great Lakes region of Turtle Island and the territory of the Anishnaabek, Haudenosaunee, Lūnaapéewak, and Chonnocton peoples. I am grateful to my spouse, Rejan Royer, for his unconditional support. Kelley Matthews (Department of Pathology, London Health Sciences Centre [LHSC] for her secretarial assistance; Kathilyn Allewell (Department of Pathology and Laboratory Medicine [PaLM] at Western University) for the preparation of the figures in the blunt trauma chapter; Brooke Day, former undergraduate student at Western University for handling and managing numerous references and editing the reference style; Dr. Edward Tweedie (Regional Forensic Pathology Unit, London, Ontario, Canada) for his contributions of figures; Dr. David Ramsay for his contribution to figures and his review of the blunt trauma chapter; Dr. Elena Tugaleva (Regional Forensic Pathology Unit, London, Ontario, Canada) for her collegial support; bioethicists Launa Elliott and Daniel Wyzynski (LHSC) for their thoughtful review of the death investigation bioethics chapter; Dr. Christopher Sherrin (professor and associate dean in the Faculty of Law at Western University) and Mark J. Sandler (criminal defense counsel at Cooper, Sandler, Shime & Schwartzentruber LLP) for their critical review of the principles of courtroom testimony chapter; Dr. Subrata Chakrabarti (Chief of PaLM at LHSC) for his help and encouragement; guest authors for their insights; Drs. David King, Chitra Rao, Michael Pollanen, Michael Shkrum, and the late Dr. John Fernandes for fostering my interest in forensic pathology; the coroners, legal counsel, judges, and various police agencies in Ontario for their contributions to death investigation; pathology staff with whom I have worked with over the years in Ontario for their dedication to the medicolegal autopsy service; the many individuals associated with the publisher, Springer. I especially want to thank those who have died and given me gifts of knowledge.

Contents

Part I Principles of Medicolegal Death Investigations

1 **Medicolegal Death Investigations and the Autopsy** 3
Rebekah Jacques and Liz Siydock

2 **Death Investigation Bioethics** 53
Rebekah Jacques

3 **Principles of Courtroom Testimony** 95
Rebekah Jacques

Part II Medicolegal Postmortem Examination

4 **Sudden and Unexpected Natural Deaths in Adults** 127
Kris Cunningham and Qi Zhang

5 **Drug-Related Deaths** 161
Karen Woodall

6 **Physics 101 and Classification of Injury** 185
Rebekah Jacques

7 **Blunt Trauma** 189
Michael J. Shkrum

8 **Sharp Force Injuries** 233
Rebekah Jacques

9 **Asphyxia & Anogenital Injuries** 249
Rebekah Jacques

10 **Firearm-Related Injuries** 283
Rebekah Jacques

11 **Environmental Injuries** 303
Rebekah Jacques

12 The Negative Medicolegal Autopsy ... 319
Rebekah Jacques

Part III Medicolegal Death Investigations of Special Populations

13 Pediatrics ... 339
Rebekah Jacques

14 Maternal Deaths ... 369
Joseph A. Prahlow and Theodore T. Brown

15 The Pathology of Elder Abuse and Neglect ... 397
Rebekah Jacques and Qi Zhang

Index ... 431

Part I
Principles of Medicolegal Death Investigations

Chapter 1
Medicolegal Death Investigations and the Autopsy

Rebekah Jacques and Liz Siydock

Death Investigation Systems

Death investigation systems have implications for bereaved families, public health, social policy, child welfare agencies, organ procurement organizations, law enforcement, and the legal system. A core function of the death investigation system is to certify the identity, cause, and manner of death of individuals who die within the jurisdiction of the regional death investigation system. Properly funded and independent death investigation systems can also function as a public service. The system can offer a variety of public service benefits from the information and knowledge obtained from deaths to many stakeholders including law enforcement, public health departments, the public, and bereaved families. Judiciary stakeholders and law enforcement depend on the death investigation system to prosecute crimes and guide investigations. Public health departments rely on the system for disease monitoring and data collection. Bereaved families rely on the death investigation system to identify their loved ones, provide clear explanations for the cause of death, and screen for hereditary diseases. Organ procurement organizations rely on death investigation systems to permit postmortem organ and tissue donation.

Government-sponsored medicolegal death investigation is an important function to understand why its citizens die in order to prevent future premature deaths. Central to determine how citizens die is through the medicolegal autopsy. The medicolegal autopsy is performed on the instruction of the legal authority responsible for the investigation of sudden, unexpected, or unexplained deaths. The circumstances that warrant a medicolegal autopsy are variable from nation to nation and even

R. Jacques (✉)
London Health Sciences Centre, London, ON, Canada
e-mail: rebekah.jacques@lhsc.on.ca

L. Siydock
Office of the Chief Coroner and Ontario Forensic Pathology Service, Toronto, ON, Canada

R. Jacques (ed.), *Forensic Pathology*,
https://doi.org/10.1007/978-3-031-42038-2_1

region to region. This is in part because the authority to investigate deaths by a legally qualified administrator depends on the jurisdiction. The legal authority is variable across the globe and includes coroner, medical examiner, and continental systems (Fig. 1.1).

One of the primary functions of the death investigation system is to certify the identification, cause, and manner of death for individuals whose deaths fall in their jurisdiction. The cause of death can be determined by the performance of an autopsy on the decedent. The autopsy is authorized by statute for the greater public good. Under the legal authority, a medicolegal autopsy can be ordered without the permission of bereaved relatives. However, the autopsy is performed by a physician qualified to do so, usually a forensic pathologist. Although the final product of the death investigation systems is to produce a medical death certificate, the administration and processes differ between the systems.

The majority of deaths are caused by natural diseases that have been diagnosed by a physician. Usually, these deaths do not fall under the jurisdiction of the medicolegal death investigation system. Unexplained natural deaths and deaths caused by injuries or drugs are typically investigated. These deaths must be reported to and investigated by the representative authority of the medicolegal death investigation system, which can be a coroner or medical examiner (Fig. 1.2). The percentage of

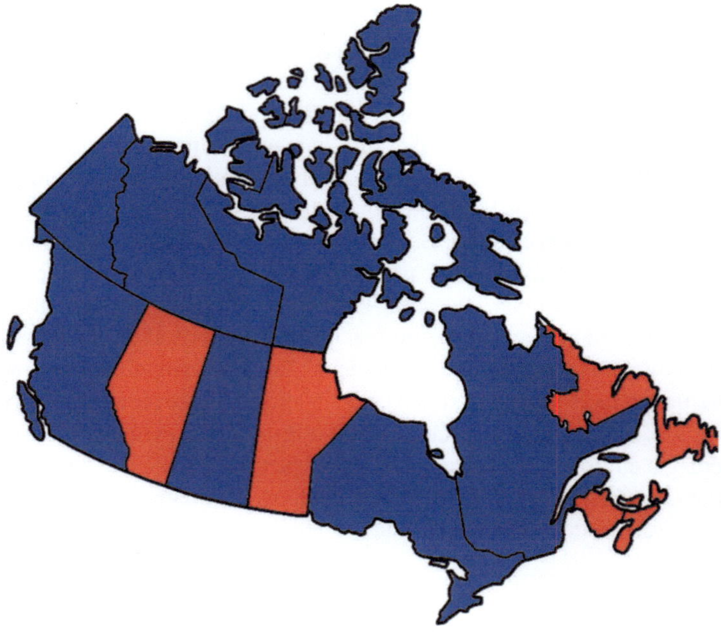

Fig. 1.1 Canadian Death Investigation systems by province and territory are largely divided into a coroner system (lay and medical) and a medical examiner system. Continental systems are absent

Coroner	Medical Examiner
Citizen	Physician
No specified training	Pathologist forensic board certified (usually)
Administrator or Law enforcement	Public Health Role
Elected or appointed	Appointed (usually)

Fig. 1.2 General comparison of coroner and medical examiner. Exceptions are not noted here

deaths investigated is variable. In Canada, this can range from 7% to 45% annually [1].

Coroner System

A coroner is a public official who certifies death. The origins of the coroner system are centuries old and arose in Great Britain. A coroner, or *crowner*, was an official of the court and representative of the King, with no medical training, who investigated deaths, namely, investigating the deaths of those found guilty of murder as the coroner had to distribute the property associated with this death [2]. The coroner system was adopted by British colonies and remains in place in many of these jurisdictions.

Today, there are marked variations in coronial training. For example, in the United States, there are 16 states that do not have laws requiring coroners to have specific training requirements and four states require them to be physicians, though not necessarily pathologists [3]. Coronial systems are subclassified into two types—a lay coroner and a medical coroner system, with the former being more common. The lay coroner may come from a variety of different backgrounds including journalism, law enforcement, law, and so on. The medical coroner system requires that the coroner be a physician but not necessarily a pathologist. Coroners provide administrative capacities and have the legal authority to order an autopsy but are not qualified to perform autopsies. Consequently, coroners rely on pathologists and forensic pathologists to assist in their investigation by performing autopsies and sometimes attending death scenes. In performing the autopsy, forensic pathologists can provide an accurate cause of death and gather postmortem data for identification. Involvement by forensic pathologists and other forensic experts provides this system's medical and scientific investigations.

In criminally suspicious deaths, young pediatric deaths, or homicides, there are two, non-competing, but concurrent investigations performed by the coroner and by law enforcement. In the coroner investigation, the coroner seeks to certify the identity of the deceased, the surrounding circumstances, the manner of death and the cause of death. The investigation by law enforcement is to determine whether a criminal offence has occurred. If the police investigation reveals that a criminal offense has occurred their role is to bring to justice those responsible.

The coroners' system usually has a provision for going beyond an investigation of the death to a public "inquisitional" hearing, often referred to as a coroner's inquest. The primary purpose of this type of hearing is to develop recommendations by a panel, of a variable number, of jurors for the prevention of similar deaths without making findings of fault. A coroner, instead of a judge, typically oversees these formal court proceedings; however, the coroner usually has access to legal counsel.

In the United States, there was a movement in the middle of the twentieth century to replace the coroner systems with medical examiner systems [4]; however, this change from a coronial system to a medical examiner has slowed in recent years [5].

Medical Examiner

The medical examiner system is an American invention and is just over a century old. This system was developed as a means to avoid the risk of political interference [5]. This system combines the medical and scientific examination of death but typically does not have a public "inquisitional" hearing like the coronial death investigation system.

Medical examiners are typically medical doctors who have training in pathology, medicolegal death investigation, and the performance of medicolegal autopsy. Their medical specialty is forensic pathology. The medical examiner has the overall responsibility for the operations, professional, and medical practice of the death investigation. This system mirrors other areas of medicine, in which the medical experts are the leaders of the system. This system strongly aligns accountability with responsibility in death investigation.

In criminally suspicious deaths, the investigation by law enforcement is also required to determine whether a criminal offense has occurred.

Continental System

This system is a police-initiated and -oriented process where a law enforcement agency inquiry is sometimes combined with a medicolegal, scientific, and judicial investigation.

Death Certificate: Certifying the Identification, Cause, and Manner of Death

One of the products of a death investigation system is the death certificate. A death certificate certifies the identification, cause, and manner of death. This, in turn, is officially filed as required by the state and is coded for mortality data that can be compared between regions and countries. In the death investigation system, the coroner or medical examiner who has officially investigated a person's death completes and signs the death certificate. Death certificates exclude stillbirths. Stillbirths need to be separately certified on a fetal death certificate, or a similar document, if the fetus is at least 20 weeks gestation. A fetus that is considered to be less than 20 weeks is usually classified as a product of conception. Stillbirths may be investigated by the death investigation system if the circumstances warrant an investigation (i.e., a stillbirth following an assault of a pregnant person). However, not all jurisdictions permit the investigation of stillbirths.

Many countries that are member "states" of the World Health Organization (WHO) must agree to their various rules and regulations. One of these items includes a standardized method of collecting the cause of death information via a standard death certificate model [6]. The standard death certificate requires two parts to the cause of death statement. The cause of death is coded by a nosologist. The nosologist codes the cause of death according to the World Health Organization's "International Statistical Classification of Diseases and Related Health Problems." This information can be used to monitor death rates and make other comparisons between countries. The death certificate should be completed objectively utilizing the known circumstances and facts to author an accurate death certificate.

Identification

The method(s) of identification used is determined on a case-by-case basis and starts at the death scene. Identification is divided into comparative and non-comparative methods. Non-comparative, or non-scientific, methods include visual identification of human remains, either directly or by photograph, circumstances, scars, age-related diseases, physical attributes, acquired and congenital anomalies, the decedent's clothing, and personal effects. In death investigations that involve multiple fatalityies marked decomposition/skeletal remains, or truly unidentified human remains without a tentative identity, non-comparative methods largely function as supportive data points and comparative or scientific mean is often used. Comparative or scientific means include comparative dental analysis of dental records and radiographs, fingerprints, radiographs, DNA, and the medical record. Tattoos are debated to fall in both categories. A limitation of the comparative methods used is that a prior existing record needs to exist and be available to compare with the postmortem findings, except for DNA. DNA profiling is a direct comparison made from human remains and a profile obtained from a close biological relative.

The other concept used in determining identification is the nature of the search universe. The search universe is a concept used to determine who composes the population of human remains. There are two types of search universes:

1. **Closed population**: The number of dead bodies aligns with the number registered to a fixed, identifiable group. The advantage of a closed population is that exclusionary criteria can be used to make an identification where there is no comparative method to identify human remains. This concept can be used in plane crashes, house fires in multi-generation families, or school fatalities.
2. **Open population**: The number of dead bodies does not equal those registered or there is no registry. In this search universe, all human remains need to be individually identified.

There are ethical, humanitarian, and legal reasons for the establishment of the identity of human remains include the following:

1. The need to know, especially by families, the individuals who have died
2. To establish the fact of death for legal and statistical reasons
3. To record the identity for administrative reasons related to the death certificate and other official records
4. To record the identity for ceremonial and burial rites purposes
5. To allow for legal proceedings

Cause of Death

Cause of death is defined as a disease and/or injury, which initiated a train of events, that, no matter how brief or prolonged, led to a fatal termination. The concept of cause of death is grounded in the philosophy of causation. From a cause-of-death perspective, two views of causation by philosophers David Hume and John Stuart Mill can be contrasted [7]. For Hume, his reductionistic notion of causation is equivalent to the causal chain [8]. The causal chain is a linear series of events that are temporally ordered and mechanistically linked such that each event is bound to the events before and after it. This reflects the common-sense notion of cause and effect over time [8]. From a cause-of-death perspective, the cause of death is the causal chain, starting with the initial event, and all linkages to events due to an actual physical event(s). In other words, event A leads to event B, and event C leads to death (Fig. 1.3). This philosophical perspective fits nicely in the WHO recommended method of capturing Part 1 of the cause of death statement, whereby the initiating event is the underlying cause of death. Subsequent events are either the immediate or intermediate cause(s) of death. An immediate cause of death is the final disease, injury, or complication that resulted from the underlying cause. Sometimes, the mechanism of death is captured in the immediate cause of death, but is not necessary. The intermediate cause(s) of death is an intermediary event(s). For some deaths, the sequence of disease or injury involves conditions that occur between the underlying and immediate causes of death is the intermediate cause of death. In summary, the underlying cause of death and intermediate and immediate events have a temporal cause-and-effect relationship that is stated in Part 1 of the cause of death statement. They are placed such that the most recent condition, the immediate cause of death, is at the top with each antecedent condition being listed below sequentially such that the underlying cause of death is on the lowest line. This contrast to Mill's holistic notion of causation, where interacting causal variables do not operate in a linear causal chain. Mill's approach to complex causation scenarios is useful when there are significant interactions between disease, injury, toxicological effects, and circumstantial events (Fig. 1.4).

Part II of the cause of death statement is (are) condition(s) that co-existed or preexisted prior to death and contributed to death but do not result in the underlying cause of death. These can include risk factors for the underlying cause of death.

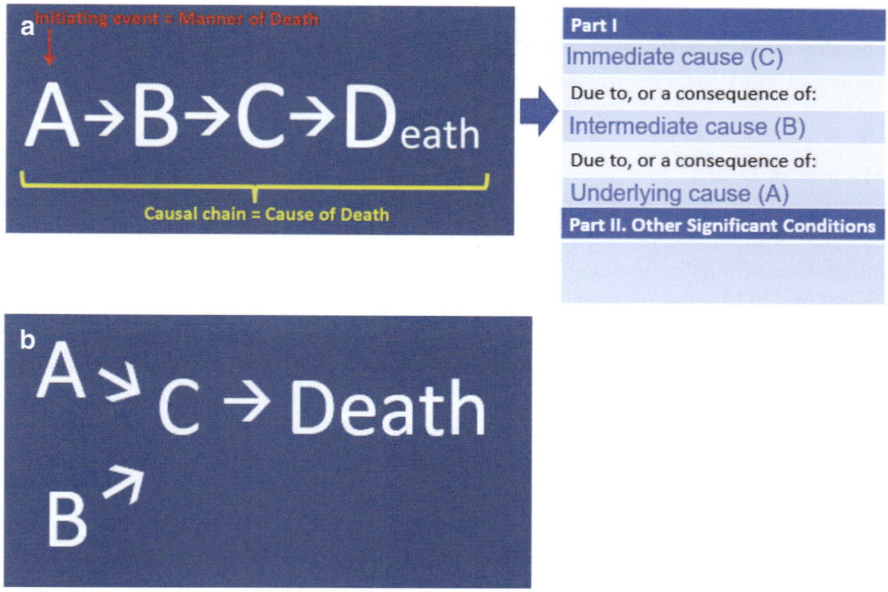

Fig. 1.3 Contrast the formulation of causation using differing philosophical perspectives. For Hume, (**a**) causation is equivalent to a causal chain and fits easily in the WHO-recommended format. Mill (**b**) had a holistic notion of causation

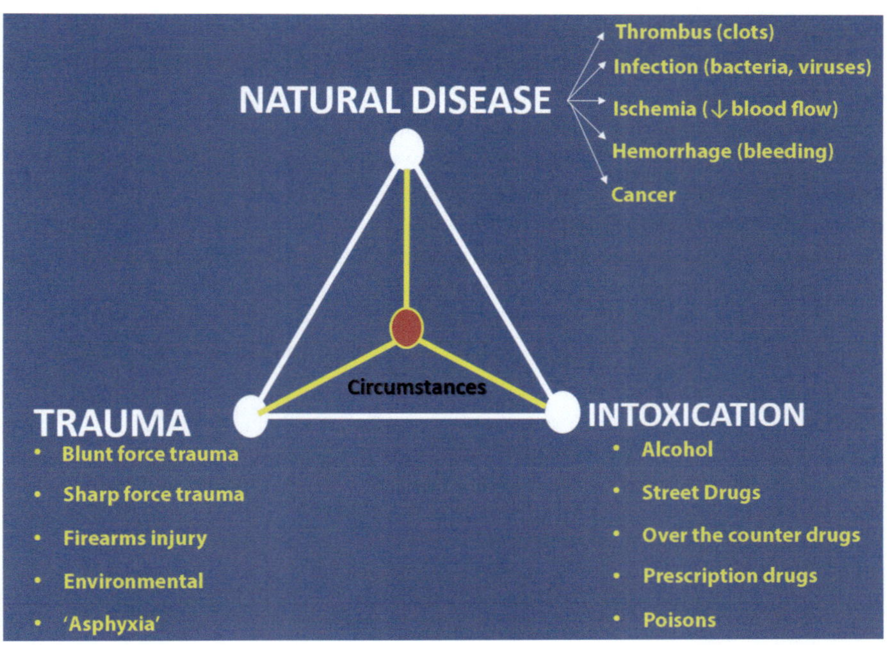

Fig. 1.4 Deaths that involve the interactions between disease, trauma, and intoxication with substances complicate a linear causal chain. (Image modified. Courtesy: Ontario Forensic Pathology Service)

There is no best method to author a cause of death statement. Using unambiguous statements can facilitate accurate reporting of the cause of deaths. There are a variety of guidelines for formulating the cause of death [9].

Manner of Death

Manner of death explains how the cause of death came about. It is based on the integration of the circumstances and factual evidence [10] of the initial event of the causal chain. Manner of death is dependent on circumstantial explanations based on the death investigation, which provides the broader background surrounding the death. It is by convention and is not legally binding. The primary role of the manner of death is for vital and descriptive statistics in public health surveillance that can assist in societal problems of crime, pandemic/epidemic diseases, and worker safety. Secondary uses include financial purposes such as insurance payouts and veteran's benefits.

Around the world, there is variation among countries that have adopted manner determination [10]. Unlike the cause of death, the World Health Organization format for death certificate does not include manner. The determination of the manner of death on the death certificate was first standardized in the United States in 1910 [10]. Many jurisdictions use five manners of death: natural, accident, suicide, homicide, and undetermined (Fig. 1.5). In select jurisdictions, therapeutic complication is an additional option [11]. There are a variety of definitions associated with each manner of death depending on the jurisdiction.

Determining the manner of death can sometimes be challenging because death can occur in complex circumstances that require the interpretation of death scene findings, multiple injuries, toxicology, and natural disease. Determining the manner of death does not utilize a scientific framework. Given the multiple iterations of death and the circumstances surrounding death, there are some deaths that do not fit easily into one category, resulting in ongoing discussions [10]. The coroner or medical examiner typically author the manner determination; however, in some jurisdictions, other authorities may author some manners of death. For example, in the United Kingdom, homicides may be determined by legal proceedings [10]. Deaths that undergo coroner's inquests the determination of the manner of death is

Manner	Definition/Explanation
Natural	Death that is solely due to a natural disease or complication
Accident	Death due to an incident/injury that occurs without foresight/expectation
Suicide	Death resulting from the intentional act of taking one's own life
Homicide	Death at the hands of another
Undetermined	There is uncertainty about the cause of death, lack of evidence, conflicting evidence/alternative interpretation of facts or an unnatural manner cannot be excluded.

Fig. 1.5 Summary of manners of death

performed by the jurors. These processes integrate local and societal values that can also contribute to individual variability [10].

Homicides are defined as a death that has occurred at the hands of another. Homicides can be either culpable or non-culpable. Intention and culpability are legal determinations, not medical. Non-culpable homicides could include those that occur in self-defense or in-custody deaths. Culpable homicides include murder and manslaughter. Murder and manslaughter are legal terms that are erroneously used interchangeably with homicide. Murder is defined as the intentional use of physical force or power, threatened or actual, against another person, or community that results in death [12]. The criteria applied to be classified in one manner over another are variable. Consequently, it can be difficult to measure differences and make comparisons between countries over time.

Accurately determining the manner of death is important for the decedent's family, police investigation, research, and public health policies. Although the manner of death may have legal implications, as it can have a quasi-judicial role. If the manner of death is not homicide, the person's death may or may not enter the legal system.

Mechanism of Death

The mechanism of death is the physiological and/or biochemical process by which the death came about. These include cardiac arrest, cardiac arrhythmia/dysrhythmia, respiratory arrest, exsanguination, pulmonary edema, hemorrhagic shock, hypoxic-ischemic encephalopathy, and multisystem organ failure. It is not a requirement of the death certificate as the mechanism of death is usually not specifically related to the disease process; it merely attests to the fact of death. For example, hypoxic-ischemic encephalopathy may be due to sequelae related to trauma, drugs, or natural diseases. Therefore, the mechanism of death provides no additional information on the cause of death but can be useful in providing additional details to paint a picture of the mechanism related to the cause of death.

Death

The unit of analysis for the forensic pathologist is the dead body. Consequently, understanding different concepts of death is relevant as death investigation systems authority often only arises after death, with few legislative exceptions such as permission for organ and tissue procurement decisions of impending and expected deaths.

Simply put, death is the irreversible cessation of life. Death can be classified from a hierarchical perspective of the different tissues and organs that have irreversible discontinuation of function at differing rates. There is debate from a sociocultural, religious, ethical, medical, and sometimes legal perspective, as to what constitutes death. From a medical perspective, death can have a hierarchical arrangement that reflects the way human biology is organized. Death can be organized from the level of a single cell, called cellular death. **Cellular death** is the irreversible cessation of metabolic respiration. Once metabolic respiration ceases postmortem changes such as autolysis and decomposition follows. This arises at different rates because cells have variable functions, which can impact the various cellular metabolism. For example, fibroblast cells remain metabolically active and can even be cultured days after somatic death, whereas a neuron (brain cell) dies after a few minutes of hypoxic-ischemic (oxygen-blood flow) deprivation. Death can also be defined by an organ, such as **neurological determination of death**, which is the death of the brain. Neurological determination of (brain) death arose as a result of the advances in medical resuscitation such that the use of ventilation and pharmacological intervention would result in the survival of patients who would have otherwise died from cerebral hypoxic-ischemic injury or other cerebral injury. These cerebral insults would have injured the brainstem and cause a sequence of events that would result in a cardiorespiratory arrest. Modern resuscitation efforts interrupt this causal pathway and can lead to a variety of outcomes including recovery, loss or altered level of consciousness with or without the ability to breathe, and even brain death. The Academy of Medical Royal Colleges (2008) published a "Code of Practice for the Diagnosis and Confirmation of Death" that instructs that death is the "irreversible loss of capacity for unconsciousness, combined with irreversible loss of the capacity for consciousness, combined with irreversible loss of the capacity to breathe." Clinically, key to the description of the term irreversible is to distinguish death from anesthesia, transient coma, and the effects of alcohol, or other substances. Consciousness is based on two criteria: awake and awareness. The spectrum of awake and aware classifies disorders of consciousness into coma (absent awake and awareness), vegetative state (awake present but absent awareness), and minimally unconscious state (awake with minimal awareness). Brain death and somatic death indicate that one is neither awake nor aware. **Somatic death** is death at the level of the human body.

Many countries do not have a statutory definition of death and leave this determination to medical experts. However, legal proceedings may arise when there is a conflict between sociocultural determinations of death and brain death.

Postmortem Changes

Following death, there is a continuum of changes that occur to the dead body. There are many variables that can impact postmortem changes and the rate of these changes. These changes include the following:

Livor mortis: Gravity-dependent accumulation of blood pooling in the skin and organs creates a purple-red discoloration. Following the cessation of circulation, there is a settling of blood in the dependent parts of the body with blanching in gravity-dependent areas of the body that come into contact with firm surfaces (Fig. 1.6). The distribution of livor mortis can provide information on the position of the body at the time of pooling but also raise the consideration of position-dependent causes of death, such as positional asphyxia, in some cases. The color

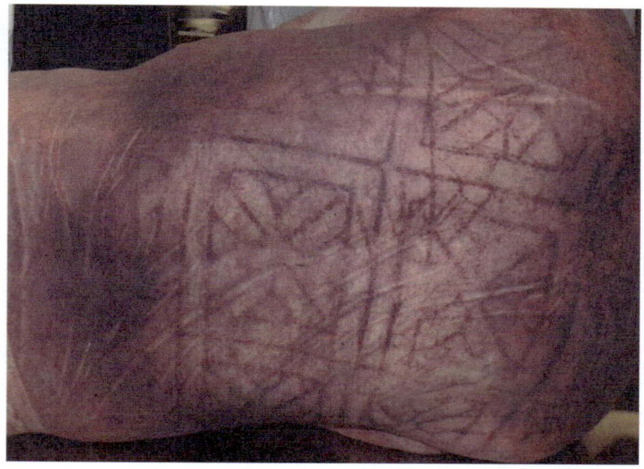

Fig. 1.6 Patterned dorsal lividity demonstrating the tiled floor the body was discovered on

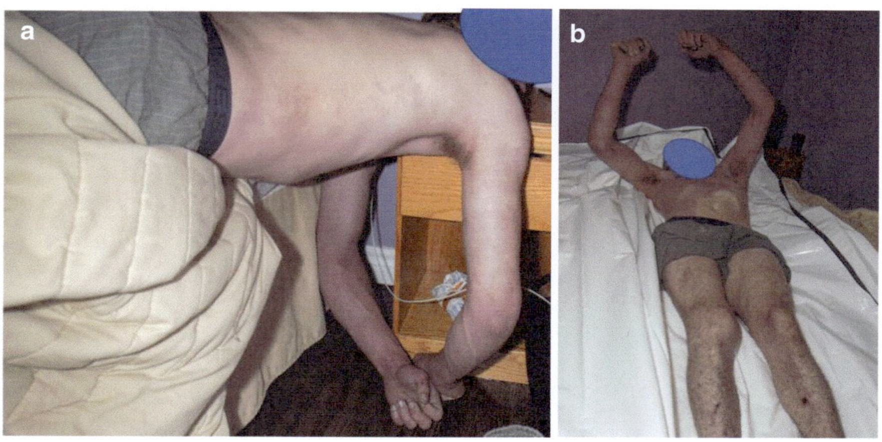

Fig. 1.7 Antigravitational rigor can indicate the position the body was in at the scene during the development of rigor mortis. (**a**) Original position at the scene. (**b**) The upper extremities remain above the body despite the effects of gravity once the body is moved and turned over

of livor mortis may indicate a cause or mechanism of death. For example, brown livor mortis may raise a primary or secondary methoglobinemia as a cause of death and diminished livor mortis may indicate exsanguination as mechanism of death.

Rigor mortis: Postmortem stiffening of the body is due to depletion of the energy-carrying molecule (adenosine triphosphate) and accumulation of lactic acid. Glycogen stores are rapidly depleted postmortem (in death) and therefore prevent the energy-dependent breakage of sarcomere contraction. It can provide information on the position of the body at the time of development (Fig. 1.7). This is a transient postmortem change that is typically divided into three phases: onset, peak, and dissipation.

Algor mortis: This is postmortem cooling of the body to ambient temperature.

Decomposition: Decomposition is the breakdown of organic matter into simpler forms of matter. The final common pathway is skeletonization. The type and rate are environment-dependent. Decomposition is largely classified as follows:

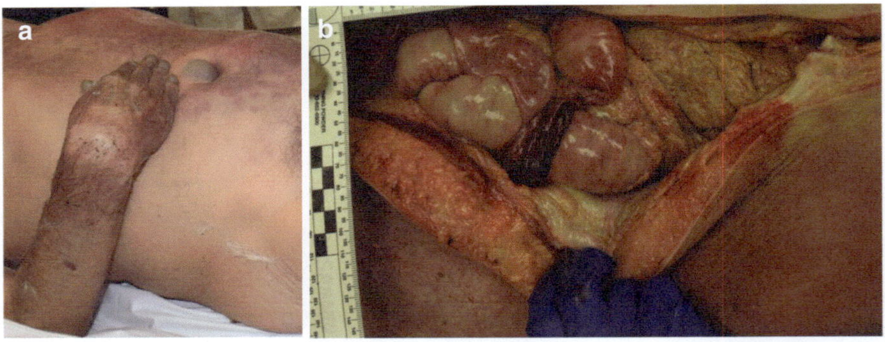

Fig. 1.8 Atypical putrefactive decomposition of the umbilicus (belly button) due to an umbilical hernia that brings the intestine closer to the skin surface at the umbilicus (belly button). Putrefactive decomposition usually arises in the right lower abdominal quadrant first because of the proximity of the cecum to the abdominal wall. (**a**) External surface of the abdomen showing a green discoloration of the umbilicus. (**b**) Internally, the bowel was incarcerated in the umbilical hernia

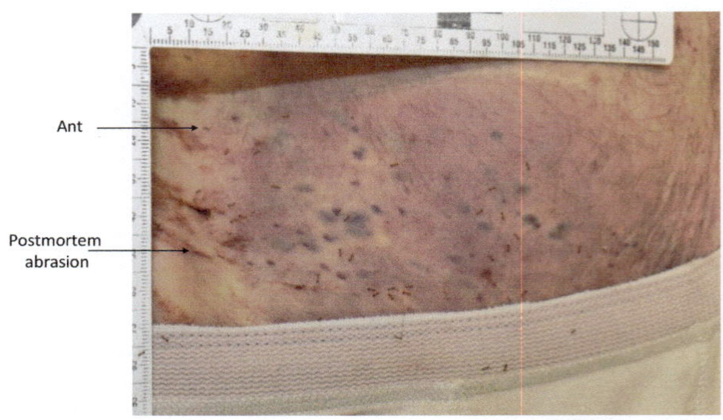

Fig. 1.9 Postmortem predation of ants leaving small cutaneous (skin) abrasions. Tight clothing can offer some protection from postmortem injury

Autolysis: It is an aseptic breakdown of tissues due to the release of intracellular enzymes.

Putrefaction: It is the most common form of decomposition due to the local and hematogenous spread of intestinal bacteria and other microorganisms. It arises in warm and humid environments. It results in liquefaction and gaseous transformation of organs and tissues. Atypical putrefaction may suggest a localized infection or trauma (Fig. 1.8).

Mummification decomposition: Typically, arises in a warm or cold but dry environment that results in the desiccation of tissues.

Adipocere formation (saponification): It is also referred to as grave wax because it typically arises in damp and oxygen-free environments. In these environments, a wax-like organic substance is formed by anaerobic bacterial hydrolysis of fat to oleic, palmitic, and steric acids.

Maceration: It is an aseptic autolysis of the stillborn fetus in utero.

Taphonomy: It is the environmental influence on the body after death, including insect activity (Fig. 1.9), postmortem animal predation (Fig. 1.10), and human intervention.

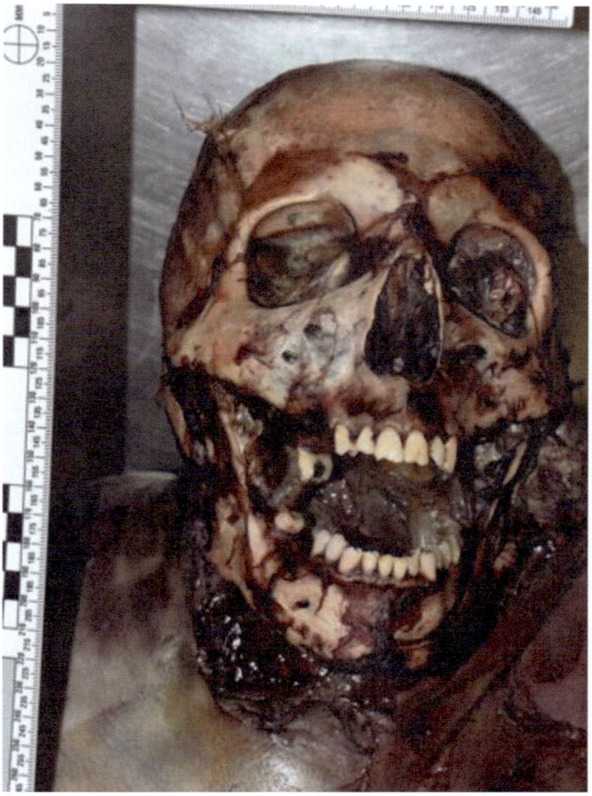

Fig. 1.10 Postmortem predation of the tissues of the head and proximal neck from a pet dog that is supported by the paucity of bleeding (vital reaction) along the distal neck

The Autopsy

Central to the medicolegal death investigation system is the autopsy. The autopsy essentially is not only an examination of a dead body and an indispensable tool to determine the cause of death but also serves other functions including a source of evidence for criminal matters, a data source to generate knowledge that may aid in medical science, and a wide variety of other needs [13]. The etymology of the term autopsy comes from the Greek term *autopsia*, which means seeing with one's own eyes [14]. This term has been used interchangeably with the terms necropsy, which means to look at the dead, and postmortem examination. Unfortunately, this medical procedure is associated with misconceptions and myths by the public as well as physicians [15]. There is no substitute for the autopsy because there is no procedure that can provide the same quality and type of information. The type of information that comes from the autopsy includes accurately establishing the cause and manner of death, replacing conjecture with facts, confirming/correcting antemortem diagnosis, and identification of new or re-emerging diseases as a means to protect public health and improve the accuracy of vital statistics and assuage grief for bereaved families.

The autopsy is the pathologist's tool to discern disease and injury. The autopsy is performed by a medically qualified specialist practitioner in the field of pathology—a pathologist or a subspecialist—a forensic pathologist. In deaths that arise in criminally suspicious circumstances, the objective of the autopsy is also to collect medicolegal evidence from the decedent's body to corroborate, and sometimes discredit non-medical evidence, aid in the police investigation, and ascertain the truth around a person's death, and the prosecution/defense of the accused. The pathologist who performs the autopsy is expected to provide competent evidence, collect exhibits, determine the extent of the injury, and provide an objective documentation of physical findings. The autopsy offers a different source of evidence and information related to medical facts and interpretations, collection of exhibits, and holistic assessment.

The autopsy is a methodological approach using a thoughtful and scientific investigation of disease, toxicology, and injury that led to death. Determining an accurate cause of death can benefit the decedent's family, society, legal system, and healthcare system. Performing autopsies is also a method to protect public interests and provides information necessary to address legal, public health, and safety issues. The autopsy is a powerful tool and can be a source of training, research, and function as a medical audit.

The value of the autopsy can be broken down into benefits for families, criminal justice system, public health, and medicine. The benefits for **families** include (1) identifying pathologies as a means to explain death; (2) identification of familial diseases so that healthcare and reproductive guidance can be provided to genetically close surviving family members; (3) forming a factual basis to counsel relatives to assuage grief; and (4) opportunity to benefit from the altruism associated with organ or tissue donation for transplantation, research, and education. The value to **medicine and public health** is that there is an accurate cause of death that contributes to accurate mortality statistics on which government health policy, and research funding are allocated to prevent premature death, evaluate new medical therapies, and surgical procedures, better characterize poorly understood diseases and possible adverse effects, and serve as an early warning in public health and safety to prevent future disease and injury. The value to the **criminal justice system** is that the autopsy provides objective medical evidence and the confirmation of identity that are fundamental to the proper administration of both civil and criminal justice systems wherein these systems decide issues related to matters of injury and death. The autopsy and the accompanying understanding of death, injury, and disease are fundamental to the proper administration of civil and criminal matters. The autopsy can also help to ensure the public that the deaths of vulnerable individuals who die in institutions are being thoroughly investigated.

Autopsies are largely categorized into two types (Fig. 1.11). Procedurally, they are similar, but the differences are largely regarding the authorization of the post-mortem examination and the focus of the examination. The autopsy is unique in medicine in that the physician—the pathologist—performing the procedure has less to do with obtaining authorization. Permission is given by the next of kin for the hospital autopsy and is sought by the treating clinicians. In medicolegal autopsies, the authorization to perform the examination comes from a statutory authority.

Hospital	Medicolegal
Performed by a hospital pathologist	Performed usually by a forensic pathologist
Has had a medical investigation	Has a medical death +/- police investigation
Person died as a patient in hospital (controlled environment)	May come from hospital, majority do not
Most are natural: - Family may want piece of mind - Education - Research - "Correct" diagnosis - Genetics: future pregnancies	Often unexplained deaths or criminal element
Performed under authorization of next of kin	Performed under legislation
No exhibits collected	Exhibits may be collected

Fig. 1.11 Comparison of the hospital and medicolegal autopsy. The procedures between hospital and medicolegal autopsies are procedurally similar, but the focus differs

The clinical, academic, or hospital autopsy: This autopsy is performed with the *authorization* of the decedent's next of kin. The purpose is to arrive at a diagnosis that could not be achieved during treatment or to confirm a diagnosis when there is doubt. The hospital autopsy is predominantly focused on clinicopathological correlation (provision of correlations between clinical diagnoses and symptoms to pathological findings), research, educating medical personnel, and quality assurance.

The medicolegal or forensic autopsy: This autopsy is performed on the instructions of the legal authority in circumstances relating to sudden and unexpected deaths, obscure deaths, and suspicious/criminal deaths. The autopsy is done on behalf of the state and as such does not require the authorization of relatives of the decedent. The state takes possession of the body for the protection of the public interest. The body is released following a complete investigation into the circumstances around a death. Autopsies and storage of material occur without family authorization at the request of a judicial authority, such as a coroner, procurator fiscal, examining magistrate, and so on. The medicolegal autopsy is primarily focused on determining a cause of death and other medicolegal opinions.

The clinical autopsy rate has been declining for quite some time [2]. However, the medicolegal autopsy rate varies by country. A Canadian study found that the medicolegal autopsy rate rose, up to 62%, while the clinical autopsy rates fell to 0.69% [16, 17]. The medicolegal autopsy is performed on individuals wherein the cause of death is uncertain, typically in the case of sudden, unexpected, and unexplained deaths. The majority of these cases are non-criminal in nature. The minority of cases have an element of foul play suspected or are criminal in nature. Other forms of autopsy include the "Military" autopsy and the "private" autopsy. The "Military" autopsy flows from military law and is often performed on soldiers who have died overseas in conflict or peace keeping missions. A "private" autopsy is one for which families not only authorize but also pay for.

Forensic Pathology

Forensic pathology is a branch of a field in medicine called pathology. Pathology is the study of disease, including its causes, pathogenesis, and the ways in which the disease process affects the body. Forensic pathology was only recognized as a medical specialty in 1959 in the United States and 2003 in Canada. Knowledge in forensic pathology is the ability to recognize and diagnose disease and injury. The pathological findings must take into account the medical history and circumstances of death of the decedent, and the disease concepts that are established from observations of many individuals suffering of a similar nature. Forensic pathologists identify changes in morphology at the macroscopic and microscopic levels, toxicological findings, and biochemical alterations in body fluids. In addition, they use a variety of molecular, histologic, and immunologic techniques to understand the biochemical, structural, and functional changes that occur in cells, tissues, and organs to render diagnoses.

Forensic pathology is the application of science and medicine to problems of law. This subspecialized area of medicine is considered to be part of a larger area of medicine referred to a forensic medicine (Fig. 1.12). Unlike forensic pathology, forensic medicine does not limit its scope to death investigation. The unit of analysis in forensic medicine is living people. A related subspecialized area of clinical medicine is forensic psychiatry. Outside of medicine, there are other forensic disciplines in which the unit of analysis is physical things rather than human bodies. These forensic disciplines can be used in death investigations.

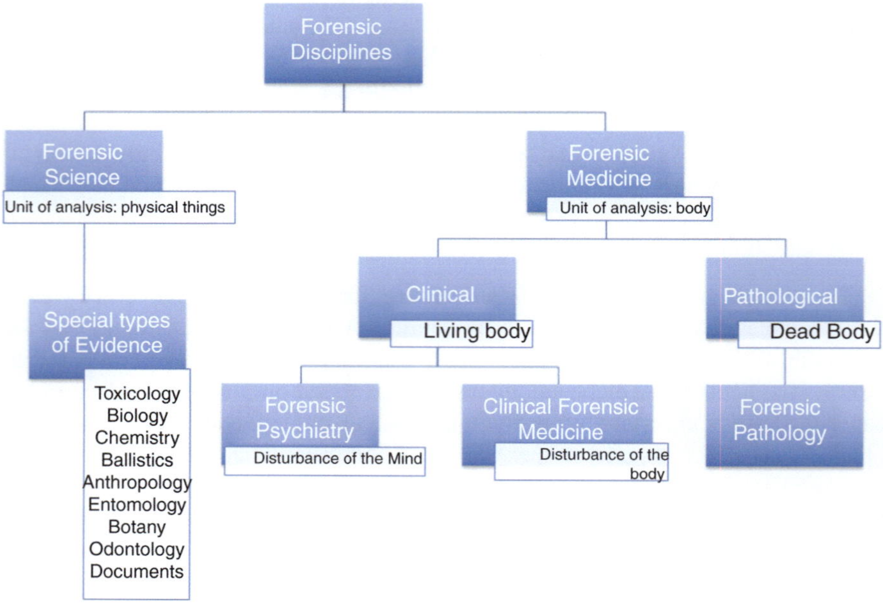

Fig. 1.12 Summary of common forensic disciplines

Steps of the Autopsy

The steps of the autopsy mirror a physician's clinical interaction with patients that starts with obtaining a history, a physical exam, and ancillary investigations to arrive at a diagnosis for the patient's main complaint (Fig. 1.13). During an autopsy, it is up to the pathologist to determine the appropriate extent of diagnostic measures necessary to formulate an expert opinion and be prepared to support that opinion. Following the completion of the internal examination, the body should be reconstructed with all major organs and tissues returned to the body. In particular, the face and hands should be readily viewable by family at the funeral arrangements following the postmortem examination.

Step 1: History

The first step of the autopsy is gathering information about the scene(s), circumstances, and history of the events surrounding a death. History documented in the autopsy report should include relevant facts and does not have to be an exhaustive recall of all details, unless necessary. This can include medical and social history. The scene information can provide the position of the body, the clothing of the decedent, postmortem changes, medications, illicit drugs, and the presence of weapons or blood.

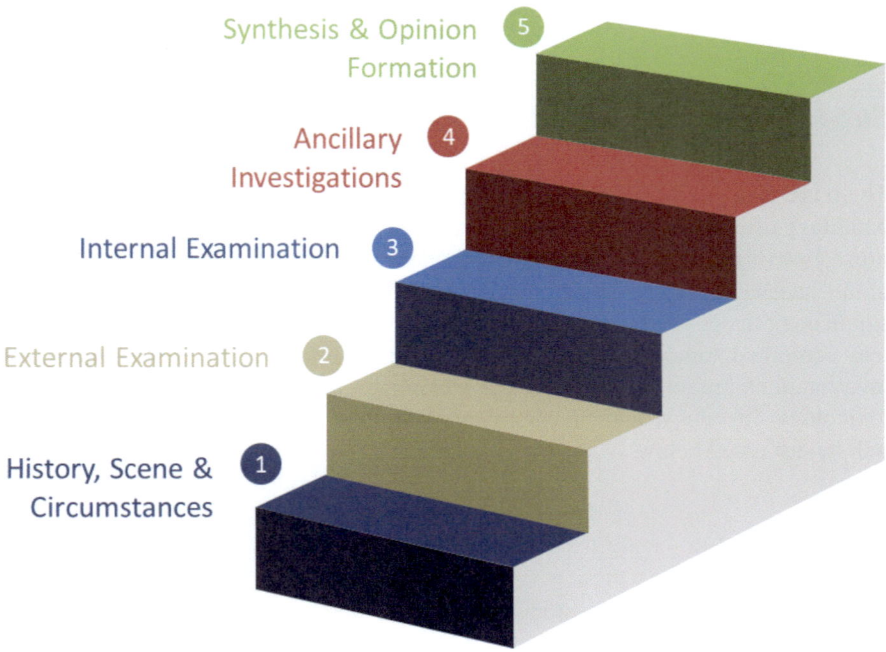

Fig. 1.13 The steps of the autopsy

Step 2: External Examination

The pathologist performs a head-to-toe examination, collecting information about the potential cause of death, i.e., examination for the presence or absence of natural disease, injury, medical and surgical intervention, organ procurement surgery, and postmortem changes. The presence or absence of clothing, jewelry, and personal effects need to be documented. This step also includes the collection of physical evidence and biologic samples. Examination of the clothing can not only provide information on the pattern and nature of underlying injuries but may also inform the circumstances.

Step 3: Internal Examination

The internal examination typically starts with an *in situ* examination of the intracranial, thoracic, abdominal, and pelvic cavities before and following the removal of organs. The anterior neck structures are also examined and may occur following the removal of the brain and viscera. The purpose is to identify, or rule out, signs of disease, injury, and therapy. An internal examination may require special dissections such as layer musculocutaneous dissection of the anterior and posterior neck, anterior and posterior torso, and limbs. Exhibits, such as bullets, may also be recovered in this step. The internal examination may not be necessary in all deaths, especially when all of the questions of the death investigation can be answered without the internal examination and families have coconscious objection to the internal examination.

Step4: Ancillary Investigations

There are wide variety of ancillary investigations that can be performed. Forensic pathology uses evidence-based methods that were introduced centuries ago with the prosection of the decedent and written documentation that is supplemented by diagrams and photography. There have been advances in ancillary investigations that supplement the postmortem examination; these are largely in the realm of postmortem computed tomography (PMCT), toxicology, and genetic testing. Ancillary investigations are not always necessary. Common ancillary investigations include toxicology, histology, and biochemistry. Histology, biochemistry, and radiology will be discussed below.

Histology

Histology is the microscopic study of tissues. In autopsy practice, histology is the microscopic assessment of representative tissue samples obtained from major internal organs and from abnormal findings. This tool can assist in (1) confirming the macroscopic impression; (2) detecting or excluding histopathological findings; (3)

establishing a cause of death; (4) creating a permanent, reviewable histological record of disease; (5) dating injuries; (6) screening hereditary heart disease (i.e. cardiomyopathies); and (7) offering diagnostic refinements. The selection and interpretation of histological findings occur in conjunction with the macroscopic autopsy findings and historical information. Complementary investigations, such as enzyme and immunohistochemical, *in situ* hybridization, and electron microscopy, and molecular pathological investigations are even less frequently applied.

The role of histological examination in medicolegal autopsies is a subject of debate in terms of the need to maintain a high volume of histology countered by a call for a more rationalized evidence-based approach [18, 19]. Histology does increase costs and turnaround times and may be unnecessary in some deaths [20]. The standards for the practice of forensic pathology proposed by the Forensic Pathology of the College of American Pathologists indicate that the extent of histologic sampling of autopsy tissues is at the pathologist's discretion [21]. The National Association of Medical Examiners recommends that histological sampling occurs in all medicolegal autopsies with no gross anatomical cause of death unless the remains are skeletonized [22]. Inadequate sampling or lack of tissue may lead to erroneous final interpretations in some cases [20]. A retrospective study that compared the provisional report based on the gross findings, to the final reports, after histological examination, found that histological evaluation commonly altered macroscopic findings in the lungs, liver, and kidney. In particular, these macroscopically normal organs showed microscopic abnormalities.

Vitreous Biochemistry

Vitreous fluid of the eye is used to test for biochemical changes but can also be used in toxicology when no blood is available, the blood is contaminated, or the decedent is embalmed. The biochemical indicators are similar to plasma levels. Ranges depend on laboratory standards (Fig. 1.14).

The initial postmortem changes include an increase in potassium and a decrease in glucose. As a result, hyperkalemia and hypoglycemia cannot be proven using a postmortem sample. Sodium and chloride followed by urea and creatinine are more stable [23]. There are six common abnormal biochemical patterns:

1. Uremia/renal insufficiency: Elevated urea and creatinine levels in the setting of normal sodium and chloride.
2. Hypernatremia: Elevated chloride and sodium levels in the setting of normal urea.
3. Hyponatremia: Decreased chloride and sodium levels in the setting of normal urea. This is often seen in individuals who are dependent on ethanol. Ketones may also be elevated. Given that sodium and chloride can decline with postmortem interval, the state of the remains and level of potassium are considerations to interpret this pattern.

Electrolyte or other element (units in brackets)	Physiological Normal Ranges*	Postmortem Changes**
Glucose (mmol/L)	4-7	↓↓↓
Potassium (mmol/L)	3.5-5	↑↑↑
Sodium (mmol/L)	135-145	↓
Chloride (mmol/L)	97-110	↓
Urea (mmol/L)	2.9-8.9	Fairly stable
Creatinine (umol/L)	62-120	Fairly stable
Ketones	Negative	Fairly stable

* Ranges are laboratory dependent

** Quantity of arrows indicate degree of instability

Fig. 1.14 Vitreous biochemistry ranges and associated postmortem changes

4. Dehydration: Elevated chloride and sodium levels in the setting of elevated chloride and urea.
5. Diabetes mellitus: Elevated glucose and ketones.

Radiology

Conventional radiographs in the form of X-rays are indicated in young children and infant deaths, namely, skeletal surveys, penetrating injuries (i.e. firearm-related deaths and stabbing injuries), identification purposes, SCUBA-related deaths, and severely burned and markedly decomposed bodies. Many institutions routinely use postmortem computed tomography (PMCT) scans. PMCT is a complement to the autopsy and has many applications. PMCT scans are a fairly rapid, reviewable record that shows excellent spatial resolution for visualization of the skeleton, foreign bodies, and gas. Its major limitation is soft tissue and solid organ resolution. Many natural diseases such as meningitis, encephalitis, cardiomyopathies, and fatal coronary artery diseases are difficult to ascertain on PMCT. Other limitations to PMCT are related to the impact of interpretation of postmortem changes, particularly in the lung, make it challenging to distinguish pathologies from normal findings. Contrast studies are challenging to perform in the non-physiologic state of dead bodies due to the lack of circulation, which is normally used clinically to better study a particular organ or blood vessel. Imaging that better characterizes soft tissue and solid organ pathologies is magnetic resonance imaging (MRI), but their acquisition times, approximately, 2–3 h for a body region, such as the head, hinder routine use. In addition, MRI utility is dependent on the body temperature to differentiate different tissue types. As algor mortis is a normal postmortem change and refrigeration is used to preserve bodies, this technology can be limited in the postmortem context.

Step 5: Summary and Opinion

The fifth step is an integration of the four prior steps to use factual evidence and logic to arrive at an opinion about the cause of death and other relevant medicolegal opinions. This is also an opportunity to summarize the pertinent negatives and positives of the postmortem examination. The opinion must explain the basis of the main medicolegal opinions (i.e. cause of death, timing of injuries, and implement used to cause injury) that the pathologist is prepared to offer at trial. This ensures transparency of the pathologist's opinion and facilitates the understanding of the report by the prosecution and the defence counsel, before legal proceedings [24].

Medicolegal opinions should follow an empirically gained knowledge base that is tested by an analysis of case series or experimentation rather than an outdated approach of anecdotal evidence and experience. Using an evidence base in forming opinions ensures the practice of forensic pathology aligns with other areas of medicine and assures quality forensic pathology work. Furthermore, caution must be used to ensure that the pathologist does not place inordinate weight on the historical data, as it may be a source of confirmation bias. Although the background circumstance of the case must be known to the pathologist, the history cannot bear the entire burden of the expert opinion. The evidence-based framework consists of the following main analytical domains:

1. **Fact correspondence**: Opinion corresponds to empirical data.
2. **Consideration of first principles**: Opinion accords with the basic principle of pathology and pathophysiology. For example, expert opinion of the timing of injuries should correlate with the presence or absence of an inflammatory reaction, hemosiderosis, or evidence of healing such as granulation tissue.
3. **Coherence with the evidence base**: The diagnosis should also cohere with the published literature and not represent a novel theory of causation or a personal theory of the pathologist.
4. **Consideration of counterexamples or alternate explanations**: Opinion must consider case reports as alternative explanations or counterexamples of a phenomenon. This balances the perception that no two cases are identical and the challenges of applying traditional study designs in medicine to forensic issues.
5. **Fairness and truth-seeking**: The opinion is reasonable and balanced and represents what is believed to be the truth. This includes limitations and issues of uncertainty, which can highlight unknowns in science and medicine [24].

Testimony

Sometimes, a forensic pathologist is subpoenaed, or summoned, for legal proceedings to provide oral testimony that describes observations on the body and interpretations in addition to providing expert opinions. This is a means to legally test the forensic pathologists' opinions and also present the pathological findings, sometimes in the form of autopsy images. This is sometimes considered the sixth step of the autopsy.

Autopsy Report

The report of postmortem examination is a medicolegal report that is prepared and written with care. This report constitutes the medical evidence and may form the basis of any oral evidence that may be given in the future. While testifying, the report may serve as the basis of a script to provide testimony. Once the autopsy report is completed, it may be reviewed by multiple stakeholders, including family members but also researchers. Interpretations and opinions must be formulated after consideration of all available information that has been obtained. The basis of most reports lies in the notes and/or voice recordings made at the time of postmortem examination. These notes, in addition, to the postmortem report can be admitted into the court.

The anatomy of the report includes a heading with the details of the decedent, including autopsy number, name, location of autopsy, date of autopsy, and date death pronounced. All attendees, assistants, and any other persons present at the time of the postmortem examination need to be included. The pathologists' qualifications and work address need to be included. Often the postmortem report mirrors the steps of the autopsy. The first step of the autopsy should include the relevant history, scene, and circumstance, which includes the pathologists' disclosure of their relevant independent review of the scene images and possible scene visits. The observations made from the four steps of the autopsy and the interpretations and opinions derived from them need to be described in the postmortem report that paints an image of the observed phenomenon and its implications (Fig. 1.15). The ability to describe is as essential as the skills related to the dissection. The basis of the pathologist's opinion and report should be based on facts. The postmortem report may be anticipated to become evidence for the courts. This report should be carefully scrutinized by the authoring forensic pathologist to avoid errors such as typographical errors and laterality errors. After signing the report, the authoring pathologist considers requesting a peer review of the report and all other relevant materials.

Like all medical records, the finalised postmortem report is a legal document, and pathologists ought to resist attempts to alter or delete portions of the report without disclosure. Instead, if opinions have changed or other changes are required (i.e. proper speeling of the decedent's name) an addendum should proceed and the reasons for this change. These changes should be disclose in the amended report.

History	Differentiate between what you were told and what you observed Identify what your information sources were Identify what your information sources were before and after the subsequent Use precise terminology Maintain objectivity
External Examination	Use precise terminology Maintain objectivity Disclose special procedures and exhibit collection
Internal Examination	Use precise terminology Maintain objectivity Disclose special dissections & evidence collection
Ancillary Investigations	Detail all specimens, consultations and exhibits collected Detail all retained organs and tissues
Summary and opinion	Stay within your field of expertise Differentiate observations from interpretations Write only what you would be comfortable saying in court Highlight limitations (ie decomposition), where appropriate Use simple and precise language
General	Author your report to mirror the steps of the autopsy and as your template/transcript for giving oral evidence Include attendees

Fig. 1.15 Guiding principles in authoring autopsy reports

Photography

The observations of the autopsy require a visual examination of the entire body. As the autopsy is an inherently destructive process, an externally reviewable record is warranted. Consequently, photodocumentation is an essential component of the postmortem record and like the handwritten notes becomes part of the factual record. The photographs are a representation of the gold standard, which is the physical examination. The photograph is the adjunct to the forensic pathologist's examination of the original injury [25] and other observations. Photography can supplement contemporaneously documented descriptions and drawings. The benefits of photodocumentation includes an independent review of the body that allows for accountability and peer review of injuries and other observations, evidence in courts, and discussion points with families. In legal proceedings, autopsy photographs of injuries and other findings may be used to provide evidence for court, utilized to refute or support interpretations, and to serve as part of the medicolegal record. Autopsy images may also be used in publications or teaching.

Photographic evidence obtained during the autopsy should use proper photographic techniques, including proper lighting, proper framing and angles, use of scale, and avoidance of extraneous materials such as autopsy tools and the exclusion mortuary staff faces [26]. The images taken during the autopsy should be complete and include the police seal, the identification tag, in addition to anterior and posterior overalls, three views of the head in the Frankfurt plane (Fig. 1.16), and personal effects [27]. In addition, other images may be taken as needed. The images should be an accurate representation of the factual evidence. Photographs should minimize alterations that can falsify aspects of the original appearance due to (1) technical distortions of color, lighting, and depth, (2) interpretive error that can occur when interpreting a 2D image of 3D complex anatomy, (3) quality of photographic images which varies with the camera and competence and experience of the photographer, (4) deterioration of data, and (5) digital manipulation of images when the chain of evidence and secure is an issue [25, 28, 29].

Photographs of the body should be taken with a scale. The scale, with a unique case number, should be placed in the same plane and as close as possible to finding without obscuring details. The scale should be a linear measuring device that is validated and adheres to validated standards such as the National Institute Standards and Technologies [30]. Common scales used in autopsy images include Bureau Reference Scales and the ABFO No. 2 Scale. The latter is a smaller L-shaped scale for photographing possible bite marks. Qualities of high-quality images include consideration of composition, focus, lighting, color, distortion, and exposure. The subject in the images should fill the frame and ensure that the camera is parallel to the subject and focal plane. The subject should be in focus. This requires an understanding of the focal plane of the subject. The focal plane is the distance between the camera lens and the perfect point of focus in an image. The scale should be at

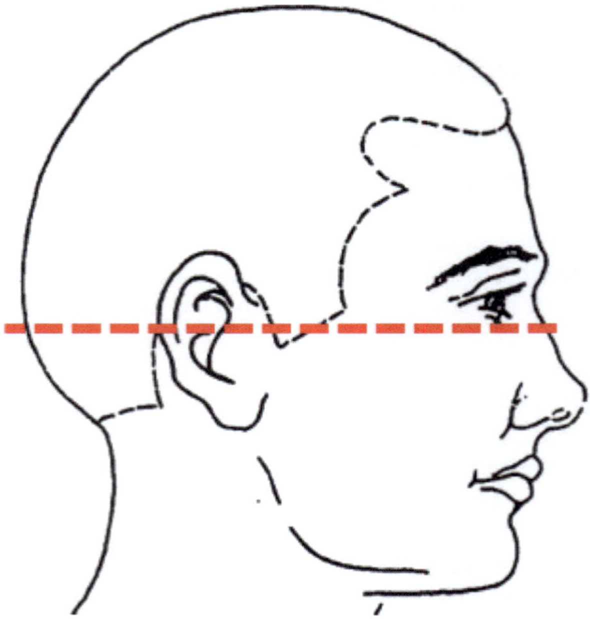

Fig. 1.16 The Frankfurt plane is the anatomical position of the skull based on a horizontal plane that passes through the inferior margin of the left orbit and the upper margin of each ear canal

the focal plane so that its measurements are also in focus. The depth of field refers to the greatest area of focus in the image. This is controlled by the size of the aperture opening and the image sensor of the camera.

The unique case identifier on the scale is advised to minimize the misfiling of images into non-related cases. The unique case number can be a printed adhesive label or a single-use printed scale. When using the former, care must be taken not to obscure the unit of measure on the scale with the label. A subsequent image may be taken without scale, if necessary. If images are unacceptable, re-photography is required. Any images taken should not be deleted.

Digital cameras are widely used in forensic work, and the images produced are accepted in the legal system, specifically, relevant, properly authenticated digital images that accurately portray a finding. However, the choice of which images are admissible in a legal proceeding is up to interpretations of the law. Photographs taken at autopsy are by digital cameras, which are complex optical electronic devices that perform multiple functions each time the shutter button is pressed. Unlike analog cameras that capture images by exposing photographic film to light, digital cameras record the image in a series of binary numbers that a computer can read. Once the shutter button is pressed, the image is captured on a digital sensor, which is a digital version of the film. This small silicon chip holds millions of pixels, which are tiny light-sensitive elements that receive individual particles of light. This light is converted into an electric charge by the sensor which is then converted by the camera's processor. The processor converts this signal into a binary form that the computer can read. This file is saved to a memory card, which is a small removable storage device in the camera. It is this data that must be kept in its raw form. The computer can convert the binary data into images.

An understanding of the technical knowledge of photography can facilitate the production of high-quality images. A camera is a complex piece of optical equipment that utilizes light and the interactive relationship of the light exposure trio to create images. Without light, an image will not be captured. The light exposure trio is the shutter speed, aperture, and ISO (Fig. 1.17). The camera's aperture controls the quantity of the light reaching the camera's sensor. The aperture is a diaphragm composed of a set of blades that creates an octagonal shape on the lens that controls how much light will enter the camera by widening or narrowing. The size of the aperture is referred to as an f-stop—the higher the f-stop number, the smaller the hole created by the blades. The aperture also controls the field of depth. The shutter speed determines the duration of the exposure of light to the sensor. The shutter speed is determined by the time duration between the opening and closing of two blinds over the sensor. The first blind opens to expose the sensor and the second one closes to end the exposure. A longer shutter speed exposes the sensor to more light. The ISO indicates the sensitivity of the sensor to light. The higher the number, the more sensitive.

A legal prerequisite to the admissibility of any evidence is that it can be authenticated. Authentication requires that there is sufficient evidence that the exhibit is

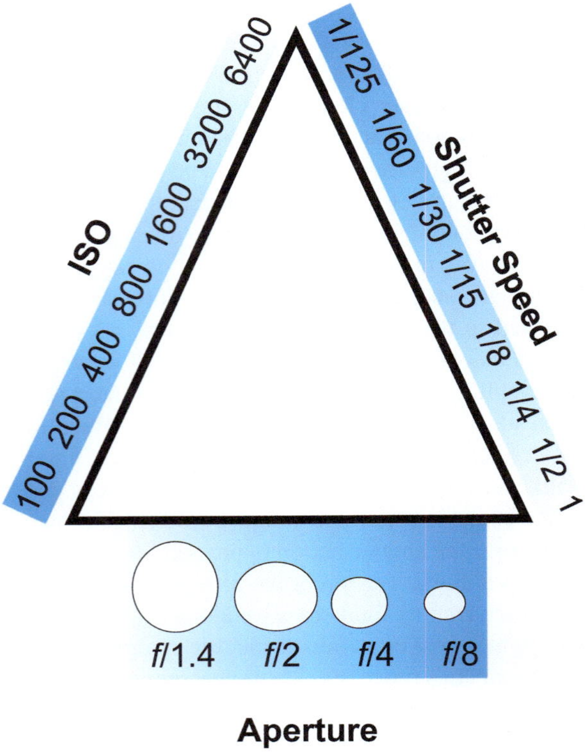

Fig. 1.17 The light exposure trio: aperture, shutter speed, and ISO. Between the lens and the sensor are two barriers—the aperture and the shutter that work to control how much light reaches the sensor of the digital camera. The larger the aperture and the longer the shutter speed, the more light will hit the sensor

what the proponent claims to be. If this is challenged, the proponent needs to show that the image or data of the image is not altered. This is not to say that images cannot be altered, but rather the alterations need to be disclosed. Common alterations include the following enhancement techniques, which are used to improve the appearance of the image: cropping, white balance, color balancing/correction, brightness, and contrast adjustments. Furthermore, no images obtained during the postmortem examination must be deleted. These include mistaken images of the autopsy floor.

During a postmortem examination, photographs are taken. The photographer may be the pathologist, ancillary pathology staff, police officer, or dedicated biomedical photographer. High-quality training in forensic pathology photography includes technical knowledge of camera operation and subject matter knowledge of anatomy and pathology. Communication and discussion can go a long way between the forensic pathologist, pathology staff, and photographer. This will allow the photographer to understand what needs to be photographed and determine how to best approach the pathological findings during the postmortem examination. Communication can bridge the gap between the anatomical subject matter of the medical staff and the photographic approach of the non-medical photographer.

Quality Assurance and Peer Review

Quality assurance is the systematic monitoring and evaluation of multiple aspects of the postmortem report and examination to ensure that standards of quality are met and protect the legal system from interpretation errors and conclusions. Quality improvement is required to maintain the death investigation system's integrity, transparency, and public confidence [31]. The major obstacle to modernizing a forensic pathology practice to incorporate a quality improvement practice is competing obligations of pathologists, understaffing, and underfunded monitoring and facilitating peer reviews.

Quality assurance includes the pre-analytic, analytic, and post-analytic phases of the postmortem examination. Part of the pre-analytic phase is to ensure that the body has been properly tagged. This typically is in the form of an official identification tag or hospital identification bracelet. It is essential to confirm the identity of the decedent, or if not identified, ensure that the official body tags are present and correspond with the Warrant for postmortem examination or other relevant official documents. Unofficial toe tags (i.e. hospital tags) as a sole means of identification in the medicolegal context are fraught with problems as they are placed on the body postmortem without known confirmation of who has placed the tag. Unofficial toe tags can also be detached easily from the body and then placed on the wrong body [32]. When the body bears no appropriate identification tagging, the best course of action is to a witness who has known the person in life, the medicolegal authority, or a police officer and formally confirm to the pathologist. Also, if the historical and circumstantial information does not correlate with the postmortem examination, there may be a pre-analytical error. For example, if the decedent's medical record indicates that there was a right-sided below-knee amputation but the decedent has both legs, either the history or the identity of the deceased is incorrect. The analytical phase of quality assurance includes disclosure of "critical values" or "critical diagnosis." The requirement of communicating critical laboratory results to reflect pathophysiological derangements was defined in 1972 as "Laboratory values which reflect pathophysiological derangements at such variance with normal as to be life threatening if therapy is not instituted immediately" [33]. This concept of critical value (significant findings) has extended into pathology but has largely been uncharacterized in the postmortem context [33]. Forensic pathologists are responsible for communicating critical diagnoses to prevent harm to others, including timely communication of the results of carbon monoxide blood testing, meningitis, unexpected toxicology results, HIV testing and other communicable diseases, suspicion of child abuse to law enforcement and child protection services and secret homicides, concerns of hereditary diseases, and unexpected fatal injuries. The nature of the message dictates that the person to disclose this information can action on this message. Further consensus on what signifies a critical diagnosis in medicolegal autopsies is required [33].

The different quality assurance measures in forensic pathology include the following:

1. Physicians who are properly trained and qualified in forensic pathology
2. Maintenance of certification in forensic pathology as part of continuing professional development and Professional Regulatory control
3. Formal expert witness training for practitioners
4. Maintenance of a Registry of Forensic Pathologists as part of managerial oversight
5. Managerial oversight of standards of practice
6. Use of maintained standard operating procedures and standards of practice related to autopsy performance and reporting
7. Caseload management
8. Practice audits: peer review of autopsy reports and expert witness testimony
9. Postmortem examinations performed subsequently or with the defense pathologist in attendance

In the post-analytic phase, amending postmortem reports and peer review are considered. Amendment is a simple process and is encouraged when warranted. Most amendments may include the correct spelling of the name. Amending a cause of death may require direct communication with stakeholders. Peer review is the standard for clinical, scholarly, and accreditation processes [34]. Peer review can function as an accepted gatekeeper for objectivity and accountability [34]. Peer review provides accountability, enhances the quality and integrity of the work, improves competence, disciplines methodology, and safeguards justice [34]. A formal system of quality assurance that includes peer review of autopsy reports by a second forensic pathologist contributes to the validity and reproducibility of autopsy interpretations [35]. A peer review in forensic pathology ensures accurate interpretation of findings and determination of cause of death. The goal of peer review in forensic pathology is to maintain the overall quality of the report of postmortem examination to assess for reasonableness of opinions and accuracy of interpretation of findings including errors of misinterpretation, lack of recognition of significant findings, errors of omission, and failure to pursue relevant ancillary investigations. The utilization is dependent on the nature of the case and the resources available.

The objectives of the peer review are to determine the following:

1. Reviewability: can the autopsy report be independently reviewed by another forensic pathologist?
2. Expert opinions: are expert opinions about the relevant medicolegal issues, such as the cause of death given and whether are they balanced, reasonable, and substantiated by the available evidence?
3. Opportunities for disagreement and learning.

Peer review can be prospective or retrospective. Prospective peer review entails a review of a draft of the postmortem report, review of autopsy images, scene images, and relevant ancillary investigations. This allows oversight and ensuring accuracy of a report before it enters the court system. This is also an opportunity for interaction between the original pathologist and peer-reviewing pathologist permitting them an active role in the oversight process. In addition, this also allows the original pathologist to inform the reviewing pathologist of subtleties that are not readily apparent in reviewed materials. Given this interaction, it is difficult to have a blinded peer review and therefore does have some risk of conflict of interest. Any perceived conflict of interest should be avoided but if they cannot be avoided should be disclosed. Retrospective peer review can be performed in trial transcripts and reports [36]. Ideally, the testimony could be reviewed in real time or prior to presentation in court to ensure quality and accuracy [34].

Social Determinants of Health

People of higher social position live longer and remain healthier than those of a lower position in society and therefore less likely to enter the death investigation system. The difference in morbidity and mortality is largely due to socioeconomic differences, prejudice, and discrimination against oppressed groups of people [37]. Social determinants of health are the socioeconomic conditions that impact the quality of health of individuals and communities. These social determinants can result in premature deaths due to social inequality among many [38]. The social determinants including income, Indigenous and other ethnicities, gender, and housing, among others, cause some populations to experience a disproportionate burden of morbidity and premature mortality. A social determinant of health approach identifies the impetus of death as a consequence of how society distributes economic and social resources. Groups seeking equity are disproportionality and adversely impacted by the institutions and processes that determine access to healthcare [38]. In particular, murdered Indigenous women and girls are overrepresentation in the death investigation system. Suicide rates among Indigenous peoples around the world are much higher than in the general population due to the harmful impact of colonialism [39]. Consequently, the medicolegal death investigation can play a pivotal role in providing knowledge of the egregious and persistent disparities in the community that it serves. Social policy guided by mortality research that is guided by conceptual frameworks of procedural justice can guide insights into the origins of disparities in mortality status. These can improve access to healthcare and health-related behaviors and reduce systemic oppression for racialized groups.

Second Autopsy and Exhumations

Forensic pathologists may be needed to examine human remains after burial. Exhumation (also referred to as disinterment or disentombment) is a rare practice in forensic pathology that refers to the recovery of a buried dead body from a grave for medicolegal purposes typically to perform a first or repeat postmortem examination [40]. The frequency is dependent on the country, that is considered dependent on political and religious convictions, and autopsy rates [41]. Exhumation is the last resort to examine a dead body of an unexplored or improperly explored death [40]. Exhumation requires following local disinterment laws and cooperation from those requesting disinterment, the funeral director, cemetery administrator, and anthropologist. There are three guidelines that need to be considered and fulfilled when considering performing a postmortem examination following disinterment: (1) the needs or questions can only be answered from the postmortem examination; (2) the questions or needs cannot be answered without (re-) examination of the exhumed body; in other words, a review of medical records, history and postmortem examination, stock pot, slides, and histology, if available, cannot answer the question; and (3) there is a reasonable likelihood that the needs and questions of postmortem examination can be answered when considering the decompositional changes, previous autopsy artifacts, embalming, or other body preparations. In other words, what is the probability of success [42]? The purposes for exhumation include identification, concerns of an unnatural death, and unlawfully interred bodies [43].

The ability of the postmortem examination to answer the questions proposed depends on the nature of those questions and the condition of the body. Exhumation has been shown to be worthwhile for living relatives whose loved ones were buried in mass graves following wars in places such as Serbia, Croatia, and Yugoslavia [44]. If there are toxicological considerations, collection of soil samples around the body should be considered [42].

Funerary Artifacts

Forensic pathologists sometimes are requested to examine embalmed human remains. Embalming is meant to preserve the body and minimize risks of communicable diseases to the community. Understanding the embalming process and associated artifacts is necessary to avoid misinterpretation of the body. Funeral home practices vary, but it is not typical for funeral directors to obtain photographic or other visual records of the bodies that are prepared for burial—in addition, documentation of the type of embalming fluids used, procedures used, and selection of arterial and venous access. The components of the embalming fluid typically include preservatives, anticoagulants, perfuming materials, surfactants, active dyes, modifying agents, and vehicles [42]. Among the preservatives, these include formalin, paraformaldehyde, acetaldehyde, dialdehyde, glutaraldehyde, methanol, phenol, and ammonia compounds [42]. The embalming fluid is injected under pressure into the arterial system, and blood is drained from the venous system. As the embalming fluid is injected into the vascular system, the blood will drain from the venous system. The embalming injection sites will vary in number and location to ensure adequate perfusion. Typical injection sites to access major arteries and veins include the following: (1) anterior base of the neck, posterior to the sternocleidomastoid muscle, (2) overlying the clavicle, (3) upper medial upper arms, and (4) in the groins. These access sites are typically sutured or glued following embalming. There may be other incisions, to remove pacemakers and for the insertion of the trocar within the abdomen. The trocar is typically a long metal tube with a sharp point that has two functions: (1) to aspirate material from the thoracoabdominal, and pelvic cavities and (2) to inject embalming fluid. The challenges with performing postmortem examination in embalmed bodies include limitations of toxicology, interpretation of funerary artifacts, and lack of flexibility of tissues due to formalin fixation. The limitations of **toxicology** relate to the fact that much of the blood has been drained, and tissues have embalming fluids. This requires cautious and careful interpretation of toxicology analysis, if performed, ideally, with a sample of the embalming fluid as a control. The limitations related to the interpretations of the funerary **artifacts** is usually straightforward as the embalming incisions and trocar puncture site are typically easily identifiable (Fig. 1.18). Other artifacts include postmortem bruising and enhancement of antemortem bruising. Postmortem bruising typically occurs before arterial embalming, when there is still blood in the vasculature, at the embalming site. If not recognized immediately during embalming, the postmortem bruise can become extensive. Antemortem bruises can appear or enlarge during the extravasation of the embalming fluid into the bruised area. In addition, postmortem clots that remain in the vasculature following embalming may be misinterpreted as antemortem thromboemboli. Histological evaluation of the "clot" should be helpful in differentiating an antemortem thromboembolous from a postmortem clot. **Flexibility of tissues**: Typically, the mouth is wired shut, making examination of the oral cavity challenging unless wires are cut. Also, tissues are now formalin-fixed, and palpation to detect early pneumonia is less reliable.

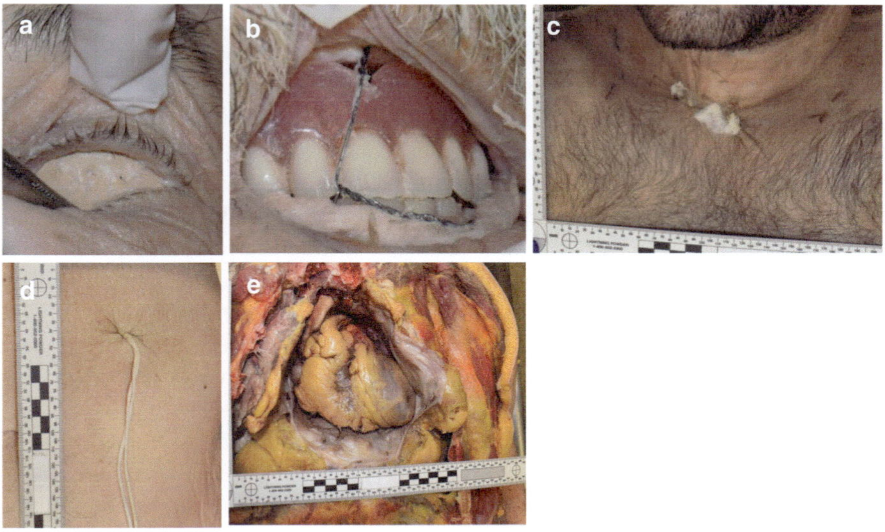

Fig. 1.18 Common embalming and funerary artifacts. (**a**) Corneal caps of the eyes to give structure to the globe. (**b**) Sutured jaw with wires to prevent a gaping mouth once rigor mortis passes. (**c**) Sutured injection sites for the delivery of embalming fluid and removal of intravascular blood. (**d**) Suture trocar incision of the abdomen (belly button to the left of the ruler). (**e**) Puncture sites from the trocar into the heart

Humanitarian Forensic Action

Given the etymology of the term "forensic" which is the application of an area of expertise to law, a common conception is that forensic pathology and other forensic sciences are crucial in the criminal justice system. However, forensic pathology and related sciences can have applications in a new field called humanitarian forensic action. Humanitarian forensic action is the application of the knowledge and skills of forensic sciences and medicine to humanitarian activities. Specifically, forensic work can alleviate human suffering and protect the dignity of all victims of armed conflict and catastrophes. This work is often framed under International Humanitarian law [45] and is carried out in a neutral, impartial, and independent, free of cost to the victims and their families. Forensic assistance can function in the following ways: (1) providing dignified management of human remains, (2) identifying human remains, and (3) resolving the uncertainty of who remains missing. Identifying human remains has humanitarian implications for the bereaved and is an ethical cornerstone of forensic practice [46]. In the setting of climate change resulting in increased frequency and intensity of natural disasters, the demand for humanitarian forensic action is likely to grow.

Understanding the Experience of Loss

The sudden unexpected death of a loved one is not an unusual experience. Many families have this "turn on a dime" experience where life as you know it changes in a moment, rocks the very core of your existence, and makes you question your identity and your place of safety in the world.

Being a member of the death investigation team often requires having conversations with families regarding the sudden unexpected death of their family members. Breaking bad news is not easy and requires skill in addition to an awareness of attitude considering the impact this has on the individual/family in the moment and in years to come [47]. This is a task that many within the profession, if given a choice, would choose not to engage in considering that how people learn about their family members' death can have a profound impact on their ability to cope and grieve [48]. Although a task is usually undertaken by police services or victim services, regrettably, it can fall to the investigating coroner, forensic pathologist, or other members of the death investigation team.

For those faced with this task, there are many questions that inevitably come to mind. How do you engage in the conversation with the family, when and where should it happen, and by whom? What information should be shared besides telling the family that the individual has died? What happens if the person being told reacts in a negative way potentially harming themselves or someone else? How long should you stay with the person when you share this news? When should you leave? What other factors such as culture or religion need to be taken into consideration when the death notification is made? Do you do this in person, over the phone, or through another individual? These and probably many more questions may come to the mind of the person who will be sharing this news of death—news that changes the person's life as they know it and represents the beginning of life without their loved one. This information needs to be shared in a clear, caring, sensitive, and compassionate manner because the words will be etched in their memory forever. According to Ombres et al. [49], the literature unanimously agrees that the ideal death notification occurs in person; however, in practice, this may not be feasible, especially in remote areas, and notification must occur by phone. Recognizing the significance and impact of breaking bad news to families around the death of their family member protocols and guidelines should be developed to help professionals [47]. The Scientific Working Groups for Medicolegal Death Investigation (SWGMDI) has created principles for communicating with next of kin during death investigation [50]. These principles are adaptable by any individual or office and provide the medicolegal professional insight and examples of best practice approaches including a list of things not to say. Another medical model for breaking bad news is the six-step SPIKES (S—Setting up an interview, P—Assessing the patient's perception, I—Obtaining the patient's invitation, K—Giving knowledge and information to the patient, E—addressing the patient's emotions with empathetic response, and S—Strategy), and a six-step protocol as well as the BREAKS (B—Background, R—Rapport, E—Explore, A—Announce; K—Kindling, and S—Summarize) is a systematic and easy communication strategy for breaking bad news. "*They will never forget those words*."

Conversations with families that are done well can have a lasting effect and often assist them with taking the next steps toward healthy grieving. Communication that is not done well, is poorly timed, or conveys inaccurate or contradictory information can leave the family feeling undervalued and retraumatized often complicating their grief process [49]. Ombres et al. [49] suggest that complicated grief can have many negative outcomes including the potential for increased mental health illness, physiological illness, and increased mortality. It is a task that is conceivably unpleasant and one that no one wants to do. Very few professionals receive formal training in communication with families because it is perceived to be a skill that is not often used and there are other skills that are used more important and have a need to be practiced more. Although it is rare that a physician would have to share this news with a family because police services typically make the death notification it is interesting to note that, in one study, 80% of medical resident doctors indicated that they felt inadequately trained to deliver death news to families and this lack of training induced stress symptoms in them [49]. The delivery of death notification often falls to the responsibility of the police service, many of whom indicate that they do not feel they are adequately trained to deliver this life-altering information. In a study of 50 law enforcement officers, 67% of participants found death notifications very stressful or extremely stressful, citing lack of training, over-identification with the family, concern over physical or verbal aggression by the family, and labeling by other officers if they expressed emotional difficulty with the task. Communication with families requires a level of self-confidence and competency in having difficult conversations and delivering death notifications. Schepers indicates that "truth telling" is encouraged, widely accepted, and endorsed [51]. It is highly recommended that any individual who has the potential to interact with a family should be provided with the appropriate training. This would include, but would not be limited to, death notifications, grief education, cultural/religious sensitivity training, effective and appropriate language, and communication in difficult situations.

While it might feel rude or uncomfortable to say, "Your husband has died," the use of euphemisms such as "passed away" or "we lost him" does not fully process in the acutely stressed mind of a survivor. Sugarcoating the message may create unnecessary distress or confusion, and sometimes resentment, for not being more straightforward. It is important to use the words dead and died. Research shows that avoiding these words and using euphemisms shows that these common practices are more harmful to the survivors' healing process [52].

Grief, Mourning, and Bereavement

Grief and mourning, normal reactions associated with death affect people on many different levels: physical, emotional, spiritual, psychological, and behavioral. Processing the experience is necessary to move toward healthy grieving [53]. This can be a difficult task, especially in a society where death and grief are both typically denied and avoided [54]. While we all understand that someday we will die, we do not like to acknowledge it, think about it, converse about it, or recognize it as reality. Denial of death can lead to unhealthy and unrealistic expectations of grief. However, before we can begin to discuss the importance and value of communicating with families about their death experience particularly related to death investigation, it is necessary to understand the language and terminology used when discussing grief. Often, the terms grief, mourning, and bereavement are used interchangeably. However, they are distinct in their relationship to a person's experience with death (Fig. 1.19).

Bereavement is defined as the event of loss and can also be referred to as the period of time immediately following a loss. It comes from an old English word that means "rob," "deprive," and "seize". When a person dies suddenly and unexpectedly, those who remain are often left in a state of bereavement, meaning that a part of ourselves is stripped away against our will. As much as the death of an individual can disrupt our lives, it is also an event that is very natural and normal in the human

Grief	Mourning	Bereavement
-internal experience of emotions after any loss. -reaction to loss.	outward expression of grief.	-event of loss -period of time immediately following a loss, during which you experience grief and express mourning.

Fig. 1.19 The differences between grief, mourning, and bereavement

experience. In order to understand bereavement, it is necessary to understand grief and mourning.

Grief is defined as the reaction to loss. It includes a set of thoughts and feelings a person has that affect their emotional as well as their mental, physical, and spiritual responses. There is no set time for when this grief reaction can occur, and not every person experiences all grief reactions. This does not mean that the person is not experiencing grief. Grief is a unique, individual, and highly variable experience [55]. It is multi-layered and ever evolving. Grief does not have an ending. Often grief will manifest itself as disbelief, confusion, tension, anxiety, or pain. In the early days after the death, there can be an overwhelming feeling of disorganization and depression. Everything can seem surreal, and a person's sensory responses are unreliable and erratic. As well there can be a sense of euphoria with a hypersensitivity to people and events. There can often be a preoccupation with the deceased and/or the spirit of the deceased. This may present in the form of dreams, signs, or a felt presence. Grief can arouse a very wide range of emotions, including but not limited to, sadness, longing, loneliness, sorrow, self-pity, anguish, guilt, and anger as well as relief and joy. Often the bereaved may experience confusion, outrage, and a sense of injustice over the loss. There can also be a level of frustration due to the lack of control a family experience—lack of control around the investigation, the autopsy, and, in some cases such as homicide, information related to the deceased.

> *Grief has a much longer half-life than we expect, even when we understand the process and attend to it* (Devine [56]).

Mourning is the process by which a person integrates the death of the individual into their ongoing life. Mourning is the outward appearance of our grief, what we choose to show to the outside world. This can be influenced partially by social, familial, religious, and cultural norms. Some visible behaviors of mourning include the procession of funeral vehicles, wearing of black clothing or armbands, and flying flags at half-mast.

Finally, a last word regarding the word ***CLOSURE.*** In the world of grief, there is no closure. Grief is something that lasts a lifetime. The griever never gets over their grief; they come to a place where they learn to live with the experience or learn to grow around [57].

Speaking with Families and the Forensic Pathologist

> *No one ever told me that grief felt so like fear. I am not afraid, but the sensation is like being afraid. The same fluttering in the stomach, the same restlessness, the yawning. I keep on swallowing. At other times it feels like being mildly drunk, or concussed. There is a sort of invisible blanket between the world and me. I find it hard to take in what anyone says. Or perhaps, hard to want to take it in. It is so uninteresting. Yet I want the others to be about me. I dread the moments when the house is empty. If only they would talk to one another and not to me.* (C.S. Lewis, A Grief Observed)

C.S. Lewis epitomizes the experience of death from the perspective of fear—fear of the unknown, fear of the acknowledgment of death, and fear of the recognition that death of another reflects our own mortality. He continues with fear of not knowing the meaning of life, of consciousness being self-deception, and of losing a clear memory of his love [58]. He also identifies the confusion and disbelief that encompasses the death experience and the conscious desire not to hear the information being shared [58].

Death communication is not a novel concept, but rather something that has always been present, yet historically avoided [54]. In death investigation, the discussion or conversation around death and speaking with families is not a new phenomenon. Today, in some investigation systems, the forensic pathologitsts are engaged in formal discussions through programs such as Next of Kin Clinics [59]. From this perspective, it is extremely important to be mindful that families who have had the experience of sudden unexpected death have additional layers of challenges and emotions and have not chosen to be "here"—unlike the forensic pathologists who has spent multiple years obtaining education and preparation in medical school, residency, and specialty training; become familiar with the sights, sounds, and smells of the autopsy suite; and developed a foreign language to tell the story about the death. For these reasons, it is critical to set a compassionate, sensitive tone with families at the time of death investigation. The family relies on the honest, insightful, knowledgeable direction of the coroner, medical examiner, and forensic pathologist.

If we recognize that the experience of grief related to the death of an individual is a unique experience unlike anyone else's, we must realize that the approach we take with each family member of the deceased must also be unique. There is no scripted cookie-cutter approach to speaking with and sharing information with families about the unexpected death of their loved one. The approach that you take will very much become a part of their personal history with the event of their loved one's death. Despite the significant impact it has on families, very few empirical studies exist regarding appropriate methods for death notification [49].

Families recall vividly not only what is said but also how it is said.

> *I've learned that people will forget what you said, people will forget what you did, but people will never forget how you made them feel.* (Maya Angelou)

Cultural/Religious Issues and Autopsy

Sensitivity and respect for cultural and religious considerations should always be considered and accommodated for within what death investigation can permit. Varying beliefs, customs, and traditions surrounding death and death practices are common to all cultures and religions, and often these beliefs may come into conflict regarding autopsies.

Although many cultures will indicate opposition to autopsy, citing religious beliefs as the reason, most religions and cultures are accepting of autopsy with a few citing objections (i.e. Islam and Judaism), suggesting that the dissection violates the sanctity of maintaining the completeness of the body. In these situations, special techniques (i.e. waterless autopsies) are used and, if possible, a minimally invasive autopsy is performed.

The main issues surrounding the objection of autopsies that are cited are delayed burials, "harm" caused to the body, and the removal of body parts [60]. These concerns do not differ across religions. The benefits, however, are also perceived to be similar: autopsies can lead to scientific advancement, discovery of important medical diagnoses, enhanced education, and establishing cause of death.

The following is a brief overview extracted from the Multifaith Information Manual [61] of cultural and religious beliefs around death and autopsy, which may assist the forensic pathologist in their consideration of accommodation for families with cultural or religious requests (Fig. 1.20).

Islam (Muslim)

Although the Qur'an does not directly discuss autopsies, the Islamic population objects to them indicating that the deceased should be buried as soon as possible, preferably within 24 hours. Authorization occurs when the benefits outweigh the damages such as in the case of the medicolegal autopsy.

Islam (Muslim)	Judaism	Hinduism	Buddhism	Christianity	Jehovah's Witness	Indigenous/ First Nations/Native Americans
-Qur'an does not directly discuss autopsies -Buried preferably within 24 hours -Authorization: benefits > the damages	-Generally opposed -If required: consider only examining organs that must be examined -All fluids, organs and any materials used must be buried with the body -Buried preferably within 24 hours -May request rabbi to be present at autopsy	Disapprove of autopsies but will comply, if necessary, by law. Jains & Sikhs have no religious objection to the autopsy.	No objection to autopsy May request time be given for the soul to leave the body	Christianity considers autopsy an act of charity to help others. Catholics & Protestants have no objection to autopsy. -Understand the value related to medical education	-Autopsy is mutilation to the body however, they will consent when required by law. -request that no organs be removed	-Customs for handling of a body, dissections, removal of body parts and delay in burial - Concerns related to colonial intrusion

Fig. 1.20 Accommodation consideration examples based on religion and culture

Judaism

Autopsies are generally opposed by Jewish people because of their belief that man is created in God's image and therefore desecration of the body is desecration of God's image. If an autopsy is to be performed, it should involve only those organs that must be examined. In addition, all fluids, organs, and any materials used during autopsy must be buried with the body. Additionally, the autopsy should be performed as soon as possible allowing for burial within 24 hours. Some families may request the presence of a rabbi either at the autopsy or in the building where it is taking place.

Hinduism

Hindus believe that an autopsy may be disturbing to the soul and ultimately disapprove of autopsies but will comply, if necessary, by law. Jains and Sikhs have no religious objection to the autopsy.

Buddhism

Buddhists have no objection to autopsy. They believe that they can be of benefit to the medical community in determining diagnoses as well as bringing justice to a criminal. The only request of this religion is that an appropriate time be given for the soul to leave the body.

Christianity

Catholicism/Protestantism

Catholics and Protestants have no objection to autopsy. They see it as valuable and agree with medical education and organ retrieval/transplant. Christianity considers autopsy an act of charity to help others. Although there are no limitations at autopsy, it is expected the body be handled with respect.

Jehovah's Witness

The objection Jehovah's Witnesses have to autopsy is mutilation to the body; however, they will consent when required by law. They request that no organs be removed and the body be handled respectfully.

Indigenous/First Nations/Native Americans

The major concern regarding autopsy and Indigenous peoples is customs for handling of a body, dissections, removal of body parts, and delay in burial.

Whether it be in the clinical or medicolegal setting, by understanding the influence various belief systems have on autopsy, pathologists will be better equipped to communicate with next of kin, minimize emotional trauma, and facilitate the grieving and burial process. Sometimes, minor changes to practices such as prioritizing an autopsy or having a recording of religious chanting can make a difference for the people within the cultures and religions.

Providing Information to Families

Due to the unexpectedness of the experience of loss when families receive the news of the sudden, unexpected death, they have difficulty processing and remembering the verbal information being provided to them. There are a variety of appropriate and inappropriate behaviors that can be displayed to families (Figs. 1.21 and 1.22). Besides keeping the information simple, it is necessary to provide this information in a variety of formats besides verbal such as a written pamphlet or a link to the organization's website. The most important information being shared should be given in writing; this would include such things as the coroner contact information and the location of the body. This helps to demystify the experience and offers a level of transparency to the forensic process. Other things to take into consideration are the use of an interpreter including sign language, non-English speaking and deaf families, and translated written information in the language that is appropriate for your family. It is important to anticipate that the family will have questions. Some of the more frequently asked questions are as follows: how did this happen? Where

- **Do acknowledge the loss**
- **Do use the name of the person who died**
- **Do be aware that children grieve differently from adults and from each other**
- **Do listen as much as you can; talk less**
- **Do accept emotional expression**
- **Do show empathy**
- **Do intervene to stop harmful behaviors when there is a safety concern**

Fig. 1.21 The "Do's" of family interactions

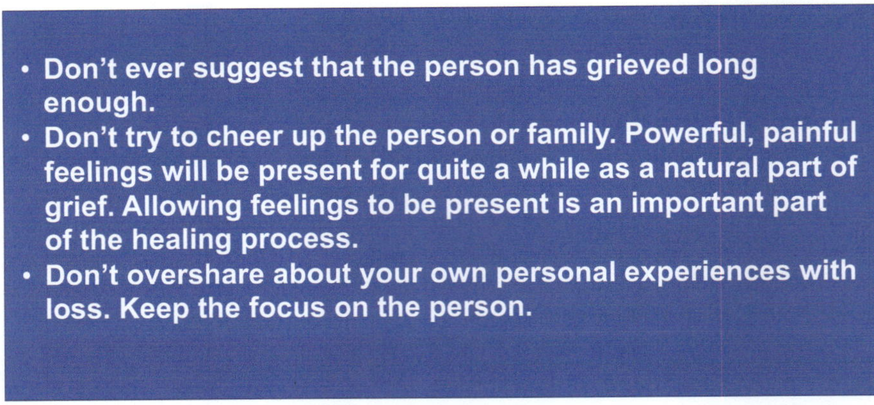

Fig. 1.22 The "Don'ts" of family interactions

is the body? Can I see the body? Did they suffer? Why do you have to do an autopsy? Will we be able to have an open casket after the autopsy?

The following are some suggestions from the Dougy Center [62] around words and actions that offer support and comfort and words and actions that do not.

Words and Actions That Offer Comfort and Invite Communication

Can you tell me more about what this has been like for you?
What kinds of memories do you have about [insert decedent name]?
What sorts of things have you been thinking about [insert decedent name] since he/she/they died?
How is your family doing? What kinds of concerns do you have about them?
I don't know what to say, but I know this must be very difficult for you.
I can't imagine what you are going through or simply, I can't imagine.
I'm so sorry or I am so sorry for your loss.
(If crying) It is so natural to cry at this time.
One of my favorite memories of [insert decedent name] is…
Do you feel like talking for a while?
I'm here for you, whatever you are feeling right now.

Words and Actions That <u>Do Not</u> Offer Comfort

I know how you feel. (You can't know exactly.)
You must feel [insert emotion].

Time will heal you.
Just be happy that he/she/they is/are not in pain anymore.
Be strong. You're holding up well.
Keep busy.
[Insert decedent name] was suffering. Now he/she/they is/are in a better place.
Now you have an angel in heaven.
It could be worse, you still have [insert survivor(s)].
You'll be stronger because of this.
I know this must be difficult, but it's important to remember the good things in life as well.
You'll need to be strong now for your family. It's important to get a grip on your feelings.

A grieving person is in a place that is usually foreign to them. Even if they had other losses, each loss is new and unique. Just a phone call (without ever expecting a response) saying that you care is thoughtful and comforting.

A final word about communication. Requesting or choosing one family member as a primary point of contact is highly suggested. This will minimize misunderstandings or misinterpretation when sharing information or direction for the next steps.

Viewing the Body

As previously mentioned, truth telling is extremely important including sharing with the family the condition of the deceased person's body [51]. Many people draw their knowledge and experience from television and anticipate that the deceased will look as they do when they are sleeping. We know that this is not always the case, especially with decomposition, dismemberment, severe injury, or charring from fire deaths. Preparing the family for the condition of the deceased will assist them in setting realistic expectations for viewing and final arrangements (i.e. open or closed casket). In some situations, funeral homes have staff who can reconstruct the face of the deceased to a more recognizable resemblance of who they were in life.

If the body of the deceased is severely decomposed, charred, or dismembered, the likelihood is that the funeral home will not encourage them to view the body. If it is a family's informed wish to view the body, they should be given the opportunity to view it in an appropriate environment that is conducive to viewing it with compassionate, supportive preparation to ensure that they have all of the necessary information to make an informed decision with minimal risk of re-traumatization. This experience will minimize fantasy thinking, assisting the families in accepting the reality of the death and moving forward in their steps toward healthy grieving. Families should be provided with clear, concise direction of what is and is not acceptable within the viewing environment (i.e. Please do not bang on the glass, kick or punch walls or you can hold your baby, but you will need to sit in this chair when you do so).

If there is any risk that viewing of the body would compromise the integrity of an investigation, or expose the family to any risk, this should be explained to the family, and they should be asked to wait until the body has been prepared by the funeral home before viewing. It should be noted that, in some cases, the family will not have the opportunity to view the body of the deceased. This would include situations where there is a risk of infection or chemical exposure.

There may be cultural or religious rituals and ceremonies that the family or community needs to perform soon after the death. Accommodations should be made for these practices to the extent that is possible.

In the event that a compassionate viewing is being provided for the family, the suggestion is to have this happen after the autopsy, so the body of the deceased is prepared and presentable, as well there is no concern with delaying the medicolegal process.

At some point in time in the investigation, it will be necessary to have further conversation with families about the progress of the investigation, preliminary autopsy results, potential organ retention, and so on. It is important to convey only information that is known. Providing hypothetical information will create confusion and cause families undue stress. Remember that they are not processing in the same way that we are.

Organ Retention and Disposition

On occasion at the time an autopsy is conducted, the pathologist may request to retain an organ(s) for further examination. This occurs whenever the pathologist believes that the retention of the organ(s) is necessary to further investigate the cause and manner of death or seek expert consultation. Families should be made aware of the reason and necessity for retention and how this helps to inform the cause and manner of death. Families should be provided information about the options for disposition after the investigation is complete. If the family is going to incur any costs related to the disposition of the organ, they should be made aware of this prior to the agreement for retention. There may be religious/cultural or social reasons that families may express with regard to the burial or cremation of the body not in its entirety. If it is an option to hold the body until the organ can be repatriated to the body, then this option should be presented to the family. Documentation and indication of the length of time that organs will be retained prior to disposition is strongly suggested.

Visual Identification

As previously indicated, families may derive a lot of their knowledge from television. This can set the coroner or forensic pathologist up for unrealistic expectations because much of what is portrayed on television is not what happens in the lived experience. For example, the family may expect to be taken to the location of the body to identify the deceased or taken to the morgue to have the door opened, the tray pulled out, the sheet drawn back, and identification happened. Ideally, scientific/comparative methods are the preferred process for the identification of the deceased with a visual identification by a family member as a last resort. Families should be provided information about the process of scientific identification and how this process ensures greater accuracy and minimizes the risk of traumatizing the family. As a mechanism for processing, their grief families may also want to "do" something to assist with the identification process. In these situations, families could be asked to assist the coroner to obtain dental records, medical information, and so on to assist.

An important point to remember at this time is that, if the deceased is not positively identified, there may be limited information that can be provided to a family member. This can be upsetting for families, so it is necessary to have a further discussion about the risks of sharing confidential information, the impact on the family, and the death investigation.

Resources and Supports

As conversations continue with the family in the early stages of the investigation, the coroner or medical examiner will begin to have a greater understanding of the family's support systems. If a family is lacking in the areas of support, this would be a good time to offer resources and supports. It is suggested that supports are specific to the manner of death and the relationship with the deceased. For example, the family member who has the experience of a child who dies by suicide should be provided information specific to that of a parent who experiences the death of a child by suicide. Connecting like with like or, now more commonly referred to as, peer to peer creates a common ground and normalizes the grieving person's experience.

Reports

In both the coronial and medical examiner systems, reports related to the death of the deceased are generated. In some jurisdictions because of privacy laws, not all reports are provided to family. It is ensured that families understand what they are entitled to receive. Information on how to obtain the reports, any documents that need to be completed for this process, as well as a time frame in which they can expect to receive the reports should be provided to them. Often families need these reports for financial and/or legal reasons. Families should be made aware of the process for asking questions or clarification about reports and that the reports; in particular, the autopsy report is best explained by the pathologist that authored that report. Families may assume that photographs are part of the content of reports. In most institutions, this is not the case. Guidelines should be established when requests for photographs are made. A practice that works well is having the family member(s) attend to an in-person location that is convenient for all to review the photos and answer any questions the family may have related to the photos. Then after the viewing of the photos, the family can make an informed decision as to whether they want to receive the photos. Photographs would then be printed and ink-marked with the organization's logo.

Personal Effects/Belongings

At the time of their death, individuals may have items on their person, referred to as personal effects or belongings. These can include anything from a cell phone, a wallet, identification, to loose change in a pocket, or jewelry items. Any items should not be discarded regardless of perceived "value." Families cling onto any connection with the deceased including things such as paper receipts. If these items remain at the pathology unit, a process that ensures transparency is to document, itemize, and photograph the items. This helps avoid any discrepancy with family. Depending again on the jurisdiction, the police service may take these items into their possession and later release them to the family. These items may also serve as evidence in legal proceedings. The procedure in your unit/agency should be understood to ensure accurate conveyance of the procedure.

Children and Grief

The mere thought of children being subjected to grief as a result of death invokes a need to protect them. There is a perceived belief that children should be shielded and not exposed to the events and customs that death brings. Because death is a natural life event for children, it is inevitable that they will be exposed to it at some point in their lives. How a child processes death is dependent on their age and developmental understanding of death and loss.

When interacting with young children, it is important to remember that they are very ego-centric and may believe that something they did caused a person's death. It is important to ensure that they understand they did not. In the field of thanatology, when working with children, we speak of the 5 Cs; the most common five concerns that children have at the time of the person's death. Did I ***cause*** it? Can I ***catch*** it? Can I ***cure*** it? Who's going to take ***care*** of me? And how will I stay ***connected***? Answering these questions will ensure that their concerns are addressed.

It is important to always remember that everyone including children grieve differently. A child's work is play, so often after the death of their person, children will play to process the event. They will ask questions and, when satisfied, will return to their play. If a child is not satisfied or does not believe the adult providing the information is telling the truth, they will return with more questions.

Be mindful that children will mimic or model the behavior of the adults in their world. Expressing emotion and talking about the deceased provide permission for the child to do the same.

Truth Telling

Truth telling is always important with everyone but especially with children. It is widely accepted and endorsed when explaining death to children [51].

Often at the time of death, coroners or pathologists will imply that the deceased did not suffer, died quickly, or had a peaceful death in hopes of making the family feel better.

It is better to tell the truth, as families will process the information in their own way that is often embedded in their values and/or belief system. For example, a delay in death may be viewed by family as an opportunity for the decedent to engage in spiritual considerations.

In his book, Being Mortal, Dr. Atul Gawande shares a story of regret about a woman who at his suggestion spent the remaining 2 weeks of her life in treatment instead of going to the beach and spending time with her grandchildren. He says the reason he regrets this is "because I knew it was a complete lie. I just wanted to have something positive to say [63]."

NOK (Next of Kin) Clinic Meeting/Post Autopsy Family Conference

As mentioned earlier, most families draw their information/education from television, so understandably after families have received reports related to their person's death, they may have questions and concerns or even disagree with the cause and/or manner of death. It is considered best practice to offer/provide a Next of Kin Clinic meeting or Post Autopsy Family Conference [59]. This is an opportunity to educate families about death investigation as well as police investigation and other investigations occurring simultaneously as well as dispel the fallacies and mistruths that arise because of a lack of knowledge. This meeting can be arranged either in person or virtually with all the parties involved in the death of the individual including but not limited to the forensic pathologist, investigating coroner, family liaison, police service, emergency medical service, healthcare representative, fire marshal office, and so on plus family members and their supporting people. Families should be asked to submit their questions and concerns in advance of the meeting. These should be distributed to all participants and the most responsible person be assigned to answer the question(s). Families should be invited to bring a photograph of the person who died, and an opportunity extended at the beginning of the meeting to share about their person. If permissible, scene photographs, autopsy photographs, imaging photographs, anatomy photographs, and so on should be provided during this time if this family has requested. An opportunity to record the meeting should be extended to the family if all parties agree. Meetings should be limited to a 2 hour time frame with an invitation extended for future meeting(s) if needed.

Family Liaison Units

Some jurisdictions and provinces have the services of Family Liaison Units or persons to assist families in navigating through death investigation. These units/persons are designed to help demystify the experience of death investigation and advocate for and encourage communication and inclusiveness of family throughout the process. The establishment of a Family Liaison Coordinator in Ontario was from a recommendation from the Goudge Inquiry [64].

Family Indigenous Liaison Unit (FILU)

In 2016 in every province and territory across Canada, Family Indigenous Liaison Units (FILUs) were established. These units were designed to provide specialized services to families of missing and murdered Indigenous women and girls and work parallel with the work of the National Inquiry into Missing and Murdered Indigenous Women and Girls.

FILUs assist families in accessing available information about their missing and murdered loved ones from many government sources. Receiving information about their missing or murdered person is important for their healthy grief journey.

If families need additional support, FILUs make connections between family members and cultural advisors, elders, or counseling services and programs, depending on the family's wishes.

Summary

Just as forensic pathologists are the principal medical arm of the death investigation system, so too is the autopsy the principal method of analysis. In communicating with families, it is important to be mindful that the words we use instantly change the life of the family member who must learn to live with the absence of their person. The art of healing begins and ends with communication.

References

1. Statistics Canada. Canadian coroner and medical examiner database. 2006-2008. Annual report.
2. Wood MJ, Guha AK. Medicolegal autopsy rates in Halifax, Nova Scotia. Why the difference? A historical perspective. Arch Pathol Lab Med. 2001;125:924–30.
3. Centers for Disease Control and Prevention. Coroner training requirements. http://www.cdc.gov/phlp/publications/coroner/training.html. Updated 1 Jan 2015. Accessed 18 Apr 2021.
4. Hanzlick R. The conversion of coroner systems to medical examiner systems in the United States: a lull in the action. Am J Forensic Med Pathol. 2007;28(4):279–83.
5. Hanzlick R, Combs D. Medical examiner and coroner systems: history and trends. JAMA. 1998;279(11):870–4.
6. Hanzlick R, editor. Cause of death and the death certificate. College of American Pathologists; 2006. ISBN: 093030490X
7. Cordner SM. Deciding the cause if death after necroscopy. Lancet. 1993;341:1458–60.
8. Pollanen MS. Deciding the cause of death after autopsy—revisited. J Clin Forensic Med. 2005;12:113–21.
9. Hanzlick RL. Cause of death statements and certification of natural and unnatural deaths. College of American Pathologists; 1997. Available from: https://netforum.avectra.com/eweb/DynamicPage.aspx?Site.NAME%26WebCode.DeathCert.
10. Oliver WR. Manner determination in forensic pathology. Acad Forensic Pathol. 2014;4(4):480–91.
11. Gill JR, Goldfeder LB, Hirsch CS. Use of "therapeutic complication" as a manner of death. J Forensic Sci. 2006;51(5):1127–33.
12. WHO. World report on violence and health. Geneva: WHO; 2002.
13. http://www.austlii.edu.au/au/other/lawreform/ALRC/1977/7.html#Ch_13Heading2.
14. Lane M, Vercler CJ. AMA J Ethics. 2016;18(8):771–8.
15. Plattner T. The response of relatives to medicolegal investigations and forensic autopsy. Am J Forensic Med Pathol. 2002;23(4):345–8.
16. Burton JL, Underwood JC. Necropsy practice after the "organ retention scandal": requests, performance, and tissue retention. J Clin Pathol. 2003;56(7):537–41.
17. Turnbull A, et al. Hospital autopsy: endangered or extinct? J Clin Pathol. 2015;68(8):601–4.
18. Byard RW, Winskog C. Histology in forensic practice: required or redundant? Forensic Sci Med Pathol. 2012;8(1):56–7.
19. Molina DK, Wood LE, Frost RE. Is routine histopathologic examination beneficial in all medicolegal autopsies? Am J Forensic Med Pathol. 2007;28(1):1–3.
20. Bernardi FDC, et al. Histological examination has a major impact on the macroscopic necropsy diagnoses. J Clin Pathol. 2005;58:1261–4.
21. Randall BB, et al. Practice guidelines for forensic pathology. Arch Pathol Lab Med. 1998;122:1056–64.
22. National Association of Medical Examiners. Forensic autopsy performance standards. Am J Forensic Med Pathol. 27(3):2006, 200–225.
23. Coe JI, Am J. Forensic Med Pathol. 1993;14:91–117.
24. Pollanen MS. Forensic pathology and the miscarriage of justice. Forensic Sci Med Pathol. 2012;8(3):285–9.
25. Brennan PAW. The medical and ethical aspects of photography in the sexual assault examination: why does it offend? J Clin Forensic Med. 2006;13:194–202.
26. https://books.google.ca/books?id=SYqsCQAAQBAJ&pg=PA280&lpg=PA280&dq=Melvin+A.+Shiffman,+Code+of+Professional+and+Ethical+Conduct,+in+Ethics+in+Forensic+Science+and+Medicine:+Guidelines+for+the+Forensic+Expert+and+the+Attorney&source=bl&ots=QucoeDTVYO&sig=ACfU3U1rXNLLLLLIxGNx96hhMtzc0fCT6w&hl=en&sa=X&ved=2ahUKEwi2xu6G363wAhVTV80KHUiqB5QQ6AEwBHoECAYQAw#v=onepage&q=Melvin%20A.%20Shiffman%2C%20Code%20of%20Professional%20and%20

Ethical%20Conduct%2C%20in%20Ethics%20in%20Forensic%20Science%20and%20Medicine%3A%20Guidelines%20for%20the%20Forensic%20Expert%20and%20the%20Attorney&f=false. p. 236.
27. OSAC 2021-S-0013 Standard guide for postmortem photography.
28. Nayler JR. Clinical photography: a guide for the clinician. J Postgrad Med. 2003;49(3):256–62. https://www.jpgmonline.com/article.asp?issn=0022-3859;year=2003;volume=49;issue=3;spage=256;epage=262;aulast=Nayler.
29. Forensic photography certification requirements. International association for identification. http://www.theiai.org/certifications/imaging/requirements.php. Accessed 18.05.12.
30. Ferrucci M. et al. Dimensional review of scales for forensic photography.
31. Obenson K, Wright CM. The values of 100% retrospective peer review in a forensic pathology practice. J Forensic Legal Med. 2013;20:1066–8.
32. Rutty GN, Burton JL. Chapter 6: The external examination. In: Burton JL, Rutty GN, editors. The hospital autopsy. 2nd ed. London: Arnold; 2001. p. 42–51.
33. Lundberg GD. When to panic over abnormal values. MLO Med Lab Obs. 1972;4:47–54.
34. Welner M, et al. Peer-reviewed forensic consultation: safeguarding expert testimony and protecting the uninformed court. J Forensic Psychol Pract. 2012;12:1–34.
35. Byard RW. Unexpected infant death: lessons from the Sally Clark case. Med J Aust. 2004;181(1):52–4.
36. Obenson K. Wright CM. The value of 100% retrospective peer review in forensic pathology practice. J Forensic Legal Med. 2013;20:1066-8
37. Buka SL. Disparities in health status and substance use: ethnicity and socioeconomic factors. Public Health Rep. 2002;117:S118–25.
38. Raphael D, editor. Social determinants of Health. Canadian perspective. 3rd ed. Toronto: Canadian Scholar's Press Inc.; 2016. p. 11.
39. MacNeil MS. An epidemiologic study of Aboriginal adolescent risk in Canada: the meaning of suicide. J Child Adolesc Psychiatr Nurs. 2008;21(1):3–12.
40. Nouma Y, et al. Forensic examination after exhumation: contribution and difficulties after more than thirty years of burial. J Forensic Legal Med. 2016;44:120–7.
41. Grellner W, Glenewinkel F. Exhumations: synopsis of morphological and toxicological findings in relation to the postmortem interval. Survey on a 20-year period and review of the literature. Forensic Sci Int. 1997;90:139–59.
42. Hanzlick R. Embalming, body preparation, burial and disinterment. Am J Forensic Med Pathol. 1994;15(2):122–31.
43. Akhiwu WO, Nwafor CC. Exhumations: rarely done procedure but useful in many circumstances—a review of 47 cases in Nigeria. Egypt J Forensic Sci. 2019;9:67, 9 p.
44. Mirza FH, et al. J Forensic Legal Med. 2012;19:337–40.
45. Cordner S, Tidball-Binz M. Humanitarian forensic action—its origins and future. Forensic Sci Int. 2017;279:65–71.
46. ICRC Report. The missing and their families. Chapter II Executive Summary (ICRC/TheMissing/01.2003/EN/10). https://www.icrc.org/eng/assets/files/oth-er/icrc_themissing_012003_en_10.pdf. Accessed 18 Aug 2022.

Understanding the Experience of Loss References

47. De Leo D, Zammarrelli J, Viecelli Giannotti A, Donna S, Bertini S, Santini A, Anile C. Notification of unexpected, violent and traumatic death: a systematic review. Front Psychol. 2020;11:2229. https://doi.org/10.3389/fpsyg.2020.02229.
48. Lord JH. 2008. I'll never forget those words: A practical guide to death notifications. Compassion Press.

49. Ombres R, Montemorano L, Becker D. Death notification: someone needs to call the family. J Palliat Med. 2017;20(6):672–5. https://doi.org/10.1089/jpm.2016.0481.
50. Scientific Working Group on Medicolegal Death Investigation. Increasing the Supply of Forensic Pathologists in the United States: A Report and Recommendations. December, 2012. http://www.swgmdi.org/images/si4.fpsupplyreportpublisheddecember2012.pdf.
51. Schepers S. Commentary: Fifty Years of Development in Pediatric Psycho-Oncology Research and Practice: How Far Have we Come? Journal of pediatric psychology. 2019. 44. https://doi.org/10.1093/jpepsy/jsz043.
52. Jabr A. Death communication: what we've failed to teach. EMS World; 2021.
53. Worden JW. Grief counseling and grief therapy: A handbook for the mental health practitioner (2nd ed.); 1991. Springer Publishing Company.
54. Baker AW, Keshaviah A, Horenstein A, Goetter EM, Mauro C, Reynolds C, Zisook S, Shear MK, Simon NM. The role of avoidance in complicated grief: a detailed examination of the Grief-Related Avoidance Questionnaire (GRAQ) in a large sample of individuals with complicated grief. J Loss Trauma. 2016;21(6):533–47. https://doi.org/10.1080/15325024.2016.1157412.
55. Kübler-Ross E. On death and dying. Bull Am Coll Surg. 1975;60(6):12–7.
56. Devine M. How long does grief brain last? Refuge in Grief. 2022. https://refugeingrief.com/2022/03/11/how-long-does-grief-brain-last/.
57. Tonkin L. Growing around grief: another way of looking at grief and recovery. Bereavement Care. 1996;15(1):10. https://doi.org/10.1080/02682629608657376.
58. Lewis CS. A grief observed. Faber & Faber; 2015.
59. Vanezis P, Leadbeatter S. Next of kin clinics: a new role for the pathologist. J Clin Pathol. 1999;52(10):723–4. https://doi.org/10.1136/jcp.52.10.723.
60. Weaver K, Beal S, Burton E. Religions and the autopsy. Medscape. 2020. https://emedicine.medscape.com/article/1705993-overview.
61. Ontario Multifaith Council on Spiritual and Religious Care. Multifaith information manual. 5th ed. Webcon; 2014.
62. The Dougy Center for Grieving Children and Families. https://www.dougy.org/.
63. MLA. Gawande. Being Mortal: Medicine and What Matters in the End. New York: Metropolitan Books, Henry Holt and Company, 2014.
64. Goudge Inquiry. 2007. http://www.goudgeinquiry.ca.

Chapter 2
Death Investigation Bioethics

Rebekah Jacques

Ethics and Morals

"If morality is "the science of the good", ethics is the study of that science…" [1]. The terms "ethics" and "morals" are often used interchangeably but can have different meanings. **Morals** is focused on the *practice of morality,* and ethics is the *theory of morality*. **Morality** is a broader term that refers to the right and wrong about human conduct that is largely agreed upon to allow for a stable social contract for a functioning society. Collectively, morality encompasses norms to guide human behaviour and includes moral principles, rules, ideals, rights and virtues. Common norms that humans evaluate themselves and others include: to tell the truth, do not punish the innocent, keep your promises, do not kill, do not steal and obey just laws. **Ethics** is the systematic study of morality and provides a philosophical account of *justified* behaviour and belief. It is also a means of decision-making that requires knowledge, skills and practice. Thus, ethical decision-making is grounded in a body of knowledge of ethical theories, which can be used in medical disciplines, including forensic pathology.

In medicine, the ethics of the physician's role dates back to the Hippocratic maxim to "do no harm". More recently, this has evolved into the field of bioethics because Hippocratic ethics was not well equipped to handle developments in health sciences, biology and biomedical technology. In particular, it was challenged to address issues of informed consent, privacy, access to healthcare, public health responsibilities and research involving human subjects. To meet these challenges, a modern era of ethics arose—the field of bioethics. Bioethics provided a body of scholarship that was produced by philosophers, theologians, medical-care providers, lawyers and judges that have identified shared values that provide the basis for normative principles and precepts of modern medicine [2] and focus on substantive

R. Jacques (✉)
London Health Sciences Centre, London, ON, Canada
e-mail: rebekah.jacques@lhsc.on.ca

R. Jacques (ed.), *Forensic Pathology*,
https://doi.org/10.1007/978-3-031-42038-2_2

answers regarding principles, rules and ideals of good and bad. These normative principles have been derived largely by John Stuart Mill and Immanuel Kant and their interlocking ideas about morality and human behaviour.

Professional Ethics

Prior to medical school, a person's notion of right and wrong is based on "common morality", which outlines universal core norms that are acceptable to all people, in all places, living a moral life [2]. These norms are rules, standards and moral character traits (virtues) shared by all individuals committed to morality which include honesty, fidelity, trustworthiness and integrity [2].

Once an individual enters medical school, to become a physician, their moral universe is altered. This is because common morality is insufficient to address the ethical dilemmas that arise in medicine [2–4]. Professional ethics is employed to address these issues. Professional ethics is the ethics of a group of practitioners, which are often encapsulated in a code of ethics, and also lends itself to creating higher standards for physicians compared with others outside of medicine. In medicine, the basis of the professional ethic is embedded in the notion of privilege and the reciprocity between the public and physicians [3, 4]. The practice of medicine is permitted by a social contract that allows the responsibility of physician services in exchange with the high ideals associated with the medical profession. The purpose of social recognition of this privilege reflects a common judgement that the public interest is better served when privileges are allotted to some. Society can benefit when doctors have special privileges related to specialized knowledge for public purposes. Physicians have an agreement with society, wherein society permits physicians privileges, but, in return, physicians must accept the associated obligations of professional ethics, namely competency, trustworthiness, and self-regulation. A doctor who strays from the high ideals expected of physicians will not be tolerated by society. These privileges are revocable if there is an inability to meet these responsibilities or for reasons of exploitation, abuse, or neglect. These privileges are special liberties that are justified at the expense of the rights and liberties of others. Similarly, the performance of the autopsy [5] and expert testimony is the practice of medicine that benefits society [6]. Therefore, physicians who practice medicine in the post-mortem context are also bound by this social contract, which includes duties to maintain trust and competency. However, beyond these duties, the normative boundaries of professionalism in forensic pathology are not well defined.

Death Investigation Bioethics

Bioethics is a foundational component of professionalism in medicine [7]. Many medical training programmes have standardized their training in ethical issues that arise in a particular medical practice or specific specialities [7]. This is because the unit of analysis, relationships, and processes differ between medical specialities. Many of the ethical issues forensic pathologists face differ from other physicians because death investigation functions laterally to the paradigm of modern bioethics, resulting in an ethical morass. Treating physicians (i.e. non-pathologists) have a patient-centred approach with emphasis on the patient's diagnosis, well-being, and treatment of illness and disease that is exclusively grounded in clinical knowledge, confidentiality, principles of beneficence, non-maleficence, and respect for autonomy. Pathologists, like all physicians, are also held to a very high ethical and professional standard by medical accreditation, licensing boards and the public. Yet the nature and context of the medical practice for pathologists differ from other physicians, and therefore ethical issues in pathology differ. Furthermore, bioethics training programmes in pathology and forensic pathology are lagging behind other medical specialities [7]. In many training programmes, there is a lack of formal ethics training among pathology residents [8, 9] and forensic pathology fellows [7]. The programs that offer ethical training in forensic pathology appear to be case-based when opportunities arise. Unfortunately, not all common ethical dilemmas may arise during training and may lead to gaps [7]. Intentional ethical training specific to ethical issues that arise in death investigation is a strategy to fill these gaps [7]. Training on the ethical issues specific to the practice of pathology in general can serve as a starting point to death investigation bioethics because of the following shared issues:

1. **Duties**: Pathologists have duties to a wider group of stakeholders than other physicians [10]. This is in part due to a systemic manifestation of the institutional design in which pathologists are often separated from the people they serve resulting in less to no direct patient interaction. Despite duties to multiple stakeholders, the content and nature of these duties are not established and there is no ethical guidance to assist pathologists when conflicts arise between duties to different stakeholders.

The duties of a forensic pathologist extend beyond those of a pathologist because forensic work can exist outside of the healthcare system (Fig. 2.1). Forensic pathologists operate in the death investigation system, which houses the interface of healthcare and legal systems, in addition to organ procurement organizations and public health agencies (Fig. 2.2). In the legal system, forensic pathologists have a role as an expert witness. In this role, the forensic pathologist has a duty to the court, specifically a duty of objectivity, to provide independent, impartial, and unbiased evidence to the court. However, it is unclear whether forensic pathologists also have a duty to the accused and what the content of that duty is. In the healthcare system, autopsy suites and pathologists are often housed in healthcare institutions, such as hospitals, highlighting that the autopsy is part of medicine. The work of a forensic pathologist can also include the discovery of impropriety or incompetence on the part of the clinical team or institutions. When this occurs, the pathologist has an obligation to tell the truth in order to prevent similar deaths and excuse themselves from being an accomplice. In this way, the pathologist is the "conscience of medicine" [11]. In addition, pathologists have duties to the pathology assistants, and others that are in atten-

Fig. 2.1 The duties of the forensic pathologist to different stakeholders and institutions. Duties to different shareholders can sometimes conflict, and the duty to the accused, if any, is unclear. The intertwined and complexity of relationships are not demonstrated

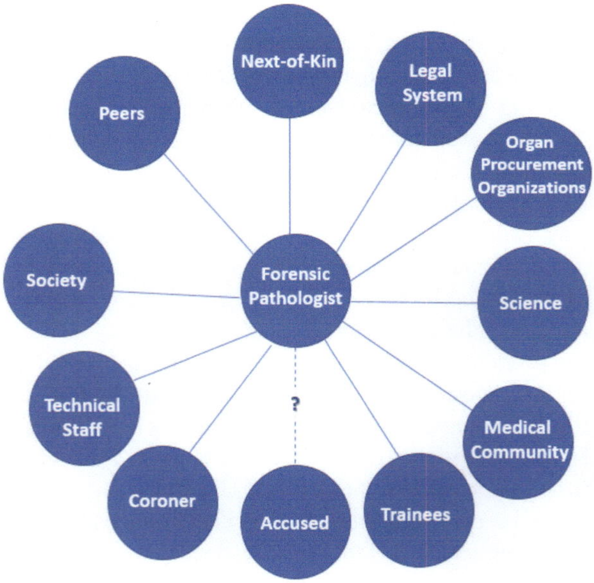

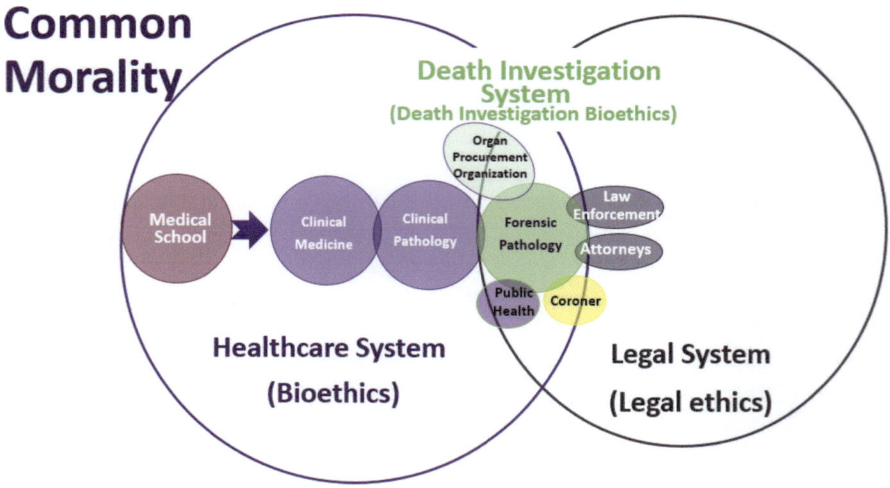

Fig. 2.2 Summary of the ethical paradigms and institutional relationships that can be applied in death investigation

dance of the autopsy, not to expose them to risks, in particular transmissible diseases, and toxic substances, that they are not willing to take themselves or would be inappropriate to expose others to when there are reasonable alternatives.

2. **Role of procedural trust**: Much of the pathologist's work is based on procedural trust by colleagues and other stakeholders, rather than personal trust, compared with other areas of medicine. This is because a pathological diagnosis is a

significant medical act that requires specialized expertise, which is not easily transferrable to non-pathology areas of medicine. In the healthcare system, it is the pathologists' diagnosis of cancer that results in the treating physicians in the healthcare system to offer life-preserving therapies, such as surgery, chemotherapy and radiation, to the patient. The autopsy is also a pivotal medicolegal act with ethical implications. In particular, the discovery of a concealed homicide by the forensic pathologist would result in further investigations, and even potential arrests, by law enforcement.

3. **Non-traditional physician–patient relationship**: Pathologists spend their time studying and diagnosing diseases in tissues of patients (living bodies) rather than discussing treatment options to patients and obtaining medical histories from patients. This systemic separation of pathologists from patients by the institutions that the pathologist operates in results in a departure from the traditional physician–patient relationship. The nature of the work of the forensic pathologist, which is performing autopsies on human remains (dead bodies) under legal authorization, is a significant departure from the traditional physician–patient relationship.
4. **Pathologists are the "guardians of the tissues"**: Given the finite nature of human tissues, pathologists have duties to ensure human tissues that are recovered from surgeries [12] and autopsies are used appropriately. This includes organ retention, implications for genetic testing and both the disclosure and disposal of human tissues. Decisions on organ retention require the retention and treatment is founded in medical and ethical reasoning such that human dignity is upheld. Genetic testing of tissues removed from patients during surgery and decedents during autopsy can yield sensitive and potentially relevant data including unsolicited findings [13] about the decedent and their biological relatives. Ethical values of autonomy, beneficence, and non-maleficence need to be considered when proceeding with genetic testing. Biological samples are collected and used for a variety of purposes. In the clinical setting, patient tissues are primarily obtained for diagnostic purposes and may secondarily be used for quality assurance and research purposes. The fate of these tissues will vary depending on the patient's consent or the nature of the research study. Most tissues are eventually disposed of as medical waste. Diverting tissues for secondary uses, such as research, requires clinical research guidelines and may depend on patient's consent [14]. Tissues collected from patients occur under the authorization of patient consent; however, tissues collected during medicolegal autopsies occur under the authorization of the law rather than an individual's autonomy.

"Pathology ethics" has developed into a small area of scholarly work that can inform our thinking in death investigation bioethics but does not address common issues in forensic pathology that are centred around the autopsy (Table 2.1). One of the fundamental differences between pathology and forensic pathology is that the former is focused on helping patients by diagnosing diseases in their tissues that were obtained by consent. In contrast, in forensic pathology, there is no benefit to the decedent in making a post-mortem pathological diagnosis via the

Table 2.1 Ethical issues reflected in the phases around the medicolegal autopsy

Pre-autopsy	Autopsy	Post-autopsy
Conduct at scenes	Dignity and respect for the decedent	Genetic testing
Indications for an autopsy	Organ and tissue retention	Disclosure of results: public health, relatives, media, medical error
Discussion with families	Handling personal effects	Family communication
Family objections/ accommodations	Documentation	Report writing, forming opinions
Organ and tissue donation	Role for research and teaching	Peer review/second opinions/defence work
	Resource allocation	Expert witness
	VIP/prioritized autopsies	"Critical values/diagnosis"

medicolegal autopsy. The autopsy is for the benefit of others, and the authority to perform the autopsy is from law rather than autonomy. Consequently, many ethical challenges related to the autopsy are not captured in pathology ethics but would be addressed in death investigation bioethics. Death Investigation Bioethics is an area of scholarly work that examines the ethics around the phases of the medicolegal autopsy.

The need for ethical perspectives around the autopsy has independently emerged through two public inquiries in two separate countries—the Bristol Inquiry in the United Kingdom and Canadian Inquiry into paediatric forensic pathology in Ontario (referred to as the "Goudge" Inquiry). The former was a public inquiry into children's heart surgery at Bristol Royal Infirmary, which led to the Bristol Inquiry Interim [15] and the Redfern Reports [16]. The Bristol Inquiry revealed that over a long period of time, tissues and organs had systematically been removed during the post-mortem examination of children who had died following surgery. These tissues and organs were used for a variety of purposes including audit, medical education, research or simply storage [17]. The parents of the deceased children were typically unaware of the fact that the body of their child, whom they buried or cremated, was missing a(n) organ(s). This inquiry led to reform about organ retention in the United Kingdom and other jurisdictions. The Goudge Inquiry, which also examined deaths in children, recommended that forensic pathologists in Ontario Canada have a code of ethics (http://www.attorneygeneral.jus.gov.on.ca/inquiries/goudge/report.pdf).

A scholarly area of ethics around the phases of the autopsy needs to be done to move beyond organ retention policy and a code of ethics recommendation, such as death investigation bioethics, which is a nascent field of pathology ethics [18]. While there have been individual contributions, through scholarly or institutional work, to the role of bioethics in medicolegal death investigation, mainstream bioethics has largely neglected this area of medicine. This blindspot in death investigation systems has led to a lack of scholarly development, policy and frameworks on how death investigation systems ought to treat human remains and develop consensus on bioethics professional values and standards.

Furthermore, there is a lack of consensus among forensic practitioners about using medicolegal autopsies and tissues derived for research and education [19]. This lack of consensus not only challenges the creation of ethical guidelines but also reflects the intricacy and complex realm of a medicolegal practice in death investigation [19].

Forensic pathologists routinely encounter ethical complexities in their medicolegal practice that are not neat or easily solved. Characteristics of pathologists including self-scrutiny and reflection are not only essential skills in assuring excellence in forensic work but also help foster optimal ethical reflection and rigorous decision-making. Pathologists require the following skills for an ethical medicolegal practice:

1. The ***ability to recognize*** the ethical considerations that arise in death investigation. This requires not only an awareness of ethical dilemmas that occur around the autopsy but also a working understanding of ethical concepts such as virtues, beneficence, relational autonomy, respect for persons, all forms of justice beyond criminal justice, non-maleficence and privacy as they apply to situations that arise in death investigation.
2. The ***capacity to honestly examine*** one's own values and biases as it relates to death investigation. Being attuned to one's own uncertainty is one component of this essential ethics skill.
3. The ***ability to identify one's areas of competence*** and as a corollary, to identify the limits of one's competence. This is essential because it is linked to bioethical principles of beneficence and non-maleficence, which are fundamental to the public's trust that pathologists will do what they can to serve the public's interest. In situations, where one is likely to be stretched beyond one's ability or expertise, it is imperative to make every effort to enhance one's abilities and expertise by consulting other forensic pathology experts. As an expert witness, this means stating areas of uncertainty and also that the question is outside of your expertise when it is.
4. The ***ability to identify specific situations that are likely to give rise to problems that are ethical in nature***. To actively anticipate and engage in these issues and, where possible, prevent their emergence. However, when the ethical issue appears irreconcilable, further understanding of the reasons and perceptions of others for deciding a course of action can help resolve conflict by using ethical frameworks. In addition, ethical theories can inform our thinking by considering values, principles, theories and approaches in bioethics but are not meant to offer clear-cut answers to many of the ethical dilemmas that arise in death investigation. Rather, ethical theories provide perspectives and guide our own reasoning process towards conclusions, which not everyone will necessarily agree, but which can withstand close scrutiny and open dialogue with others. Working through ethical issues with wise colleagues who are candid, clear-sighted and knowledgeable. Depending on the complexity of the scenario, an ethical issue may also require consultation with a bioethicist. Since most bioethicists work in healthcare institutions, rather than the death investigation system, reciprocal knowledge exchange with the bioethicist may be necessary to understand the facts of the ethical dilemma.

Ethical Dilemma

Awareness of ethical issues requires recognizing ethical dilemmas. The four components of an ethical dilemma include the following:

1. A **moral agent**: A person who has the ability to make ethical decisions based on what is right or wrong. In death investigation, this may be the forensic pathologist or others that work in death investigation.
2. An **action or choice**: The ethical dilemma demands that the moral agent adopt the moral obligations of each of two or more alternatives, but incompatible actions, such that all required actions cannot be performed.
3. A **consequence or outcome**: The action or choice of the moral agent can be both anticipated and unintended but are embedded in ethical or value perspectives.
4. The **context**, which are the circumstances that form the setting of the dilemma. In general, the context of the death investigation system sits at the intersection of healthcare and the legal systems, wherein the autopsy is central and the entrenched values in each institution are further embedded in the social, political and cultural considerations. The context outlines the roles of the stakeholders and the rules for interpersonal behaviour, where the experiences of the bereaved family can also be recognized. It is often the context that gives ethics a reputation of being non-reproducible. This is because the context can affect the other parts of the ethical dilemma resulting in completely different reasoned decisions and outcomes.

The components of the ethical dilemma can be highlighted in the classic trolley dilemma [20]. The trolley dilemma (Fig. 2.3) is a thought experiment in ethics in which a fictional situation has an onlooker, who has an opportunity to save five people in danger of being hit by a trolley, by diverting the trolley with a lever to hit one person instead. In this dilemma, the onlooker is the moral agent, the lever represents the choice or action, the number of individuals killed by the trolley is the outcome and the context can be a wide variety of things including the characteristics

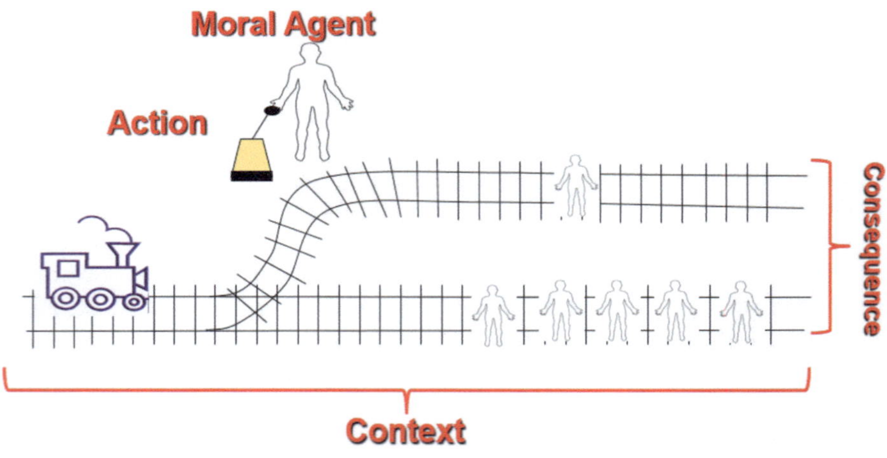

Fig. 2.3 The components of the ethical dilemma highlighted by the trolley dilemma

of the people on the tracks. A utilitarian ethical analysis would reason that the right course of action is for the onlooker to move the lever such that one person dies to save five people. This theory justifies that the best actions are those that result in the greatest good for the greatest number of people. In other words, saving five people is the greatest good. Alternatively, employing deontological theory to this ethical dilemma would result in a different choice. This ethical theory argues that the action is inherently wrong, regardless of the consequences, and thus the onlooker ought not to move the lever. There are variations on this dilemma, which largely change the context, in attempts to better understand normative behaviours.

Ethical Theories

Practicing forensic pathologists cannot be engaged in professional medical practice without consideration of how to guide our conduct and decisions using a bioethical lens. In a professional ethical practice, ethical theories and ethical frameworks can be used to guide decision-making and when used can result in better ethical decisions because both are rooted in epistemology and knowledge. Ethical theories try to identify and justify ethical norms or principles. Each theory focuses on a different aspect of the ethical dilemma. The various analytical approaches and methodologies in ethics can serve as a starting point for the development of norms of ethical conduct and approaches specific to death investigation bioethics (Table 2.2).

Virtue Ethics

Virtue theory focuses primarily on the moral agent and their intentions of acting functions as the basis of normative expectations for professionals [21]. Virtue is a quality, a state of character, which enables one to make the right decisions when confronted with a moral dilemma. To be virtuous requires balancing between two vices to arrive at the golden mean, which is the desirable middle way between two extremes, one of excess and the other of deficiency (Fig. 2.4).

In death investigation, this requires an exploration of the normative qualities that are expected of the virtuous forensic pathologist who has the moral and intellectual disposition to act habitually for the good, out of the right motives and intentions. Some of the characteristics of the virtuous forensic pathologist include honesty, fidelity, and intestinal fortitude. Honesty is a normative expectation given the weight of procedural trust that is allotted to pathologists. Forensic pathologists must tell the truth regardless of the outcome for the accused and the potential harm to families who want to know the truth about how a loved one has died. Fidelity is also an important virtue because pathologists need to understand the possible repercussions of a pathological opinion. A cause of death that speaks to the manner of being non-natural has implications for insurance companies, the liberty of others, and parental custody. In addition, forensic pathologists also need to act ethically, even if our

Table 2.2 Summary of common analytical approaches and methodologies that guide ethical behaviour

1. **Descriptive**: What do we actually say is the right and good?
   (a) Describes the ethics of individuals or communities
   (b) Examines how ethics actually are expressed
   (c) Attempts to reconcile the "is-ought" chasm in traditional philosophical analyses
   (d) Utilizes empirical methods
2. **Theoretical:** How do we justify our judgements of the right and good?
   (a) Analytical questions are philosophical rather than empirical.
   (b) Largely concerned with justification.
   (c) Main schools of ethics theory:
   - **Virtue ethics**: The good is based on the character of the moral agent and its development
   - **Deontology**: The good is known by its consistency with ethical principles.
   - **Consequentialism**: The good is known by its consequences.
   - **Principilism**: Approach for justification of right action to move towards normative standards by balancing four principles: autonomy, justice, beneficence and non-maleficence.
   - **Communitarian/feminist ethics**: It overlaps with consequentialism and deontology but is embedded in community rather than an individualistic perspective. The good is that which balances benefits and harms between the powerful and vulnerable. Guided by duties and obligations, which are in keeping with the nature of interdependent relationships.
3. **Normative**: Arguments for how we ought to choose rightly and act good.
   (a) Draws upon descriptive and theoretical considerations as necessary to formulate concrete advice
   (b) Judgement requires an articulation of the ethical dilemma and balancing values at stake in decisions

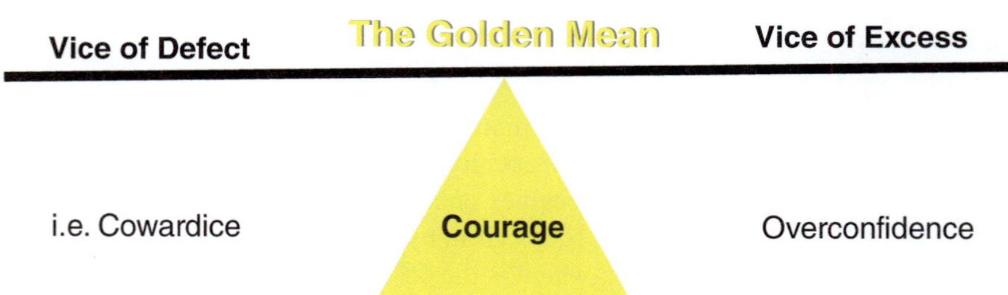

Fig. 2.4 The golden mean target for the virtuous moral agent

self-interests are at risk. This includes disclosing when we have made a mistake, correcting the error, and having the courage to do so. These virtues have implications as some pathological opinions may not be popular or favourable and require intestinal fortitude to ensure that fidelity and honesty are maintained.

Like all theories, there are shortcomings with virtue ethics. First, virtuous individuals who are well intentioned remain vulnerable to making bad decisions because virtue alone is insufficient to make the right decisions. For virtue theorists, the desire to do good and have good intentions also requires knowledge and practice that create habits of virtuous action. Good actions that lack a virtuous disposition can result in moral failure. Second, virtue-based theories do not state which virtues are necessary and sufficient to be virtuous. Third, the theory is based on a circular argument that the good is done by the virtuous person. Nevertheless, the existence of virtue theory and its implication on intentions, motives and actions seem intuitively right to have a role in death investigation.

Deontology Ethics

Deontological theories are duty-based theories focused on the decisions or actions of the ethical dilemma, wherein there are intrinsic actions or aspects of actions that make them wrong or right. Deontology is rooted in a nineteenth-century doctrine of the writings of Immanuel Kant's Categorical Imperative wherein a moral agent acts as if their behaviour were a universal law in ethics. Kant argued that the moral agent should always tell the truth because this is an inherent universal good and would result in the collapse of society if this was not the standard. The actions themselves are contextually defined to determine the harm and benefit of that action. For forensic pathologists, always telling the truth is also a universal law due to the weight of expert opinions, the role of procedural trust in forensic work. and its implications for stakeholders. Kant is also credited for the creation of autonomy and argued that humans ought to be treated with respect, as ends in themselves, not as means to another individual's ends [4]. Kant also argued that each human being's potential capacity for "moral action" is for acting on the basis of impartial rules derived from reason. Kant also had thoughts on our duty to treat the dead with dignity as a specific duty that derives from human goodwill. Unlike the Kantian universal law, this duty is for specific people—namely relatives, friends and local authorities [22].

The shortcoming in deontological theory arises in the assessment of the rules. For example, when the rule "physicians should never kill" is tested in contexts involving euthanasia, it has been argued that physicians should not abandon their patients during their time of greatest suffering [23]. Similarly, forensic pathologists promise to tell the truth, the whole truth and nothing but the truth, but the addition of a voir dire to their testimony prevents the expert from telling the truth as they view it. In addition, from an autonomy perspective, the decedent's body functions as a *means to an end* in death investigation whereby an autopsy is performed so that knowledge gathered from the post-mortem examination is useful to others including the bereaved family, legal system, law enforcement, and medicine.

Consequentialism Ethics

Consequentialist theories focus on the outcome of a decision or action of the moral agent. A leading proponent of this theory was Jeremy Bentham who proposed a way to measure consequences, whereby the impact of decisions on the well-being of all affected individuals should produce “the greatest happiness of the greatest number” [24]. This measure of well-being is described as “utility” and his doctrine as “utilitarianism”. Utilitarianism asserts that decisions be judged by their consequences, in particular by their effect on the sum total of individual well-being. In this theory, all individuals’ utility levels should count and count equally. The doctrine indicates that the rightness of an action is not intrinsic but determined by the “hedonic calculus” by adding up the pleasure and pain that a decision produces. A decision is to be judged by its effect on the sum of an individual’s levels of well-being by measuring and adding up these magnitudes. The right choice is viewed as the one that produces the most gain. The maximum good is to be obtained and bad to be avoided. The central notion of utilitarian theory is that the overall goal is to achieve social good by maximizing “utility”. Decisions should be made that maximize social good. For utilitarians, maximizing utility or social good leads to the answer to what action is right.

In general, the death investigation system operates in this theory as the performance of the autopsy is for the benefit of the common good. This is because society can benefit from the knowledge of why its citizens die through the performance of an autopsy so that similar deaths can be prevented by research and public health initiatives. Furthermore, the death investigation system infringes on the basic rights of the individual (and their relatives), to be free of intervention, in favour of the rights of society. The rights of society are not a mere force but a matter of right and ethical justness. The common good in death investigation potentially has superior claims to which the individual good is sacrificed.

This ethical theory is commonly used in organizational ethics such as public and institutional policy discussions. A policy is to be judged by its effect on the sum of an individual’s levels of well-being. Post-mortem genetic testing on the decedent, rather than testing each surviving family member and trying to obtain a cardiac phenotype, maximizes the social good as the additional costs associated with testing all first-degree family members would exceed simply testing the decedent as a form of familial screening.

This method has practical and philosophical problems in guiding policy decisions regarding health status. First, this method can ignore individual and cultural variations in attitudes towards mortality. The theory implies that the community is homogenous and differences are minimal. Second, some individuals may be harmed, while others benefit to achieve the greatest utility. Specifically, minority groups are vulnerable to harms. This is particularly important because equity-deserving groups are over-represented in death investigation systems. Third, consequences are interpreted by the values of the groups harmed and those benefitted from decisions; therefore, the consequences are not necessarily measured on the same scale.

Principilism

Principilism is a normative framework for justification of right action to move towards normative standards. It is designed for practical decision-making for conflicts that arise in medicine. Although the approach lacks a foundational theory, it employs practical judgement instead. The approach is to start from where people generally do agree and use practical judgement in decision-making. Principilists argue that moral principles cluster under four principles, which serve as a framework for professional duties and provide a normative guidance for professional ethics. These clusters also align with the moral norms and values of Western society. These principles have informed, guided and shaped professional decisions and behaviours in healthcare.

The components of the framework include the following:

1. **Respect for autonomy** is respecting persons and their autonomous decisions. This principle is grounded in the Kantian value that personal freedom with minimal interference from others will maximize individual capacity to flourish. This includes treating others with dignity and promoting their independence and personal responsibility, which are rooted in the democratic political tradition. In professional work, this principle defines professional obligations to respect confidences, communicate honestly and practice informed decision-making. This principle is a staple in the healthcare setting, in which the physician–patient relationship is central in this context. This principle considers that individuals have the right to determine what happens to their bodies. This is commonly manifested through informed consent and confidentiality. Departures from autonomy would be considered battery or medical neglect.

At death, the "rights" of individuals, including autonomy, are largely "extinguished" in the absence of specific legislation to extend them. Furthermore, in death investigation systems, forensic pathologists, medical examiners and coroners have supremacy over autonomy when they exert their authority to perform autopsies over the objection of families. The rationale for this supremacy stems from previous conflicts about performing autopsies when families object to postmortem examinations. This conflict was resolved in favour of forensic pathologists and coroners because their authority was congruent with the public interest. The public interest in knowing the cause of death is such that knowledge gained from the autopsy can lead to steps that prevent similar deaths [25], including homicides. However, these powers are not limitless and should be invoked with both legal and ethical considerations.

2. **Beneficence** is meant to provide benefits over harms in professional actions and decisions. In death investigation systems, this can include permitting postmortem organ donations for the purpose of transplantation for those waiting for life-preserving measures, rather than ensuring that the integrity of the body, for the sole purpose of the autopsy, is maintained. Other examples of beneficence in the post-mortem context of performing the autopsy include identifying new or re-emerging diseases, identifying and reporting heritable diseases, accurate reflection of the causes of death to improve the mortality and morbidity of the population, advancing medical knowledge and replacing conjecture with facts.
3. **Non-maleficence** is meant to avoid harms in professional actions and decisions. In death investigation systems, the lack of autopsy access may result in harm in certain situations. Not performing the autopsy could negatively impact other institutions (i.e. criminal justice, healthcare and public health) and the lives of others (i.e. accused and families).

4. **Justice** denotes the concept of fairness and guides decisions about what is owed to others in a manner that is appropriate, equitable, and fair. This also includes resource allocation in which death investigation is apportioned when health and financial resources may be limited. However, there are different types of justice. In the death investigation system, criminal justice, which is the just infliction of punishment, is prioritized over other forms of justice. The supremacy of criminal justice in death investigation system may lead to inappropriate consideration and balancing of other ethical principles.

Sometimes, these four principles are in conflict and are not readily reconcilable. The rules for how to manage these conflicts are as follows:

1. Infringing one principle requires a realistic prospect of realizing the best ethical course of action.
2. Infringement is necessary to the resolution.
3. The infringement is the least possible and commensurate with achieving the best ethical course of action.
4. The negative effects of the infringement are minimized.
5. Decision is impartial (i.e. morally irrelevant information is ignored).

The shortcoming of principilism is that this approach is limited to assisting in the subjective world of motives, intentions, emotions, and beliefs. Specifically, the principles are not guides to action but rather a collection of matters to consider when dealing with an ethical dilemma. The principles lack a systemic relationship with each other, and the approach lacks a unified theory to assist with conflict that often happens between principles. This approach has also been critiqued for its focus on autonomy and its inability to address core issues of relationship and community [26]. In death investigation, these limitations are magnified because the notions of autonomy and justice differ in the post-mortem context. Autonomy, in its traditional form, has a limited role in death investigation because respect for self-determination and bodily integrity is largely extinguished post-mortem. However, the role of privacy and confidentiality can persist. Furthermore, justice, specifically criminal justice, has a larger role in medicolegal death investigation than other forms of justice, which was not the intended form of justice in this approach.

Communitarian Ethics

Communitarian ethics focuses on the community context of the ethical dilemma, specifically origins of duties and obligations that individuals have to their community. The focus is to create a good society and produce individual's rights for that society. Communitarian viewpoints are found among Greek philosophers, such as Plato and Aristotle, and more contemporarily in feminist ethics, which has made great contributions to expand concepts on community. The feminist perspective is grounded in the ethics of care, whereby the underlying assumption is that humans are interdependent and interconnected rather than autonomous individuals who are to leave each other alone. This position contrasts with other ethical frameworks, which focus largely on an individualistic level. Furthermore, the notion of relational autonomy is introduced in this theory and certainly has value in death investigation as it provides a contextual approach to autonomy that meets the needs of the complexity of the post-mortem context by highlighting the social context of the end of life. Relational autonomy aims to maintain autonomy while incorporating insights into socially embedded notions. Specifically, in death investigation, this is a means to balance the relational autonomy of families and the efforts of the death investigation system to determine the cause of death and other medicolegal opinions that may require autopsy, specifically dissection, organ retention and research to advance knowledge in the field of forensic pathology, medicine and science.

The foundational viewpoint in communitarians is who decides what is virtuous. These are largely centred on two views: one view is a relativist communitarian which is every community defines its own norms [27]. In this view, ethics are inherently contextual, lacking a universal place to stand outside any cultural context. In contrast, universalist communitarians' view is that a single true form of a good society and its associated virtues.

In death investigation bioethics, communitarian ethics may have a role. If community norms have value, then attempts to inoculate these norms and limit deviance from them are appropriate. Communities are central to the work in death investigation. For example, using autopsies to identify familial causes of premature death is a societal and familial virtue. The challenge is to balance promoting community values from becoming repressive. Furthermore, when disagreements occur within a community, the issue is to determine who decides what the community's values really are.

Ethical Frameworks

Many practical questions would remain unanswered using a general ethical theory. In contrast to theoretical ethics, applied (practical) ethics utilizes norms and other moral resources in deliberating about problems, practices, and policies in professions, institutions and public policy. A framework differs from a theory in that the framework is a heuristic tool to aid in more systematic reflection concerning ethical decision-making. Ethical theories offer a comprehensive, coherent and consistent account of normative considerations, including metaethics. Frameworks are meant to guide non-ethicist physicians in the identification and resolution of ethical dilemmas. In general, the frameworks lay out a series of steps that an individual could follow to arrive at a resolution of an ethical issue encountered in a death investigation or organizational context. As an example, an ethics decision-making framework might include the collection of facts relevant to the case, the identification of relevant ethical principles, the identification of options and the choice of action by the application of ethical principles.

Here is a list of common ethical decision-making frameworks:

1. IDEA framework: This framework is divided into four steps that include: (a) identifying the facts, (b) determining the relevant ethical principles, (c) exploring the options, and (d) making a decision that is acted upon [28, 29].
2. A4R: Accountability for Reasonableness is a framework for priority setting especially at the organizational ethics level. This framework forces consideration of procedural fairness, equity, and transparency when priority setting in which the guiding principles include relevance, publicity, appeals and revisions, enforcement, and leadership are utilized [30].
3. Structured Learning in Clinical Ethics (S.L.I.C.E.): This provides a template to help medical professionals identify their own reflective ethical practice [31]. The advantage of this framework is the laws that govern the medicolegal autopsy can be explicitly utilized.
4. The Markula Center for Applied Ethics—a framework for thinking ethically. This online app provides viewing an ethical problem from six ethical lenses (a framework for ethical decision-making—Markkula Center for Applied Ethics (scu.edu)).

Theories That Apply in the Forensic Context

The field of bioethics has largely been dominated by issues of clinical care and research. Bioethical theories used in medicine are largely rooted in the liberal individualism of the patient. It is a challenge to simply import these bioethical theories and frameworks that were designed to address conflicts between the clinician and the patient into the death investigation system. A framework is needed that is attentive to the nature and content of the duties of the forensic pathologist and values of death investigation. An ethical framework in medicolegal death investigation system must begin with a recognition of the values at the core of death investigation, not simply a modification of values that are created to guide other kinds of healthcare interactions. Unfortunately, relatively less theoretical development and metaethics of death investigation exist. Death investigation bioethics, like the field of death investigation, has focused more on practice and particular cases than on theory, with the result that some concepts, methods and boundaries remain largely undefined [32] despite that death investigation exists to promote human welfare.

Although there are constraints with the current state of bioethics in addressing ethical issues in death investigation, all is not lost. There are areas of established ethical principles that have value in death investigation. For example, the value of confidentiality and privacy, which flows from the principle autonomy, of the decedent remains a primary duty of physicians and arguably continues after a person has died. Disclosing the findings of an autopsy may also be justified when others are at risk of serious harm associated with it such as reportable communicable infections, suspected child abuse, and heritable disease. These breaches are justified in the public interest of public safety for the administration of justice. However, breaches of confidentiality due to the celebrity status of the decedent are doubtfully justified [5]. Like other physicians, forensic pathologists must always anticipate having to justify any decisions or actions taken if there is an unwarranted breach of confidentiality.

Code of Ethics

Professions are composed of persons with unique expertise that are grounded in ethical ideals and trust. In medicine, physicians have a professional morality that specifies general ethical norms for the practice of medicine. The medical profession is characterized by competence, commitment to devote itself to social values, and reliance on the practice of medicine. This devotion allows trusted physician autonomy. The special roles of physicians, and their relationship in medicine, require rules that may not be necessary or even be appropriate outside of medicine. These rules may undergo formal codifications of instruction and standards in detailed statements to avoid the vagueness of traditional standards of professional morality and publicly stated values. A profession's code of self-governance is an important articulation of ethical standards and is stated in a code of ethics. The codes of ethics specify rules of etiquette and rules of ethics. Codes of ethics are not mere reiterations of common morality but embody a professional standard whereby an institution outlines its expectation of conduct for individual professionals. A code of ethics should embody a theory about the relationship between the profession and the community it serves. In addition, it outlines that members respect certain normative values.

All major professional institutions have a code of ethics which binds their members to conduct that fosters respect and fidelity of the institution and its members to society. Consequently, these codes behold the ethical elements particular to the profession and highlight the different ethical standards that are applicable to a discrete group of physicians. As the duties, obligations and values of forensic pathologists differ from other physicians, a code of ethics in medicolegal death investigation should speak to this distinct group. Before a code of ethics becomes operative, members ought to have the opportunity to have input and discussion [33] that are based on the standards of the forensic pathology discipline. This gives merit to the code of ethics as these professional codes can foster and reinforce member identification when they effectively incorporate defensible moral norms. However, if they oversimplify moral requirements, or are indefensibly rigid, with regard to unwarranted claims of their completeness and authority, the code will not be beneficial.

Examples of organizations that have made steps to establish and promote the ethical conduct of forensic experts are as follows:

1. American Academy of Forensic Sciences (AAFS) code of ethics:
   (a) Forbids distortion of data and credentials, including misrepresenting education, training, experience, area of expertise and data upon which experts base their opinion [34].

   (b) Created a committee on Good Forensic practice that has developed aspirational guidelines for forensic experts that are meant to go beyond the code of ethics minimal standards [35]. An important criterion is that experts should possess independence that would protect their objectivity.

2. National Association of Medical Examiners' bylaws on ethics focuses on misrepresentation of education training, experience and data rather than specific behaviours or testimony [36, 37].
3. Ontario Forensic Pathology Service: code of ethics based on the fundamental duties of the forensic pathologist [38].
4. Australia's Civil Procedure Rules: code of conduct that indicates the expert's general duty to the court as follows as expert witnesses have an (a) overriding duty to assist the court impartially on matters relevant to the expert witness's area of expertise; (b) paramount duty is to the court and not to any party to the proceedings (including the attorney retaining the expert witness); and (c) expert witness is not an advocate for a party [39].

Codes of ethics are the minimum professional obligations, but individual professionals ought to strive for aspirational ethics. Physicians may think that they are satisfying all relevant moral requirements by following the code of ethics, but this is only one tool in the ethical toolkit. Furthermore, a code of ethics cannot address every ethical dilemma and the dominant ethical approaches within an organization may not provide a clear resolution to ethical dilemmas [40].

Ethical decision-making based on frameworks or codes of ethics alone cannot always resolve complex ethical dilemmas.

Moral and Legal Status of Human Remains

Prior to death, a person's body is inseparable from who the person is [41], and therefore living individuals have moral status and personhood. **Personhood** are individual *beings* who are part of the moral community and deserve moral consideration. These can include adult humans, foetuses and animals. **Moral status** is a common ethical perspective used to determine if others have moral obligations, and what the nature of these obligations are, to special *beings*. To have moral status means that others have moral obligations to the special *being*. The nature of these obligations may be dependent comparatively where some beings have more or less favourability than other entities with different statuses [42]. The rationale for determining moral status is that those with moral status are vulnerable to harm or wrongdoing. Following death, the "person" is gone but their body remains [41]. If the dead body has moral status, this requires respecting their autonomy, considering the person's prior preferences regarding disposition and treatment of their body following death [43]. This behaviour of respecting the autonomy of persons, once dead, is a normative practice that is demonstrated in organ donation practices, funerary practices, and honouring the decedent's last will and testament [43]. Furthermore, wills not only provide a mechanism for living people to carry out the decedent's last wishes but also reflect other values such as promise keeping and reciprocity. Fulfilling the decedent's last wishes by the living is necessary in order to trust that their own wishes will be implemented when they are dead themselves [1].

The determination of moral status and personhood is based on establishing what a being needs to possess to be a member of the moral community and deserving of moral consideration. There are two criteria that could support that a dead body has moral status and personhood. First is the **genetic criterion** that by virtue of a dead body's unique human genetic code, it is this genetic code that is the basis for all the significant traits that are common to persons, indicates that this dead individual has moral status [44]. This is an argument used in the abortion context but emphasizes a particular concept about what constitutes personhood, which is a consequence of genetic constitution. Arguably, dead bodies have genetic constitution and on this basis have personhood. The genetic criterion seemingly has a low threshold and would be overinclusive of a single human cell (i.e. skin cell) that would not ordinarily include as having personhood. The second criterion is the **social criterion**, which uses the social aspect of personhood wherein a being has personhood whenever society recognizes an individual as a person [45]. A dead body would require moral consideration when it morally matters to someone, namely surviving family members. This mattering of human remains is manifested in society's respect for the person by acknowledging the body's history with that person by considering the person's preferences and values, including culture, religion, treatment and final rites of their body following death [41]. The manner in which the person's remains are handled and treated flows from the fact that their body had once been the body of a living person [41]. The respect and care the living have for who that person was extends to their remains [46]. This is demonstrated through widespread funerary practices. Respecting the history of the body also contributes to the well-being of relatives so that families can honour that person's preferences, values and previously expressed wishes [41]. The value of these actions is that it is beneficial for the living, whereby honouring the wishes of living persons posthumously maintains trust [47]. To do the opposite can generate harm (i.e. anxiety, anguish and distress) to the relatives [41]. This notion of respect for persons is the fundamental basis of modern ethics involving humans and is endorsed by philosophical literature. In upholding funerary rites, society demonstrates that this respect for persons continues post-mortem. The criticism for the social criterion is not all dead bodies matter to others and therefore would not have moral status.

Arguments that deny the moral status of human remains are based on the **consciousness criterion**, which asserts to have personhood is the ability to consciously experience pleasure and pain [48]. Human remains lack consciousness and therefore would not be eligible for moral status by this criterion, but this would also include individuals in comas, which would normally be considered having moral status. In addition, there is an unresolved, complex, philosophical debate on whether the dead can be harmed [41]. Ethical analysis of moral status among those who are "brain-dead" suggests that these individuals have moral status and therefore can be harmed with respect to precedent autonomy and surviving investment interests [49].

Regardless, whether human remains can or cannot be harmed is not equivalent to saying that some actions are not wrong because they do not harm human remains. There can be other reasons some actions are wrong that do not include harm to human remains. The manner in which decedents are treated has ethical significance due to the intrinsic value of a dead body. We can show disrespect to a person, who is now dead, by not considering the values embedded in human remains by forensic pathologists, families, other stakeholders, and society.

Alas, there is no prevailing view of the moral status and the personhood of human remains. This is largely due to controversy about when moral status and personhood start and stop. The paradox of bodily value is not new [50] and extends into the legal realm. From a legal perspective, common law allows individuals to dispose of property after death. This notion of property rights for the body has also been used as an attempt to resolve post-mortem issues. Property, in a legal sense, refers to the rights associated with the property, including the right to possess, use and dispose of [51]. The implications of the property model in the notion of ownership are that consent based on ownership authorizes the unrestricted right to the "owner", which is where the property notion of human remains falls short. Given the abolition of slavery as recognized in the Universal Declaration of Human Rights, it is now recognized globally that no person can own another human [52]. Ownership of human tissues, ante-mortem and post-mortem, has been unsettled [53]. Unlike other forms of property, a dead body cannot be auctioned off like other worldly goods [50]. Importantly, denying human remains the status of property does not lessen its value compared to inanimate objects but rather highlights its immeasurable value [50]. Regardless of the law's position about property regarding human remains, the law recognizes the right of custody, control and disposition, which are attributes of ownership [54]. The issues of property and ownership have been reaffirmed in one area—anatomical gifts [55]. For example, in the United States, each state has adopted a version of the Anatomical Gift Act of 1968 [55]. This Act essentially puts the doctrine that a person has no property rights to another human body including their own, by allowing testamentary organ donation [55]. Furthermore, non-authorized donation by surviving next of kin of certain tissues, such as corneas, was considered legally permittable. Next of kin rights depend on the purposes for which the organs/tissues were removed [55]. Another argument for the property rights of human remains is that, if the human tissues have been modified for a specific use, such as used to make a microscopic slide, there can be property rights over these tissues because they become part of the medical record [54, 56]. However, human remains are not equivalent to other parts of the medical record, which can be reproduced by photocopying. Ultimately, property rights of human rights has limitations when used in the postmortem context. An alternative consideration to property rights is the individual's entitlement to certain treatment. This entitlement is reflected in an individual's entitlement to a decent burial, also known as the right of sepulchre [55]. Proper disposal of the body also has benefits for society by ensuring bodies do not lead to widespread infection. It also aids in the prevention of the mishandling of human remains and allows next of kin the right to make arrangements for disposition. Further, the social expectation that the right to possess the body includes all reasonably foreseeable organs [54].

Finally, rights possession protects human dignity by permitting the right of an individual to a decent burial [57]. In the death investigation system, pathologists, at most, have a quasi-ownership role in that they have stewardship duties to human tissues and temporary possession of human remains. This stewardship duty allows pathologists to perform their role as it is necessary to examine tissues and organs but does not extend to owning the human remains of others who have died that were accessed through the privilege of being a pathologist.

Ethical Tensions Related to the Autopsy

The presence of human remains that fall under the jurisdiction of the death investigation system, brings with it several interests that must be considered. These include family interests where the decedent belongs to them as a member of their family. Families are also the guardians of the family's and the decedent's values, which may be based on religion, culture, or even personal convictions. The body continues to represent the memories of that person, and there is often a need to bereave near the body and sometimes death scene. The performance of a medicolegal autopsy on a dead relative may cause conflict between different stakeholders in the death investigation system, including pathologists, surviving family members, police and attorneys. This is because there may be competing interests and different views of the value of an autopsy. A family's objection to a medicolegally indicated autopsy can sometimes reflect the tension between the ethical values of relational autonomy of the family versus the advancement of criminal justice in the legal system. Also, the objection can reflect the ethical principle of beneficence wherein the aim of the death investigation system is to serve the public by discovering why an individual died in order to benefit society by using the knowledge from the autopsy to prevent similar deaths in others, including bereaved family members. Previously, such actions taken by the state were justified to advance the public's interest in the death of its citizens regardless of the context of the death. However, this may impinge on values by members of groups within society and cause sociocultural offense.

All societies honour and protect its dead. Ignoring these duties that bereaved families have in relation to the decedent should be avoided in the death investigation system as it is normal for families to have a gaze of the decedent that is overlapping or different from other stakeholders in death investigation (Fig. 2.5). For the pathologist, human remains are both a biological and forensic material, which can lead to objectifying and theorizing perspective of the decedent [58]. The pathologist, and other members in the death investigation system, cannot know the essence of the person from the postmortem examination [58]. This discordance can cause pathologists, and other members in the death investigation and legal systems, to overlook the families' perspective in the pursuit in trying to achieve or demonstrate the truth for the courts. On the contrary, the subjective perspective of the decedent's family may be to protect the decedent's body as it is a moral, spiritual and cultural representation of the person [58]. Memories and promises of that person are associated

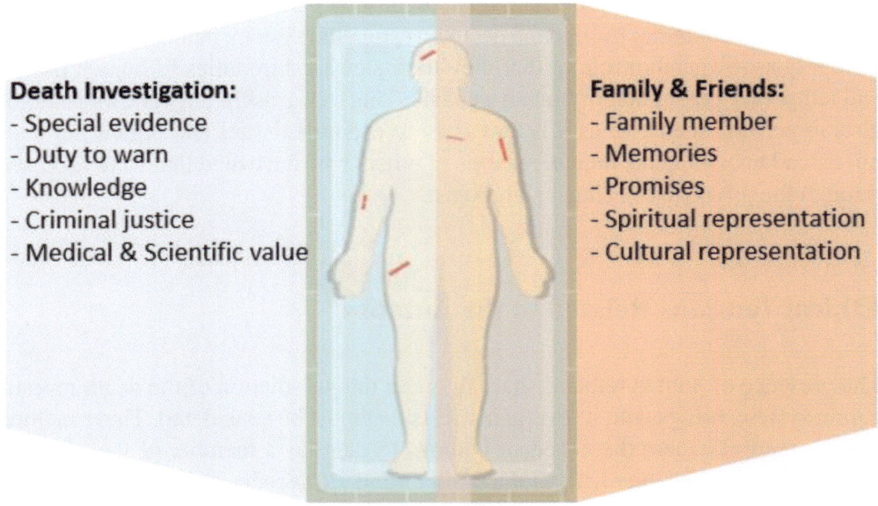

Fig. 2.5 The opposing and shared perspectives of the value of the autopsy of the decedent from the death investigation system and family

with that body [46, 58]. The family response to the phenomenon of death and its appurtenances play an important role in the death investigation system perceived needs for investigation of deaths that are typically sudden, unexpected, unexplained and not readily accountable. The objections by families can be variable, often based on religious, and cultural reasons, but not always. It may include the historical use of the "public autopsy" as a means to punish criminals or rooted in misconceptions of the autopsy [59]. Failure to respect prior preferences can result in anxiety and distress in the living [43]. The living tend to feel obligated to carry out the wishes of the dead because they usually align with other values that they hold important [60]. How death investigation systems treat family members in death can impact the welfare of the living family and friends of the decedent [50]. It also demonstrates respect for surviving relatives who have a strong connection between the body and the decedent [47]. The interests of relatives are recognized in courts to prevent the mistreatment of decedents [47, 61]. Perspectives of mistreatment is influenced by cultural norms and forensic investigators need to be sensitive to cultural differences to avoid perceptions of mistreatment of the decedent. However, even the performance of the autopsy may be viewed as mistreatment. Ultimately, the value of the dead body is a vital source of memories, a form of evidence and knowledge. It is the embodiment of memories of the decedent that lends us to respect who that person was and respect the person's remains. This link leads the living to keep promises, such as executing wills. This continued value of the decedent's identity, in relation to the decedent's body, highlights the scientific and ethical importance of the moral status of the body and the performance of the autopsy [46]. The decedent's memory is preserved through relatives. Through this link, relatives perceived desires, wishes and sociocultural beliefs are analogous to surrogate decision-making [46]. The value of the decedent's body can extend beyond the body as an object to collect evidence and knowledge, and the decedent's identity is preserved through relatives [46]. Forensic pathologists, trained as physicians, carry with them a duty that is owed to the decedent that is engrained from their years of medical and ethical training in caring for and treating patients. The World Health Organization proposes that the two bases of this duty include: one is that pathologists have a duty to the memory/reputation of the decedent that the true cause and circumstance of death be revealed and the other is that the forensic pathologist has a fiduciary duty to community, including the decedent's family, and the integrity of the medical profession to arrive at the truth of the decedent's death [62].

A study that examined family members, who had their deceased relative undergo a medicolegal autopsy, showed that their reasons for objection fell into four categories: First, the autopsy would disturb the peace of the decedent. Second, the decedent would not have wanted an autopsy [63]. This objection is based on the societal value that we honour promises, even in death, as demonstrated through the practice of honouring wills, which is a means to honour the wishes of the decedent [63]. The third category is fear of bodily mutilation, and the fourth category is religious reasons [64]. However, the majority of family members were in favour of an autopsy where the cause of death and circumstances were not readily apparent [64]. In particular, family members were interested in the autopsy findings. The value of the knowledge gathered from the autopsy can assist relatives in coping with the death of their loved one [64] and provide information for quality improvement and evidence for criminal prosecution (or freedom).

Forensic work is invariably attached to families and counselling families about the nature of the work is necessary, especially during objections. Death investigation operates in a pluralistic society with multiple perspectives of death and imposing a singular view that the decedent is an object to collect evidence and determine the truth about someone's death and ignoring sociocultural views of the decedent can potentially harm families whose beliefs may differ [46]. When a family objects to an autopsy, the death investigation system needs to give weight to these objections and in doing so reconcile the public interest, where possible. Unfortunately, there is often a lack of clear participation rights in the process of death investigation for surviving family members and the range of support for bereaved families is woefully inadequate [65]. The Bristol Inquiry [15] and the Canadian Missing and Murdered Indigenous Women (MMIW) Inquiry [66] make clear that the current death investigation systems do not provide proper support for the bereaved. Bereaved families are not reliably and systematically provided information on autopsy decisions, inquests or other processes. Many families are unfamiliar with the death investigation system and processes that they are often suddenly and expectantly involved in. Furthermore, the death investigation system struggles to be sensitive to their distress and properly inform families. This failure translates to a paucity of reliable responses to the wishes, culture and religious beliefs of surviving family members, especially members of minority communities. On the rare occasion, when families have exercised their right to objection by appealing to the relevant court, the courts in some jurisdictions, where family opposition to the autopsy has been tested, have invariably ruled in favour of the families' wishes and no autopsy was performed to respect their wishes [67]. Death investigation systems ought to be aware of this ethical issue and have a system to take actions to reduce harm, including offense and unnecessary distress, where possible. This includes notifying families of the death, scene conduct, post-mortem examination, tissue sample, organ storage, disposal and return; all require ethical consideration. Death Investigation Navigators for families could be helpful in minimizing objections and also to better serve bereaved families. Ignoring the family's objections or concerns significantly deviates from the practice of medicine and the role of relational autonomy. The pathologist not only has an obligation to acknowledge the family's belief systems, regardless of its origins, but also has a role in informing the family members of the value of the autopsy as the general public has a very vague concept of what an autopsy entails, including the purpose of the autopsy [59]. Death investigation systems ought to consider the wishes of next of kin and where possible accommodate those wishes to the greatest extent possible that is compatible with their legal obligation to act in the wider public interest. For example, an objection to the autopsy may be attributed to concerns about a delay in the release of the body for funerary purposes. Although an autopsy performed within 2 days of the death will not typically delay funeral arrangements, a forensic autopsy unit should be able to accommodate families who request that the autopsy be conducted on the day of death for religious or cultural reasons. If there is a delay in the release of the body these delays may result in additional emotional stress and trauma to the family [41]. By accommodating the family, where possible, the death investigation system can honour the spiritual and sociocultural perceptions of death and the respect for persons and autonomy of the family. However, when there are criminal justice implications, where the autopsy could lead to the prosecution or conviction of a person accused of causing harm to the decedent, including relatives, forensic pathologists ought to be permitted to investigate suspicious deaths without interference from relatives, who are unable to use substituted judgement due to their own self-interest or potentially involvement in the death. However, the public and state's interest in death determination is weaker beyond public health and legal measures, whereby the public health concerns are often robust and outweigh the rights and interests of the family. The role of medicolegal autopsy is fundamental to the proper administration of civil and criminal justice systems where the issues to be decided are related to matters of disease, injury, and death [68].

There are diverse meanings about the dead that are inscribed in different spaces and relationships to the human remains and how we enact them. This multiplicity of meanings and functions includes medical and scientific value, in addition to the familial and socio-cultural aspects. In the mortuary, the scientific gaze is the dominant gaze to allow for the objective prosection of the dead. In the forensic context, human remains also function as a special piece of evidence. In the familial context, the decedent represents the memories held by relatives and families. Furthermore, it is generally agreed among members of society that the bodies of decedents should be treated with the principles of respect [43], dignity and promise-keeping. The Bristol inquiry has illuminated that decedents remain sociocultural attributes. From a sociocultural perspective, the decedents' body embodies sentiment and spirit. Human remains have familial and socialized aspects characterized by its lived identity, pre-existent personhood and ethereality [69]. The respectful handling and treatment of human remains are linked to the fact that these bodies were once living persons [43]. However, given the plurality of community, standards of respectful treatment of human remains are variable over place, space, time and families. To outline what is respectful requires knowing what is the disrespectful treatment of a dead body. The context, intent and objective play a role in determining whether a particular action is disrespectful [43]. Also, respectful treatment of human remains varies with time, culture, groups and individuals. The difference is the perspective of whether they violate the principle of respect [43]. As a means to respect the deceased persons and their families, the death investigation system ought to accommodate their values and preferences, where possible.

Organ and Tissue Donation for Transplantation

Many people die due to the shortage of available donor organs and tissues [70]. Transplantation has become the standard for end-stage organ failure. The death investigation system can have a powerful role in increasing the availability of organs and tissues for transplantation but is often an overlooked component of donation. In particular, coroners, medical examiners and forensic pathologists have a huge impact on the availability of donor tissues and organs. This is because individuals whose deaths are subject to a medicolegal death investigation are a major source of organs and tissues for transplantation. Approximately 70% of suitable donors fall under the jurisdiction of the coroner [71], and the release of these organs and tissues for donation is often based on the legislative power of the coroner and forensic pathologist [72]. There are competing interests and commitments around organ procurement for donation in the dead among stakeholders—family, physicians, organ procurement organizations and patients on waiting lists, police and attorneys. Donation denials may occur when the needs of the death investigation system come into conflict with those of the healthcare system resulting in tensions as to what would benefit the needs of the community. Death investigation systems ought to monitor how they address a conflict of commitment regarding organ and tissue donation requests such that unfounded denials do not exist (Fig. 2.6).

The burdens of organ and tissue shortage are not distributed equally when forensic pathologists and coroners do not release these organs and tissues equitably across the recipient population. For example, the paediatric population is disproportionately disadvantaged because they need organs from paediatric donors due to organ size considerations [73]. Unfortunately, despite children being in the most need, they are often the most often denied. This has been demonstrated in two studies wherein coroners and forensic pathologists have denied organ procurement in nearly three-fourths of paediatric deaths [74, 75]. Permitting post-mortem donation in the medicolegal context has the ability to give families the benefit of being able

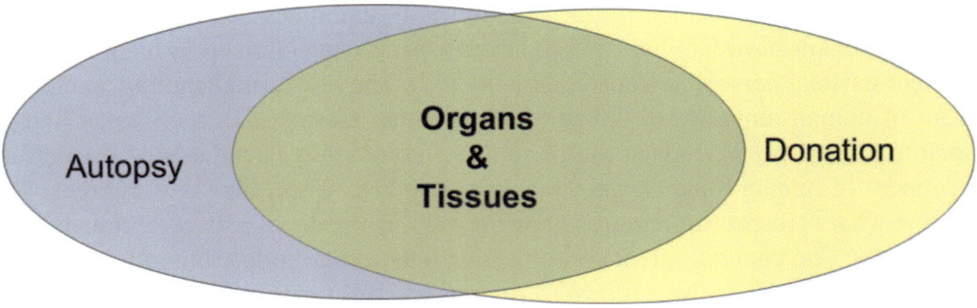

Fig. 2.6 Apparent conflict of commitment between post-mortem organ and tissue donations and the autopsy. Supporting organ and tissue donation requires balancing this against concerns that donation may impact the outcome of the death investigation

to give a life-saving gift to recipients. As a corporate citizen, death investigation systems have an interest in allowing organs and tissues to be made available for transplantation as this will can be life-extending, save healthcare dollars and provide benefits for the bereaved families and the recipient. In the vast majority of coroner's cases, including criminally suspicious deaths and homicides, it is possible to procure organs without compromising the death investigation, or civil or criminal proceedings arising from the death. This has consistently been demonstrated in other jurisdictions [76]. A means to accommodate organ donation for transplantation in a case of isolated head trauma, for example, is to request a computed tomography scan of the chest, abdomen and pelvis to be performed and interpreted before donation to maximize donations in an informed way.

Organ Retention

Retention of tissues, and occasionally whole organs, is part of the autopsy process. The importance of organ retention allows a pathologist to further characterize injury or disease and seek expert consultation, when appropriate. Organ retention is the possession of a whole organ and differs from tissue samples kept in "stock jars", paraffin blocks and as other laboratory specimens. Common organs retained include hearts, eyes and brains. A retained organ is typically submerged in formalin for proper fixation to reduce the risk of artefactual handling changes. This is particularly important in the examination of brains, which requires a lengthy fixation to maximize diagnostic yield and greatly enhance the detection of subtle neuropathological findings [77, 78]. Not retaining an organ could interfere with the evidentiary value provided in homicide cases. For example, a murder charge was dropped because the infant's brain was no longer available for further examination [79].

Prior to the Bristol Inquiry, retaining organs removed at autopsy, without explicitly informing the next of kin, was a customary practice among pathology departments. The public discovery that hospitals throughout England and Wales have been retaining organs for years emerged during the Bristol Inquiry. This Inquiry examined the circumstances around the removal, retention and disposal of human tissue, including children's organs, without the explicit knowledge of the next of kin. Many organs, tissues and even foetuses were retained in institutions that performed hospital and medicolegal autopsies [17]. Organ retention without disclosure to the next of kin was a means to avoid harming families. The medical community considered that approaching recently bereaved families about retaining body parts would be unseemly and inappropriate. It was considered unnecessary and potentially distressing to discuss organ prosection and retention [80]. Furthermore, the public seemingly did not want to know about the associated procedures related to death [80]. The solution was "benevolent paternalism", which aims at protecting a person's good by hindering their autonomy. Thus, retaining organs without the family's knowledge prevented potentially harmful information from being shared with the next of kin. The consequence of benevolent paternalism affected the public's trust of physicians, impaired a family's ability to work through bereavement and violated religious and cultural freedom. Family members believe that they have let their dead relative down by failing to ensure that they have safeguarded their values [81]. The public discovery of this practice also demonstrated the breakdown in procedural trust between institutions, pathologists and current and future relatives of decedents. One of the most serious outcomes was a decrease in the number of organ donations for transplantation [80]. The inquiry also showed that the public did want to know more about the process that occurs after death, including fuller explanations of the procedures and treatment of bodies at autopsy [80]. Retention of organs and tissues is considered ethical under the right circumstances, whereby the reasons are connected to the public good and the good of individuals to explain death and prevent future morbidity and mortality [1].

The findings of the inquiry resulted in systemic changes around post-mortem organ retention policies and practices in multiple countries. These changes emphasized the obligation of pathology and forensic institutions to engage in the full disclosure of autopsy details and procedures to bereaved relatives [82]. Recommendations from the inquiry are that organs are not to be retained unless relevant to establishing the cause of death [17]. Families have an option to delay the funeral, while the pathologist fixes and examines organs, to enable the return of the organs to the body for burial or cremation [17]. The obvious disadvantage is that this can delay funerary arrangements and impair storage space in the morgue. The other option for the family is to release the body for a funeral, without the return of the organs, in which case, the family shall be invited to authorize respectful disposal [17].

Pathologists, and the institutions they operate in, function as custodians and stewards of the human body, tissues and retained organs. They operate as stewards of the tissues obtained from medicolegal autopsies and hold these tissues *in trust* for the benefit of the decedent's families and society. In this role, there are certain responsibilities attached including deciding appropriate collection of tissue and organs that have critical diagnostic and medicolegal implications. This includes safekeeping of samples, transfer to third parties and eventual disposal. It is the duty of the pathologists to obtain what is necessary to establish the cause of death and any other relevant medicolegal purposes. This aligns with the pathologist's duties of keeping and guarding the integrity of tissue-containing paraffin blocks and glass slides [12] and formalin-fixed tissues in stock pots. These specimens must be maintained in good order and be readily available if further review is required. The determination to retain the organ is based on the pathologist's judgement and standard of practice. In this determination, the burden is placed on the pathologist to have a defendable and justified position. This includes ensuring that retained organs and tissues are used legitimately and ethically [1]. This position balances the responsibility of performing a comprehensive and accurate post-mortem examination and the values of both families and society. To ensure fidelity requires a transparent and accountable process. To achieve this requires documentation of all aspects of autopsy practice. Detailed technical aspects of the autopsy can be obtained from publications [83, 84]. However, removal of small tissue specimens for histology, microbiology, toxicology, special dissections and a wide range of tests, if occurred, should be disclosed in the autopsy report for transparency and reviewability.

Ethics and the Expert Witness

Very less has been published in the forensic pathology literature on the ethics of being a retained as an expert witness. Although the ethical minimum in law is not to lie under oath, there are a vast range of behaviours that, while legally permissible, may not be acceptable as ethical among forensic pathologists but can sometimes be considered expected services by legal counsel. Also, the ability to tell the truth may be limited by issues beyond the expert's control including rules of evidence, judicial rulings on admissible responsively, the attorney's line of question and phrasing of questions [85].

Ethical issues are sometimes legal issues. Much of what a forensic pathologist does is based on a legal and ethical framework; however, sometimes law and ethics diverge. Furthermore, law and medicine belong to separate institutions with their own ethics, culture and values. Consequently, this can result in the potential for conflicts and misunderstandings. A pathologist may find themselves concerned about a conflict between the duty to comply with the law and the ethical obligations of medicine. This can arise when the legal obligations appear to conflict with a perceived ethical acceptability about a particular course of action.

There are differences between legal, policy and ethical expectations (Fig. 2.7). Ethics are guidelines that are not established in legislation, but are imposed by the medical community and voluntarily assumed by the medical profession. Consequently, these differences can give rise to ethical tensions between medicine and the law. Forensic pathologists bring their ethics of the medical profession into the legal system. Bioethics is engrained in medical training; to abandon this training in forensic work would not align with what it means to be a physician. The legal system is based on a set of ethics that does not necessarily consider the value systems of medical ethics. In particular, forensic pathologists are experts who are trained in

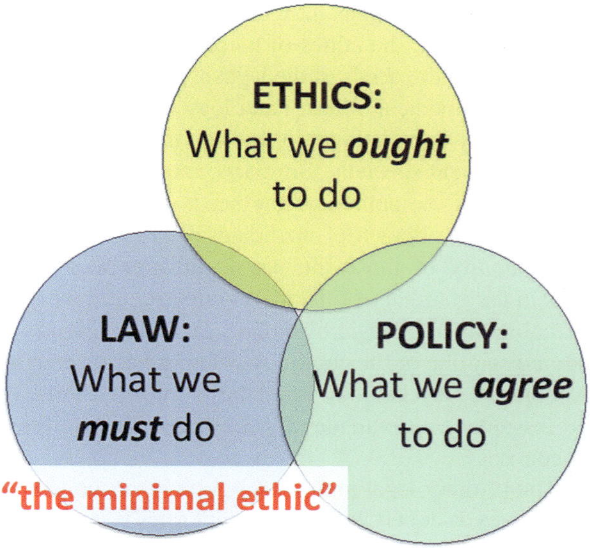

Fig. 2.7 The role of ethics, law and policy in decision-making. (Image courtesy: Dr. M.F. McKneally as adapted by M. McDonald)

medicine, which is designed to help and serve patients and the public. Policy is what we agree to do, such as organ retention procedures. Conflicts between law and medicine can be minimized through honesty, truthfulness and objectiveness.

In the context of an expert hired by an attorney, Saunders views expert witness ethics as having two competing roles: (1) the expert is an educator who informs the legal counsel about the strengths and weaknesses of a case and (2) as part of a team working with a legal counsel to achieve a goal [86]. Ultimately, if a forensic pathologist is hired as an expert, they are being paid for their time, not their opinions.

The ethical imperative of a forensic pathologist to be honest and a truth-teller has its own ethical imperative [2]. A forensic pathologist enters into a special relationship in which there is an understanding, both explicitly and implicitly, between different parties/stakeholders, that this carries with it the understanding that special duties are imposed. When authoring reports and communicating with police, attorneys and families, forensic pathologists ought to avoid all forms of deception. Forms of deception include intentional, equivocation, evasion and benevolent deception, by being "economical with the truth" or abstaining from correcting a misunderstanding [87]. This should not be confused with the virtue of plain speaking, especially in front of a jury. As physician experts, forensic pathologists need to evaluate our words and actions for what it truly is and leave an honest impression with the trier of the fact. So not only do forensic pathologists have as much of a duty as everyone else to be honest, but they also have a special duty to ensure the maintenance of the fiduciary relationship. Truth-telling permits the community to preserve trust and the importance of preserving trust because of the extraordinary difficulty of restoring this fiduciary relationship in the community once lost/destroyed. In the words of Roger Higgs: "If truth is the first casualty, trust is the second" [88].

Forensic pathologists have dual roles and owe allegiance to more than one institution. However, the ethics of medicine applied to forensic pathology may not be well suited to the needs of the legal system because this will utterly corrosive to the integrity of medical ethics. Pathology is not defined by the purposes we put to it. Competency in pathology depends on the knowledge and methods that are specific to this medical specialty. Similarly, medical ethics is not defined by convenience, the needs of the courts, or the needs of the state. Ethics of medicine, in which pathology is a branch of medicine, is based on the vulnerability, dependence and exploitability of those the physician attends. Pathologists, as physicians, must remain the guardians of the moral integrity of the profession and its ethics [89, 90]. Pathology is not a legal discipline, and although it is used to serve the courts, it is not a discipline of the courts. As such, it has its own set of values and ethics that a pathologist must embody when they serve the courts. When pathologists forgo their professional physician identity, they allow themselves to become agents of the state or counsel.

The primary legal and ethical purpose of the trial is to ascertain the truth [39]. Physicians as expert witnesses, adopt roles that are contrary to the role of their own professional ethics. In Sanders' discussion of expert witness ethics, he argues that an approach to be used in the expert's duty to tell the truth is an epistemological approach of when an expert can state that they know something [39]. The epistemological approach to answering that one knows something/knowledge is the interplay of the following three factors: belief, truth and justification [39]. Belief is defined as a person's subjective perspective concerning the truth of a proposition [39]. The absence of belief is ignorance [39]. Truth is the reality of a proposition and is independent of belief [39]. The lack of truth is classified as an error [39]. Justification is the quality of the reasons for a particular belief [39]. Lack of justification is a mere opinion [39]. This is interplay of belief, truth and justification also operates in pathology opinions in post-mortem reports, and court room testimony. A standard for considering authoring the cause of death statement, is that one needs to be prepared to provide lengthy testimony justifying your cause of death opinion on what you believe to be true based on the facts and interpretation. This is not to say that opinons can change to reflect a change in facts.

Both Pollack and Diamond [91, 92] utilize ethical tools to navigate the ethics of expert testimony, namely honesty and transparency as the foundation of forensic experts. Honesty is truthfulness and avoiding deceit. Transparency requires explaining what facts and logic are used to arrive at a conclusion and the uncertainty that may be associated with it [93]. This helps the trier of fact, such as the jury, to make a determination of your opinion and its relevance to the case. These are common ethical values in medicine and law. This also guards the forensic pathologists' credibility and community standing. In a medicolegal context, the virtue of a forensic pathologist is to seek truth from knowledge and the virtue of a judge is to strive towards justice.

Ethical Case Study

In 2015, for the first time in Canadian history, a retained body part was admitted as evidence in a murder trial. The legal rationale was that the actual tissue represented real evidence and would better assist the jury with understanding the nature of the injuries. The autopsy images were reportedly too dark and fell short of demonstrating the vaginal injuries [94]. The judge admitted the evidence, indicating that the probative value outweighed the prejudicial effect [95, 96]. The body part that was brought into the courtroom was pelvic tissues that were removed during the autopsy of Cindy Gladue. Cindy Gladue was an Indigenous woman, who had died from an 11-cm vaginal injury that led to blood loss. The accused, a non-Indigenous man who hired Cindy Gladue for sex work, confirmed that he did inflict this injury with his hand, which would indicate that the mechanism of injury was blunt force trauma. However, the stated mechanism of injury was in doubt because it was not supported by the initial observations made at the time of autopsy by the forensic pathologist. Consequently, the pathological evidence became pivotal in determining if the accused was telling the truth, making the issue of consent irrelevant. However, the initial forensic pathologist's (referred to as prosecution pathologist for simplicity) expert opinion regarding the mechanism of the fatal injury was in conflict with that of the pathologist hired by the defence attorney (referred to as the defence pathologist). This was relevant to the prosecution's case as the mechanism of injury spoke to the accused's narrative. The prosecution's pathologist indicated that the vaginal injury was due to a sharp force injury, while the defence pathologist opined that the injury was a laceration due to blunt force trauma. Essentially, the opinion of the prosecution's pathologist was not supportive of the accused's claim. During the trial, the retained body part was brought into the courtroom and each pathologist took turns demonstrating the vaginal injury to the jury, and other members of the court, and indicating their opinion on the nature of the injury. The actual tissue was behind an opaque screen but was projected on an overhead projector.

The acrimony that followed not only reflects the larger failure of bioethics in death investigation systems to resolve the tension and duties forensic pathologists have to the courts, and the society it serves but also reinforces that human dignity does not end with death. Although forensic work is obligated to criminal justice, this should not occur at the expense of professional and medical ethics. Pathologists serving forensic roles are bound by medical ethics or in time will be the focus of public condemnation. This action also reflects the tension between law and ethics, whereby an action that is legally permissible does not imply that it is ethical. The ethical issue is should a forensic pathologist bring in a retained body part from an Indigenous woman for the sole purpose of achieving criminal justice in a public courtroom? An approach to examining the ethical oversights is to examine the components of the ethical dilemma and weave different ethical theories into each component of the ethical dilemma:

Moral Agent

The moral agent includes the role of the forensic pathologists but can also include others in the legal system who are also moral agents. The focus here will be on the role of the pathologist rather than those of the law profession because they do not share the same ethical norms to which physicians are expected to uphold. Pathologists as expert witnesses are obligated to justice but not at the cost of the ethics of the medical profession. Guiding ethical principles in medicine include human dignity and the pathologist's role as guardians of human tissue. The role of human dignity is reflected in medicine via the clinical practice of "draping with dignity", which denotes that intimate parts of the body of the patient must be covered with clothing/sheet to restore dignity during physician examination. Human dignity is a concept that is an expression of ideas about ethical propriety, particularly elements of respect, autonomy and empowerment [97]. Often, this clinical practice still continues in many autopsy suites whereby the genitalia is covered with a towel following the external examination, or the unclad body is covered with a sheet during breaks of an extended post-mortem examination. Therefore, the presentation of an intimate body part in a courtroom is directly counter to norms of physician behaviour. In short, medical ethics creates boundaries between what is public and private, essentially defining what counts as autonomy.

Pathology ethics also describes the pathologists' duty to function as guardians of human tissue [12]. This guardianship reflects the understanding of the uniqueness and preciousness of each tissue and not to misuse the tissue. More specifically, for pathologists to permit non-relevant individuals to examine a retained body part is an abrogation of the responsibility and a disservice to the community we serve.

The burden is upon the pathologist to balance not only the rights and expectations of the families and courts with the responsibility to perform a comprehensive, accurate examination of the body and to ensure that adequate notification for extended examinations is obtained [98] but also what that examination will entail. Forensic pathologists have accepted their responsibility to society, including maintaining the highest professional standards regarding the post-mortem examination, reporting of findings and conclusions and testimony to advance the interests of justice. The pursuit of justice, through utilizing science and medicine, is done in a manner that respects the social and cultural values of affected communities. Like other areas of medicine and science, forensic pathology is also reassessing the interaction between science and society [64, 80, 99, 100].

Action

The action was a decision about the pathologist assisting the jury in making a decision about the pathological evidence as a means to fulfil the jury's role as fact finders. Any action should outline all realistic options, balance competing values, principles, obligations and responsibilities and build arguments for each option in order to make a reasoned approach. Instead of bringing human tissues into court, there were a wide variety of alternative options to consider to supplant their oral evidence that include not showing any images, improving the quality of the autopsy images and disclosing these improvements to the court, re-taking the images, using anatomical models, "hot-tubing" and computer-generated images. Furthermore, the pathologist should consider the impossible challenge for the lay jury that is expected to arrive at their own opinion when examining the actual pathological evidence in the context that two experts disagree. This is particularly challenging because the jury is expected to make an expert interpretation by the direct examination of the tissue, when the experts cannot agree. The view used in bringing human remains was a "deficit model" of jury understanding. The "deficit model" indicates that the jury lacks understanding of the pathological complexities of an issue and to correct this lack of understanding is a need for better learning by dwelling on the facts via demonstrating the tissues. As if the value of human remains drops out of the process altogether. If settling the facts will independently reveal the right decision. The issue with introducing real evidence in this scenario as a means to discuss facts as an independent first step towards fact finding is that the facts are bound up with values in ways that make it impossible to discuss the facts of the injury without implicating values on human remains. The display of a woman's body speaks to how that body is valued, the more valued the body, the less likely the body will be displayed. The values, obligations and responsibilities of bringing human tissues into a public venue, even with the best motives, will arouse feelings of humiliation for families and their communities. When human dignity, which belongs to every person even in death, is sufficiently transgressed in the name of legal justice pathologists ought to consider medical ethical principles as guidelines. The action of displaying human remains in the court added to the normalized institutionalized violence against Indigenous women. Sometimes, in medical and scientific deliberation, determining a fact between two experts requires evaluating values first, rather than the facts. Evidence is not value-free [101, 102].

Consequences

The consequences of bringing in a retained body part into the courtroom include the harm to stakeholders and the potential harm to the jury but there was also a breach of the fiduciary duty of forensic pathologists. The moral weight of human dignity that the living assigns to human remains demonstrates respect and promotion of the well-being of the living. The reassurance that one's values will be respected in death is a comfort to people while alive. This can only be sustained if they are *indeed* respected as a societal norm after death. This includes the process for informing the next of kin of organ retention and the management of expectations over the process of using retained organs. The process of retained organs includes the re-examination of retained organs in the privacy of a morgue. It is quite reasonable for the public to expect that the display of the retained organ in a public setting, such as a court of law, would not occur. Simply put, the harm to the deceased may derive from organ retention and display of organs in court might be considered desecration of the decedent's body [103]. This organ belongs to a person who is connected to their family. A failure to treat an organ with dignity, by extension, is a direct harm to that person's family. Treatment of a human organ signifies in a broader perspective social, emotional, and cultural senses. In this situation, the duty of restitution and reconciliation can involve creating a space for rearticulating mutual expectations and shared meanings, which enables an understanding of how setbacks be conveyed without destroying the relationship between medical professionals and the Indigenous community. The harm to Cindy Gladue's family includes dehumanizing the memory they carry of Cindy as a person, a mother, a daughter and a sister. Cindy's family was devastated by the judge's decision and argued their input and authorization were required to protect Cindy's dignity as an Indigenous woman [104]. Furthermore, it alienated oppressed groups, including Indigenous people, women and sex workers from the medical and legal systems. Finally, it epitomized that Indigenous women are disproportionately targeted for violence in Canada and institutional anti-Indigenous racism and sexism, which are remnants of Canada's Indigenous genocide. Permitting an organ that is associated with sex and reproduction is a direct attack on the reproductive capacities of Indigenous women. The consequences of this action were a form of collective, cultural, historical and ongoing injury against Indigenous peoples. It also had the potential of harm to the jurors as a form of post-traumatic stress disorder, which is becoming a more recognized issue.

Fiduciary relationships between pathologists and other stakeholders in the death investigation system involve trust and confidence. Trust is built and preserved by consistent, reliable transparent and truthful practices of all members and institutions within the death investigation system engaged in provision of death investigation. This includes the pathologist who retained the organs, who was entrusted to act in good faith that the retained organs would be used in a manner that is in keeping with the social expectations and the expectations of the medical profession. It is reasonable that a pathologist would not only retain an organ for re-examination in these circumstances but also examine the injury microscopically. Microscopic examination of the injury serves the public interest to better understand the time interval between the injury and death as this can inform medicolegal opinions about the survival period. Not introducing human tissue into the courts would also align with medical practices, such as "draping with dignity" that the public learns from other areas of medicine that sensitive areas of the body certainly would not be showcased in a public forum. Furthermore, it is understood that the physician pelvic exam is considered by most people with uteruses as unpleasant, embarrassing, anxiety-provoking and associated with fear [105]. The damage to the fiduciary duty is that bereaved families, or potential bereaved families, and individuals that have interests in confidentiality and privacy, raise doubts that these values will survive death where relevant. Consequently, the privilege to have custody of these organs is in jeopardy because of concerns that human remains will not be treated with dignity. Privacy does not end after death. Privacy is a core principle of autonomy. The right to respect for private life does include displaying genitals. Privacy and privilege can be conceived of as "rights" belonging to the individual, while confidentiality is a duty of the clinician to the patient within the context of the therapeutic relationship. Beyond these legal concepts, confidentiality is also grounded in the ethical principles of respect for persons, beneficence and autonomy. Further, privacy is a heterogenous construct and it is reasonable that the cause of death and other relevant findings would be disclosed in a court of law in these circumstances.

Context

The context resides at the intersection of the death investigation, healthcare and legal systems and the colonial context between Canada and Indigenous nations.

Intersection of the Death Investigation, Healthcare and Legal Systems

The history of medicine is filled with controversy related to oversight of ethical practice but none as much as that associated with examining the female body [106]. Furthermore, both medicine and law have been responsible of patriarchal practices and inappropriate sexual behaviour that victimizes a woman. These practices carry broad social import because it is nested in the inequities of the past drawing on the historical context and underscores the importance of social commentary on professional values. All three systems failed to recognize that societal values were not reflected but rather emphasized the systemic racism of the expendability of Indigenous women [66] and directly contributed to a substantive injustice of reducing Indigenous women to sexual organs.

Forensic pathologists operate in death investigation systems, which intersect with the healthcare and legal system. This intersection is highlighted structurally as many forensic pathologists operate in hospitals and as subpoenaed expert witnesses in courts of law. As physicians, the medical and ethical training of a forensic pathologist occurs in the healthcare setting. In the healthcare system, it is not uncommon for physicians to examine the bodies of others, including sensitive areas of the body when medically indicated. It is also a customary practice that physicians consult other physicians when there are outstanding questions about an observation on the body or when assistance is required. The normative expectation is that this intimate examination occurs in the privacy of hospital rooms and morgues. In the legal context, this discussion between medical experts could have been accommodated by "hot-tubing", whereby the two pathologists review the retained tissues together, have an honest discussion about the mechanism of injury and come to some sort of consensus (i.e. a vaginal injury is present) that opinion is presented to the jury and other members of the court. This would include the humility that vaginal injuries are quite rare for a forensic pathologist to assess. Instead, the introduction of retained body parts into the courtroom placed the legal enterprise above respect for the dead and human decency.

Indigenous Communities

When post-mortem tissue has been physically separated from the decedent, this prosection does not sever the family and community ties to the decedent, nor does it transect the associated cultural and historical context of these relationships. From an Indigenous perspective, the reductionistic process of removing and presenting tissue in court as abstract evidence, void of any historical or colonial context, serves as a reminder of the colonial practice of stealing and preserving Indigenous body parts for pursuing "scientific investigations", morbid curiosity but also the colonial past was brought into the present when the reproductive organs of Indigenous women were used as trophies during colonial massacres [53, 107, 108]. Furthermore, the continued practice of buying and selling the remains of Indigenous peoples implies that these communities are for putting on display, which continues to dehumanize Indigenous peoples [109]. These remains are largely from collections at holding institutions that have been complicit in colonization. In some countries there has been implementation of Federal laws, such as the Native American Graves Protection and Repatriation Act in the United States, to make efforts to return these ancestors to their Indigneous communities. In Canada, there is no Federal law and attempts to change Canadian law to return these ancestors to Indigenous communities have failed.

Indigenous women are murdered at an alarming rate and when found dead under suspicious circumstances their deaths are not as thoroughly investigated as non-Indigenous women [110]. This systemic racism has led to the National Inquiry into Murdered and Missing Indigenous Women and Girls. This inquiry affirmed that gender and ethnic inequity have led to the normalization of Indigenous women as disposable humans, which puts them at risk of exploitation. The courtroom was a place where Cindy was transformed from a human and reduced to a piece of tissue. In the face of such disparities, pathologists and others in the death investigation and the legal system need to be leaders that overcome ethnic and gender disparities, not emphasize them. Furthermore, this prevented reconciliation with Indigenous nations and was a substantive injustice by failing to protect Indigenous women, who are commonly victimized.

Research

Forensic pathologists may believe that they have an ethical and intellectual obligation to conduct research. Research in forensic pathology is important because, for some research questions, human tissues are the only means to solve certain types of equipoise. The autopsy continues to be a focus of biomedical research as a means of identifying new diseases, clarifying the mechanisms and patterns of illness and injury, exploring treatments that may ameliorate suffering and sustaining medical advances in order to improve societal welfare. In addition, the autopsy provides the opportunity to access human tissue [68]. Despite this long tradition, the hospital autopsy has declined, leaving more pressure on the medicolegal autopsy to fill this void. Unlike a hospital autopsy, a medicolegal autopsy is performed without authorization from the next of kin. Hospital autopsy authorizations will often provide opportunities to consider an approval for research, which is not a common priority in death investigation and medicolegal autopsies. A medicolegal autopsy is performed for the purposes of legal interest in determining the cause of death and other medicolegal purposes. The information that may be obtained from the autopsy can also aid medical and forensic sciences as research-related benefits such as contributing to expanding knowledge of medical treatments and novel discoveries. Despite the value of autopsy in research, consistent ethical (and legal) guidelines for research-related issues beyond the medicolegal imperatives have not been developed [19]. The ethical issues for clinician researchers are clearer than they are for forensic pathology researchers, largely in part because the research participant is alive. Forensic pathology continues to lag behind other medical specialities in its research, research ethics and the development necessary to build the evidence base for its practice. This is in part because forensic pathology is a boutique area of medicine and is comparatively disadvantaged when compared with other areas of medicine that have much higher rates of publication, such as medical genetics and oncology. Furthermore, forensic pathology is not a priority for health-care research funding bodies and the nature of forensic pathology research requires study designs that are different from the typical randomized clinical trials. This has also led to a lack of growth in the development, conduct and application of research ethics in forensic pathology. The research–practice dichotomy in forensic pathology is complicated by the interaction with next of kin, the legislative powers, and law enforcement agencies.

Conclusion

The medicolegal autopsy is an act of moral, medical and legal significance. The purpose of the autopsy is for the benefit of medical knowledge, education, the legal system, the public health system, society and the decedent's family. Accepting and performing an autopsy is entering a commitment of trust with all of those that the forensic pathologist has an obligation to. The fidelity of this trust is an ethical requirement that is as binding as the physician–patient relationship [11]. Education in science and medicine does not protect from ethical failures [111–113]. A solution is to utilize ethical concepts to inform our thinking by considering values, principles, theories and approaches in bioethics. The wisdom that exists in bioethics and ethical decision-making can be used to facilitate the resolution of ethical dilemmas in death investigation. However, ethical issues in forensic pathology are not just a subset of healthcare ethics but require its own normative ethical theory for this medical subspecialty to consider the implications of forensic pathology, which are not covered in other places in healthcare ethics. Forensic pathology is embedded in unique ethical dilemmas in which forensic pathologists are concerned with factual and corroborative information; they perform autopsies with an emphasis on objective diagnosis and classification of injury and disease for societal interests, rather than individual patient interests, by providing expert testimony that advances the interests of justice and society. As medical professionals, they are torn between different considerations and exposed to seemingly incompatible expectations from their surroundings. Unless forensic pathologists regulate their profession through ethics, we are open to new abuses and diminish our ethical commitment as physicians. This needed body of work is called death investigation bioethics and requires three areas of development. First, a full set of ethical principles and complementary ethical theories germane to death investigation should be developed. Second, we must better understand how explicit attention to ethical concerns impact decision-making in death investigation. Third, new ethical analytic approaches that contribute to constructive death investigation decision-making should be developed. Although death investigation is a rational, goal-oriented activity and a means to solve death investigation using scientific and medical evidence, decisions in death investigations are also complex and value-laden.

References

1. Harris J. Law and regulation of retained organs: the ethical issues. Leg Stud. 2002;22:527–49.
2. Beauchamp TL, Childress JF. Principles of biomedical ethics. 8th ed. New York: Oxford University Press; 2013.
3. Appelbaum PS. Psychiatric ethics in the courtroom. Bull Am Acad Psychiatry Law. 1984;12:225–31.
4. Appelbaum PS. The parable of the forensic psychiatrist: ethics and the problem of doing harm. Int J Law Psychiatry. 1990;13:249–59.
5. Fowler DR. Public figures, professional ethics, and the media. AMA J Ethics. 2016;18(8):839–42.
6. Foucar E. Pathology expert witness testimony and pathology practice: a tale of 2 standards. Arch Pathol Lab Med. 2005;129:1268–76.
7. Denton JS. Ethics education in forensic pathology fellowship training: is there a need? Acad Forensic Pathol. 2013;3(3):312–6.
8. Domen RE. Ethical and professional issues in pathology: a survey of current issues and educational efforts. Hum Pathol. 2002;33(8):779–82.
9. Bruns DE, Burtis CA, Gronowski AM, Task Force IFCC, on Ethics. Variability of ethics education in laboratory medicine training programs: results of an international survey. Clin Chim Acta. 2015;442:115–8.
10. Pellegrino ED. The autopsy. Some ethical reflections on the obligations of pathologists, hospitals, families and society. Arch Pathol Lab Med. 1996;120:739–42.
11. Pellegrino ED. The autopsy: some ethical reflections on the obligations of pathologists, hospitals, families and society. Arch Pathol Lab. 1996;120(8):739–42.
12. Mills SE, et al. Guardians of the wax and the patient. Am J Clin Pathol. 1995;104:365–7.
13. Vos S, et al. Ethical considerations for modern molecular pathology. J Pathol. 2018;246(4):405–14.
14. Emanuel E. Reform of clinical research regulations, finally. NEJM. 2015;373(224):2296–9.
15. https://webarchive.nationalarchives.gov.uk/20090811143822/http:/www.bristol-inquiry.org.uk/final_report/the_report.pdf.

16. https://assets.publishing.service.gov.uk/government/uploads/system/uploads/attachment_data/file/229155/0571_i.pdf.
17. The Royal Liverpool Children's inquiry report (the Redfern report), London, 2001.
18. Jacques R. Death investigation bioethics as a NEW subdiscipline. The role of bioethics in AI and emerging health technologies: activator, inhibitor or collaborator. Book of Abstracts. Canadian Bioethics Society; 2020.
19. Roberts LW, et al. Perceptions of the ethical acceptability of using medical examiner autopsies for research and education: a survey of forensic pathologists. Arch Pathol Lab Med. 2000;124:1485–95.
20. Thomson J. The Trolley problem. Yale Law J. 1985;94(6):1395–415.
21. Pellegrino ED, Thomasma DC. The virtues of medical practice. New York: Oxford University Press; 1993.
22. Liosi S. Our duty to the dead. Philosophy Now. 2018;126.
23. Quill TE. Doctor, I want to die. Will you help me? J Am Med Assoc. 1993;270(7):870–3.
24. Bentham J. The principles of morals and legislation. Oxford: Clarendon Press; 1996.
25. Jason D. The role of the medical examiner/coroner in organ and tissue procurement for transplantation. Am J Forensic Med Pathol. 1994;15:192–202.
26. Clouser KD, Gert B. A critique on principilism. J Med Philos. 1990;15(2):219–36.
27. Donnelly J. Cultural relativism and universal human rights. Human Rights Q. 1984;6(4): 400–19.
28. Toronto Central Community Care Access Centre. Community ethics toolkit. 2008. Accessed online 4 Jan 2010. http://www.jointcentreforbioethics.ca/partners/documents/cen_toolkit2008.pdf.
29. Jonsen A, Seigler M, Winslade W. Clinical ethics: a practical approach to ethical decisions in clinical medicine. 5th ed. McGraw-Hill Inc.; 2002.
30. Daniels N, Sabin JE. Setting limits fairly: can we learn to share medical resources? Oxford: Oxford University Press; 2002.
31. Logarajah S, Roff S. Structured learning for clinical ethics in anesthesia. Clin Ethics. 2016;11:200–9.
32. Ethics. Acad Forensic Pathol. 2013;3(3):272–336.
33. Coe JI. President's message: ethics for the forensic pathologist. Am J Forensic Med Pathol. 1980;1(4):367–8.
34. American Academy of Forensic Sciences. Code of ethics. Colorado Springs, CO.
35. American Academy of Forensic Sciences Committee on good forensic practice. Standards of good forensic practice. Acad New. 2000;30(1):33.
36. Melinak J. The ethics of working as a retained forensic expert. Acad Forensic Pathol. 2013;3(3):281–8.
37. https://www.thename.org/code-of-ethics
38. Ontario Forensic Pathology Service. Practice manual for registered pathologists. 2022.
39. Sanders J. Expert witness ethics. Fordham Law Rev. 2007;76(3):1539–84.
40. Rosner R, Weinstock R, editors. Ethical practice in psychiatry and the law. New York: Plenum Press; 1990.
41. Wicclai MR, DeVita MA. Oversight of research involving the dead. Kennedy Inst Ethics J. 2004;14(2):143–64.
42. Horta O. Why the concept of moral status should be abandoned. Ethic Theory Moral Pract. 2017;20:899–910.
43. Wicclair MR, DeVita MA. Oversight of research involving the dead. Kennedy Inst Ethics J. 2004;14(2):143–64.
44. Noonan J. An almost absolute value in history. Cambridge: Harvard University Press; 1970.
45. Laitinen A. Hegel and respect for persons. Roots of respect. 2017.
46. Lane M, Vercler C. Is consent to autopsy necessary? Cartesian dualism and its limitations. AMA J Ethics. 2016;18(8):771–8.
47. Pentz RD, et al. Ethics guidelines for research with the recently dead. Nat Med. 2005;11(11):1145–9.

48. Singer P. Practical ethics. Cambridge University Press; 1993.
49. Nair-Collins M. Can the brain-dead be harmed or wronged? On the moral status of brain death and its implications for organ transplantation. Kennedy Inst Ethics J. 2017;27(4):525–59.
50. Brazier M. Retained organs: ethics and humanity. Leg Stud. 2002;22:550–69.
51. Haden-Pinneri K, Weedon VW. Organ and tissue retention. Acad Forensic Pathol. 2013;3(3):294–300.
52. United Nations. The universal declaration of human rights. New York: United Nations; 1948. Available from: http://www.un.org/en/documents/udhr/. Accessed 16 Jun 2022.
53. Public Hospitals Act, RRO 1990, Regulation 965, ss 20(2)3, 31(1), 31(2).
54. Whaley K. Disputes over what remains: bodies, burial, ashes and new developments. Whaley Estates Litigation; 2012. p. 10-1–10-38.
55. Klaiman MH. Whose brain is it anyway? Legal Med. 2005;26(4):475–90.
56. Dewar S, Boddington P. Returning to the Alder Hey report and its reporting: addressing confusion and improving inquiries. J Med Ethic. 2004;30:463–9.
57. Haden-Pinneri K, Weedn VW. Organ and tissue retention. Acad Forensic Pathol. 2013;3(3):294–300.
58. Stempsey WE. The penetrating gaze and the decline of the autopsy. AMA J Ethics. 2016;18(8):833–8.
59. Wood MJ, Guha AK. Medicolegal autopsy rates in Halifax, Nova Scotia. Why the difference? A historical perspective. Arch Pathol Lab Med. 2001;125:924–30.
60. Callahan JC. On harming the dead. Ethics. 1987;97:341–52.
61. Nelken D, Andrews L. Am J Law Med. 1998;24:261–92.
62. Cordner S, El Nagel M, Lineham B, Wells D, McKelvie H. Ethical practice in laboratory medicine and forensic pathology. WHO Regional Publications Eastern Mediterranean Series 20. WHO Regional Office.
63. Berg J. Grave secrets: legal and ethical analysis of postmortem confidentiality. Conn Law Rev. 2001;34:81–122.
64. Plattner T. The response of relatives to medicolegal investigations and forensic autopsy. Am J Forensic Med Pathol. 2002;23(4):345–8.
65. Berry C, Heaton-Armstrong A. A review of the coroner system in England and Wales. Clin Med. 2005;5:455–9.
66. Interim report of the national inquiry into missing and murdered indigenous women and girls: our women and girls are sacred. ISBN: 978-0-660-09755-8. p. 12
67. Lynch MJ. Forensic pathology: redefining medicolegal death investigation. JLM. 1999;7:67–74.
68. The Royal College of Pathologists of Australasia. Autopsies and the use of tissues removed. CMAJ. 2017; https://doi.org/10.1503/cmaj.120565.
69. Norwood F. The ambivalent chaplain: negotiating structural and ideological difference on the margins of modern-day hospital medicine. Med Anthropol. 2006;25:1–29.
70. United Network for Organ Sharing. Data. https://www.unos.org/data/. Accessed 14 Feb 2021.
71. Culimore E. At last minute, 3 babies are denied donor organs. Philadelphia Inquirer. 11 Mar 1993.
72. http://www.attorneygeneral.jus.gov.on.ca/inquiries/goudge/report/v3_en_pdf/Vol_3_Eng.pdf, p. 580.
73. Pinckard K, et al. Acad Forensic Pathol. 2013;4:497–504.
74. Shafer TJ, et al. The impact of medical examiner/coroner practices on organ recovery in the United States. JAMA. 1994;272:1607–13.
75. Strama BT, et al. Criminal investigations and prosecutions not adversely affected by organ donation. A case law review. Newsletter Med Law Comm. 1994:15–21.
76. NAME position paper on the medical examiner release of organs and tissues for transplantation. 2006.
77. Black M, Graham DI. Sudden unexplained death in adults caused by intracranial pathology. J Clin Pathol. 2002;55:44–55.

78. Katelaris A, et al. Brains at necroscopy: to fix or not to fix? J Clin Pathol. 1994;47:718–20.
79. http://www.cbc.ca/news/canada/newfoundland-labrador/brain-missing-matthew-rich-thomas-michel-murder-charge-dropped-1.3360899.
80. Carvel D. Controversies concerning human tissue retention and implications for the forensic practitioner. J Clin Forensic Med. 2002;9:53–60.
81. Brazier M. Organ retention and return: problems of consent. J Med Ethics. 2003;29:30–3.
82. Drayton J. Organ retention and bereavement: family counselling and the ethics of consultation. Ethics Social Welfare. 2011;5(3):227–46.
83. Randall BB, et al. Practice guidelines for forensic pathology. Arch Pathol Lab Med. 1998;122:1056–64.
84. Hutchins GM, et al. Practice guidelines for autopsy pathology: autopsy performance. Arch Pathol Lab Med. 1994;118:19–25.
85. Holmgren BL. Ethical issues in forensic testimony involving abusive head trauma. Acad Forensic Pathol. 2013;3(3):317–28.
86. Saunders J. Expert witness ethics. Fordham Law Rev. 2007;76(3):1539–84.
87. Jackson J. Telling the truth. J Med Ethics. 1991;17:5–9.
88. Higgs R. On telling patients the truth. In: Lockwood M, editor. Moral dilemmas in modern medicine. Oxford: Oxford University Press; 1985.
89. Pellegrino ED. Guarding the integrity of medical ethics: some lessons from Soviet Russia. JAMA. 1995;273:1622–3.
90. Pellegrino ED. The Nazi doctors and Nuremberg: some moral lessons revisited. Ann Intern Med. 1997;127:307–8.
91. Pollack S. Forensic psychiatry in criminal law. Los Angeles: University of Southern California Press; 1974.
92. Diamond BL. The forensic psychiatrist: consultant vs activist in legal doctrine. Bull Am Acad Psychiatry Law. 1992;20:119–32.
93. Katz J. "The fallacy of the impartial expert" revisited. Bull Am Acad Psychiatr Law. 1992;20:141–52.
94. R v Barton, 2015 ABQB 159 (CanLII).
95. White Burgess v Haliburton, 2015 SCC 23 (CanLII) (para 54).
96. R v Sekhon, 2014 SCC 15 (CanLII) (para 46).
97. Griffin-Heslin VL. An analysis of the concept dignity. Accid Emerg Nurs. 2005;13(4):251–7.
98. Dyer C. New bill will regulate the retention of tissue. BMJ. 2003;327:1304.
99. Williams ED, Crews JD. From dust to dust: ethical and practical issues involved in the location, exhumation and identification from mass graves. Croat Med J. 2003;44(3):251–8.
100. Hudson ML. The impact of Maori cultural values on forensic science practice in New Zealand. J Forensic Sci. 2008;53(2):380–3.
101. Biller-Andorno N, et al. Evidence-based medicine as an instrument for rational health policy. Health Care Anal. 2002;10:261–75.
102. Norheim O. Role of evidence in health policy making a normative perspective. Health Care Anal. 2002;10:309–17.
103. Weedn VW, Holdsworth MT, Barron AM. Legal and ethical considerations in forensic pathology research. Acad Forensic Pathol. 2011;1(3):288–301.
104. Death and Life of Cindy Gladue by Kathryn Blaze Carlson, 15 May 2015. The Globe and Mail.
105. O'Laughlin D, et al. Addressing anxiety and fear during the female pelvic examination. J Prim Care Community Health. 2021;12:2150132721992195. https://doi.org/10.1177/2150132721992195.
106. Brennan PAW. The medical and ethical aspects of photography in the sexual assault examination: why does it offend? J Clin Forensic Med. 2006;13:194–202.
107. Razack SH. Gendering Disposability. Can J Women Law. 2016;28(2):285–307.
108. Smith A. Conquest: sexual violence and American Indian genocide. Durham, NC: South End Press & Duke University Press; 2015.

109. Simkin J. Creating a new reality: repatriation, reconciliation and moving forward. Ottawa, ON: Canadian Commission for UNESCO's IdeaLab; 2020.
110. Reclaiming power and place: the final report of the national inquiry into missing and murdered Indigenous women and girls.
111. Martinson BC, et al. Scientists behaving badly. Nature. 2005;435:737–8.
112. Saks MJ, Koehler JJ. The coming paradigm shift in forensic identification sicience. Science. 2005;309:892–5.
113. Foucar E, Wick MR. Evidence-based medicine and tort law. Semin Diagn Pathol. 2005;22:167–76.

Chapter 3
Principles of Courtroom Testimony

Rebekah Jacques

Introduction

Expert testimony makes up a small, but significant, portion of the work of a forensic pathologist. Yet, compared with many other physicians, forensic pathologists and medical examiners testify more frequently; this is intrinsic to a medicolegal practice. Furthermore, during the performance of an autopsy on a criminally suspicious death, a forensic pathologist considers early on the importance of photodocumentation and dissection, among other decisions, in part, because they inform the pathologist's ability to form relevant opinions but also to present those opinions to the courts.

The legal process is very different compared with the practice of medicine. This is in large part due to the different cultures, training, specialised terminologies, different ways of communication, paradigms and epistemologies between law and medicine. In contrast to specialised areas of medicine where physicians have additional training in different areas, judges are generally not specialists in murder trials, and therefore a vast array of experiences can exist among judges. Furthermore, during court proceedings, judges can have multiple roles including trier of fact (in cases that do not involve a jury) or gatekeepers of the evidence (determine the admissibility of expert evidence). In contrast, physicians typically have a small amount of formal education in civil law (i.e. tort law) but have little to no formal education in criminal law or in being a medical witness.

Legal proceedings have a different approach from medicine to problem-solving. Medicine is predominantly a helping profession in which physicians are expected to help others, primarily patients, and their families. The practice of medicine is focused on making diagnosis and treating or ameliorating disease. The legal system is chiefly concerned with resolving disputes and maintaining social order. Once a

R. Jacques (✉)
London Health Sciences Centre, London, ON, Canada
e-mail: rebekah.jacques@lhsc.on.ca

R. Jacques (ed.), *Forensic Pathology*,
https://doi.org/10.1007/978-3-031-42038-2_3

legal decision is made regarding a conflict between parties, there is little room for revisions and, subject to restrictive rights of appeal or review, is essentially final. This principle of finality is foreign to physicians because the immediacy of decision-making to achieve a legal "finality" runs counter to the principles of science and medicine [1]. Physicians are accustomed to dealing with the gap between current knowledge of science and medicine—a gap that is constantly changing due to the effects of ongoing research and evidence-based medicine. In other words, there is no finality of knowledge. Much like other physicians, forensic pathologists utilise a holistic approach to resolve medicolegal issues by utilising the five steps of the autopsy to develop a hypothesis or tentative causes of deaths, which are tested and revised as additional data, facts and information come into play with each step or over time as new facts emerge. Pathologists practice in an environment in which hypotheses are evaluated with tests designed to yield precise and accurate interpretations. The difference in forensic pathology, as compared with most areas of medicine, is that the pathological diagnosis and conclusions can be part of the investigation of a criminally suspicious death, legal remedies, and testifying in court proceedings. The pathological diagnosis does not actually assist the decedent, but the knowledge gathered from the autopsy can be used to assuage grief among the bereaved family.

The commonality of both law and medicine is their truth-seeking function as a shared foundational principle to resolve issues. Over time, law and medicine are subject to mutual adjustments as there is a continuous exchange of knowledge and methodologies. Law and medicine have shaped each other throughout history and likely will continue to do so.

Structure of the Court System

Each country has a different organisation of its court system and accompanying laws that guide decision-making. There are many different courts, and the venues for testimony vary based on each country. Forensic pathologists may testify in adversarial or inquisitorial processes but typically deliver their oral testimony on criminal issues (Fig. 3.1). Sometimes, forensic pathologists may be called to testify in civil matters, such as cases of wrongful deaths. Court structure is typically complex and physicians' experience when attending court will vary depending on which court and which jurisdiction they attend. Regardless of the nature of the court, forensic pathologists must remember that their oral testimony is recorded and can be referred to in higher or subsequent court appearances for a particular case. If there is uncertainty about the process in a particular court, the pathologist is well

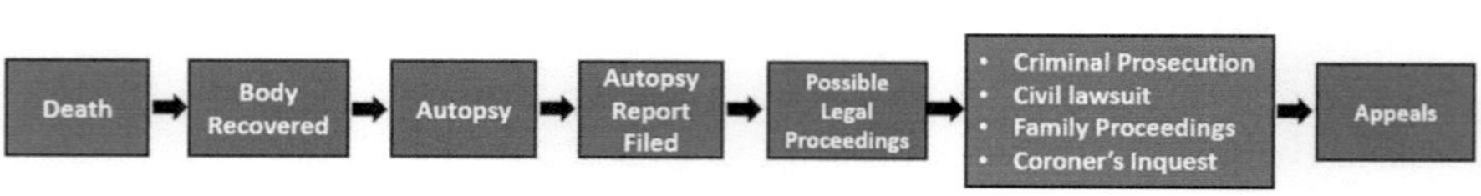

Fig. 3.1 Timeline to potential legal proceedings

advised to seek clarity from those who are parties to a particular proceeding, particularly from those who are requesting that the pathologist testify.

In many countries, the origins of their courts are based on the Anglo-Saxon model, which is an adversarial system. Typically, there is a hierarchical arrangement of the courts composed of lower and higher courts, usually ascending to a final appellate court, often referred to as a supreme court. Essentially, the supreme court is at the top of the hierarchy. There may also be courts that are specific to content or appeals. Most criminal cases enter the court system at the lower courts and may move up to higher courts. Decision-making by judges in Anglo-Saxon-based courts of law is bound by "doctrine of precedent" whereby prior judgements on questions of law determined in one court are generally binding on lower courts. Collectively, decisions based on judge-made law are referred to as "common law" or "case law" decisions. Judges may also be asked both to interpret statutes (i.e. laws created by legislatures) and pre-existing judge-made laws. Furthermore, the nomenclature of the judge(s) may be dependent on the level of court. In Canada, the judges of the lower courts, such as the provincial court, are referred to as "Your Honour". In the Supreme Court, "Justice" is the appropriate term to address the judge. Some jurisdictions in Canada have dispensed with more traditional references to "My Lord" or "My Lady"—elsewhere, these labels continue to exist. Forensic pathologists are well advised to ascertain, in advance of testimony, how judges expect to be addressed in the jurisdiction and level of court in which they will appear.

An inquisitorial process where forensic pathologists may testify in Ontario and other jurisdictions are Coroner's inquests. These inquests are designed to find facts about an event and make recommendations to avoid similar deaths rather than assign blame. A Coroner's inquest has a panel of jurors and is presided over by a coroner rather than a judge. In addition, the decedent's family can have "standing" at coroner's inquests whereby family members have the opportunity to directly ask the forensic pathologist and other witnesses questions.

Criminal Versus Civil Cases

The legal proceedings in English models of law that a forensic pathologist will be involved are largely divided into criminal and civil cases based on the relevant legal issues, which are reflected in the different legal remedies, nomenclature, standard of proof and processes applicable to each. Other legal proceedings include regulatory and administrative proceedings such as disciplinary proceedings that consider human rights tribunal or labour relations. The criminal system involves the investigation into and potential prosecution of statutory crimes or offences. In the vast majority of cases, it is the state that investigates and, where applicable, prosecutes alleged offences and deals with conflicts between the government and individuals. Criminal cases involve offences that are against public interests, and thus "the state" acts as an agent for the public. The main legal remedies in criminal cases are liberty, and in some jurisdictions—life, for the accused; however, in civil cases, finances or property maybe in jeopardy. The role of the court in civil cases is to resolve conflicts fairly between individuals or individuals and institutions that are not criminal in nature. The nature of the remedy that may be imposed on an individual or institution is often compensatory in nature—i.e. designed to restore the position of the successful claimant to that which was held prior to the actionable event. Sometimes, financial damages awarded may include a punitive component. Forensic pathologists most commonly testify in criminal cases but may also be involved in a variety of other legal proceedings, such as a civil action based on allegations of medical negligence contributing to a death or family law proceedings involving custody or access issues based on allegations relating to a parent of a deceased child.

The differences between criminal and civil cases are also reflected in nomenclature. In criminal court, the prosecuting authority is generally referred to in Canada as the Crown, and the case is described as His Majesty the King versus the named accused. The individual lawyer who conducts the prosecution is referred to as the Crown Attorney, Assistant Crown Attorney, Crown counsel or the prosecutor. The person or entity charged may be described as the defendant or the accused, although it is always preferable for witnesses to refer to the defendant by name so as not to subtly erode the burden of proof. To perhaps state the obvious, the defendant should also not be referred to in homicide cases as the assailant or perpetrator—that determination is for the trier of fact, whether judge or jury, to make, not the witness. In civil cases, the parties are generally referred to as the plaintiff, the person or entity claiming relief and the defendant. This nomenclature can become more complicated based on the nature of the civil case. In both civil and criminal legal proceedings, the counsel attorneys will often address each other in court as "my friend" or "my learned friend". This is not only a form of respect but also convenient to avoid the embarrassment of forgetting the opposing counsel's name.

Given the potential impact that a finding of guilt may have on a defendant's liberty in criminal cases, the prosecution must prove its case on the highest standard of proof—i.e. proof beyond a reasonable doubt. It also follows that a defendant need not prove innocence but is presumed innocent unless and until guilt has been proven beyond a reasonable doubt. Although reasonable doubt is composed of common words, together these words have a specific legal context [2]. In R. v. Starr, the Supreme Court of Canada explained that proof of probable guilt is insufficient. Proof beyond a reasonable doubt "falls much closer to absolute certainty than to proof on a balance of probabilities" [3]. The trier of fact must be "sure" that the defendant is guilty although proof of a "mathematical certainty" is not required and rarely attainable. Note that the legal term "beyond a reasonable doubt" is a legal standard with no scientific or medical correlation and should not be used in the formulation of forensic pathology opinions [4]. The standard of proof in civil cases is lower than in criminal courts and, generally, proof on a "balance of probabilities" suffices. This standard means that a claim will succeed if established to be more likely than not to be true.

Given these differences, it is not surprising that the legal proceedings of the civil courts differ from the criminal courts. The civil process starts with pleadings, followed by discovery, then pre-trial conference and finally trial. There may be a mediation step between the pre-trial conference and trial. Pleadings are formal written statements by each of the party's claims in a civil case whereby they define the issues that need to be decided. The discovery is a pre-trial phase in a civil action in which each party investigates the facts of the case.

The criminal process often, though not invariably, commences with the arrest of a defendant, and related bail proceedings to determine if the defendant should remain in custody pending trial or be released with or without conditions. The charges against the defendant are contained in "an information" which is converted to "an indictment" if the case proceeds to a higher trial court. Early in the process, the prosecution must provide "disclosure" to the defendant or the defendant's legal representative, consisting of the relevant evidence in its possession pertaining to the charges. Unlike civil cases, the defendant need not provide disclosure to the prosecution, except in limited circumstances. As a criminal case proceeds further, there are a series of meetings between counsel or pre-trial meetings with a judge to narrow the issues and potentially resolve the case. For homicide cases that generally must be tried in the higher trial court, the defendant may have a preliminary inquiry. A preliminary inquiry or hearing is a court proceeding presided over by a judge, typically in the lower courts, to determine if there is sufficient evidence to set the matter for trial. Although the threshold required to "commit" a defendant to trial is low, the preliminary inquiry may afford the defendant an opportunity to hear from and examine some of the prosecution's anticipated witnesses, including the forensic pathologist. The process of a preliminary inquiry and trial for the witness is similar and should be treated with similar seriousness by the forensic pathologist. Testimony of the preliminary hearing by the witness is transcribed, available to the parties, and may be used to either refresh the witness's memory or challenge the witness at the trial where alleged inconsistencies exist.

Both civil and criminal legal proceedings have an appeals process that may be accessed, in the higher courts, by either party that requests a formal change to a prior court decision. The appellant may initiate a post-conviction relief process based on fresh evidence, including re-interpretation of the post-mortem findings. This process allows for error correction as well as clarifications and interpretations of the law.

Criminal and civil proceedings are not mutually exclusive and there are incidents wherein both types of proceedings, criminal and civil may follow, typically with the civil action following the criminal procedures.

Trial and the Adversarial System

In common law jurisdictions, achieving justice is generally based on revealing the truth using an adversarial process rather than an inquisitorial process. The adversarial process is based on the premise that the oppositional presentation of the relevant evidence before an impartial decision-maker allows for truth-seeking, while other goals of the legal system, such as treating parties fairly, are met [5]. The trial procedure is based on the adversarial system in which contestants seek to establish, through relevant supporting evidence, before an impartial trier of facts, those events, which form the bases of their respective positions. Decisions are based on evidence adduced by parties, not by the judge, who are presumed to be best able to advance their case. The judge functions as a neutral arbiter. This is distinguished from an inquisitorial system in which the court is actively tasked to investigate the facts of the case and is not an impartial referee between the contestants. For forensic pathologists, trained as physicians and medical scientists, the adversarial system is an unfamiliar entity that deviates from medical training and the inherent inquisitive nature of medical practice.

Doctors as Witnesses

Doctors may be subpoenaed to court, like any other citizen, such as being a happenstance witness to a criminal act and giving evidence about the event in a court of law. Doctors most often become involved with the law simply because of their professional skills, knowledge or experience. Consequently, doctors may have an important role in the legal system by providing medical evidence as a fact witness or expert witness. Prior to testifying the physician must know and understand their role as a witness because the differences between these two types of witnesses limit the nature of one's testimony. An expert witness is allowed to give opinion evidence, while a fact witness is not. Typically, there are orders that exclude witnesses with the common exception of the officer in charge of the investigation, who may be required to testify first. The other exception is often made for defence experts, so they can listen to the testimony of the Prosecution/Crown's expert and possibly other Prosecution/Crown witnesses.

Regardless of the physician's role in the legal system, their overriding duty is to give evidence to assist the court; in addition, they must act independently and be honest, trustworthy, impartial and objective. Their testimony must be accurate and precise. Furthermore, the evidence that the witness provides is only one part of the entire body of evidence and may be congruent or incongruent with other evidence. Consequently, forensic pathologists can be credible sources of evidence that may be used in the legal system to support claims of truth.

Fact Witness

A fact witness testifies to what that person saw, heard or experienced. The witness cannot offer opinions with some exceptions (i.e. provide distances or estimations of time). Physicians can be a professional fact witness in which they offer factual evidence on medical findings, observations and actions and sometimes the reasons for them. They can provide factual medical evidence of a diagnosis, such as a fractured bone, but no opinion is provided (i.e. the amount of force required to fracture a bone). Their report or testimony deals with the relevant medical findings on a factual basis.

The fact witness highlights the difference between the witness and the trier of fact. Fact witnesses testify to facts, such as what they observed, heard, and so on, while the trier of fact forms opinions and draws conclusions based on the testimony of witnesses [5].

Expert Witness

Due to the widening knowledge gap between laypersons and experts, the role of experts in courts of law has become increasingly important. Courts of law recognise that triers of fact are not easily able to form opinions on some matters and are unlikely to reach the correct inference from facts alone [5]. The need for medical experts to testify originated in English common law [6]. The concept that specialised knowledge can assist the trier of fact to understand the evidence, or to determine a fact, allows for the admittance and utilisation of an expert witness with relevant knowledge, skill, experience, training and education to provide testimony on their opinion [6]. Consequently, expert witnesses are increasingly needed as knowledge continues to expand such that the courts progressively rely on their expertise in achieving their noble goal of determining the truth. This is because ordinary citizens are placed in an important role when they serve as jurors where they are expected to make critical decisions on the basis of highly technical, medical and scientific information. However, the incorporation of expert medical witnesses into legal proceedings does result in additional costs and complexity of the legal system [7]. Furthermore, the high cost of retaining a medical expert can be a barrier to accessing justice and the fairness of the legal system [5]. This barrier further emphasises why experts must remain impartial in their role.

Expert witnesses are individuals who are permitted to express opinions but only on matters that are based on their area of expertise gained through a specialised area of knowledge, skills, training or experience. The acceptability to offer opinions in certain areas of expertise is exclusively that of the judge. In practice, the parties may agree on those issues and the judge will concur. In other instances, when the parties disagree on whether the witness can give expert testimony or if agreeable to give testimony but disagree on the scope of the testimony a "voir dire" may be used. A "voir dire" is an opportunity for the opposing parties to outline proposed evidence, explore it and argue about its admissibility. Further exploration of the expert's qualifications may be conducted. A voir dire can facilitate a judge's decision in determining admissibility and the witness may be examined and cross-examined. However, the expert has a duty to self-regulate the limitations of the testimony where warranted. The forensic pathologist testifies to what the death is and to the medical facts of that death without trying to ensure that the accused is either convicted or acquitted. Attempts to sway the trier-of-fact are the role of the counsel, not the medical expert witness.

The duty of the expert witness is to provide impartial testimony that assists the court so that the court can use a reasoned application of the law to the facts. In addition, to upholding their duty to tell the truth, medical expert witnesses need to provide the medical facts so that the trier of fact can reach an accurate fact-based inference. This is typically on issues where the trier of fact's knowledge base is unlikely to make that inference [5]. Expert medical witnesses are essential in explaining medicine, including complex and controversial areas in medicine [7] into readily understandable information to non-medically trained members of the court. In this way, the expert functions as an educator to the lay persons on scientific and medical terms that are critical in their decision-making.

As experts are permitted to give opinions, they need to be explicit about the facts and reasons underlying these opinions and where possible refer back to the literature [8]. One of the concerns that the courts have regarding hearing opinion evidence is the risk of attornment because the trier of fact cannot critically assess opinion evidence. A contributor to this is that forensic pathologists can have impressive credentials that may sway the trier of fact and counsel [5]. These may include forensic pathologists that also have leadership roles, such as the medical director, which is an administrative role and does not necessarily indicate specialised knowledge in medicine. Thereby, the authoritative title may overly sway the trier of fact. In addition, expert witnesses explaining their reasoning allow the trier of fact to understand the basis for their opinion and detect biases, errors and/or assumptions. Also, when the medical and pathological data and legal issues are aligned, forensic pathologists ought to be able to address them when asked (i.e. the cause of death). But the converse is true, some questions are best answered on non-medical evidence (i.e. who caused the gunshot wound).

The medical evidence is just one component of a death investigation and legal process. Consequently, it is not up to the pathologist to singly determine the "truthfulness" of the accused's position and circumstances of a person's death. If the pathological evidence from the post-mortem examination was to solely decide the verdict, then the pathologist would be held responsible for the "ultimate issue", which is the determination of guilty or not guilty of the accused. Determining the "ultimate issue" by the expert witness is an area of controversy as there are concerns that doing so would compromise the impartiality of the expert medical witness. It is argued that this is the responsibility of the trier of fact to use objective medical evidence and place it in the context of all available information to make a decision on the "ultimate issue". However, there are some cases that experts are permitted to testify on the "ultimate issue" but the courts exercise more caution in these circumstances. The court requires proof "beyond reasonable doubt" for a criminal offence that is usually not provided by the medical evidence alone. Admittedly, this position is considered controversial, as it could be argued that an expert could testify on the ultimate issue if within their expertise and scope of testimony.

The Inquiry into Paediatric Forensic Pathology in Ontario, Canada (also referred to as the Goudge Inquiry), identified that utilisation of medical experts in court systems is vulnerable to miscarriages of justice when the expert does not recognise their role in the legal system. Consequently, the legal system requires safeguards in the admissibility of expert evidence; however, precautions do not shield from all scenarios that arise in forensic pathology. This is because counsel and judges, who are experts in law, frequently lack scientific literacy that scientists develop through years of education and experience [9]. Consequently, the medical expert witness has an active and collaborative role in addressing questions that are asked of them by counsel that are outside of their area of expertise. Specifically, the expert needs to indicate that the question is outside of their area of expertise. The expert can suggest which other expert their question would be better suited, where relevant. In an ideal legal system, third-party medical experts, separate from court trials, would independently guide the legal system on how expert testimony could be used. The advantage would be that the courts could maximise forensic pathology wisdom to include medicolegal issues beyond the cause of death.

Expertise in pathology, medicine, and science does not lend itself to expertise in law particularly the legal culture, ambiguity, and nuance of the law. Forensic pathologists are usually not trained as lawyers, so having a fulsome knowledge of the law, and the implications of their testimony is not always known. At a minimum, expert witnesses function as educators and impartial truth-tellers. There are limitations of testimony by expert witnesses including that they may not testify outside of their area of expertise, generally to legal conclusions (i.e. the "ultimate issue") and to the credibility of other witnesses, as this is the role of the trier of fact. Forensic pathologists while testifying must accept a healthy measure of restraint on their service to the counsel/attorneys where appropriate. Erroneous medical judgment can result in miscarriages of justice and risk undermining society's expectations about the benevolent use of medical skills. Furthermore, expert witnesses are not partisan advocates for the prosecution or defence, and should identify plausible alternative theories where relevant and not overstate their level of confidence [8]. It is the forensic pathologist, not the lawyer, that swears "to tell the truth, the whole truth and nothing but the truth". Although legal procedures around evidence admissibility may effectively prevent experts from telling the "whole" truth, the forensic pathologists' duty is to ensure that their evidence is appropriately contextualised so as not to mislead the trier of fact of the truth in the face of the legal procedures. Forensic pathologists need to do their best to be objective to facilitate a fair legal outcome and defend against unrecognised bias and blindspots of other hypotheses.

'Defence' Pathologist

For pragmatic reasons, the forensic pathologist is typically "called" by the prosecution to give oral evidence relating to their autopsy findings of the decedent in a criminal trial. The forensic pathologist may also work as a consultant for the defence counsel. In this consultant role, the forensic pathologist is typically referred to as the "defence pathologist" to differentiate their role from the forensic pathologist that performed the post-mortem examination and is "called" to testify by the prosecution. The defence pathologist is consulted by the defence counsel, often to provide the opinions and medical explanations to the defence lawyer (Table 3.1). The defence pathologist may review a variety of materials including the scene and autopsy photographs, medical notes, the autopsy report, ancillary reports, microscopic slides and relevant literature. These items can serve as a means for the defence pathologist to provide medical opinions in a variety of ways, including verbal communication with the defence attorney, preparation of a report, and courtroom testimony. In addition, the defence pathologist may attend court to listen to the testimony of the pathologist, at the request of the defence lawyer. This auditory practice allows the defence pathologist to advise the defence lawyer about questions that can be asked of the medical witnesses. The opinions and reports of the defence pathologist are considered "privileged" information, which means that the defence lawyer does not have to release this information to other parties involved in the legal proceedings unless the defence pathologist is called as witness.

Inclusion of a defence pathologist may create or exaggerate an adversarial atmosphere in legal proceedings. In reality, honest, and legitimate differences of opinions are commonplace among physicians. There are a variety of different reasons for differences of opinions, which may include differences in theoretical foundations, analyses of data, interpretation of information or inherent research biases.

Regardless, if a defence pathologist is involved or not, the forensic pathologist that performed the medicolegal autopsy and is being called to testify by the prosecution should be available to discuss the autopsy findings with the defence counsel. This is because the forensic pathologist should not adopt a side in a legal case but is obliged to serve the courts and tell the truth. Forensic pathologists may promote the

Table 3.1 The role of medical experts in court proceedings

Testimonial
Author post-mortem reports
Oral testimony
Consultative
Provide legal counsel an understanding of the opposition's position
Assess the validity of the opposing opinion
Assess the pathological evidence available
Provide a rebutting opinion of the opposing expert
Provide medical knowledge to test the opinions of the opposing experts
Provide questions to ask the opposing expert
Address new issues that may have arisen since the post-mortem examination
Determine if other evidence is required
Assist in the wording of questions

interests of the prosecution or the defence but only when the medical and pathological facts support it.

Notification of Court Appearance

When requested to appear as a witness for the court, it is the witness' duty to comply. When summoned to appear as a witness for court, the notification for appearance is usually in writing via a subpoena or summons. This written document is a court order signed by a judge, or other court official, that compels a witness to appear in court to provide oral evidence and informs the recipient of the name of the accused, the criminal charges and the level of court. In addition, the recipient will be directed to a specific time, date(s) and place to be available for testimony. It typically will not indicate the involved decedent, requiring further inquiries. After receiving a subpoena, follow-up communication with the requesting attorney to solidify the date of testimony and a meeting about the testimony before the court appearance occurs. The courts have the authority to compel attendance even with other commitments of the witness and can hold the witness in contempt of court and be fined or face imprisonment for not attending. Most courts and judges are reasonable, and usually, the instructing counsel and expert witness can arrive at an understanding to accommodate other commitments. Implementation of flexibility and advanced notice by both sides usually can result in successful scheduling of a court appearance. However, scheduling is a balancing act trying to predict how long a witness's testimony will last. Even if scheduled for a particular time, there may be delays.

Anatomy of the Courtroom

Many forensic pathologists are familiar with the layout and functions of a hospital and mortuary; however, the organisation of a courthouse has its own layout and functions. Like hospitals and mortuaries, courthouses vary in their layout reflecting the historical context and needs at the time the building was designed. The courthouse can be simple or complex structures but is typically composed of multiple areas including a security area, one or more courtrooms, office areas for counsel and administrative staff, deliberating rooms for jury members, waiting areas, bathrooms, and judge's chambers/suite. Some newer courthouses may even have a cafeteria. Upon entering the courthouse, usually, the first space encountered is the security area, which is reminiscent of airport security areas where there are metal detectors. In the security area, individuals and their accompanying personal effects are searched by court security officers.

The courtroom is the area in which witnesses testify. The anatomy of the courtroom reflects the adversarial process of the legal system and is reminiscent of the layout of many churches (Fig. 3.2). Once the witness is instructed to enter the

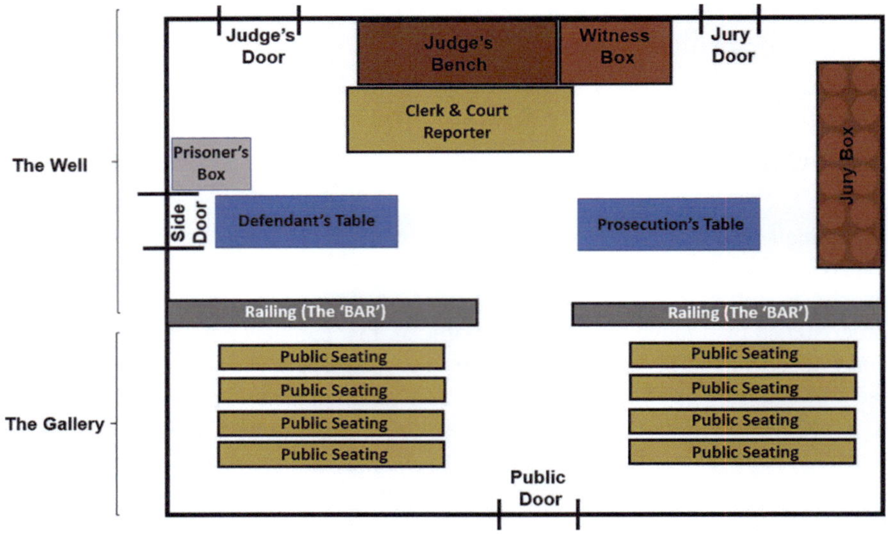

Fig. 3.2 Layout of the courtroom in general

courtroom, the witness will enter, and later exit, from the rear through the public door. The courtroom is divided into two spaces called the gallery and the well. The rear half of the courtroom is the gallery and contains seating for the public, including journalists and family members of the accused and decedent, to observe the judicial process. Depending on the case, the gallery may be filed with observers or even completely empty. The gallery is separated from the well by a railing, referred to as "the bar". The significance of "the bar" relates to the success of law students passing their licensing exam to become an attorney. This is referred to as "passing the bar" signifying that attorneys no longer have to sit in the gallery with the public but have joined the legal profession. Counsel, court employees, paralegals, articling students, the investigating officers and those who have been given permission may traverse the bar. In the rear of the well, there are at least two counsel tables that face the judge's bench. The lawyers and their clients (unless in custody) sit at these tables during the court proceedings. The defendant's table is typically adjacent to a side door where the accused, if in the custody of the police, will be escorted by police to enter and exit the courtroom through the side door. If the accused remains in custody that will be required to sit in the prisoner's box, which can be variably positioned in the courtroom. The prosecution's/Crown's table is closest to the jury box. The jury box is placed along one side of the well and contains seating for 12 jurors. The jury members typically have their own door to exit and enter the courtroom so that they can travel to another room for deliberation. At the front of the courtroom is the judge's bench, which is a raised desk for the judge. Adjacent to the bench is the judge's door, where the judge and courtroom personnel can enter and exit the courtroom. The judge typically exits the courtroom to access the judge's chambers. The judges' chambers are an office area that serves multiple functions. The clerk or registrar maintains order in the courtroom and announces "all rise" as the judge enters and exits the courtroom. The announcement of "all rise" indicates to everyone in the courtroom to stand up as a means to show respect to the judge and the court. Directly, in front of the judges' bench is a work area for the courtroom clerk and court reporter. The clerk manages the exhibits and paperwork, performs the oath/affirmation process with the witnesses and provides drinking water for the witnesses. The court reporter records testimony, which is also referred to as the "record". Essentially, the "record" is a concurrent recording of the oral testimony (done in a variety of ways) to permit a reviewable transcript to be prepared or evidence to be read out in court if there is a dispute about what was said. The record can also include other items beyond the transcript, such as exhibits and indictments. The witness box is located between the jury box and the judge's bench. This can be located on either side of the judge's bench depending on the layout of the courtroom. This is where the witness testifies.

Trier of Fact and Trier of Law

The trier of law is the judge whose role is to interpret and apply legal rules and principles to the procedures during the trial. The role of the trier of fact is to adjudicate aptly when medical experts called by opposing parties differ in their interpretation of the same evidence [7]. The trier of fact is a judge unless there is a jury sitting with the judge they will take on this role. The judge and jury are presented with evidence upon which they will make a determination of the facts of the case to which the law is applied.

Juries consist of a panel of 12 lay persons who are chosen randomly from the community in which the offence allegedly occurred. Jurors are laypersons who have an important legal role in trials where they are expected to hear and see evidence and then evaluate the reliability and credibility of the presented evidence in order to make a decision on the ultimate issue. These jurors are expected to bring community standards to the legal process. They make the determination of guilty or not guilty of the accused in the context of the law as determined by the trier of law.

Preparation for Testimony

The forensic pathologists should prepare themselves prior to attending court (Table 3.2). The pathologist needs to bring all of the relevant notes, reports, a few copies of the current curriculum vitae and reports of post-mortem examination with attached ancillary reports to the courtroom. These should be organised so that the relevant documents can be readily identified while on the stand.

Forensic pathologists ought to prepare their knowledge around the case, including the post-mortem report, autopsy images, scene images, and pertinent relevant literature. They should also prepare to answer questions that avoid medical and scientific jargon such that the trier of fact would understand and clarify their usage

Table 3.2 Guiding principles in giving oral evidence for expert witnesses

Beforehand	Prepare Review materials Obtain contact information of instructing lawyer/counsel or other designated contact person Be available to meet with both prosecution and defence Document pre-trial/discovery conversations including contents of discussion, date and time, who you spoke to Review prior courtroom testimony transcript
Day of giving testimony (oral evidence)	Bring folder with copies of current curriculum vitae and autopsy report Arrive early Dress business conservative Head nod/non-verbal respectful acknowledgement of jury members Listen carefully Speak clearly Use simple and precise language Stay within your field of expertise Separate observations from opinions Provide impartial, unbiased and objective evidence
Following testimony	Contact instructing lawyer immediately if you need to correct something in your testimony

of terms that may be used in the ordinary sense (i.e. choking versus manual strangulation). Potential areas of questioning should be anticipated and prepared. This includes contemplating how to translate complex medical concepts into plain language for the trier of fact by simplifying concepts that the average person, without medical training, could comprehend. If medical terminology must be used, this should be supplanted with simple explanations (i.e. laceration can also be referred to as a tear). In addition, the expert's courtroom transcript from previous testimony ought to be sought and reviewed prior to trial testimony.

Pre-Testimonial Meeting

Typically, legal counsel will want to meet with the expert before providing courtroom testimony and after the post-mortem report is signed. The forensic pathologist ought to make themselves available to both prosecution and defence counsel. This gives counsel the opportunity to know what the pathologist is going to say when asked about general areas of interest and in response to specific questions. This is also an opportunity for counsel to explore their line of questioning and hypotheticals. In addition, this also allows the expert witness to be prepared for potential questions and answer them with an opportunity for thought to best answer a question when on the witness stand. The expert can assist in how the counsel should best frame questions and go through the findings of the post-mortem report. The attorney should understand the pathologists' opinions and the basis for these opinions. The strengths and weaknesses of each opinion can be explained. This is a good opportunity to correct any preconceived ideas that may be wrong or highlight certain aspects or implications that may not be recognised. Also, the central issues of the pathology evidence can be explored. For example, sometimes, the central issue is the toxicological issue rather than the nature of the injuries. If any errors in the post-mortem report are identified, this needs to be raised to the instructing counsel and can be brought up in testimony. This is where additional new facts about the case or theories may be disclosed. The limits of the expert testimony should be established during this meeting. In addition, the use of demonstrative evidence, such as autopsy images or diagrams, can be decided with input from the pathologist that aligns with the instructing counsel's line of questioning. The pathologist has a better idea of which images are more instructive.

These meetings between experts and counsel, both instructing (i.e. prosecution) and non-instructing (i.e. defence), are opportunities for counsel to test hypotheses and test legal theories. This means that the expert witness should refrain from sharing the legal theories and merits of strategies of opposing counsel. The contents of the conversations between counsel and pathologists can be documented by the pathologist. These notes; however, may be discoverable by either counsel. During this meeting, obtain the instructing attorney's contact number in case of an emergency or unexpected traffic delays on the day of testimony. Have an agreed time to attend court and be early. Expect that the instructing, and sometimes the non-instructing counsel, may have questions for the expert witness on the day of the testimony, just prior to testimony.

Day of Expert Testimony (Oral Evidence)

Prior to day of testimony, the expert witness should be prepared and know the contents of the autopsy report and review all the information that was used to compose the autopsy report prior to testimony. In addition, all other relevant information including transcripts of the expert's own testimony, if present, should be reviewed. The autopsy folder and its entire content, including a few copies of the post-mortem report and expert's curriculum vitae should accompany the forensic pathologist.

The medical expert should arrive early and appear before the court in a manner where the dress, appearance and demeanour demonstrate the authority of their role as a physician and align with the seriousness of the court's work (Table 3.3).

Table 3.3 Courtroom etiquette

1. Turn off personal electronics
2. No gum, food or beverages (water is provided by the clerk)
3. Consider head nod at the "Bar" upon entry and exit into the courtroom while facing the judge's bench as a sign of respect
4. Answer questions when looking at the jury to obtain non-verbal feedback of comprehension
5. When the judge enters and exits the courtroom, everyone in the room must rise, be quiet and show respect
6. Refer to individuals in the court formally, including referring to the judge as "your honour" or "justice" depending on the level of court
7. Wait outside the courtroom until instructed to enter the courtroom
8. Remain silent throughout the proceedings until questions are asked of the witness

Professional, conservative business attire is appropriate and displays personal grooming. Clothing, jewellery and other personal effects that draw attention to the dress should be avoided. The demeanour of the medical expert is polite and exhibits equanimity by maintaining their composure in giving expert opinions and not allowing the behaviours of others to affect their composure or expert opinion. The oral testimony is delivered in a clear, balanced and dispassionate manner to the trier of fact. The pathologist is expected to make direct eye contact with counsel (or judge) who is asking questions but look upon the jury when answering the question. The expert's eye contact to the jury can provide non-verbal feedback to the expert their comprehension of the oral evidence. Explaining complex medical and scientific terms by simplifying terms and words can go far in helping the trier of fact do their work. Verbal descriptions of injury should not be couched in obscure anatomical terminology. Instead, injuries should be described in an informative and non-condescending manner. The answers are spoken in a clear articulate and confident voice with a reasonable pace that is deliberate to allow the judge, counsel and jurors to make notes. Furthermore, the contents of the response should answer the question being asked in a succinct, full answer and then stop and wait for the next question. If there are unreasonable attempts to reduce answers to "yes" or "no" answers for complex questions, the expert should politely decline and explain the reasoning behind this decision. If a yes or no is warranted, it should be provided followed, if necessary, by an explanation. Witnesses should avoid answering questions that they have not been asked. Witnesses who do not follow this basic rule may not be regarded as impartial because they appear more intent on advancing a position than responding to questions. The caveat being that witnesses must ensure that their answers are not cut off in a way that can leave their answers potentially misleading.

Sometimes, there may be language interpreters that need to meet with the expert witness before their oral evidence. Typically, the interpreters want to understand the autopsy report as many interpreters are fluent in their language but may not be fluent in the medical terminology in their language. Furthermore, if interpreters are involved, the pace of speech of the expert needs to be even slower than normal oral testimony to allow the interpreters to perform their role accurately and precisely.

Before entering the courtroom cell phones, pagers and other electronics should be turned off. When it is the expert's turn to testify, they will be called into the courtroom. Once the witness enters the courtroom, they will be evaluated as a professional. If the jury is present, it is okay to acknowledge them with a nod or polite smile as the expert walks by the panel of jurors. When the judge enters and leaves the courtroom, all persons in the courtroom will be instructed to "all rise". This means everyone needs to stand, remain silent and remain standing until the court clerk states that all persons in the court can sit. All individuals must be addressed formally and avoid first names unless referring to young children or otherwise instructed; this is a means to show respect and promotes the appearance and reality of impartiality, rather than undue familiarity. While sitting in the witness box, there is a need to demonstrate good posture, pay attention and show responsiveness.

At the end of the testimony, the judge will inform the witness that they are excused. Once dismissed, the witness should collect their materials and leave the courtroom directly through the gallery. Turning to perform a slight head nod at the bar and at public door while facing the judges' bench. This is considered a means of showing respect when entering and exiting the courtroom but there is not complete consensus that this is necessary as it is judge dependent. When in doubt, it is usually best to demonstrate respect.

Oral Testimony

Oral testimony is a form of evidence that is sometimes considered the sixth step of the autopsy. Although debated by some, providing expert testimony is considered the practice of medicine [10]. In the 1990s, the American Medical Association (AMA) resolved that expert testimony is the practice of medicine and therefore is subject to peer review [6]. Furthermore, the AMA indicates that it will assist medical organisations in disciplining physicians who testify falsely against their colleagues [6]. Complaints can be reported to licensing boards [6]. Case law in this area, although minimal, suggests that American medical professional boards can revoke the medical license of a medical expert who gave false testimony in a medical malpractice lawsuit [6]. As such, expert testimony should align with medical practice standards [10]. In addition, it behooves the physician expert to ensure their liability coverage supports expert witness work [6].

The extent and details of testimony depend on not only the details of the case but also the training and style of the attorney. Providing oral testimony is considered a form of evidence and has a formalised structure of speaking that differs from everyday conversation. The etiquette of speaking in court is different in eight fundamental ways. There is also a variety of legal terms used during court proceedings that may not be familiar among medical experts (Table 3.4).

First, there is typically a previous discussion, with at least the instructing attorney, about what the expert will state in their testimony and the structure of providing evidence.

Second, the structure of oral testimony is unidirectional. Legal counsel, and sometimes the judge who typically asks questions for clarification, ask the witness questions, and the witness answers those questions. The witness does not ask questions of counsel; however, the witness can ask for the question to be repeated. Similarly, if there is a substantive error (i.e. laterality error) in the question, it is appropriate to courteously correct counsel.

Third, the role of eye contact when the witness receives and answers questions differs from everyday conversation. In everyday conversation, the person who asks the question is typically the same as the person the answer is directed to. However, during testimony, when the witness is being asked a question by legal counsel the witness usually answers the questions when looking upon the jury rather than counsel. Once the question is answered by the witness, it is not uncommon for periods of silence to occur, especially during cross-examination.

Table 3.4 Common legal terms and phrases in court proceedings

Term/phrase	Meaning
To tell the truth, the whole truth and nothing but the truth	1. Everything said will be true. 2. That the witness will not omit something that could alter the effect and impact the evidence. 3. The witness will not add something that is not true to the truth
Trier of fact	A person (i.e. judge in the absence of a jury) or a group of people (i.e. jury) who determines what the facts are available, how relevant and probative the facts are in a legal proceeding, such as a trial.
Trier of law	The judge, whether sitting alone or with a jury, decides on the applicable law.
Ultimate issue	This is the factual or legal issue that will, in the case at hand, determine guilt, or lack thereof, of the accused.
Part heard	The legal proceeding is not completed yet, and the matter has only been partly heard by the court. As an expert, if there is a break during testimony, the witness is unable to answer questions during the break depending on the stage of the proceedings. If the witness is still in direct examination, the instructing counsel can still ask questions during the break but about questions not yet covered. The opposing counsel is free to ask questions to the witness. During cross-examination, the instructing counsel cannot speak to the witness, other than formal proceedings.
Voir dire	This legal phrase means "speak the truth" and is a mini-trial within a trial that serves to resolve a single issue.
Reasonable doubt	A legal standard of proof that must be met for guilty verdicts in criminal cases with no scientific or medical correlation and should not be used in the formulation of medical opinions.

Fourth, is the role of the "record" is to capture the oral evidence in written form. The cadence of speech should be reasonably paced with a stable tone of voice that allows for proper recording of answers by court staff for the record. When a medical term is used in the expert's answer, and if the term is not in the autopsy report, the expert witness will often spell it out for the courtesy of the court reporter. Furthermore, if an image or diagram is used, this visual testimonial aid is described verbally for the purposes of the record. Often the expert will gesture to their own bodies as a convenient anatomical model to convey anatomical locations. For example, the forensic pathologist may point with their own hand to their own head to demonstrate the gunshot wound of entry that is located behind the ear. This demonstration should also be described for the purposes of documenting a written record.

Fifth, is the tendency for some of the oral content to be presented as though the expert witness is giving a lecture in science and medicine to undergraduate or medical students. Given the inherent nature of the specialised language and knowledge used by medical experts, it is likely that the members of the jury may find their testimony difficult to understand. Many individuals in the courtroom, especially the trier of fact, usually lack medical training, and are relying on the forensic pathologist's testimony to facilitate knowledge transmission. This can be done by using simplified language and terminology that the trier of fact (and accused) will understand and conveys the truth.

Sixth, the notion of "part heard" is when court proceedings have started but are adjourned to a later time or date. The implication for the witness is that they may have started their testimony but are not finished. During this time period, the witness is unable to answer questions during the break depending on the stage of the proceedings. If the witness is still in direct examination, the instructing counsel can still ask questions during the break but only about questions not yet covered. The opposing counsel is free to ask questions to the witness. During cross-examination, the instructing counsel cannot speak to the witness. Furthermore, if a juror or family member is observed outside of the courtroom, it is best to avoid discussion about the experts testimony and findings during that time period, but arrangements to meet with family members following the completion of the legal proceedings can be made.

Seventh, during the line of questioning, counsel may object to a question being asked or object during the expert's answer by saying "objection". The witness needs to stop speaking as the court sorts out the legal grounds for the objection. The witness should not weigh in on the issue as it is being debated, unless asked. If this occurs, wait until the judge makes a ruling (i.e. decision). If the judge sustains (i.e. upholds) the objection, the question is not to be answered. If you have already given an answer, the judge will instruct that the answer is to be stricken from the trier of facts determination. If the judge overrules (i.e. rejects) the objection, an answer may be given or the previous answer stands.

Eighth is the function of the "***voir dire***", which can limit what is said by the expert. A *voir dire* is a legal phrase the means "to speak the truth" and is a mini-trial within a trial that serves to resolve multiple issues at the same time. The *voir dire* can have multiple outcomes, including exposing a lack of qualification of the expert witness but also making the expert opinions limited or inadmissible in some format. A *voir dire* is not supposed to influence the trial as the judge is assumed to ignore what was heard in the *voir dire,* and if a jury is present, they are excused from the court room. The witness may be excused or have to testify during the *voir dire*.

It is now typically permitted that the expert may use their autopsy report as a testimonial aid to ensure the accuracy of details. There are various testimonial aids, beyond the autopsy report, that can aid the expert witness during legal proceedings and typically include a variety of visual aids that are used to demonstrate a fact or opinion. Autopsy images have traditionally been a common visual aid. The selected images should balance fairness versus emotive impact or prejudicial impact. The concern related to prejudicial impact is the implication that the jury hates the injuries observed on the decedent and projects that emotion onto the accused. Although this decision is often a legal determination, using autopsy images, if deemed necessary, should be "displayed with dignity", whereby the injury may be shown, but the sensitive areas of the body are cropped out and the alteration is disclosed. Furthermore, post-traumatic stress disorder is becoming a recognised problem among jurors and the use of autopsy images may contribute to this phenomenon. Consequently, other visual aids such as diagrams with explanatory legends, computer-generated images and anatomical models may be a preferred method of explaining autopsy findings. Sometimes, the expert witness's own body is used as a convenient example to explain concepts and anatomy. If using an anatomical model, beware that the courts may want to retain this as an exhibit, so discussion with counsel prior to testimony can help prevent this or alternatively counsel may purchase a pathologist-approved anatomical model to be submitted as an exhibit. When using visual aids, there need explicit oral descriptions of the visual aid for the purposes of the "record". Having the expert simply point to an injury on an image, or other visual aid is insufficient because it lacks clarity for the "record". A common method is to orient the findings using analogue clock positions. If using laterality terms such as right and left of the decedent, ensure to clarify that what is being referred to is the decedent's body rather than the right or left of the image.

There are a variety of questions and various styles of questioning that can be used by counsel (Table 3.5). Common questions include those that are outside or intersect with other areas of expertise, common knowledge, and hypotheticals. Regardless of the nature of the questions being asked, the expert must maintain a professional composure during expert testimony. In return, an expert witness should expect to be treated with professional composure and respect by counsel. Like any exam, the expert should understand and answer the questions being asked. However, unlike an exam, the expert does not have to know the answer to the question being asked—it is absolutely appropriate to answer "I don't know" when this is the truth. Remember that experts do not guess, even if trying to be helpful. Physicians are accustomed to trying to be helpful, but there are limits to knowledge, even in their own specialty. It is also reasonable to state that a question is outside of your expertise. Some questions may fall in an area that overlaps with another expert but still allows some form of an answer by the pathologist to assist the courts, but it is the expert's responsibility to make clear that the matter is outside or partly of your expertise. When answering questions about common knowledge, the expert needs to be careful in answering that the trier of fact does not put the weight of an expert opinion on common knowledge. Putting the weight of expert opinion on common knowledge is misleading and inappropriate, but answers should focus specifically on issues related to medicine and science. The experts' answer can be prefaced as having common notions of knowledge. Counsel may ask questions that present hypothetical scenarios or other facts in the court during the examination. Hypothetical questions and situations may be composed of evidence, but not necessarily, introduced in the case. These are often artificial and sometimes cumbersome hypothetical constructs, put to the pathologist. Often the answer to these questions may be framed as possibilities and probabilities. It is reasonable for a pathologist to consider these hypothetical situations, and sometimes new facts, in combination with the existing medical evidence, and if appropriate accept that, in view of this potentially different basis, one's conclusion may change. Clinging to previous opinions in the face of evidence to the contrary is not serving the court. Similarly, if a question has been answered and the expert has changed their perspective on their answer, the expert has a duty to ensure the court is aware of this new perspective. This can occur while the expert is still testifying and will be part of the record. However, if, after the witness has been dismissed,

Table 3.5 Common court questions

Initial questions:
1. Would you like to swear or affirm?
2. Could you please state and spell your name?
Qualifying questions:
1. Where did you receive your medical training?
2. Have you ever been qualified to testify in court?
3. How many times have you testified?
4. How many medicolegal autopsies have you performed?
5. How many medicolegal autopsies that you performed were considered homicides?
6. Where is your medical practice?
7. How many years have you been a forensic pathologist?
8. What is forensic pathology?
9. Which courts have you previously testified?
10. Other questions related to your curriculum vitae.
Direct examination, cross-examination and re-examination
1. What information were you told prior to the commencement of the post-mortem examination?
2. What is a post-mortem examination?
3. What is the anatomical position?
4. What is the cause of death?
5. What is the mechanism of death?
6. What is the mechanism of injury?
7. What amount of force was required to cause the injury?
8. What was the fatal injury?
9. What are defensive injuries?
10. Would the decedent survive the injuries if the injury occurred while in hospital/had immediate medical care?
11. Was it possible that the decedent fell on a knife?
12. What was the position of the body when the decedent was injured?
13. What is the post-mortem interval?
14. Could the injuries have been caused by more than one individual?
15. Could the decedent do this to themselves?
16. What is a ligature?
17. How do (conjunctival) petechial haemorrhages arise?
18. Can people survive strangulation?
19. What are recent injuries?
20. What is the pathological range?

the expert is required to inform instructing counsel of this change, in turn, counsel should immediately inform others of this change, namely the other party, judge and jury. In the rare instance, that the instructing counsel refuses to follow through on informing of the changed position, it is the responsibility of the expert to inform the court. If the expert is uncertain, they can ask the court or obtain legal advice.

The outcome of an adversarial system can lead to a dichotomous variable—a winner and a loser. The role of the expert is to neither win nor lose the case at hand but to tell the truth. As an expert witness, the truth means ensuring factual accuracy, asserting principles relevant to shared understanding, ensuring honesty and a truthful appearance, and ensuring faithfulness to medicine and science.

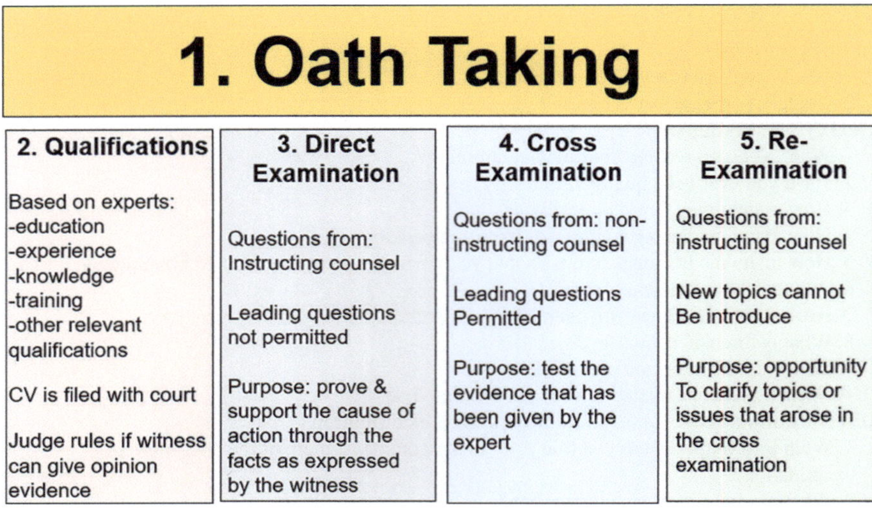

Fig. 3.3 Summary of the parts of oral testimony

Steps of the Examination

The five routine steps of expert witness testimony in a criminal court include the 1. Oath taking, 2. Qualifying the Expert, 3. Direct Examination, 4. Cross Examination, and 5. Re-examination (Fig. 3.3).

Oath Taking

In this step, the witness publicly promises "to tell the truth, the whole truth and nothing but the truth", not just the parts of the truth that help the instructing counsel. Therefore, the witness must answer each question asked with care and honesty. The implications of oath taking are to render the individual liable for criminal prosecution of perjury if lying occurred. In oath-taking, the witness can choose to swear or affirm "to tell the truth, the whole truth and nothing but the truth". Taking this oath with a religious text, such as the Bible, is swearing an oath. In the absence of a religious text, this promise-keeping is referred to as "affirming". Whichever the witness chooses, the obligation of truth-telling and the legal effect is the same.

Each portion of the statement "to tell the truth, the whole truth and nothing but the truth" has a subtle nuance (Table 3.2). For example, if the forensic pathologist is asked about the absence of a "hilt mark" adjacent to a stab wound, the answer should entail that there is no hilt mark and this is observed in stab wounds when the handle of a knife hits the skin, indicating that the entire knife blade entered the body. However, the absence of a hilt mark does not mean that the entire blade did not enter the body. Excluding the latter portion in one's explanation would be an example of not telling the "whole" truth, as long as the rules of evidence allow the pathologist to answer the question fully.

Qualifying the Expert

Prior to offering oral evidence, the witness must be qualified via a voir dire as an expert to give an opinion in a particular field. At this stage, qualifications are examined and accepted by the judge before the expert can offer opinions. To be accepted as an expert witness, the court must establish that the witness fits the criteria in a specific area of expertise. It is not necessary that the witness has been previously qualified, although this may be asked. The court makes this determination for itself by ensuring that the witness has the required education, experience and/or other relevant qualifications to provide opinion evidence in the legal proceedings. This is also an opportunity for the instructing counsel to elicit information regarding the expert's knowledge, training, skill or experience that is capable of assisting the trier of fact to resolve factual issues as they pertain to a legal matter. The instructing counsel may go through relevant highlights in the expert's curriculum vitae. This is typically through questions about the witness' education and experience. For forensic pathologists, it is an opportunity to be clear that their training and competence in pathology have been scrutinised by an independent national organisation. During this step, the opposing counsel has an opportunity to cross-examine on the issue of qualification and this may proceed via a voir dire. The presiding judge ultimately rules whether the witness can give opinion evidence, what area(s) and if there are limitations. During this stage, the expert's curriculum vitae is typically filed as an exhibit.

Once qualified, the permitted experts' testimony is dependent on rules around admission, the judge and counsel. In addition, it is critical that the medical expert witness also self-regulate their opinions during testimony to areas in which they are qualified because it is not uncommon to be asked questions outside of the experts' area of expertise. This is because both lawyers and judges are knowledgeable in law but are not experts in medicine and may not understand the medical issues adequately to consider the appropriate questions [6]. In addition, counsel may want to elicit information and the forensic pathologist seems like the person most likely to give an answer.

Direct Examination

The attorney that has called the witness to court is the instructing counsel, and they will be the first to examine the expert witness under oath. This is called "direct examination" or "examination in chief". The line of questioning typically flows from the organisation and contents of the autopsy report. Therefore, forensic pathologists can author and use their post-mortem report as a guide for their script. The nature of questioning is variable and may take on the form that permits open-ended answers or yes-or-no answers. These questions may be expanded to include the opinions that have been expressed in the autopsy report; however, additional opinions may be sought. One way of approaching this step is to start with the cause of death and then follow the steps of the autopsy, as outlined in the autopsy report. This methodology allows the trier of fact to know the experts' opinion as to the cause of death and then how the expert arrived at that opinion.

In this step, leading questions can be permitted on uncontentious questions. Leading questions are a type of question that is phrased in such a way that it prompts the respondent towards an already-determined answer. For example, a leading question: Was the colour of the decedent's bruise yellow? A non-leading question: What colour was the decedent's bruise?

Cross-Examination

Once the direct examination is complete, the non-instructing counsel (i.e. typically the defence lawyer) will have an opportunity to question the witness during the "cross-examination". In some legal proceedings, there may be more than one defence counsel present and each of them are given opportunity to ask the witness their questions. The purpose of the cross-examination will vary depending on the issues in the case. For example, if the defence takes no issue with the witness's evidence, cross-examination may be designed to elicit or highlight helpful evidence. If the defence challenges the evidence, the cross-examination may be designed to demonstrate bias, frailties in the opinion expressed, limitations or qualifications on the opinion expressed that may prompt the trier of fact to have a reasonable doubt about guilt. Or the cross-examination may elicit evidence that the opinion is based on underlying assumptions about the facts, such that alternative facts would change the opinion. This type of cross-examination assists defence counsel in creating a foundation for the defence.

Expert witnesses may be prone to give poor evidence if they fail to focus on answering the questions asked, but instead of trying to figure out the defence counsel's strategy. Most problematic is an unduly defensive posture by the witness, demonstrated by failing to acknowledge obvious limitations or qualifications on the opinion, anger or animosity towards the questioner or failure to admit error when exposed.

Effective cross-examination requires knowledge of both expert's subject matter and the basic principles of the scientific method [8, 11]. The purpose of this line of questioning is to test the evidence that has been given by concentrating on parts of the evidence that are damaging to the instructing counsel's case and those that may facilitate the non-instructing counsel's case. This is achieved by identifying gaps in the expert's testimony, considering alternative hypotheses and methodological or logical weaknesses associated with the evidence. The defence counsel will examine inconsistencies, inaccuracies or weaknesses in the prosecution's case with respect to the pathological evidence. The defence lawyer may cite academic journals, books and technical manuals. If the expert witness is presented with documents or other evidence, the witness should request a reasonable amount of time to read, consider and examine these materials before accepting or rejecting if the source is authoritative (i.e. valid and reliable). The defence lawyer(s) can also enter their own evidence, which can include the opinions of a defence pathologist.

The line of questioning during this stage of the testimony does not typically follow a particular method of organisation. The line of questioning often lacks the organisation and flow of the direct examination as questions often jump around the pathological evidence. In addition, leading questions by the non-instructing counsel are permitted. The opinions of the expert must continue to remain valid and accurate and highlight any limitations or other scientific uncertainty.

A vigorous cross-examination is thought to be an essential safeguard to ensure the quality and reliability of evidence [7]. Unfortunately, this judicial safeguard may not expose all improper expert testimony [6].

Re-Examination

Once the "cross-examination" is complete and the non-instructing counsel has no further questions, the instructing counsel has an opportunity for the "re-examination". This provides the instructing counsel the opportunity to clarify topics or issues that arose in the "cross-examination" but cannot introduce new topics. The goal is to clarify matters raised for the first time in cross-examination and not to repeat testimony given earlier.

Pathological Evidence

Evidence given by a forensic pathologist is typically oral testimony and a written document in the form of the post-mortem examination report but can include autopsy images, anatomical models and other material objects that are accepted by the courts as evidence of the facts. These items can be admitted as evidence before or after presentation by the expert. Therefore, forensic pathologists need to have a discussion with counsel before using departmental anatomical models as presentation aids, rather than being admitted as evidence. The admissibility of expert evidence has emerged as a complex body of law to ensure that evidence submitted is relevant and falls within the standards of evidential reliability and trustworthiness [6].

Testimonial evidence is an oral description of the post-mortem examination by an expert witness while under oath. Oral testimony is a verbal account of the findings and opinions of the post-mortem examination and is often accompanied by demonstrative evidence so that the trier of fact can better understand the oral testimony. Demonstrative evidence is evidence that is a representation of an object. Common examples include autopsy images, anatomical models, computer-generated images and diagrams. Demonstrative evidence can be used to explain an injury and can also be used to direct to a particular implement such as patterned injuries. Real evidence can accompany the oral testimony of the pathologist. These items form part of the physical evidence, such as the actual microscopic slides, and must be demonstrated through the chain of custody, unless the chain of custody is admitted. In addition, counsel may show the pathologist real evidence and ask for opinions related to this evidence. For example, a potential weapon could be shown to the pathologist.

Autopsy images are not always necessary as demonstrative evidence during testimony, as there are other alternatives. But when sought to be introduced, the court must balance the probative value with the prejudicial effect, particularly when shown to a jury. The probative value will depend, in large part, on the nature of the evidence, the live issues in the trial and the judge's assessment of the impact of the evidence on the trial as a whole. The basic rule of evidence is that all relevant evidence is to be received by the trier of fact unless the evidence is subject to an exclusionary rule [12]. In homicide trials, it is often argued that graphic autopsy photographs of the deceased may evoke emotive prejudice in the jury. The concern is that these images can impair the ability of the jury to objectively focus on the issues at hand. The judge may decide that admissions made by the defence obviate the need to introduce such photographs—as they are unlikely to assist the jury in what issues are in dispute. Or the judge may decide that some photographs are necessary to explain the pathologist's findings and opinion, but that they should be limited in number.

Autopsy images may potentially assist in the following ways: (1) illustrate facts on which experts have based their opinions; (2) illustrate the steps by which the expert arrives at their opinions; (3) demonstrate the nature and extent of the wounds; (4) corroborate testimony and provide a picture of the evidence to assist the jury in determining its accuracy and weight; (5) link the injuries in the decedent to an implement; and (6) assist the trier of fact to determine the truth of the hypothetical put forth by the prosecution or defence [13]. Ultimately, the images should be used to assist the trier of fact in comprehending the medical and scientific issues on the trial. Therefore, during the autopsy, care should be taken to ensure that images that may be used to inform the jury are taken with proper lighting, a scale and minimise blood and other distractions. During the autopsy, phtodocumenting blood may be important for other reasons and should be taken but additional images that show injuries and are not obscured by blood are also necessary part of documentation. Each image selected for presentation in the courtroom ought to be reasoned, coherent and justifiable. In addition, sensitive areas of the body should be given special consideration. For example, if the decedent's genitals have been captured in the best image of the forearm injury. It is completely reasonable to crop the genitals from the image before displaying it in the court. Cropping of the image needs to be disclosed to the court. Reasons for cropping can also be sought. This action balances the needs of the court and the bereaved family. Also, in the spirit of telling the whole truth, an explanation of post-mortem changes (i.e. lividity is not a bruise), to avoid trier of fact confusion, is warranted when using autopsy images that exhibit these changes.

In many Commonwealth countries, there are various measures to ensure that experts are aware that in giving opinion evidence their overriding duty is to the courts. In Ontario, the *Rules of Civil Procedure* require experts to sign an acknowledgement that their duty is to provide fair, objective, and non-partisan opinion evidence and their duty is to the court [14]. This declaration may be in the signed autopsy report. Expert witness offering opinions has a duty to assist the court that overrides their obligation to the party calling them. Opinions must reflect an objective assessment of the questions at hand is the product of independent judgment, uninfluenced by who has retained them and does not unfairly favour one party's position over another. Furthermore, the opinions of the expert need to be evidence-based. Five features of evidence-based expert opinions include the following [15]:

1. Fact correspondence: The opinion corresponds to empirical data. Caution must be used with secondary and tertiary historical data.
2. First principles: The opinion accords with pathology and pathophysiology. In addition, the methodology and reasoning should be robust and transparent.
3. Coherence with the evidence base: The opinion aligns with peer-reviewed literature.
4. Counter-examples: Valid causes of death are derived from considering and excluding alternative explanations for death.
5. Fairness and truth-seeking: The opinion is balanced, reasonable, and represents what is believed to be true.

Scientific Uncertainty (Science Versus the Law)

Forensic pathology opinions need to be grounded in science, using an evidence-based approach, rather than solely anecdotal evidence and authoritative claims based on personal experience. The evidence-based approach requires examination of the autopsy findings that are viewed through the medical literature and application of logic and reason to make a diagnosis. This allows verifiable empirical data as the foundation of a pathological opinion. Although forensic pathology opinions are now grounded in medicine and science, there are limitations of this knowledge base that can have particular significance in the courts. As new medical and scientific discoveries occur and knowledge grows exponentially, this will lead to changes in science and the practice of medicine, including forensic pathology. This scientific progress can lead to previously correct theories and diagnoses being questioned and sometimes rejected. An example of this includes the obsolete diagnostic quintet of asphyxia [16] or the controversy surrounding the "triad" of pathological findings that were traditionally considered diagnostic of "Shaken Baby Syndrome"; however, biomechanics research suggests that the force required to produce the triad was not reproducible in experimental models leading to doubt that shaking is the sole mechanism of injury [17]. Uncertainty in the mechanisms of injury surrounding forensic pathology practice lies in (1) the inability to perform experimental studies (i.e. does shaking infants cause subdural bleeds) due to obvious ethical problems, (2) lack of surety in scientific studies, and (3) application of these studies to specific cases [18]. The latter lies in problems of incommensurability and the difficulty of applying abstract criteria to specific cases. These shifts and debates are part of the scientific milieu, but in the legal system, these new discoveries and breakthroughs can cause doubt on previous opinions or alter the confidence of opinions previously held. Any scientific and medical uncertainties related to a forensic pathology opinion must be shared explicitly with the court. Despite scientific uncertainty, forensic pathology continues to be of value to the courts because, as science and knowledge continue to grow, the legal system can continue to rely on areas of medicine that over time will result in a body of knowledge that will settle and be considered reliable.

"Hot-Tubbing"

There may be a genuine disagreement between experts and uncertainty in science that may resolve with future studies but the needs of the court are immediate [1]. However, when experts do not agree on the central issue this puts the trier of fact in a difficult position in trying to choose between opposing accredited experts [7]. One method to overcome disagreements between opposing expert witnesses has been described as "hot-tubbing", though probably better referred to as "judicial colloquia". This is an opportunity for the experts to meet and come to a consensus on all or certain aspects of the case in an open forum, which is a marked departure from the adversarial process. The lawyers and judges have an opportunity to bear witness to the open dialogue between the opposing sides' experts. This allows for the courts the educational insight and assistance in decision-making [19]. It is argued that this method may make the court identify and deal with the medical issues in a case in a more expeditious fashion, making fact-finding easier in the absence of contradictory expert testimony, and when this occurs in civil matters, fewer cases proceed to court [7].

"The CSI Effect"

The success of numerous scientifically based crime-solving television shows and other media venues has resulted in a skewed perception of resources available and results to be expected in the medicolegal death investigation system by would-be jurors, judges and attorneys [20]. Popular media depictions of criminal investigations can misrepresent reality. Although these shows have stimulated interest among the public in forensic disciplines as a potential career, the media may propagate forensic science myths by portraying scientific techniques that may be experimental or non-existent [20]. The impact of these shows was encapsulated in a new term coined called "The CSI Effect" which is based on the common usage of Crime Scene Investigation (CSI) in many television shows [21]. The CSI effect encompasses the impact these shows have on the juries' expectations of forensic evidence and may predetermine their views of applicable tests and procedures [20]. This can place undue expectations on those who testify [20]. An American study found that trial attorneys and judges have to spend additional time discussing the forensic evidence and that juries often have an unreasonable expectation of forensic evidence [22]. In particular, prosecutors had to carefully go through the forensic evidence even after experts had discussed it. As expert witnesses, forensic pathologists should be aware of the CSI effect [22]. Importantly, their expert testimony and presentation need to be clearly explained so that jurors comprehend the evidence and can carefully weigh all the evidence, including both the reliability and presentation of the expert witness [23].

Summary

Intrinsically, the medical and legal systems have areas of dissimilarity due to the intrinsic nature of each of their processes. The legal system utilises an adversarial system to resolve conflicts and medicine focuses on helping by using a scientific approach. However, what is common is that both systems are interested in getting to the truth.

References

1. Foucar E, Wick MR. Evidence-based medicine and tort law. Semin Diagn Pathol. 2005;22:167–76.
2. R. v. Lifchus, 1997 CanLII 319 (SCC), [1997] 3 SCR 320. http://canlii.ca/t/1fqzt.
3. R. v. Starr, 2000 SCC 40 (CanLII), [2000] 2 SCR 144. http://canlii.ca/t/525l.
4. Holmgren BL. Ethical issues in forensic testimony involving abusive head trauma. Acad Forensic Pathol. 2013;3(3):317–28.
5. Lacobucci F, Hamilton G. The Goudge inquiry and the role of medical expert witnesses. CMAJ. 2010;182(1):53–6.
6. Bal BS. The expert witness in medical malpractice litigation. Clin Orthop Relat Res. 2009;467:383–91.
7. Jackson B. The doctor as expert witness—help or hinderance. Med Sci Law. 2007;47(4):277–87.
8. Goudge ST. Inquiry into pediatric forensic pathology in Ontario. Toronto, ON: Ontario Ministry of the Attorney General; 2008.
9. Iacobucci F, Hamilton G. The Goudge inquiry and the role of medical expert witnesses. CMAJ. 2010;182(1):53–6.
10. Foucar E. Pathology expert witness testimony and pathology practice: a tale of 2 standards. Arch Pathol Lab Med. 2005;129:1268–76.
11. Gold AD. Expert evidence in criminal law: the scientific approach. Toronto, ON: Irwin; 2003.

12. R. v. Seaboyer, [1991] 2 S.C.R. 577 at 609-11, 66 C.C.C. (3d) 321.
13. R. v. Barton, 2015 ABQB 159; R. v. Schaefler, [1993] O.J. No. 71 (C.J. Gen. Div.).
14. Rules of Civil Procedure, amending Reg. 194 of R.R.O. 1990, O. Reg. 438/08, s.48
15. Pollanen MS. Forensic pathology and the miscarriage of justice. Forensic Sci Med Pathol. 2012;8(3):285–9.
16. Adelson L. The pathology of homicide. Charles C Thomas, Springfield. 1974
17. Duhaime AC et al. The shaken baby syndrome. A clinical, pathological, and biomechanical study. J Neurosurg 1987;66(3):409–15.
18. Beresford EB. Uncertainty and the shaping of medical decisions. Hastings Center Rep. 1991;21:6–11.
19. Pinsky LS. Comment: The use of scientific peer review and colloquia to assist judges in the admissibility gatekeeping mandated by Daubert. Houston Law Rev. 1997;34:1–42.
20. Durnal EW. Crime scene investigation (as seen on TV). Forensic Sci Int. 2010;199:1–5.
21. Dowler K, Fleming S. Constructing crime: media, crime, and popular culture. Can J Criminol Crim Justice. 2006;48(6):837–50.
22. Robbers MLP. Blinded by science: the social construction of reality in forensic televisions shows and its effect on criminal jury trials. Crim Justice Policy Rev. 2008;19(1):84–102.
23. Holmgren JA, Fordham J. The CSI effect and the Canadian and the Australian Jury. J Forensic Sci. 2011;56:S1. https://doi.org/10.1111/j.1556-4029.2010.01621.x.

Part II
Medicolegal Postmortem Examination

Chapter 4
Sudden and Unexpected Natural Deaths in Adults

Kris Cunningham and Qi Zhang

Introductory Remarks

The classical postmortem examination remains the gold-standard medical examination to investigate sudden and unexpected death, assessment of medical or surgical complications, many emerging public health concerns, and novel pathophysiological conditions. The postmortem examination (otherwise known as the autopsy) is always performed as part of a clinicopathological exercise, i.e., it is *not* an exercise in merely outlining the anatomy and pathology identified. Moreover, not all is revealed when you open a body for examination. Any major or minor pathological findings must be interpreted within a detailed clinical and social context, or at least as much as possible. Technologies such as computed tomography (CT) scanning, postmortem angiography, or molecular genetics assessment represent useful investigative adjuncts when evaluating a deceased individual and increase the armamentarium of ancillary tests available to the pathologist (including tissue microscopy, toxicology, microbiology, vitreous fluid biochemistry, serology, and electron microscopy, amongst others). However, it becomes easy for individuals to lull themselves into thinking such ancillary testing can replace an autopsy examination. For example, important detail is often missed from CT scanning, and histological correlates relevant to the timing of disease processes and critical phenotypic data are

K. Cunningham (✉)
Department of Laboratory Medicine and Pathobiology, University of Toronto, Toronto, ON, Canada

Ontario Forensic Pathology Service, Toronto, ON, Canada

Q. Zhang
Department of Pathology and Laboratory Medicine, London Health Sciences Centre, Western University, London, ON, Canada

R. Jacques (ed.), *Forensic Pathology*,
https://doi.org/10.1007/978-3-031-42038-2_4

often otherwise insufficient when trying to interpret genotypic information that flows from genetic testing.

The following thoughts represent a few comments and recommendations for a pathologist to keep in mind when performing a postmortem examination. These remarks arise from common questions that have been posed by pathologists or clinicians or family:

1. It is important to ascertain the stated questions for the pathologist. This not only clarifies what questions the clinical team or family wants to be addressed but also permits the pathologist to manage expectations. It is not uncommon for non-pathologists, such as clinical physician colleagues, families, or other stakeholders (e.g., insurance companies) to have expectations that the autopsy can sort out much that it cannot. What is poorly understood amongst non-pathologists are the limitations of the autopsy procedure. What the pathologist thinks the issues are when investigating a death is not always what clinicians or others desire, even after a detailed review of the clinical record. Pathologists also have to opportunity to manage expectations at the outset, such as establishing the time needed to complete the examination and subsequent analysis; describing what dissections are performed as part of the autopsy; outlining what facts can actually be ascertained from the procedure; detailing what other specialists might be needed; and so on.
2. For the pathologist, what are your goals in performing the autopsy? Is the autopsy for the purpose of discovery (i.e., what is the cause of death?) or is it an autopsy for the purposes of documentation? Or both? Your approach to the autopsy and ancillary testing may differ given your endpoints. One common misperception is that every autopsy utilizes all dissections and ancillary tests available (it does not). Each autopsy is tailored to particular clinical questions, just like the approach in every other area of medicine.
3. Assume you are working with an incomplete dataset. There is often unknown information that would change how you view and approach the case and not everyone is completely honest or accurate with their recollection of the signs, symptoms, timing, severity, cause, or recollection of events. I know this seems obvious when practicing medicine and working with a multitude of different members of the public, but it commonly catches pathologists in interpretive errors. Remember that the pathologist is typically working from second- or third-hand medical information that some other medical professional obtained, perhaps following different questions that the pathologist would have asked the family. A limited dataset can also bias the pathologist when interpreting the relative significance of a pathological finding. Be clear about what you assume from the history and circumstances when you undertake your clinicopathological correlation so that others who consume your report have a complete context and can follow your opinions.
4. Think of death as a process and not a discrete event. This correlates with the nature of the pathology observed (e.g., development of vascular congestion and pulmonary edema in lungs).

5. When an individual dies, all physiological processes essentially stop (e.g., thrombosis, inflammation, infarction, etc.). You are capturing a snapshot of the pathology at a unique point in time. This is not always understood by non-medical professionals.
6. Oftentimes to ascertain what a particular pathological process is, one needs to look back at multiple points in time to see how the disease process evolved. This requires a careful evaluation of the clinical (historical) record available (e.g., echocardiograms, X-rays, CT scans, etc.)
7. Understanding the pathological stages of processes such as healing, inflammation, infection, thrombosis/fibrinolysis, necrosis, fibrous organization, formation of hemosiderin, and selective neuronal necrosis for example, can allow a pathologist to address issues related to the timing of a pathophysiological process (and the limitations therein). Timing often becomes very important when reconstructing clinical events.
8. Following a complex hospital death and autopsy, a pathologist must often sort out those pathological findings that were (a) pre-morbid conditions, (b) those findings representing the new intervening pathological process, (c) those findings that were iatrogenically created during their hospital stay, (d) those findings representing complications of disease or treatment and ultimately, and (e) those findings seen as part of the dying process. All of these physical changes will manifest at the time of autopsy and may necessitate a detailed review of the clinical record to reconstruct clinical observations over time. Sorting out the many physical findings will not always be possible for non-pathology colleagues and family when they evaluate the autopsy report.
9. Do not forget to review nursing, pharmacy, or physical/respiratory therapy notes as these often have valuable information not captured by physician colleagues.
10. Not every case of shock is due to sepsis, not every fever or rise in neutrophils is due to infection and some blood tests performed after death (or even post-arrest) are not interpretable as they would be in life (e.g., K^+, troponins, complete blood count, etc.). The uninterpretable nature of these tests may require an explanation in the autopsy report.
11. Fragments of partially digested food in the airway are not typically caused by aspiration but by passive translocation of gastric contents after death from the body being moved. Reliable ascertainment of antemortem aspiration usually requires a witnessed aspiration event or occlusion of the conducting airways at autopsy. Become familiar with all the artifacts that occur as part of the dying process, body transport processes, resuscitation, decomposition, and the technique of the morgue technologist performing the autopsy procedure itself. Many of these artifacts can be misinterpreted as antemortem evidence of disease or injury when they are not.
12. In general, descriptors such as pulmonary edema, cardiomegaly, left ventricular hypertrophy (LVH) and cirrhosis are not causes of death per se. What others care about is what caused that physical finding? Likewise, entities such as pneumonia and pulmonary embolism are well-recognized immediate causes of

death, but what people need to understand are the underlying conditions that led to that final pathological process (e.g., for pneumonia: community-acquired infection, immunodeficiency, occupational exposure, aspiration, hypostatic pneumonia, etc., or for thrombosis: morbid obesity, coincident colorectal carcinoma, immobility, trauma, oral contraceptive pills, and genetic-induced thrombophilia, such as from genetic mutations in Factor V, etc.).

13. "Stroke," "idiopathic pulmonary fibrosis," "arrhythmia," and "sepsis" are generally not pathological, but clinical diagnoses. As pathologists, you should be able to identify an etiologically specific cause or at least a more detailed characterization of these clinical diagnoses. For example, a stroke syndrome (clinical diagnosis) due to intraparenchymal hemorrhage of the parieto-occipital lobe of the cerebrum due to cerebrovascular hypertension, granulomatous vasculitis, cerebrovascular small vessel disease (e.g., CADISIL), congophilic angiopathy, and so on.
14. Be as etiologically specific as you can. For discovery autopsies, the worst outcome is to do a comprehensive examination and tell the clinician nothing they did not already know, or at the very least, be clear in your opinion stating that, despite best efforts and careful examination, you are not able to identify major findings that were not appreciated clinically. This statement at least serves to recognize the significance of the outcome of the autopsy for the clinician and, if the family requested an autopsy for discovery, can corroborate that the nature of the care received was clinically well documented.
15. Resuscitation-related trauma is often more extensive than appreciated; you should become familiar with the patterns and extent of injury within the chest and abdomen.
16. Contraction band change in the heart is not always an indication of ischemia, as it only represents recent myocardial damage from some cause (such as reperfusion injury, drug, trauma, ischemia, inflammation, toxin, and cardiopulmonary resuscitation efforts).

How We Die a Natural Death

There are many possible causes for a natural death that could be discussed. The most common causes in lower-income countries include neonatal conditions, infections, ischemic heart disease, and stroke as well as diarrheal diseases [1]. It is notable that many of the top ten causes of death in low-income countries are communicable infections and this speaks to the value of a robust public health system in the developed world. In upper-middle income countries, the most common causes of death include chronic conditions such as ischemic heart disease/stroke, lower respiratory disease and lung-related cancers (presumably from cigarette smoking), hypertension, as well as diabetes-associated pathologies and dementias [1].

As a first step in discussing causes of natural death, it is often useful to break the type of death down into 12 general classes that an autopsy pathologist may encounter. Unless particularly obscure, most natural causes for death can be associated with the following:

1. Arrhythmic death
2. Asphyxial death
3. Infectious death
4. Obstructive death
5. Endocrine death
6. Biochemical/metabolic death
7. Immunological/inflammatory death
8. Occlusive/thrombotic/infarction death
9. Bleeding death
10. Neoplastic death
11. Medication-induced death
12. Iatrogenic death

Often multiple classes overlap, but as a general organizing principle, this list can be useful when making sense of pathological findings. In what follows, a few considerations will be mentioned about each category, but frequently, a given death will involve aspects of several categories mentioned. As the audience for this manuscript is anticipated to be other pathologists, a detailed outline of the pathological findings observed in each category of death is not provided and assumes a basic understanding of at least a junior anatomical pathologist. What this article does focus on is a few of the pitfalls and factors of each class of death to consider when evaluating these deaths at the time of autopsy (Figs. 4.1, 4.2, 4.3, 4.4, 4.5, 4.6, and 4.7).

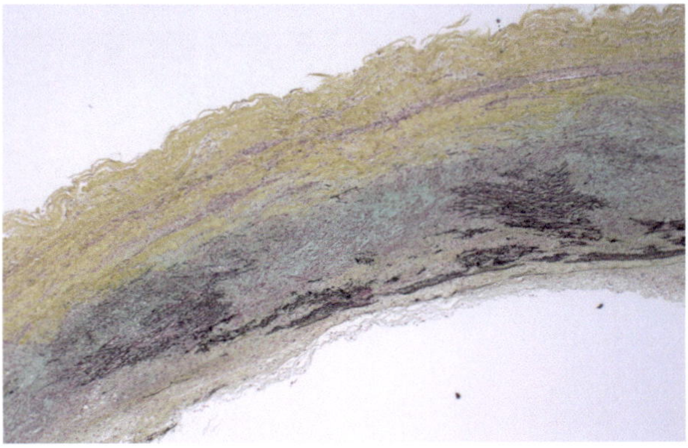

Fig. 4.1 Section shows severe aortopathy in the setting of acute ascending aortic dissection, weakening the aortic wall (Movat pentachrome: 20×)

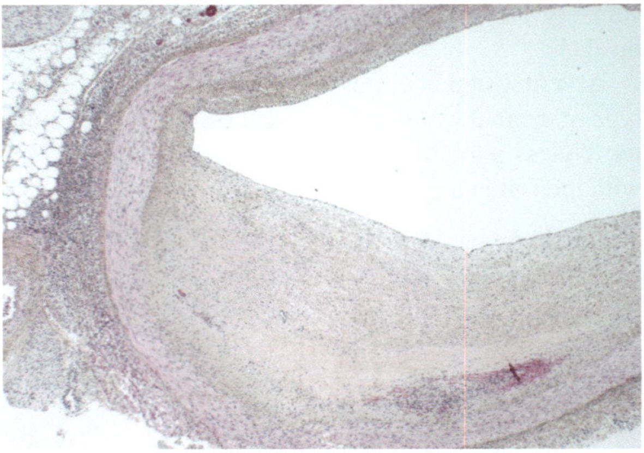

Fig. 4.2 Section shows Behcet's arteritis involving epicardial coronary artery, which increases the risk of in situ thrombosis (Movat pentachrome: 20×)

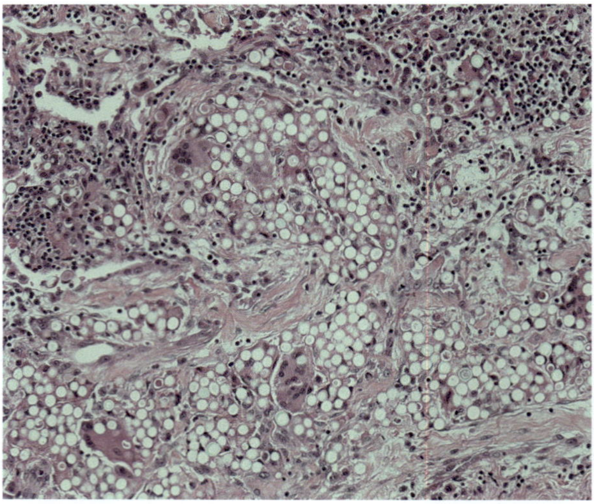

Fig. 4.3 Pulmonary blastomycosis (H&E: 100×)

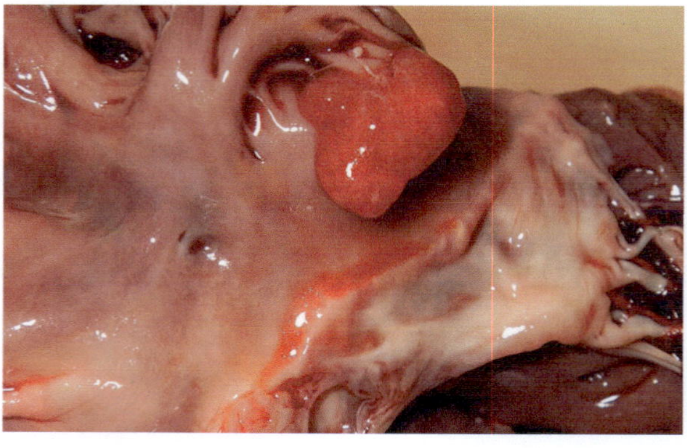

Fig. 4.4 Right atrial cardiac myxoma

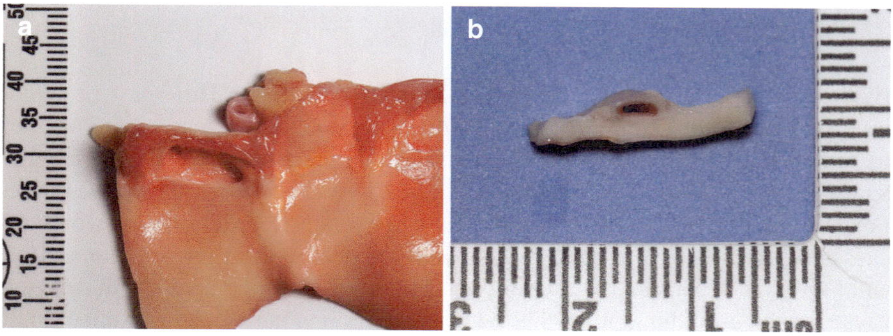

Fig. 4.5 Coronary artery anomaly: Note both ostia originate from the same aortic sinus (**a**) with the left main coronary artery coursing at an acute angle so that there is both an intra-arterial course (**b**) and inter-arterial course between aorta and pulmonary artery

Fig. 4.6 Large, non-malignant gastric ulceration in the setting of lethal upper gastrointestinal hemorrhage

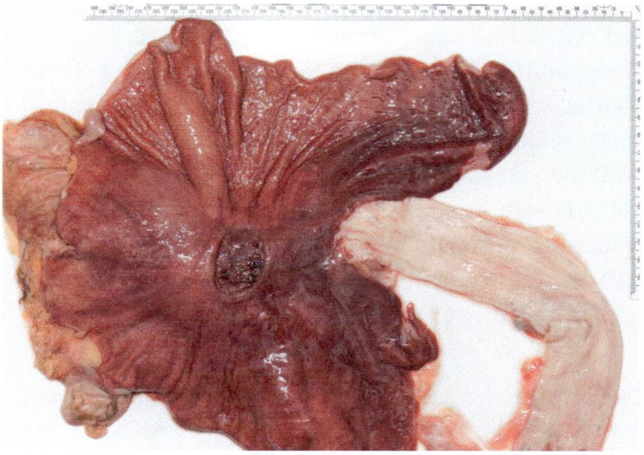

Fig. 4.7 Polycystic adult kidneys—may have an underlying genetic contribution to disease

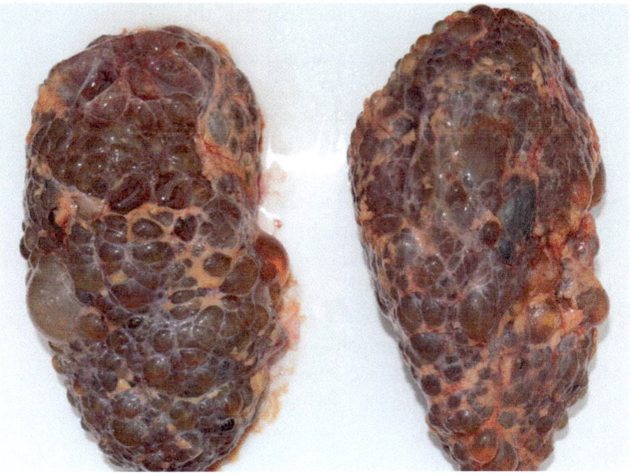

Arrhythmic Death

Evidence of a prior arrhythmia cannot be seen at autopsy. This must be either inferred from antemortem functional studies (e.g., electrocardiogram and telemetry) or inferred from the context of the scene and circumstances with a suitable pathological substrate (e.g., severe heart disease) and no likely alternative cause. For the autopsy pathologist, arrhythmias can be due to functional or structural causes. If functional, the heart will typically appear normal (or near normal) at autopsy, which represents a relevant and important negative, and the underlying cause for the arrhythmia may only be identified following a careful evaluation of the clinical record (Table 4.1). Alternatively, the autopsy pathologist may be the first person to uncover a primary arrhythmia syndrome. Where the pathologist can make a significant contribution is the identification of structural substrates for arrhythmogenesis, which are sometimes subtle and can predispose to arrhythmias and sudden cardiac death. Anything that can disrupt the normal electrical–mechanical physiology can potentially lead to ventricular arrhythmia, cardiovascular collapse, and death or, at the very least, cause sufficient myocardial damage (from aborted cardiac arrest or prolonged hypoperfusion) that then can predispose to death. Common arrhythmogenic substrates include coronary artery or vascular graft stenosis/occlusion (at least 75% stenosed), usually from atherosclerosis, but other possibilities exist (such as dissection). This usually involves the principal epicardial coronary arteries, but significant stenoses in branches can also elicit arrhythmia. Remember that each person's coronary artery anatomy is different, with a significant minority of individuals having a trifurcation of the left main

Table 4.1 The following table shows possible autopsy "negative" causes of death for consideration (e.g., natural disease conditions where no findings are identified at autopsy *or* the pathological findings are very subtle at autopsy and missed by the unwary pathologist *or* require special study of the tissues). Note: interaction with medications is also considered as adverse reactions to medications may present as pure "natural" disease conditions.

Primary or secondary arrhythmia syndromes
Unsuspected toxicities
Cardiac conduction system disease
Sickle cell anemia, acute hemolytic anemia, or other blood cell dyscrasias
Malaria
Some forms of endocrine or metabolic disease
Electrolyte/biochemical anomalies
Atypical infectious locations (e.g., retropharyngeal abscess, Ludwig's angina, and epidural spinal infections)
Some forms of anaphylaxis (where a full set of signs and symptoms is not manifest)
Some paraneoplastic syndromes
Medication interactions (e.g., monoamine oxidase inhibitor toxicities, neuroleptic malignant syndrome, and malignant hyperthermia)
Rhabdomyolysis
Thrombotic microangiopathies

[a] In some instances, a pathological process may be identified but does not represent the underlying etiology explaining death (e.g., thrombotic microangiopathy and rhabdomyolysis)

coronary artery (that includes the ramus intermedius, do not forget to look for it). The principal and secondary coronary artery branches should be evaluated. The rapid growth of a plaque from intraplaque hemorrhage can be clinically significant (or silent depending on clinical history), and the coronary arteries should be sectioned at 3–4 mm intervals to catch all lesions. Too much muscle (hypertrophy) can elicit an arrhythmia. This is best assessed by assessing the weight of the heart (typically greater than 500 g, although exceptions allow for a bit bigger heart if you are particularly tall, muscular, and athletic) and can manifest from concentric hypertrophy (ventricular myocardium too thick), eccentric hypertrophy (increased muscle around an enlarged ventricular chamber) or asymmetric ventricular hypertrophy. Be wary not to overinterpret *physiological* hypertrophy in an athletic individual, but this should be mild at most and the left ventricle should be less than 2 cm in thickness and should not have markedly enlarged or bizarre-looking nuclei. It is important to remember that when echocardiographers measure ventricular thickness in life, it is often much thinner than what is appreciated at autopsy. This increased thickness at autopsy occurs for a number of reasons, but rigor and the state of contraction likely play a role. Cardiologists are typically not aware of the difference in thicknesses between the echocardiogram and autopsy and may question thicknesses obtained by the pathologist. Remember to measure the ventricle within 2 cm of the mitral valve annulus in an adult and only include the compact ventricular muscle in thickness measurements; do not include the epicardial layer or trabeculae carneae. A small amount of variability in thickness between the septum and free wall can be tolerated in an adult (say up to 0.5 cm), but any more than that should elicit careful evaluation.

Acute ischemic injury or other acute damage to the myocardium, especially if involving a significant macroscopic region of the myocardium can trigger an arrhythmic event. Rare conditions such as conduction system disease, suggested at autopsy by assessment of the AV nodal region, should be carefully correlated with potential antemortem symptomatology prior to ascribing its significance.

Scar tissue, from any cause, is potentially arrhythmogenic. To ascribe scar tissue as the most likely arrhythmogenic substrate causing death, typically, it should be more than just *mild* fibrous tissue deposition in all its manifestations (recent/organizing or mature or old), each of which can increase the risk of arrhythmic death. Remember that mild interstitial fibrous tissue deposition can be an age-related change and allowance for a little bit of fibrous tissue should be made for late middle age and elderly populations. One may potentially infer the cause of the scar tissue by patterns of fibrous tissue deposition. The subendocardium is particularly susceptible to chronic ischemic heart disease and non-transmural ischemic infarcts. How many vascular territories are involved? How does the distribution correlate with any coronary artery disease present (if any)? Is the scar tissue mostly mid-myocardial or epicardial? Is it associated with an inflammatory process? Does it appear all to be the same age or is there temporal heterogeneity? Significant concentric hypertrophy of any cause increases the risk of subendocardial scar (as the endocardium is typically the last to receive epicardial blood flow) and subepicardial scar may be seen in arrhythmogenic cardiomyopathy, myocarditis, or sarcoidosis. Sometimes, fibrous tissue deposition (whether interstitial or replacement type) is noted within the posterior-basal wall of the left ventricle, involving conditions such as moderate to severe myxomatous mitral valve disease or muscular dystrophies. Fibrous tissue deposition can often occur coincidentally with classical cardiomyopathies, hypertrophy, or vascular disease as noted above; however, idiopathic fibrous tissue deposition with no apparent pattern of deposition is recognized (e.g., from toxic, autoimmune, atypical cardiomyopathic, or inflammatory sources) and should be managed carefully.

Cardiomyopathies and primary arrhythmia syndromes require special attention. While most cardiomyopathies are secondary to systemic conditions and, in older individuals, it typically arises from acquired disease (although there are cases of classical heritable cardiomyopathies presenting later in life), pathologists do not want to miss potentially heritable processes in younger individuals (those under 50 years, especially under the age of 40 years). Most cardiomyopathic conditions can be placed within one of the classical "hypertrophic," "dilated," "restrictive," or "arrhythmogenic cardiomyopathy" phenotypes, but mixed presentations or atypical presentations of cardiomyopathy are not rare. It is particularly important to accurately characterize the phenotype well when considering heritable cardiac conditions as this may guide subsequent surveillance and evaluation of first-degree family members. When heritable disease is contemplated, it is important to flag it as such and save a DNA source. It is also important to accurately characterize cardiac enlargement/hypertrophy secondary to morbid obesity, valvular disease, or chronic toxicity (e.g., chronic alcohol usage) as others may want to ascribe the cardiac findings to heritable disease when it is unlikely. Differentiating past episodes of myocarditis against potential cases of arrhythmogenic cardiomyopathy is known to be difficult and may require specialized consultation as potential heritability is at stake.

With primary arrhythmia syndromes, the heart is normal or near normal pathologically, but this diagnosis is considered a possibility when the circumstances suggest a sudden cardiac death in a young person and no potential cause is identified following a detailed investigation. Careful consideration of personal and family history (medical and social), performance of toxicology, and recommending that first-degree family members seek consultation within a heritable heart disease clinic is highly encouraged for the autopsy report. Ensure you have indicated that a DNA source has been saved and can be made available upon request. In suspected cases, additional ancillary studies will be performed on family members (especially functional studies), pedigree analysis will be performed and genetic testing can assist the heritable heart disease clinic by increasing the dataset over what the pathologist had available, to determine if a primary arrhythmia syndrome (or a cardiomyopathy) was potentially present in the family. Regardless, if a primary arrhythmia syndrome is being contemplated (and not formally diagnosed previously), this cause of death should only be suggested as a possibility and the heritable heart disease clinic should make the final confirmatory diagnosis (or not) as they will have carriage of the family going forward.

Remember that the typical vascular watershed areas of the left ventricular myocardium include the subendocardium, the basal muscular interventricular septum, and the tips of the papillary muscles. These areas often become ischemic in the course of an aborted cardiac arrest and sustain reperfusion injury. If the patient then subsequently dies days after the initial arrest, care should be taken not to overinterpret this arrest/reperfusion-related injury as the primary cause of the original cardiac arrest. Also remember that non-structural causes for arrhythmia, unrelated to molecular cardiac aberrations, need to be excluded such as electrolyte abnormalities (K^+ and Ca^{2+}), acidosis, hypoxemia, severe hypotension, and sepsis.

Asphyxial Death

Limiting our discussion to natural disease processes, we are typically talking about any process that structurally obstructs the upper or lower conducting airways, impairs gas exchange within the lungs, or interferes with gas exchange between red blood cells and tissues. On the latter point, this would include congenital or medication-induced methemoglobinemia. Structural and obstructive disease could include oropharyngeal, nasopharyngeal and laryngeal lesions (cancer, large polyps), Ludwig's angina, retropharyngeal abscesses, tonsillar abscesses, anaphylaxis or acute epiglottitis, thyroid carcinoma, laryngeal squamous carcinoma, and other local cancers eroding into a major blood vessel leading to extensive hemorrhage into the airway, robust fibroinflammatory (granulation) tissue surrounding a tracheostomy site or a large, tenacious mucus plug occluding a tracheostomy tube, developmental anomalies in neonates (e.g., tracheal band/web, tracheal hypoplasia, and tracheomalacia), an abnormally enlarged tongue due to intrinsic tongue pathology (even considering obstructive sleep apnea) and significant extrinsic compression of the airway or erosion of the thoracic trachea by mediastinal lesions. Lower respiratory tract lesions that could impair gas exchange could include bronchogenic malignancies, infectious pneumonia, chemical pneumonitis secondary to aspiration, acute and or chronic pneumonitis, asthma, chronic obstructive pulmonary disease, cystic fibrosis, pulmonary-renal syndromes, and chronic bronchitis. Dementias, neuromuscular disorders, and other functional laryngeal pathologies require special mention because of the risk of aspiration. Mediastinal malignancies can interfere with the mechanics of breathing. Fistulas and malignancy-based erosion from lung lesions into the airway should also be noted, with secondary bleeding and aspiration of blood. Finally, disorders of breathing involving the diaphragm, chest wall, visceral pleura or loss of pulmonary parenchyma can illicit hypoxia and death.

Regardless of the method of asphyxia found, correlation with the clinical record available by assessing what signs and symptoms were exhibited of acute or acute-on-chronic respiratory failure is important. Moreover, hypoxemia decreases the threshold for arrhythmia and can lead to secondary remodeling of the lung vasculature if chronic.

Infectious Death

There are too many possible infections (e.g., bacterial, fungal, parasitic, and viral) that could cause death to be discussed herein, but a few words can be said about evaluating an infectious death and assessing the issues to consider during an infectious autopsy. Clear management of infectious deaths is particularly important for autopsy pathologists, as was seen with the recent SARS-CoV-2 infection causing COVID-19. Careful elucidation of the range of pathophysiologies observed in novel infections and how these infections impact death investigation systems (e.g., vulnerable populations) and public health systems needs to be at the forefront of a pathologist's mind and carefully communicated to clinical and public health colleagues. Most infections causing death in a hospital environment present with an infectious prodrome, positive culture results, appropriate blood tests suggesting infection in the clinical record (e.g., neutrophilia), and structural evidence of an infection at autopsy, including sequelae of an infection such as a rash, myocarditis, tissue necrosis, and so on. In other words, there are multiple lines of evidence supporting an infectious death and time for the infection to "declare itself." However, if the death is soon after admission to the hospital or in the community, the pathologist may have to infer some of these findings from the autopsy itself. Nevertheless, these deaths are not typically challenging for the autopsy pathologist to manage; yet, where an infectious death could cause trouble for an autopsy pathologist includes scenarios such as the following:

1. Fever of unknown origin—while not all fevers are due to infection, when an infection is strongly suspected, do not forget to think about commonly missed locations for an infection such as the retropharyngeal space (if pharyngeal symptoms), epidural spinal abscess (often but not always with a vague history of back pain), purulent endometritis, extensive cellulitis (sample skin) or middle ears (otitis media, which can be accessed by sampling the petrous ridges in the skull base).
2. The very young and the elderly do not always elicit a robust neutrophilic response. The absence of a robust fever or neutrophilic reaction when first assessed cannot be used to exclude an infection.
3. There is not always a localized infection to find at autopsy, where instead a generalized bacteremia may be present. This may especially be seen in younger people. Be sure to look for small breaks in the skin or other mucous membranes as sources of infection. Sample widely for histology (including multiple enlarged lymph nodes) as soft tissue bacteremia may be appreciated at autopsy (assuming there is not advancing decomposition complicating interpretation).
4. Be sure there is evidence of an inflammatory response against any bacteria observed histologically, which would suggest that the bacteria were present in life. In addition, localized advanced putrefactive decomposition may be observed in the setting of an infection.
5. Be on the lookout for genetic immunodeficiencies (most often seen in children with multiple family members having a relevant history) or acquired immunodeficiencies (usually viral).

6. Be aware of what infections are reportable to your local public health unit. For instance, *Mycobacterium tuberculosis* and *Neisseria meningitidis* are still present unexpectedly at autopsy, and contact tracing may need to be initiated. There may also be implications for infection control with autopsy personnel.
7. Sample widely (for both histological evaluation and microbiological assessment) and consider freezing tissue samples for apparently novel infections presenting as public health concerns. Your tissue and evaluation may be key to sorting out the nature of unexplained infectious entities.

Obstructive Death

There are multiple ways this mode of death can be interpreted. Ultimately, I am suggesting there may be an obstruction of a mechanical process (e.g., intrinsic or extrinsic compression affecting respiration, blood flow, and cerebral spinal fluid flow) that can disrupt normal physiology and quickly lead to death. Examples could include obstruction of the cerebral third ventricle by a colloid cyst and impairment of cerebrospinal fluid flow, obstruction of the conducting airway by tumor or granulation tissue (e.g., exuberant granulation tissue at tracheostomy site), cardiac tamponade causing collapse of the myocardial atria/ventricles, a tension pneumothorax shifting the mediastinal structures and causing cardiovascular collapse and abdominal compartment syndrome obstructing diaphragmatic excursion and collapse of abdominal vasculature. The same sort of physiological derangement is observed with marked ascites under tension causing respiratory failure with shortness of breath and limitation in diaphragmatic excursion.

Endocrine Death

This mode of death and the next noted below (Biochemical and Metabolic Deaths) are clearly related, and overlap could be readily identified between the two. However, in endocrine deaths, emphasis will be placed on the fact that a dedicated organ or endocrine tissue has failed to function normally, which leads to insufficient or excess endocrine hormone production, that can result in aberrant physiology and new pathology in multiple tissue systems (i.e., those tissues responsive to the hormone in question). Such disease processes can be profound, acute, and immediately life-threatening (thyroid storm, acute Addisonian crisis, and diabetic ketoacidosis) or chronic and insidious with vague symptomatology (e.g., chronic hyper- or hypothyroidism and myocardial disease, craniopharyngioma, and panhypopituitarism). Consider endocrine disease when patterns of symptoms and signs from the clinical history are vague or unclear and a conspicuous cause for death is not reasonably identified at autopsy (or that coheres with the history provided). After the dissection, a pathologist may orient any relevant ancillary investigations to investigate this possibility. Only some ancillary studies to investigate endocrine disease are reliable postmortem, and all results must be evaluated with caution and carefully correlated with findings at autopsy. For example, vitreous fluid beta-hydroxybutyrate for ketoacidosis or free T3/T4 and thyroid-stimulating hormone (TSH) levels often can be reliable postmortem. Remember also that endocrine failure can be secondary to other pathologies that just happen to target endocrine organs (e.g., fungal infection or malignancy and adrenal crisis, infarction of pituitary following childbirth).

Biochemical and Metabolic Death

Disruption of individual metabolic processes with the accumulation of a specific metabolic byproduct or disruption of discrete biochemical pathways can lead to significant morbidity and ultimately death. Sometimes, intermediate and discrete metabolic products accumulate within cells and their histological appearance will be the trigger for the pathologist to suspect an unsuspected aberrant metabolic process. Such products can accumulate slowly and obstruct normal physiological processes, or they may suddenly accumulate causing tissue failure and death. In general, most often biochemical and metabolic disease declares itself clinically and a thorough workup has already been performed clinically. Occasionally, however, the pathologist is the first to discover that an individual had a biochemical or metabolic condition, and careful evaluation that involves the correlation between tissue studies, the pattern of pathology observed, and ancillary toxicological or biochemical or genetic evaluation may ensue. This is particularly common within the neonate and pediatric age range, but very occasionally biochemical and metabolic diseases can present later in life. A pathologist may be asked to perform an autopsy in a known case of metabolic/biochemical disease to ascertain if a complication of that disease entity (or the therapy for management of the condition) may have caused death. The important point to remember is that, with any biochemical or metabolic condition, there is a good possibility that it could be heritable. Thus, saving a DNA source (if not performing genetic testing) may be important for the family. Also, as with any possible genetic condition, a pathologist may wish to recommend an assessment of the first-degree family members by a geneticist if the condition is completely unknown to the family and clinical team.

Immunological/Inflammatory Death

These deaths can be difficult for the autopsy pathologist to work up. These deaths can include immune deficiency syndromes, autoimmune disease (hyperactive immune syndromes) or conditions classically thought of as collagen vascular diseases. When it comes to a history of immune deficiency, obviously a clinical history supportive of repeated infections or a family history of infections can trigger consideration of this entity. A pathologist may see opportunistic infections (or their sequelae) and pathological alteration of their lymph nodes, thymus, bone marrow, or possibly spleen. The pathological findings may be subtle in some cases, and consultation with a hematopathologist may be needed. This is complicated by the rapid autolysis and putrefactive decompositional changes after death for the above-noted structures and cells. Moreover, genetic studies are becoming a mainstay in immune deficiency workup (antemortem) and may be necessary for postmortem characterization as well. One issue that needs careful evaluation is that multiple conditions may be associated with chronic wasting, repeated infections, and unexplained pathology, which may very well be due to unsuspected immune deficiency disease, but neglect and physical abuse can also present to an unsuspecting pathologist (recall the discussion about what we do not know can sometimes be a pitfall). Consultation with a forensic pathology colleague can assist in this regard. Additionally, viruses (such as HIV), toxins, or other immune system-impairing factors need to be considered and tested for in suspected cases.

When it comes to inflammatory/autoimmune/rheumatological conditions, the pathologist may again only observe the sequelae of a rheumatological condition (e.g., myocardial or pulmonary or hepatic fibrous tissue deposition), although active inflammation and tissue destruction can sometimes be seen. The challenge for the pathologist is that these pathological observations are often out of context and the pathologist must think of them to consider the pattern of tissue injury they may be presenting. Vasculitis is a helpful, if not non-specific observation. Other non-specific pathologies (e.g., nonbacterial thrombotic endocarditis) may also be observed and represent the pathologist's first clue. Moreover, you will likely see a combination of chronicity with inflammatory conditions alongside active disease, healing lesions, and scar being evident at the time of autopsy, suggesting repeated exacerbations of disease or a chronic, perhaps subacute disease progression. Although, in the developed world, myocarditis is usually due to viruses, chronic inflammatory conditions and drugs must also be considered when myocarditis is observed, particularly if there is evidence of myocardial damage occurring at different points in time. Some types of hepatic cirrhosis associated with autoimmune hepatitis or idiopathic pulmonary fibrosis are caused by inflammatory diseases, such as with UIP pattern (usual interstitial pneumonitis) or NSIP pattern (nonspecific interstitial pneumonitis) disease. One must also be aware of certain drug or medication-related changes or rheumatological diseases caused by infections (e.g., such as from viruses [hepatitis C virus]) as opposed to a primary inflammatory condition per se. These conditions are a challenge sometimes to diagnose in life and there may be a significant benefit for the pathologist to engage in consultation with a rheumatologist after the autopsy to fully explore any clinico-pathological correlation. However, it should be noted that standard rheumatological serological studies are generally not interpretable after death and may not assist in the final determination. Inflammatory conditions are difficult to characterize precisely by pathology, as one can often say a rheumatological condition is strongly suspected, but precise diagnosis is a challenge.

Occlusive Thrombotic and Infarction Death

On the surface, this type of death is usually obvious with vascular occlusion or severe stenosis by a thrombus (recent or organized) leading to downstream infarction or ischemia, physiological dysfunction, atrophy, apoptosis, or cell death within the tissue that is supplied by the affected vessel. The physiological severity may depend on the degree of collateral blood flow, nature of the organ, degree of glucose, and oxygen consumption as well as the rate of waste production and size of infarction (e.g., electrical organs such as the heart and brain are at greater risk of causing sudden death or marked morbidity). These issues are typically not a problem for most pathologists and are generally correlated to the clinical history. The issues I would like to highlight include the following:

1. If more than one vessel is thrombosed at autopsy, if there are vessels exhibiting repeated thrombosis over a longer time period (i.e., some acute and some organizing) if there are pathological findings suggestive of prior thrombosis (e.g., unexplained scars, prior episodes of pulmonary embolism or deep vein thrombosis, prior miscarriages, gangrene, prior strokes, etc.) if the individual is relatively young with no clear explanation or if there is a family history of thromboses, then genetic evaluation of inherited thrombophilia's is recommended.
2. Not all thrombotic disorders are genetic (some are functional and acquired), and a coincident pathological process may be needed to bring out an underlying susceptibility (e.g., prolonged immobilization, pregnancy, trauma, and certain pro-thrombotic medications).
3. One may have the propagation of a thrombus, where, if acute, a thrombus may become quite elongated and even course down branch vessels. Alternatively, a proximal thrombus may partially organize and a new thrombus may overlay the original over time, with thrombus of differing ages at a given location.
4. Thrombi involving both veins and arteries should prompt consideration of a heritable thrombophilia or conditions such as lupus or isolated antiphospholipid antibody syndrome.
5. While atherosclerotic plaque disruption or large calcium nodules in atherosclerotic plaques can precipitate in situ thrombosis, so too can an inflamed vessel (arterial vasculitis or phlebitis), reaction against a foreign body in the blood stream or vascular trauma (natural or iatrogenic).
6. While in situ thrombosis is quite common, thromboemboli from the heart, carotid arteries, aorta, or other large vessels from any location can also lead to significant morbidity and mortality. For instance, in older individuals, thrombi forming over complex atherosclerotic ulcerations in the aorta frequently embolize and are not recognized clinically but are observed at autopsy with infarcts typically found in the gut, kidneys, or lower extremities.
7. The timing of thrombosis and any potential fibrous organization may be important. For example, bunion surgery led to immobility 3 days prior to sudden death, and pulmonary embolism was identified at autopsy, which was attributed to deep vein thrombosis of the leg. The family wants to attribute DVT to bunion surgery

alone, but you find acute *and* organizing thrombi in lungs and lower extremity vessels. Thus, there was evidence of thrombosis preceding bunion surgery. Therefore, at most, one may only proffer that immobility may have exacerbated an already pre-existing propensity to form DVTs.

Bleeding Death

This mode of death is again typically quite obvious and not a problem for pathologists as the culprit lesion and quantity of bleeding can be identified at autopsy, but there are some pitfalls or issues the autopsy pathologist needs to keep in mind:

1. Significant blood loss leads to hypovolemic shock and death. The amount of blood in an individual is variable and dependent on sex (typically M > F) and size (height and weight). A person's ability to tolerate blood loss depends on age and comorbidities (more below). Most individuals have between 3.5 and 6.5 L of blood in them (or approximately 70–90 mL/kg), and how much blood loss could cause death is somewhat difficult to put a hard number on as individual characteristics may vary. However, as a very general guide, certainly loss of 40% of the blood volume (assuming no other comorbidities) could elicit a shock syndrome and ultimately be fatal if not addressed promptly. However, loss of greater than about 15% of blood volume could elicit the early signs of shock. Symptomatology is graded on a spectrum, and the farther one is into shock, the more irreversible it could be [2].
2. Once you have a middle-aged to older individual or someone with significant comorbidities, then the tolerance for excessive blood loss decreases. Furthermore, when significant, blood loss can cause tachycardia and prolonged tachycardia can exacerbate any underlying pro-arrhythmic cardiac condition. For example, a 75-year-old woman who had lost approximately 750 cc of blood from an intraperitoneal bleed may expire when considered in the context of her severe coronary artery disease. Remember also that someone with anemia has decreased oxygen-carrying capacity; thus, lower volumes of blood loss can have more profound physiological effects. Tissue hypoxia from low oxygen delivery can also promote arrhythmogenesis.
3. Significant tissue destruction in a short amount of time can result in significant potassium released into the circulation (e.g., rhabdomyolysis, hemolysis, tumor lysis syndrome, and large surgeries). Moreover, significant bleeding and massive transfusions over a short time period can also result in coagulopathy, especially if there is coincident acidosis, hypothermia, excessive hemodilution from fluid resuscitation, and consumption of endogenous coagulation factors.
4. If at the time of autopsy (or from history) there are strong indications that the person had bled excessively (that is not attributable to anemia), such as decreased lividity, marked pallor of organs, and decreased blood in the vasculature, but you cannot find the location of the bleeding through the typical autopsy methods, do

not forget that fractures (such as hip fractures) can bleed heavily into the soft tissues of the thigh and be very subtle externally. Alternatively, bleeding into the soft tissues of the lower back can be missed if not purposely examined. Thus, additional dissections may be required if there is a history of falls associated with their medical condition. In addition, if the bleeding originated from within the gastrointestinal tract, while some of the blood will be seen internally, much of the blood may have passed into a toilet or be present at the scene.

5. By the nature of the organ donation procedure itself, the deceased will generally be pale after donation and this pallor will be noted at autopsy. Pathologists should not necessarily overinterpret this pallor as being present prior to donation.

Neoplastic Death

Neoplastic deaths are relatively straight forward for the autopsy pathologist to identify causally, although the precise mechanism of death can be a challenge to sort out (see below). In most instances, there is a malignant neoplasm (cancer) observed with either significant, localized spread or diffuse metastatic disease. The autopsy pathologist first needs to ascertain if there is sufficient tumor burden to potentially cause death and then characterize the neoplasm as far as is necessary for the death investigation purposes. This later goal may be challenging with extensive tumor necrosis, especially if recent chemo- or radiotherapy has occurred, or with postmortem autolysis that may necessitate focusing on smaller metastases to attain viable cellularity to characterize the histological pattern of differentiation. It is often not necessary to do a full immunohistochemical workup as in life, but sufficient ancillary histological staining to at least identify the class of neoplasm should be sought if possible. Identifying the neoplasm is aided by evaluating the pattern of metastatic spread and organ/tissue of origin. Special attention to circumstances or patterns of malignancy suggestive of heritable disease (e.g., younger individual, polyposis, and multiple malignancies) would be valuable to communicate to the surviving family.

Mechanistically neoplasms could cause death through frank tissue burden complicated by paraneoplastic phenomena, fluid and electrolyte disturbances, tumor lysis, cancer cachexia, increased infections and anemia (e.g., hematological malignancies), gastrointestinal or genitourinary hemorrhage, pulmonary emboli secondary to deep vein thromboses (e.g., serous carcinomas), erosion into vital structures such as major arteries and veins leading to hemorrhage, increased intracranial pressure (e.g., glial tumors and cerebral metastases), complications of medications, and malignant pericardial effusions. While there are several structural complications that can occur with malignancies, frequently, the autopsy pathologist is presented with just a significant tumor burden and no alternative, complication explaining death. Depending on the tumor, the degree of tumor burden can sometimes be quite remarkable before it presents clinically (e.g., gastric carcinoma) or leads to rapid death after the initial unexpected presentation (e.g., pulmonary or peritoneal carcinomatosis). Rarely, benign neoplasms can also occasionally cause death when they are large or impinging on vital structures that disrupt critical physiology that can cause death. Even more rarely malignancies arising in the setting of significant, chronic immune suppression can be observed.

Medication-Induced Death

A few words will be said about medication-induced deaths at autopsy. While most drug deaths are not classified as natural per se when one considers them from an overdose perspective, the hospital autopsy pathologist should always be on the lookout for medication-induced complications, perhaps unrelated to overdose that could cause death. This could include hypersensitivity reactions and anaphylaxis, arrhythmias, renal or hepatic failure, thrombosis or hemorrhage, myocarditis, immune complex disease, seizures, neuroleptic malignant syndrome, and pancreatitis. These cases can be difficult to prove definitively and will require a careful evaluation of the medical record and reported adverse effects history of the drug and may require consultation with a pharmacist, forensic pathologist, or clinical toxicologist to help evaluate the data available. While a forensic pathologist might be recommended to manage such cases when a medication-induced death is suspected from the outset, given their medicolegal lens on the issues, these cases can sometimes present with what appears as a natural disease death (as noted above) but only then be recognized later on as complications of a particular medication. Additional challenges often arise when trying to ascertain if the medication was the most likely cause for the complication causing death versus some other natural disease process. Was the medication taken at the prescribed dosage, frequency, and route? Was the medication present actually in the body at the time of death? Could therapeutic concentrations of the medication actually lead to the complication encountered? While medication-induced complications may be straightforward for the hospital autopsy pathologist to manage, the medicolegal issues that could flow from such deaths (e.g., court testimony) might be an unanticipated outcome of the investigation.

Iatrogenic-Induced Death

Like many of the categories discussed above, there are many possible examples of iatrogenic complications that could cause death, too many to discuss here. However, a sampling of the types of iatrogenic death that an autopsy pathologist needs to consider could include: (1) acute (or chronic) medical or surgical device failure, (2) infection and bleeding, (3) erosion of foreign body into a vital structure, (4) thrombosis of a foreign body in the bloodstream or heart, (5) contrast or other injectable agents causing hypersensitivity or immune reactions, (6) unanticipated response to medications, (7) wrong surgical sites used or trauma from surgery (e.g., right leg instead of left, trocar injuries causing hemorrhage), (8) complications from percutaneous guidewires puncturing vital structures, (9) migration of devices to inappropriate places (e.g., intra-aortic balloon pumps and J-tubes draining into peritoneum), and (10) air embolism. Other examples certainly exist.

Careful documentation of any device in situ is necessary, and the pathologist should examine the device and/or the pathological site involved carefully and not delegate this to an assistant for device removal. If a surgeon was involved, including them at the time of autopsy can also assist when trying to understand the circumstances and how any such complications or errors (if there was an error) came about. While clinicians and surgeons cannot change the findings observed, it is important that they learn from their complications so that families can receive effective communication about what happened. It is important to ensure that you as the autopsy pathologist can remain a neutral party, ensure that only factual information is reported and any opinions provided are not speculative and limited to the pathological issues at hand; or at least if the pathologist is going to speculate, be clear this is the case. Other clinicians or specialists can opine about non-pathological issues as necessary. One should also use as non-inflammatory language as possible as legal ramifications may flow from the autopsy.

Nontraumatic Sudden Death Caused by Central Nervous System Disorders

Apart from the aforementioned natural causes of sudden death, central nervous system (CNS) disorders account for one-fourth of these cases [3]. Epilepsy (SUDEP), intracranial hemorrhage, neoplasm, and infection are the most common CNS pathologies reported in sudden unexpected adult deaths [4].

Sudden Unexpected Death in Epilepsy (SUDEP)

Epilepsy patients are at increased risk of premature mortality [5, 6]. This was first reported by Dr. Sieveking in his book *On Epilepsy and Epileptiform Seizures* in 1861. He stated "...we observed that the greatest mortality from epilepsy in the former case (England) falls in the decennial period from 15 to 25, in the latter (London) from 35 to 45. The greatest general mortality in England and Wales, and in London, respectively, after the first ten years of life, occurs between 65 and 75" [7].

Except a few identifiable causes, such as drowning, internal airway obstruction by a foreign body, overdose, and trauma, the majority of epilepsy-related deaths remain unexplained after postmortem examination. These cases are now classified as sudden unexpected death in epilepsy (SUDEP). The unified SUDEP definition was proposed by Nashef et al. in 2012, as "sudden, unexpected, witnessed or unwitnessed, nontraumatic and non-drowning death in patients with epilepsy, with or without evidence for a seizure and excluding documented status epilepticus, in which postmortem examination does not reveal a toxicologic or anatomic cause of death" [8].

SUDEP is the leading cause of death in young adults with epilepsy, estimated at 1.2 cases per 1000 people with epilepsy per year [9]. Despite the increased interest in research, the SUDEP rate has stayed unchanged in the last few decades (Fig. 4.8). Along with our own experiences, many studies have shown that SUDEP is more common in young adults, with peak ages between 20 and 45 years old [4, 10–13]. There is a significant male predominance in the SUDEP group between 15 and 35 years old when compared with the non-SUDEP epilepsy-related deaths [14]. Majority of these SUDEP decedents are found in the prone position in the bed or on the bedroom floor adjacent to the bed. The deaths usually occur at night and are unwitnessed.

In terms of seizure and epilepsy history, many of those patients have an epilepsy duration of 10 years or longer. Histories of generalized seizures (generalized tonic–clonic seizures or absence seizures) are significantly more common in SUDEP cases when compared with non-SUDEP cases. In epilepsy patients who succumbed to SUDEP, the following are often reported: "poor compliance" to seizure medication, worse seizure control, recent seizure deterioration, or flare. Comorbidities such as hypertension, diabetes, and cardiac disease are less commonly observed in SUDEP patients, partly due to the young age at death.

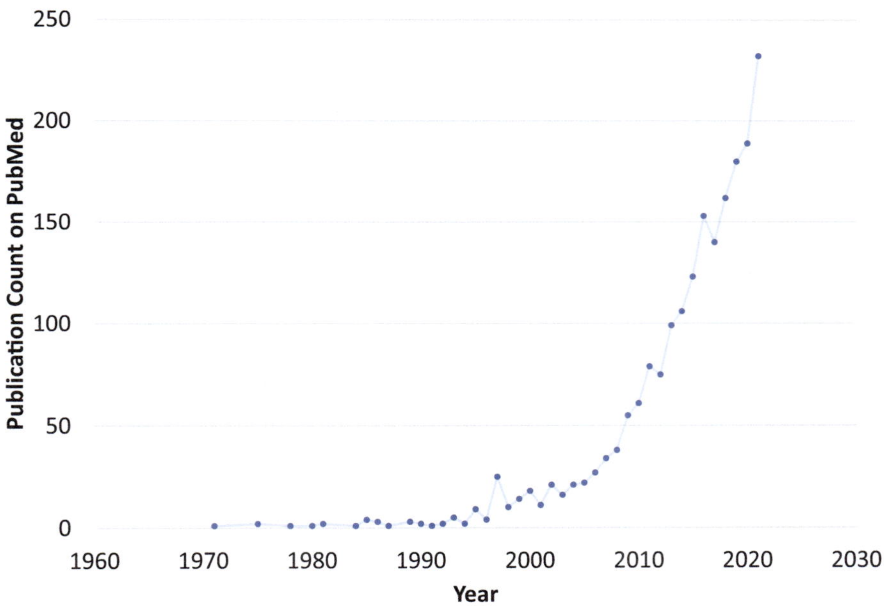

Fig. 4.8 Publications on SUDEP have increased significantly over the last decade

General Autopsy Findings and Toxicology

By definition, SUDEP is a diagnosis of exclusion. A complete autopsy is recommended for all investigations of suspected epilepsy-related death if feasible, including toxicology and Neuropathology consultation [15–17]. In addition to "routine" toxicology testing of illicit substances, antiepileptic drug (AED) concentrations should also be analyzed. Many SUDEP decedents are found to have subtherapeutic levels of AED(s). From our own experiences, multi-drug toxicity was more common than single-drug overdose in non-SUDEP epilepsy-related deaths, including antidepressant medication overdose, such as amitriptyline [14].

For most epilepsy-related death investigations, despite a comprehensive external and internal examination, there are often no structural findings identified at autopsy. Special attention, however, should be given to potential injuries sustained from recent seizures. Although not diagnostic, bite marks of the tongue and buccal mucosa are reported in 17–33% of these cases, suggestive of recent seizures [4, 14]. Other organ systems, such as respiratory and cardiovascular systems, should also be examined with special care. Pulmonary edema, bronchopneumonia, gastric contents in the airway, and evidence of drowning (overdistended lungs) are all previously reported in epilepsy-related deaths. Coronary artery disease, cardiomegaly, and myocardial infarct are also reported. Some of these findings might be significant and should be considered as competing causes of death with SUDEP (see section "Comorbidities and Competing Cause of Death"). Cardiac channelopathies are known to share similar genetic alterations of epilepsy. Genetic testing should be considered in suspected cases (see section "Molecular Pathology").

Neuropathology

For all epilepsy-related death investigations, the brain should be examined by a neuropathologist when possible. The goal of the neuropathological examination is threefold: (1) to identify potential epileptogenic lesions, (2) to document brain injuries secondary to repetitive seizures, and (3) to exclude other competing causes of death. Whole brain examination by neuropathologist(s) after formalin fixation is recommended by both the Royal College of Pathologists (the United Kingdom) and the National Association of Medical Examiners (the United States) as the "best practice" [17, 18]. However, it is recognized that this option is not always possible due to limited resources and local restrictions on organ retention.

The second option involves examining the unfixed brain in the autopsy room by a neuropathologist or forensic pathologist. The brain will be sectioned "freshly" and selected brain slices are submitted for formalin fixation and further neuropathology examination. However, this approach of slicing "fresh" brain is prone to introducing both macro- and microscopic artifacts and is considered suboptimal by many pathologists [19]. An audit of pathology practice conducted by Dr. Maria Thom and colleagues demonstrated that, for epilepsy-related death investigation, examination of fixed whole brain had a significantly higher yield in detecting relevant pathology [12].

When examining the brain, there are lesions more readily identifiable, such as tumor, abscess/infection, trauma, or vascular malformation. Other lesions, however, are subtler and require specialized training, further microscopic examination, and ancillary work-ups. These include mild hippocampal sclerosis, hippocampal malrotation, granule cell dispersion, focal cortical dysplasia, polymicrogyria, leukomalacia, and so on. Therefore, a systemic approach to examine, document, and sample all essential regions is needed for autopsies of suspected epilepsy-related death. We suggest the following:

- Any neuroimaging studies should be reviewed prior to autopsy.
- The scalp and skull should be carefully examined, for bruises or fractures possibly obtained from a recent seizure.
- Dura and leptomeninges should be examined for signs of acute or chronic hemorrhage, infection, and venous sinus thrombosis.
- The arrangement of the circle of Willis and its major branches should be examined to rule out any vascular pathology.
- Examine the external surface of the brain, for any signs of cerebral edema, focal discolorations, areas of acute/chronic hemorrhages, contusions, surgical cavities, infarcts, tumors, or vascular malformations. Brain edema in SUDEP is usually mild, where the brain appears "full" with flattening of gyri surface and effacement of the sulci. Rarely brain herniation (uncal, subfalcine, tonsillar, or diencephalon herniation) is encountered.
- Ideally, the whole brain should be fixed in formalin for at least 2 weeks and further examined by a neuropathologist at "brain cutting."
- If whole brain retention is not available, the "fresh" brain should be sliced systematically. It is well recognized that sectioning the unfixed brain, particularly the cerebral hemispheres, is technically challenging. We recommend cutting the cerebral hemispheres into "thick slices" (2–3 cm) instead of the thin 1-cm slices. Thick slides will allow neuropathologists to perform further section after formalin fixation.

  - The cerebral hemispheres are cut into 2–3 cm thick slices along the coronal plane.
  - The brainstem is separated from the cerebellum and cut into 1–2 cm slices in the horizontal plane.
  - The cerebellum is cut into 1–2 cm thick slices along the parasagittal plane.
  - All brain slices are laid out, examined, and photographed.
  - Selected brain slices are submitted for formalin fixation and subsequent neuropathology referral. In addition to any focal lesions identified on fresh brain slices, the essential slices to be submitted include coronal slices of the cerebral hemispheres at the level of anterior basal ganglia, mammillary body, amygdala, hippocampus, and calcarine; horizontal slices of the brain stem including midbrain, caudal and rostral pons, caudal and rostral medulla; and

parasagittal slices of the cerebellum including the vermis and dentate nuclei (Fig. 4.9).
- The formalin-fixed brain slices are further examined and photographed by a neuropathologist.

It is true that a substantial amount of epilepsy-related death has no identifiable structural abnormalities in the brain. Therefore, a misconception is that neuropathology examination is often non-contributory to the cause of death and is not necessary. We believe, on the contrary, that because of the subtlety of many potential seizure-related abnormalities, a thorough, rigorous, systemic examination of the whole brain or brain slices is essential in these investigations. It was shown that when the examinations were performed on fixed whole brain by neuropathologists, only 11% of the cases were "neuropathology-negative" in the setting of the epilepsy-related death investigation [12].

The techniques involved in examining fixed whole brain or brain slices are well described elsewhere. We cut the whole brain, or further section the "thick" brain slices, into 1-cm slices and layout slices for inspection and photograph. In general,

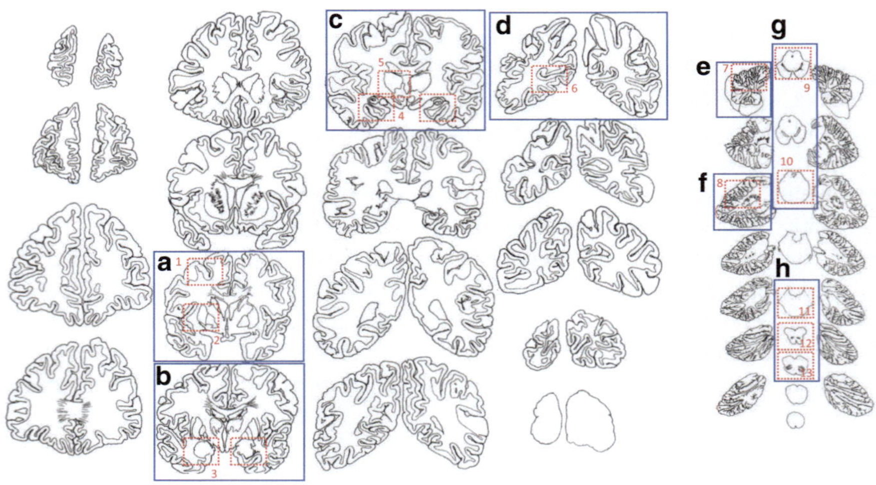

Fig. 4.9 Brain slices selected for further neuropathology examination (blue boxes), and sections submitted for microscopic examination (red boxes) for suspected SUDEP cases (in addition to any grossly identifiable lesions). Blue boxes: coronal sections of the cerebral hemispheres at the level of (**a**) anterior basal ganglia, (**b**) mammillary body, (**c**) hippocampus and lateral geniculate, and (**d**) calcarine; (**e**, **f**) parasagittal slices of the cerebellum; (**g**, **h**) horizontal slices of the brain stem including midbrain, pons, medulla. Red boxes: (1) anterior watershed, (2) basal ganglia with insula, (3) bilateral amygdala, (4) bilateral hippocampi, (5) thalamus, (6) posterior watershed, (7) cerebellar vermis, (8) cerebellum with dentate, (9) midbrain, (10) rostral pons, (11) caudal pons, (12) rostral medulla, and (13) caudal medulla

the cerebral hemispheres are sectioned into 1-cm-thick coronal sections, the brainstem into 0.5-cm-thick horizontal sections, and the cerebellum into 0.5-cm-thick parasagittal sections. Macroscopic abnormalities are documented on the diagram and photographed, such as acute/chronic contusions, hemorrhages, vascular malformations, cerebral infarct, abscess, or tumors. Special attention is drawn to the mesial temporal structures, for subtle hippocampal sclerosis or malformation (Fig. 4.10a–c).

The following regions are recommended for microscopic examination: any grossly identifiable lesions, bilateral hippocampi, bilateral amygdala, anterior and posterior watershed areas, basal ganglia with insula cortex, thalamus, representative cerebral cortex (frontal and temporal lobes), cerebellum (vermis and hemisphere with dentate), midbrain, pons (rostral and caudal), and medulla (rostral and caudal) (Fig. 4.10).

The common neuropathology abnormalities encountered in the setting of seizure-related death are listed here, organized by anatomical regions (Table 4.2). The morphological features of these entities are described in various neuropathology articles and textbooks and are beyond the scope of this chapter.

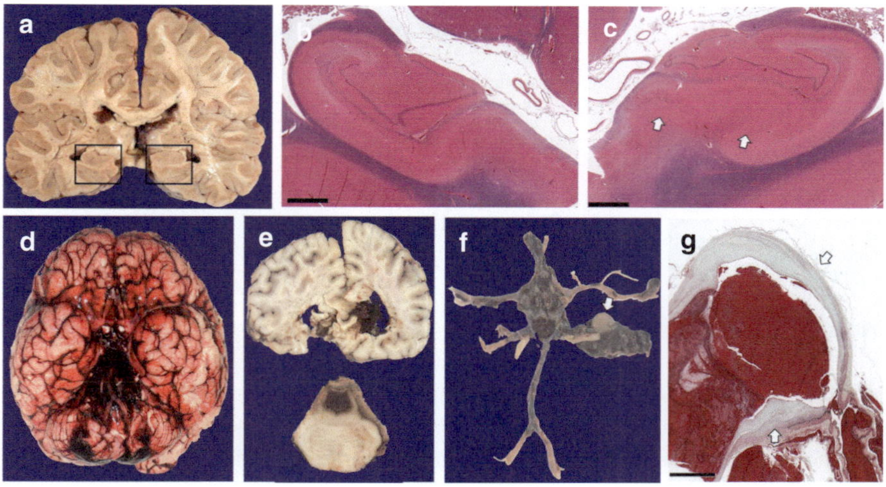

Fig. 4.10 (**a–c**) Subtle hippocampal malformation in a 2-year-old boy, who had an SCN1B gene mutation and died of SUDEP. Gross image of the coronal section at the level of pulvinar shows asymmetrical hippocampi (boxes in **a**). The left hippocampus is relatively normal (**b**). There is hyperconvoluted CA1 and subiculum of the right hippocampus (arrows in **c**). (**d–g**) A previously healthy 12-year-old girl presented with sudden onset headache and seizure and died shortly. There is massive acute subarachnoid hemorrhage on the brainstem, basal cistern, and cerebellum, extending into the ventricles (**d, e**). A saccular aneurysm is present on the right posterior cerebral artery (arrow in **f**). The vascular wall at the aneurysm is abnormally thickened, composed of endothelium and loose fibrotic connective tissue, but lacks internal elastic lamina and tunica media (arrows in **g**, Movat special stain). Scale bar: 2 mm in (**b, c,** and **g**)

Table 4.2 Common neuropathology findings in seizure-related death

Anatomical locations	Common pathology findings	References
Cerebral cortex and white matter	Cortical malformations Focal cortical dysplasia Grey matter heterotopia Polymicrogyria, ulegyria, periventricular leukomalacia, and other encephaloclastic lesions Tumors Gliomas (astrocytoma, oligodendroglioma, etc.) Glioneuronal tumors Meningioma Metastasis, etc. Vascular malformation Hypoxic ischemic injury Cortical contusions Surgical scars Old infarct Encephalitis	[12, 13]
Hippocampus and amygdala	Hippocampal sclerosis Hippocampal malformation Hippocampal asymmetry or malrotation Granule cell dispersion, bilamination, hyper-convolution, or agenesis Subiculum folding Amygdala sclerosis	[12, 13, 20, 21]
Basal ganglia and thalamus	Status marmoratus Gliosis or hypoxic ischemic changes	
Brain stem	Inferior olivary nuclei dysplasia/hypoplasia Medullary arcuate nuclei dysgenesis	[12, 13]
Cerebellum	Vermis atrophy and Purkinje cell dropout	[12, 13]

Molecular Pathology

Unlikely the well-established genetic mutation panel for sudden cardiac death investigation (cardiac channelopathy or cardiomyopathy), there are no pathogenic mutations for "SUDEP." Recent studies have identified overlapping genetic alterations in both conditions. The most frequently shared variants are the genes involved in sodium/potassium ion channel subunits and arrhythmia (familial long QT syndrome, Brugada syndrome, arrhythmogenic ventricular dysplasia, etc.). The commonly identified mutations in this group include KCNQ1, KCNH2, SCN5a, RYR2, HCN1, HCN2, and HCN4. The second group of mutations encountered in SUDEP investigations are primarily epilepsy-related, including SCN1A (Dravet syndrome), SCN2A/SCN8A (epileptic encephalopathy), and DEPDC5. Finally, chromosomal alterations, particularly chromosome 15 (isodicentric, tricentric, or triplication of chromosome 15), are also identified in epilepsy-related death. A more comprehensive list of genetic mutations can be found in many recent publications [15, 22–25].

There is no guideline on when genetic testing should be conducted for potential SUDEP cases. We suggest genetic testing for sudden epilepsy-related death when:

(1) no causes of death identified, (2) there is a strong family history, or heritable/genetic causes suspected, and (3) early onset epilepsy without known history of trauma, tumor, infection, or surgery. In addition, terminal seizures and seizures secondary to alcohol withdrawn are not indicated for genetic testing. Fresh postmortem blood or two cores of fresh tissue from the heart or kidney should be reserved for DNA extraction and sequencing.

Comorbidities and Competing Cause of Death

Diagnosis of SUDEP is often complicated by competing causes of death. For instance, a 52-year-old male with a history of poorly controlled epilepsy found dead in bed. Postmortem examination revealed moderate to severe coronary atherosclerosis with 80% luminal occlusion in the left anterior descending coronary artery. There is no evidence of acute or chronic myocardial infarct and no signs of convulsive seizures. It is almost impossible for the pathologist to distinguish cardiac arrhythmia triggered by coronary artery disease or seizures.

Recently updated classification and diagnosis criteria are proposed to capture all SUDEP cases and to solve these ambiguities [26, 27]. In brief, SUDEP cases are divided into three groups: (1) definite SUDEP, when all investigation and complete postmortem examination (including toxicology) reveal no other cause of death; (2) probable SUDEP, when criteria for definite SUDEP are met but no or limited autopsy (external examination only, extensive decomposition, etc.) is performed; and (3) possible SUDEP, when there is competing cause of death. In addition, when there is comorbidity and death may be attributed to the combination of both, a case is classified as SUDEP Plus (either definite or probable SUDEP Plus). Based on this updated classification, possible SUDEP will be the best immediate cause of death for this 52-year-old male.

Similarly, epilepsy patients with cardiomegaly, remote myocardial infarct or cardiac fibrosis, long QT syndrome, and focal bronchopneumonia could also be grouped into this possible SUDEP category. Pathologists should always take the case scenarios into consideration and weigh the probabilities of either seizure or other cause of death.

Intracranial Hemorrhage (Nontraumatic)

Intracranial hemorrhages are classified based on anatomic location, namely, epidural, subdural, subarachnoid, intraparenchymal, and intraventricular hemorrhages. Oftentimes intracranial bleeding occurs at one location and rapidly extends into more intracranial compartments. Epidural hemorrhages are almost inevitably caused by traumatic head injury, so this is true for most acute subdural hemorrhages. Acute subarachnoid or intraparenchymal hemorrhages, on the contrary, could occur spontaneously in an otherwise asymptomatic individual and cause sudden unexpected death.

Nontraumatic Subarachnoid Hemorrhage

Subarachnoid hemorrhages (SAH) are defined as extravasation of blood in space between the arachnoid and the pia membrane, which could be secondary to a head trauma or occur spontaneously. Nontraumatic rupture of cerebral berry aneurysms accounts for majority of the fatal spontaneous SAH. This is more common in sudden death of young to middle-aged adults, with a slight female predominance (41% in males versus 59% in females) [28, 29]. Other causes of spontaneous SAH include infective aneurysm, arteriovenous malformation, and cerebral amyloid angiopathy. The latter is also commonly associated with intraparenchymal hemorrhages (see below).

Although the pathogenesis is not entirely clear, berry aneurysms are considered "congenital lesions." However, they are rarely encountered in pediatric population. It is postulated that a defect of the vascular wall exists at birth, which develops into an outpouching (aneurysm) over years when there is increased blood pressure in later life. The rupture of a berry aneurysm is often preceded by physical or emotional exertions, such as heavy lifting, bending, coughing, urinating/defecating, sexual intercourse, or emotional stress. A substantial amount of these cases, however, occurred during sleep without any documented external events [28, 29].

At the time of autopsy, massive acute subarachnoid blood is typically present at the base of the brain, covering the cerebral and cerebellar surface, the brainstem, and the basal cistern. When the aneurysm is embedded within the brain parenchyma (e.g., at the bifurcation of anterior cerebral and anterior communicating arteries), acute SAH might be minimal. In these situations, high-pressure arterial blood from the rupture site may dissect through the brain parenchyma, resulting in intraparenchymal and/or intraventricular hemorrhages instead, sometimes mimicking hypertensive bleeding.

When cerebral aneurysm rupture is suspected, the pathologist should take all effort to locate the aneurysm and potential rupture site(s) at the time of autopsy, but not defer to the brain cutting after formalin fixation. Blunt dissection should be performed while the fresh blood is gently washed away. Majority of the aneurysms are at the anterior circulation, usually at the bifurcation of major branches of the circle of Willis. In about 20% of the cases, the aneurysms are on the basilar artery. Microscopically, the aneurysm is best demonstrated with an elastic stain, with attenuation of the blood vessel wall and disruption of the elastic lamina and muscularis (Fig. 4.10d–g).

Intraparenchymal Hemorrhages

In contrast to the asymptomatic younger patients seen in acute SAH, intraparenchymal hemorrhages often occur in older individuals with a history of hypertension. The bleeding commonly originates from the basal ganglia, followed by pons, thalamus, cerebellum, and cerebral white matter. In more than three-quarters of these cases, the acute hemorrhages spread into the ventricle, the subarachnoid, and occasionally subdural spaces. Cerebral edema and subsequent herniations often develop shortly after the hemorrhage. The fatality rate of acute intraparenchymal hemorrhages is high, with about 90% of the patients dying within 3 days of the bleeding [30]. Histologically, acute blood is usually seen beyond the site of origin. Hypertensive microangiopathy, in the forms of hyaline arteriosclerosis, Charcot-Bouchard microaneurysm, and expanded perivascular space, is evident. Hemosiderin-laden macrophages are also commonly seen adjacent to the small arterioles, indicating chronic bleeding.

Cerebral amyloid angiopathy (CAA) is the second most common cause of non-traumatic intraparenchymal hemorrhage. Because of the close association with Alzheimer's disease, CAA is usually seen in older individuals with a clinical history of cognitive decline or dementia. Hemorrhages caused by CAA are usually superficial, involving both cerebral cortex and leptomeninges (lobar hemorrhage), which could extend into the deep white matter. Under the microscope, the blood vessels involved usually have a "double barrel" appearance. The blood vessel wall contains eosinophilic amorphous material (amyloid), giving rise to the "rigid" appearance of the vessel. The amyloid can be readily identified by Congo red special stain or immunohistochemistry with an antibody to beta-amyloid.

Acute intraparenchymal hemorrhages rarely occur in younger individuals. This can be caused by the rupture of a vascular malformation, secondary to blood dyscrasias, sickle cell anemia, or other underlying coagulopathies. Although not considered "natural death," drug abuse, particularly cocaine, MDMA, and amphetamines misuse, is associated with acute intraparenchymal hemorrhage, often in younger individuals. The bleeding is believed to be secondary to a rapid increase in blood pressure, with or without preceding vasculitis, resembling hypertensive bleeding.

Sudden Death in Other CNS Disorders

Essentially all sudden unexpected deaths can be attributed to fatal cardiac arrhythmia, as a consequence of various cardiac or noncardiac conditions. Primary sudden cardiac death is well reported, including coronary artery diseases, cardiomyopathies, and arrhythmogenic disorders (long QT syndrome, Brugada syndrome, etc.). Lesions that disrupt the central autonomic control and subsequently lead to autonomic imbalance and cardiac arrhythmias, however, are underrecognized. In this section, we will discuss CNS lesions located in crucial central autonomic regions, that have increased risk of sudden unexpected death.

Multiple system atrophy (MSA) and Parkinson's disease (PD) are both neurodegenerative disorders characterized by abnormal accumulation of alpha-synuclein protein in neurons and glial cells. Autonomic dysfunction is frequently present for both MSA and PD, including orthostatic hypotension, cardiac arrhythmia, supine hypertension, constipation, and sexual dysfunction. Oftentimes the dysautonomia manifestations proceed to the motor symptoms in PD patients. Sudden death is the leading cause of death in MSA patients, which frequently occurs during sleep [31]. The sudden death rate in PD patients is variable, ranging from 5.3% to 43.7% of the cases [32]. The mechanisms of the sudden death in these synucleinopathies are not well understood. Laryngeal stridor and obstruction of the upper airway were previously proposed as causes of death for MSA patients. However, sudden death is not prevented even with patients who underwent tracheostomy [31]. Recently, impaired autonomic respiratory function and cardiovascular dysfunction are shown to be independent risk factors for sudden death in MSA patients [33]. In fact, Tada et al. demonstrated a marked depletion of catecholaminergic and serotonergic neurons in both spinal intermediolateral column and medulla in patients with MSA who succumbed to sudden death [34].

The pathological findings of MSA and PD are well described in the other textbooks and literature. In short, pathologists will find the characteristic pale substantia nigra and locus coeruleus in the brains of PD patients. Severe putamen atrophy and dark discoloration are often observed in MSA. However, depending on the regions involved, variable degrees of striatonigral degeneration (SND) and olivopontocerebellar atrophy (OPCA) are observed, reflecting the clinical presentation. Microscopically, in addition to the neuronal loss and gliosis, alpha-synuclein positive neuronal inclusions (Lewy bodies), dystrophic neurites (Lewy neurites), and glial cytoplasmic inclusions (GCI) can be easily identified with immunohistochemistry.

As described in MSA, **lesions involving medulla**, particularly the ventrolateral nuclear groups (pre-Bötzinger complex, preBötC) and raphe nuclei, disrupt the central regulation of cardiac and respiratory rhythm and may result in sudden death. Unexpected sudden deaths in patients with medullary brain lesions are reviewed by Jaster et al. [35]. These lesions include a wide range of neuropathologies, ranging from multiple sclerosis, infection/inflammation, hemorrhage, infarct, and tumor. Of the 9/50 cases (18%) of unexpected death in multiple sclerosis patients reported by Riudavets et al., the causes of death are attributed to demyelinating lesions involving the medulla and other central autonomic centers [36]. Chronic inactive MS was most common in these cases, with well-demarcated demyelination plaques in various brain regions, including the brainstem. Chronic active or active plaques are also seen in some cases, showing myelin loss, axonal injury, and lymphohistiocytic infiltrate.

Sudden death can also be induced by an ischemic infarct, particularly an **infarct involving the insular cortex**, with presumed autonomic disruption [37]. Although rare, rapid increase of intracranial pressure is well cited for its association with sudden unexpected death. **Intraventricular tumors**, such as colloid cyst of the third ventricle or intraventricular pilocytic astrocytoma, may occlude the foramina of Monro and lead to acute obstructive hydrocephalus, subsequent deterioration, and sudden demise [38]. Microscopically, the cyst is lined by a single layer of columnar or cuboidal epithelium with endodermal differentiation, often ciliated, mucinous, or with a goblet cell appearance. Occasionally cystic apoplexy with associated hemorrhage could also be seen.

Closing Remarks

A few more issues to consider when formulating your clinicopathological opinion within your autopsy report are as follows:

(a) Did the individual die "of" or die "with" a given disease entity? This may need to be clearly spelled out for stakeholders and families and depends on the nature of the case.
(b) How confident can you be in the results? Be explicit. Typically, your degree of confidence is not an opinion that can generally be expressed by a number (e.g., 80% confidence) but stated in relative terms. It is not uncommon that others will read into your opinion a degree of confidence that you yourself may not share, so keep this in mind when formulating your clinicopathological opinions. Thus, the avoidance of speculative comments. It is very important that you consider your audience and how your report might be utilized in the future (e.g., court and investigatory boards). Remember that it is not a failure on the part of the autopsy pathologist if a precise answer to questions posed at autopsy cannot be ascertained; there is only so much information this examination can provide.
(c) As already noted, do not speculate if possible or be clear that you are speculating if you do so and be clear when providing a differential diagnosis how far you can go when outlining your findings. Be wary of phrases such as "consistent with," as non-pathologists may interpret these phrases as indicating a level of certainty in a particular entity that you do not share.
(d) Integration of all information about the death may be needed for ultimate opinion synthesis, but be clear about where your sources of information arise, especially if there are non-pathological findings that influence your interpretations.
(e) Utilize the literature base and critically evaluate what you cite (i.e., evidence-based). Remember that obtaining pathological data and applying reason from within the body of knowledge we recognize as autopsy pathology specifically and medicine in general are what you as a pathologist can add to the investigation. Just be clear about your thought processes.
(f) Many adopt a principle of parsimony (sometimes thought of as Occam's razor) where the simplest explanation that fits the results is the one best chosen. This is likely correct much of the time, but keep in mind that, for some cases, there is more complexity than the autopsy alone can tell you about. Always question what information you do not know about and how such knowledge might affect your opinions (or not).

The quality of the information available to the pathologist when formulating their clinicopathological correlation is entirely dependent on the quality of the clinical information available to the pathologist and the skill in performing an autopsy. In many instances, non-pathologists implicitly assume the fallacy that "all is revealed" when the body is open. But by the same token, pathologists must be willing to dig for the information they require and not just rely on what is available in the immediate clinical record. Communicating with clinical colleagues or hosting case conferences with family and other investigators can be very fruitful and allow the pathologist a clear forum to clearly communicate their findings and manage expectations for what an autopsy can and cannot deliver.

References

1. WHO fact sheet. https://www.who.int/news-room/fact-sheets/detail/the-top-10-causes-of-death.
2. https://www.ncbi.nlm.nih.gov/books/NBK542273/
3. Oehmichen M, Auer RN, König HG. Forensic neuropathology and associated neurology. Berlin: Springer; 2006, 526 p.
4. Black M, Graham DI. Sudden unexplained death in adults caused by intracranial pathology. J Clin Pathol. 2002;55(1):44–50.
5. Devinsky O, Singh A, Friedman D. Deaths in epilepsy what we are missing. JAMA Neurol. 2018;75:1–3.
6. Gorton HC, Webb RT, Carr MJ, DelPozo-Banos M, John A, Ashcroft DM. Risk of unnatural mortality in people with epilepsy. JAMA Neurol. 2018:1–10. Available from: http://archneur.jamanetwork.com/article.aspx?doi=10.1001/jamaneurol.2018.0333.
7. Sieveking EH. On epilepsy and epileptiform seizures: their causes, pathology and treatment. London: Churchill; 1861, 69 p.
8. Nashef L, So EL, Ryvlin P, Tomson T. Unifying the definitions of sudden unexpected death in epilepsy. Epilepsia. 2012;53(2):227–33.
9. Harden C, Tomson T, Gloss D, Buchhalter J, Cross JH, Donner E, et al. Practice guideline summary: sudden unexpected death in epilepsy incidence rates and risk factors: report of the guideline development, dissemination, and implementation subcommittee of the American Academy of Neurology and the American Epilepsy Society. Neurology. 2017;88(17):1674–80.
10. Shields LBE, Hunsaker DM, Hunsaker JC III, Parker JC Jr. Sudden unexpected death in epilepsy: neuropathologic findings. Am J Forensic Med Pathol. 2002;23(4):307–14.
11. Zhuo L, Zhang Y, Zielke HR, Levine B, Zhang X, Chang L, et al. Sudden unexpected death in epilepsy: evaluation of forensic autopsy cases. Forensic Sci Int. 2012;223(1–3):171–5.
12. Thom M, Michalak Z, Wright G, Dawson T, Hilton D, Joshi A, et al. Audit of practice in sudden unexpected death in epilepsy (SUDEP) post mortems and neuropathological findings. Neuropathol Appl Neurobiol. 2016;42(5):463–76.
13. Leitner DF, Faustin A, Verducci C, Friedman D, William C, Devore S, et al. Neuropathology in the North American sudden unexpected death in epilepsy registry. Brain Commun. 2021;3(3):fcab192.
14. Zhang Q, Suller-Marti A, Ding JJ, Deng G, He W, Burneo JG, et al. Epilepsy-associated death in the southwestern Ontario: a clinicopathological correlation study. Brain Pathol. 2022;33:e13121. Available from: https://onlinelibrary.wiley.com/doi/10.1111/bpa.13121.
15. Thom M, Boldrini M, Bundock E, Sheppard MN, Devinsky O. Review: the past, present and future challenges in epilepsy-related and sudden deaths and biobanking. Neuropathol Appl Neurobiol. 2018;44(1):32–55.
16. Hanna NJ, Black M, Sander JW, Smithson WH, Appleton R, Brown S, Fish D. National sentinel clinical audit of epilepsy-related death report 2002. 2002. Available from: https://sudep.org/sites/default/files/national-sentinel-clinical-audit-of-epilepsy-related-death-2002-summary.pdf.

17. Middleton OL, Atherton DS, Bundock EA, Donner E, Friedman D, Hesdorffer DC, et al. National association of medical examiners position paper: recommendations for the investigation and certification of deaths in people with epilepsy. Acad Forensic Pathol. 2018;8:119–35.
18. Thom M. Guidelines on autopsy practice: deaths in patients with epilepsy including sudden deaths unique document number G175 document name guidelines on autopsy practice. 2019. Available from: https://www.rcpath.org/uploads/assets/15a26420-ce7b-4858-ad538b210328d973/G175-Guidelines-on-autopsy-practice-Deaths-in-patients-with-epilepsy-including-sudden-deaths.pdf.
19. Hammond R, Dunham C, McFadden D, Del Bigio M, Perez-Rosendahl M, Vinters HV. Postmortem examination of the nervous system: fresh vs fixed. Can J Neurol Sci. 2021;49:583.
20. Hefti MM, Cryan JB, Haas EA, Chadwick AE, Crandall LA, Trachtenberg FL, et al. Hippocampal malformation associated with sudden death in early childhood: a neuropathologic study: part 2 of the investigations of The San Diego SUDC Research Project. Forensic Sci Med Pathol. 2016;12(1):14–25.
21. Kinney HC, Poduri AH, Cryan JB, Haynes RL, Teot L, Sleeper LA, et al. Hippocampal formation maldevelopment and sudden unexpected death across the pediatric age spectrum. J Neuropathol Exp Neurol. 2016 [cited 2021 Jul 16]. Available from: https://academic.oup.com/jnen/article/75/10/981/2614387.
22. Coll M, Allegue C, Partemi S, Mates J, Del Olmo B, Campuzano O, et al. Genetic investigation of sudden unexpected death in epilepsy cohort by panel target resequencing. Int J Legal Med. 2016;130(2):331.
23. Anwar Chahal CA, Salloum MN, Alahdab F, Gottwald JA, Tester DJ, Anwer LA, et al. Systematic review of the genetics of sudden unexpected death in epilepsy: potential overlap with sudden cardiac death and arrhythmia-related genes. J Am Heart Assoc. 2020 [cited 2020 Nov 10]. Available from: https://www.ahajournals.org/doi/suppl/10.1161/JAHA.119.012264.
24. Bagnall RD, Crompton DE, Semsarian C. Genetic basis of sudden unexpected death in epilepsy. Front Neurol. 2017;8:348.
25. Tu E, Bagnall RD, Duflou J, Semsarian C. Post-mortem review and genetic analysis of sudden unexpected death in epilepsy (SUDEP) cases. Brain Pathol. 2011;21(2):201–8 [cited 2019 Apr 30]. Available from: http://doi.wiley.com/10.1111/j.1750-3639.2010.00438.x.
26. Nashef L, So EL, Ryvlin P, Tomson T. Unifying the definitions of sudden unexpected death in epilepsy. Epilepsia. 2012;53(2):227–33 [cited 2018 Jun 27]. Available from: http://doi.wiley.com/10.1111/j.1528-1167.2011.03358.x.
27. Devinsky O, Bundock E, Hesdorffer D, Donner E, Moseley B, Cihan E, et al. Resolving ambiguities in SUDEP classification. Epilepsia. 2018;59(6):1220–33.
28. Locksley HB. Natural history of subarachnoid hemorrhage, intracranial aneurysms and arteriovenous malformations. J Neurosurg. 1966;25(3):321–68.
29. Zacharia BE, Hickman ZL, Grobelny BT, DeRosa P, Kotchetkov I, Ducruet AF, et al. Epidemiology of aneurysmal subarachnoid hemorrhage. Neurosurg Clin N Am. 2010;21(2):221–33.
30. Leestma JE. Forensic neuropathology. 2nd ed. CRC Press; 2008, 97 p.
31. Shimohata T, Ozawa T, Nakayama H, Tomita M, Shinoda H, Nishizawa M. Frequency of nocturnal sudden death in patients with multiple system atrophy. J Neurol. 2008;255(10):1483–5.
32. Scorza FA, Guimarães-Marques M, Nejm M, de Almeida ACG, Scorza CA, Fiorini AC, et al. Sudden unexpected death in Parkinson's disease: insights from clinical practice. Clinics (Sao Paulo). 2022;77:100001.
33. O'Sullivan SS, Massey LA, Williams DR, Silveira-Moriyama L, Kempster PA, Holton JL, et al. Clinical outcomes of progressive supranuclear palsy and multiple system atrophy. Brain. 2008;131(Pt 5):1362–72.
34. Tada M, Kakita A, Toyoshima Y, Onodera O, Ozawa T, Morita T, et al. Depletion of medullary serotonergic neurons in patients with multiple system atrophy who succumbed to sudden death. Brain. 2009;132(7):1810–9.

35. Jaster JH, Ottaviani G, Matturri L, Lavezzi AM, Zamecnik J, Smith TW. Sudden unexpected death related to medullary brain lesions. Am J Forensic Med Pathol. 2008;29(4):371.
36. Riudavets MA, Colegial C, Rubio A, Fowler D, Pardo C, Troncoso JC. Causes of unexpected death in patients with multiple sclerosis. Am J Forensic Med Pathol. 2005;26(3):244.
37. Sörös P, Hachinski V, Sörös P, Hachinski V. Cardiovascular and neurological causes of sudden death after ischaemic stroke. Clin Neurol Sci 2012;11 [cited 2021 Jun 17]. Available from: http://www.qtdrugs.org.
38. Lagman C, Rai K, Chung LK, Nagasawa DT, Beckett JS, Tucker AM, et al. Fatal colloid cysts: a systematic review. World Neurosurg. 2017;107:409–15.

Chapter 5
Drug-Related Deaths

Karen Woodall

Introduction

A major role of a forensic toxicologist is to provide testing and interpretation of laboratory findings to assist pathologists, medical examiners and coroners in establishing whether alcohol, drugs and poisons may have played a role in the cause and/or manner of death. In many cases where there is a suspected drug overdose, toxicology testing may be able to provide identification and quantification of the drug(s) that contributed to or were the sole cause of death. Toxicologic investigations are also important even if the cause of death has already been established. In a motor vehicle fatality, drug and alcohol testing may be performed to provide information on whether impairment was a factor in the collision. In homicide investigations, the presence of a psychoactive substance may be an important issue for the investigation or during a trial. For example, if the decedent exhibited bizarre behaviour the behaviour could be attributed to drug-induced psychosis or the use of hallucinations. Deaths due to natural causes may also require toxicology testing such as acetone and beta-hydroxybutyrate in cases of ketoacidosis.

In many types of death investigations, the interpretation of toxicological results requires a thorough knowledge regarding the pharmacology of drugs and, if available, references of therapeutic, toxic or lethal drug concentrations may be a useful guide. In forensic toxicology, it is important to note that there are some important differences between data obtained from clinical studies, and therefore antemortem samples, when compared with data from postmortem samples. The interpretation of toxicological results obtained from autopsy samples requires a thorough knowledge regarding the challenges and pitfalls associated with postmortem toxicology. There are many challenges for forensic toxicologists including the ability to detect and

K. Woodall (✉)
University of Toronto, Mississauga, ON, Canada

R. Jacques (ed.), *Forensic Pathology*,
https://doi.org/10.1007/978-3-031-42038-2_5

quantitate drugs and also the interpretation of any drug findings. Some major factors that are important to consider when assessing toxicology results are shown in Fig. 5.1.

Collaboration between a pathologist and a toxicologist is essential to ensure that appropriate samples are collected at autopsy and applicable testing is performed. The final toxicology report should provide essential information for a pathologist/medical examiner and coroner who will use the results in the context of the autopsy findings and case history. Good communication with the toxicology laboratory is important to ensure information about drugs that can be reliably detected during routine analysis is accurate and information about postmortem changes has been highlighted.

The following chapter discusses some important areas of forensic toxicology: sample collection, analytical testing and interpretations of results. In addition, information regarding current issues in toxicology, novel psychoactive substance (NPS) and the opioid crisis has been included.

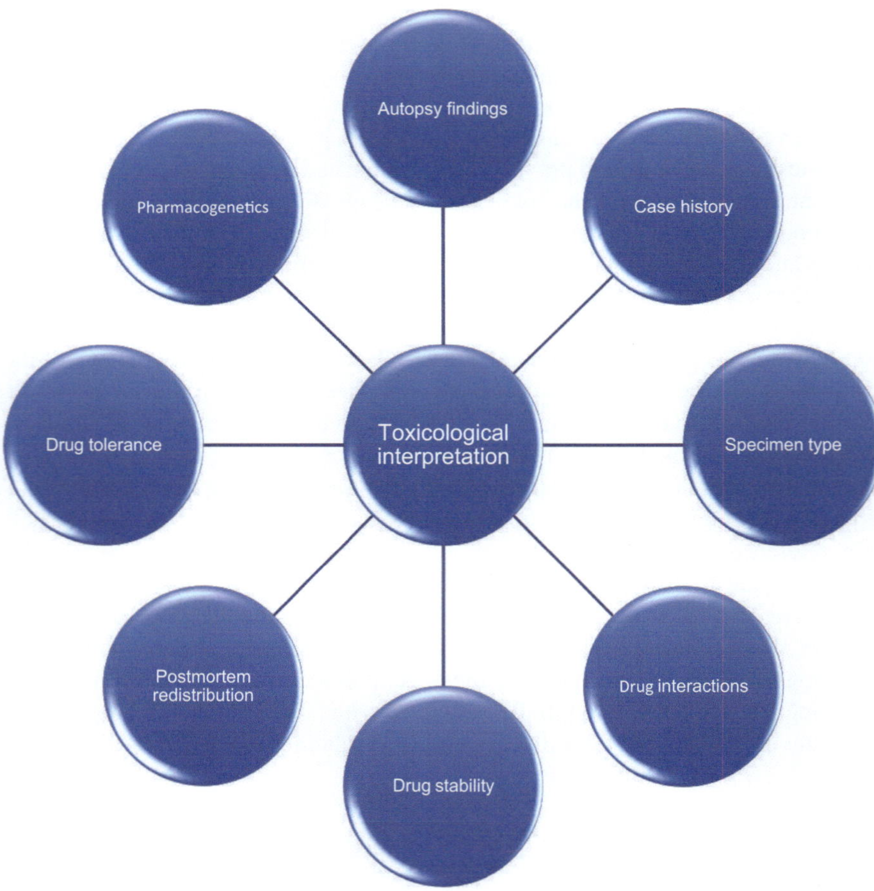

Fig. 5.1 Factors that should be considered when interpreting postmortem drug findings

History, Scene and Autopsy Findings

Indications that can direct the pathologist of a possible drug-related death include the history, scene and autopsy findings. A past medical history of drug use or a hospital urine drug screen can indicate that intoxication may have had a role in the individual's death. At the scene, there may be evidence of drug paraphernalia and rarely drugs (Fig. 5.2). These can include syringes, spoons, pipes, pieces of aluminium foil, and aluminium cans. The drugs can have a variety of appearances (Fig. 5.3). Suspected drugs should be documented and transferred into the custody of the police. During the autopsy, examination of the personal effects/belongings may also reveal drug paraphernalia and drugs. The drugs can be observed in a

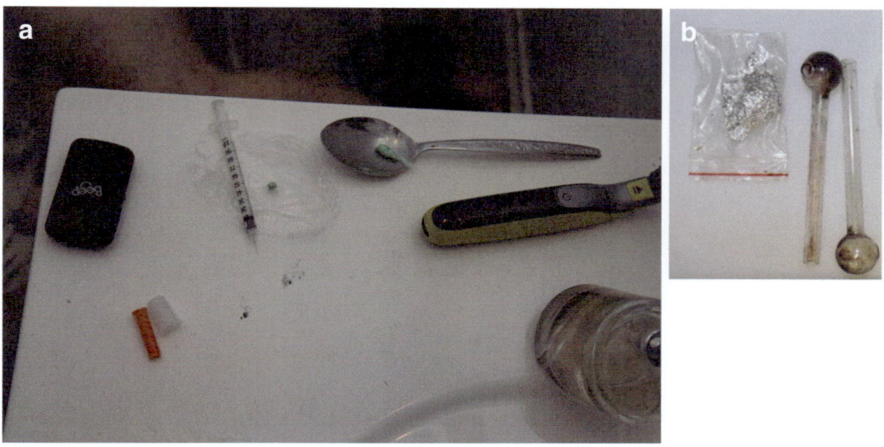

Fig. 5.2 Scene image showing suspected drugs and drug paraphernalia. (**a**) Suspected drugs on the spoon and syringe. (**b**) Glass pipe and suspected drugs in aluminium foil

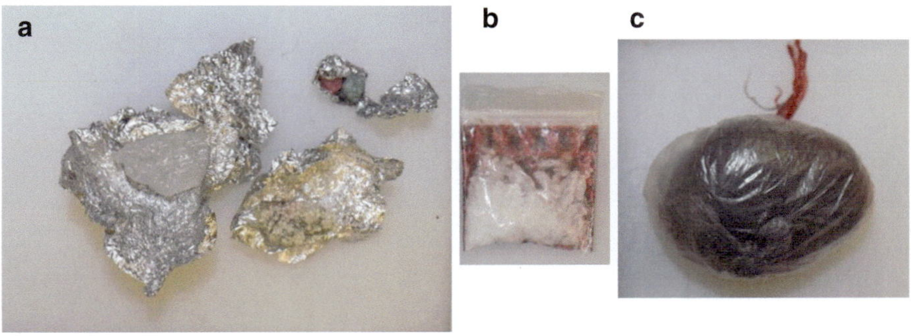

Fig. 5.3 Examples of suspected drugs recovered from the decedent's body. These need to be transferred into the custody of the forensic identification officer. (**a**) Suspected drugs wrapped in aluminium foil. (**b**) Suspected drugs in a dime bag. (**c**) Suspected drugs that were present in the rectum

variety of places on the body including pockets, hands, anorectum, vagina and so on (Fig. 5.4). This requires safety measures to avoid injuries. Externally, there may be stigmata of drug use such as needle puncture sites in the form of 'track marks', Osler/Janeway lesions due to infective endocarditis (Fig. 5.5), perforated nasal septum, callus or blister on the thumb related to repeated uses of a lighter, transdermal patch (Fig. 5.6) and so on. Internally, there may be findings, in addition to infective endocarditis of a history of drug use. These include markedly anthracotic lungs (Fig. 5.7), atypical discolouration of the bowel (Fig. 5.8) and foreign bodies of the gastrointestinal tract (Fig. 5.9). Histological examination of the lungs may show birefringent foreign body giant cells that are contaminants related to previous intravenous drug use (Fig. 5.10).

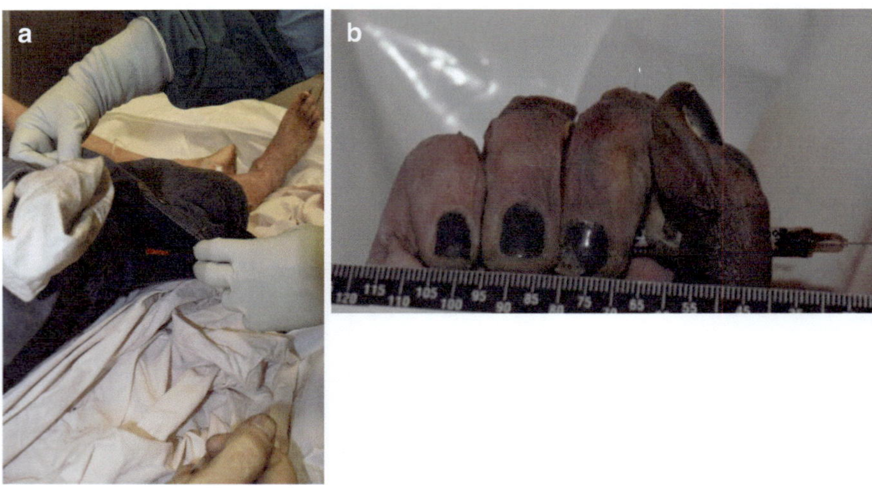

Fig. 5.4 Drugs and drug paraphernalia can be observed in the clothing and multiple areas of the body. This requires cautious techniques to avoid injury. Ideally, syringes and other items that can cause injury are removed at the scene, but that is not always possible. (**a**) Syringe in pocket. (**b**) Syringe in hand

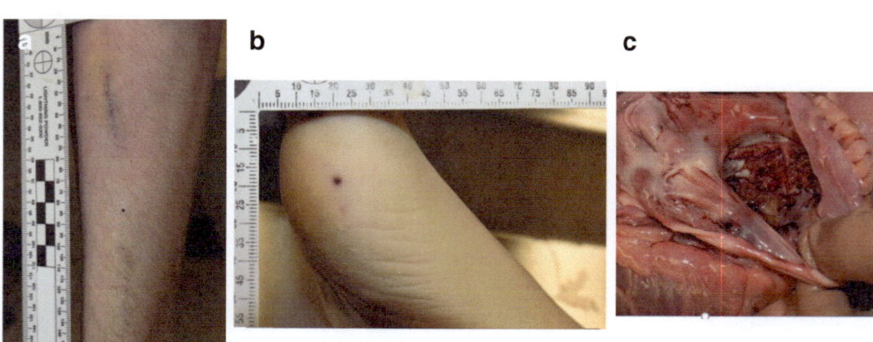

Fig. 5.5 Stigmata of intravenous drug use. (**a**) "Track marks" of the forearm represent multiple needle puncture sites, sometimes of various ages that follow the underlying vein. (**b**) Janeway/Osler node of the foot in a person with infective endocarditis. (**c**) Infective endocarditis of the heart valve

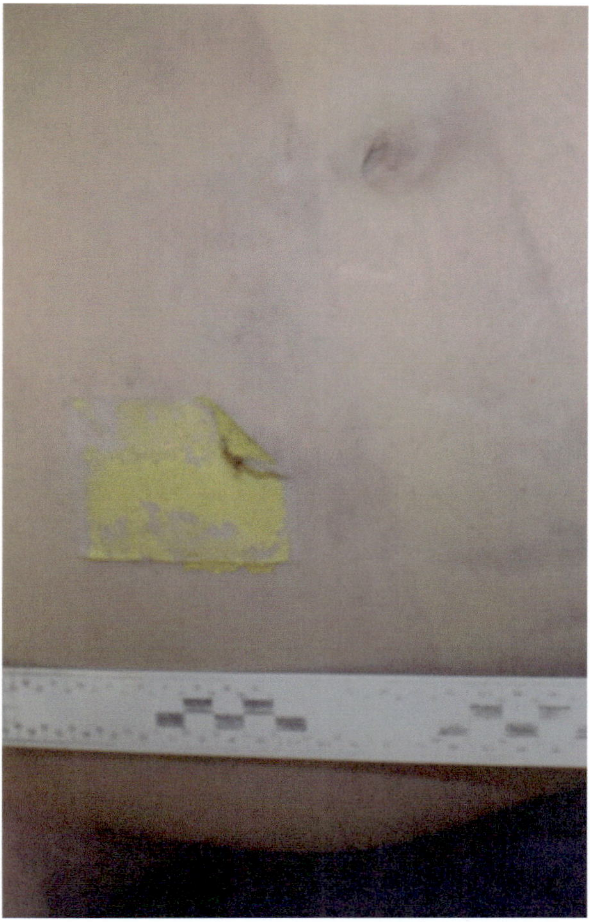

Fig. 5.6 Cutaneous patch on the abdomen. The patch was collected at the time of the autopsy as the substances associated were not known at the time of the autopsy

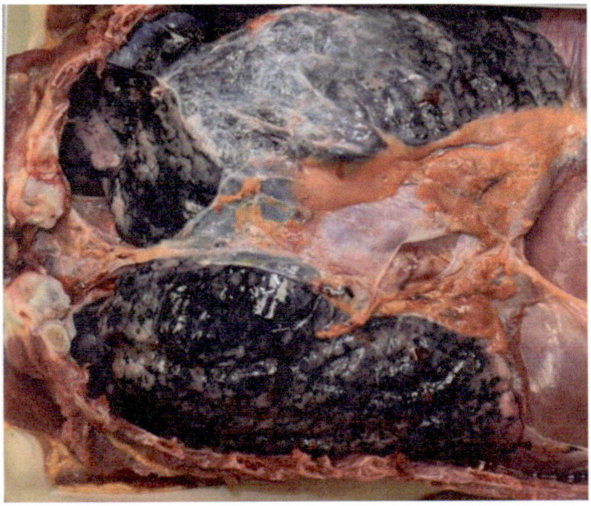

Fig. 5.7 Markedly anthracotic lungs in a young person. This finding can be observed in individuals with a history of smoking crack cocaine

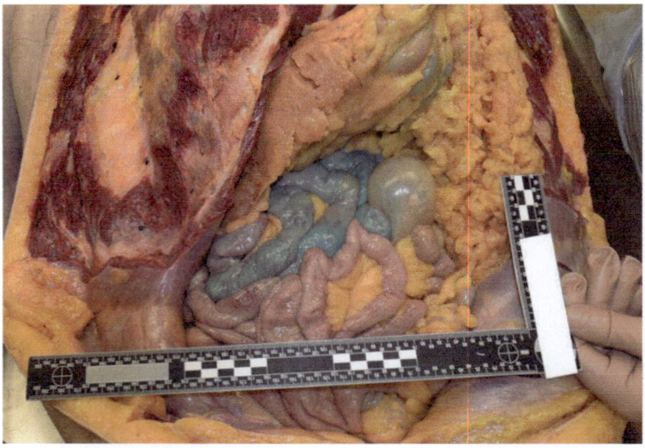

Fig. 5.8 Most drugs are ingested. There was a bottle of bathroom cleaner at the scene which was ingested to give this mint green discolouration. This discolouration is not typical for putrefactive decomposition

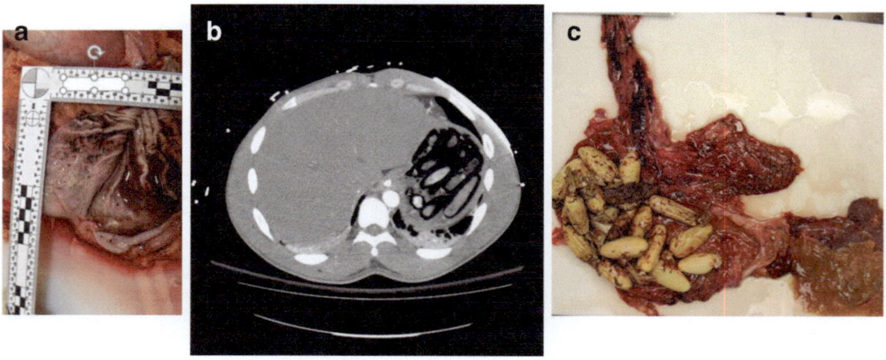

Fig. 5.9 The internal examination can show evidence of drug ingestion. (**a**) Pill residue in the stomach contents. This was collected so that, in the event the toxicological analysis of the blood was negative, the sample of stomach contents could be tested to determine the nature of the pill residue. (**b**) Computed tomography scan showed numerous foreign bodies in the stomach. (**c**) These foreign bodies were numerous latex balloons that contained cocaine. These were transferred into the custody of the police

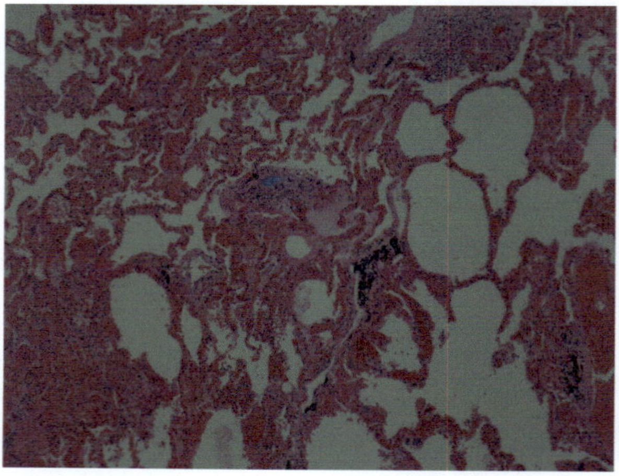

Fig. 5.10 Birefringent foreign body granuloma due to contaminants related to intravenous drug use

Sample Collection

The collection, choice of sample for testing and appropriate storage are critical aspects of forensic toxicology. The types of samples that should be collected and that are the most appropriate for toxicological analysis will depend on the case history, specific drugs of interest and analytical capabilities of the laboratory. In general, there is a hierarchy of preferred postmortem samples, the highest being the blood. The following samples are the most frequently obtained for toxicological testing; however, other sample types may sometimes be collected to assist in the death investigation.

Blood

In the majority of cases, blood within the circulation will be the most useful sample to obtain for toxicological analysis. If possible, blood samples should be obtained from a central and peripheral (femoral or iliac) source using tubes containing a preservative and anticoagulant such as sodium fluoride (1% w/v) and potassium oxalate (0.2% w/v). If subdural or epidural haemorrhage is present, blood from these sites may also be collected, as they may be useful when there is a period of time between an injury and death such as in the case of ethanol analysis. If blood is collected from a central source, it is important to note if hemopericardium or hemothorax is present for accurate interpretation of any drug or alcohol findings. This is important, especially in the context that gastric contents can intermix with chest blood. This could result in unreliable results (i.e. a markedly elevated ethanol level may be detected in the chest blood if ethanol was present in the stomach contents).

In some cases where there is limited blood volume available for analysis, drug screening should be done in an alternative sample, and then once drug and/or drug metabolites have been identified, the most appropriate quantitative analysis can be performed.

Depending on the case history, autopsy blood samples may have limited value, for example if there was hospital treatment prior to death and the presence of drugs at the time of admission is relevant to the death investigation. In cases where samples collected during an autopsy may not be directly relevant to the case then, if possible, an antemortem hospital sample should be obtained. In many cases, there will be a limited volume of antemortem blood available for drug analysis, so case history and screening of other autopsy samples may be helpful to guide the investigation.

Urine

If available, urine should be collected during autopsy. Many drugs and their metabolites are present in higher concentrations in urine than in blood and may remain in the urine for a longer time period. Urine testing can also be useful when rapid metabolism occurs, for example in deaths due to heroin, the metabolite of heroin,

6-monoactylmorphine, is easier to detect in urine and may provide evidence of heroin use prior to death. The main limitation of drug testing in urine samples is that the detection of a drug/metabolite in a urine sample is only indicative of prior drug exposure or administration. Urine findings cannot be used to determine the effects, including toxicity or impairment, of a drug on an individual at the time of death.

Liver

Liver is a useful sample for drug screening purposes when blood volume is limited. As the majority of drugs and poisons are metabolized in the liver, both the parent drug and its metabolites may be present in high concentrations when compared with blood. Care should be taken with the interpretation of drug concentrations in liver samples as postmortem redistribution of drugs can occur and concentrations may differ according to sample site [1]. If liver samples are obtained for toxicological testing, then the preferred location is deep within the right lobe of the liver to reduce the possibility of redistribution from contamination from the stomach and small intestine [2].

Gastric Contents

Analysis of gastric contents may not be required in all death investigations but can be useful in suspected overdoses. Stomach contents can provide a visual identification of the ingested drug(s) if tablets remain intact or there is pill residue. Although visual identification of tablets may be suggestive of an overdose, there are circumstances when "ghost tablets" (ghost tablets occur when formulations allow the active ingredients to be released over time but the outer pill does not disintegrate or get ingested) may be visible in the stomach at autopsy following administration of sustained-release medications. A study of oxycodone in postmortem cases reported that, in a number of deaths, numerous slow-release tablets were visually identified in the stomach but did not directly correlate to elevated concentrations of oxycodone in the gastric contents [3]. In addition, further analysis of the tablets collected from gastric contents revealed little or no oxycodone present; thus, the authors concluded that the number of tablets that are identified in the gastrointestinal tract may not be indicative of an overdose. Tablets may be collected and sent for analysis; this can be a simple visual inspection or chemical testing may be performed.

Vitreous Fluid

The location of vitreous fluid in the eye offers some protection from early putrefactive changes and microbial contamination. Therefore, this sample may be useful in cases where there are extensive changes to the body (e.g. fire deaths). Furthermore, vitreous fluid is considered an ideal sample for ethanol analysis because it correlates well with blood concentrations [4].

Sample Submission

All samples collected during autopsy should be properly labelled with the sample type, decedent identifiers, site of collection and date and time of collection as part of a high-quality death investigation. Each investigation should have a unique case or reference number to aid in tracking and for easy collaboration between the pathologist and the toxicologist. Each of the samples that are sent to the toxicologist should be sealed with a tamper-evident seal and the chain of custody document.

The pathologist should provide information about the circumstances around the death and where relevant the pathological findings. These pieces of information can be important for determining what analyses are the most relevant and also to aid in the interpretation of any drug findings. For example, a history of diabetes may warrant beta-hydroxybutyrate testing, and a cherry red colour of livor mortis may indicate the need to test for carboxyhaemoglobin or cyanide. In addition, the microscopic presence of oxalate crystals in the kidneys may be an indication of ethylene glycol exposure.

Information to provide the laboratory should include:

- Age and sex of deceased
- Unique reference number
- Seal number
- Main/relevant pathological findings at autopsy
- Postmortem interval, if known, before samples were obtained
- Medical history including any medications or illicit drug use
- Any symptoms prior to death
- Evidence of drug use from the scene (illicit, prescription and over-the-counter medications)
- Date and time antemortem samples collected

Analytical Testing

Forensic toxicology laboratories should have the ability to detect and quantitate many drugs of interest in a death investigation; however, there will be differences in analytical capabilities between laboratories, so it is important to be aware of testing capabilities (i.e. drugs identified and limits of detection) of individual laboratories. Any organization used for drug testing should follow guidelines and best practices for forensic toxicology testing, and many laboratories will be accredited as a means to ensure that the laboratory is following appropriate protocols.

Screening

Often the first step for toxicology testing is to screen samples for the presence of a wide variety of substances which will identify what additional analysis may be required. Immunoassay (IA) techniques are frequently used in many toxicology laboratories because they are a useful tool for screening purposes as this test has the capacity to test blood and urine samples for categories of drugs (e.g. benzodiazepines) or identify targeted drugs (e.g. fentanyl and acetaminophen). Most IA results will provide a dichotomous positive or negative result, but some may deliver semi-quantitative results. Although screening using IA techniques can provide a presumptive indication of drug use, it should never be used as a definitive result as there is a possibility of false positives. Screening for volatile substances, including ethanol, may be done using head-space gas chromatography. Unlike IA screening, the methods used in forensic laboratories are unlikely to result in false-positive results and are considered the gold standard for forensic alcohol testing.

The introduction of improved analytical techniques including quadrupole time-of-flight mass spectrometry (QTOF-MS) and liquid chromatography–tandem mass spectrometry (LC–MS-MS) has expanded the testing capabilities of many forensic toxicology laboratories. A technique such as QTOF-MS is increasingly used as a powerful and comprehensive drug screening tool that offers sensitivity, specificity and the ability to retroactively analyse data for the presence of new compounds when new drug data are added to a spectral library [5, 6]. This can be extremely useful in death investigations where suspected drug cases may include novel psychoactive substances (NPS). LC–MS-MS has become increasingly important in the field of clinical and forensic toxicology, especially for multi-target screening to identify and also provide quantitative results. Methods used for drug screening may be routinely updated by laboratories, so it is important to be aware of changes to ensure interpretation of positive and negative results is accurate.

Quantitation/Targeted Analysis

Following the identification of drugs during screening, additional analysis should be performed to confirm and/or quantitate drugs of interest. The use of a confirmatory/independent technique is a fundamental principle in forensic toxicology, so targeted or confirmation analysis should be performed using a separate analytical technique.

Many compounds require specific tests and should be requested in addition to standard drug screening, for example detection for gamma-hydroxybutyric acid (GHB) is not seen via routine screening procedures and has to be requested by the pathologist or be identified as relevant to the case based on the information provided as part of the case submission.

Interpretation of Results

The interpretation of toxicology results can be complicated. It requires knowledge about the pharmacology of drugs used for clinical purposes and also how drugs are used illicitly. In addition, when working with autopsy samples, there are additional factors that need to be considered that are unique to postmortem toxicology. When interpreting findings from postmortem analysis, published data are often used as a reference for expected therapeutic, toxic or fatal drug concentrations. It is important to recognize that one cannot always directly correlate postmortem results with clinical data. If possible, studies that report drug concentrations obtained from postmortem samples can be an invaluable guide for the interpretation of results. There are numerous studies that are available for many frequently detected drugs such as ethanol, cocaine and opioids and many frequently prescribed medications, although for some drugs, the data are limited, and individual case reports may be the primary source of information.

Although published data may be useful, it is important to recognize the importance of considering information from each individual case when making interpretations. Box 5.1 provides an example of how different case histories can change the interpretation of the same drug concentration. The following areas provide an overview of factors that can be important when assessing toxicological findings during death investigations.

Box 5.1 Importance of Case History

The following two cases provide an example of how the overall case history should be considered when interpreting a postmortem drug concentration.

1. The decedent was a 66-year-old male who had a history of chronic back pain. He had been using fentanyl patches (75 μg/h) for the last 18 months and his prescription history indicated therapeutic administration and no allegations of misuse. Postmortem pathological examination revealed hypertensive coronary artery disease. A fentanyl concentration of 8 ng/mL was detected in a femoral blood sample. The cause of death was listed as coronary artery disease, and the manner of death was natural.
2. The decedent was a 22-year-old male with a known history of illicit heroin use. He was found dead in his apartment, and drug paraphernalia was identified at the scene (syringe, white powder). Postmortem examination revealed acute congestion and oedema of the lungs with patchy bronchopneumonia. A fentanyl concentration of 8 ng/mL was detected in a femoral blood sample. The cause of death was fentanyl overdose, and the manner of death was concluded to be an accident.

   Note that the fentanyl concentration was the same in both cases; however, taking into consideration the background of each individual, autopsy findings, postmortem redistribution and tolerance to opioids, the final cause and manner of death differ significantly.

Postmortem Redistribution

Postmortem redistribution refers to the phenomenon that, in postmortem blood samples, drug concentrations frequently do not remain stable after death and may vary according to the collection site. This can refer to differing concentrations of a drug taken from different samples during an autopsy (e.g. femoral vs. heart blood), and also differing concentrations when comparing blood taken prior to death (antemortem) vs. blood samples taken after death (postmortem). Postmortem redistribution is a general term, and there are many factors that can influence it [7, 8]. These include:

1. Specific drug characteristics, e.g. volume of distribution, lipophilic properties and whether the drug is acidic or basic (pK_a)
2. Changes in the body after death (e.g. movement of drugs from tissue into blood and treatment of the body during resuscitative attempts)
3. Sample collection (e.g. postmortem interval between death and autopsy and type of sample)

In an ideal situation, blood samples should be obtained from multiple sites during an autopsy, and if only one postmortem blood sample can be obtained, the preferred site is a peripheral (e.g. femoral vein) blood sample. It should be noted, however, that, although a peripheral blood sample is the preferred site, it is recognized that postmortem redistribution may have already occurred, and drug concentrations may be elevated in comparison with an antemortem blood sample [9, 10]. In addition to the site of sample collection, it is often advised that forensic pathologists obtain blood from an intact ligated vessel. In practice, most pathologists collect samples using a blind stick method, when an internal examination is not performed, and a study has shown that samples drawn in this way do yield comparable drug concentrations when compared with ligated samples [11]. Another difficulty in the interpretation of drug findings from postmortem samples is that, in the majority of published literature, there is limited information regarding the collection of the samples (e.g. whether the vessel was ligated) or the time between death and autopsy, and in some reports, the actual sample site (e.g. central or peripheral) may not be noted.

Information regarding whether individual drugs are susceptible to postmortem redistribution is available for many drugs routinely encountered in forensic casework, and there are a number of drugs that are well established including, digoxin, amitriptyline and diphenhydramine. A useful resource is the comprehensive reference textbook Disposition of Toxic Drugs and Chemicals in Man, a valuable source of information for over 2000 substances [12].

Stability

Toxicological analysis is rarely performed immediately following autopsy, and it may take weeks or months before full drug testing is completed; therefore, drug stability is an important consideration in the interpretation of drug concentrations in biological samples. Changes in drug concentrations due to stability issues can occur any time after death and environmental conditions, such as temperature and exposure to light, can play an important role. Changes in the drug concentrations detected in postmortem blood may be more pronounced when compared with antemortem samples due to reduced control of environmental conditions and increased degradation due to putrefactive decomposition. Drug stability is analyte-dependent and is often determined by the physicochemical properties of the drug. Specimen collection techniques, use of preservatives and suitable storage conditions may help to mitigate some changes; however, even with precautions, changes in drug concentrations due to stability issues may occur. Examples of drugs where stability issues are well known include the following.

Cocaine

Cocaine is susceptible to both chemical and enzymatic breakdown. Cocaine undergoes chemical hydrolysis to benzoylecgonine (BE), and studies have shown that higher temperatures and pH will increase the rate of hydrolysis. In unpreserved blood samples, cocaine is hydrolysed to ecgonine methyl ester (EME) and the rate is dependent on temperature and pH of the sample [13]. When interpreting a postmortem cocaine concentration, it is important to note that, depending on storage conditions and sample pH, the concentration reported may not reflect the concentration at the time of death.

Ethanol

Ethanol concentrations may increase or decrease during storage [14]. The loss of ethanol is typically due to evaporation, oxidation or microbial consumption; however, if samples contain a preservative and are refrigerated and stored in a container that minimizes the air space above the sample, then loss of ethanol can be minimized. A more frequent problem when analysing samples obtained during an autopsy is the postmortem synthesis of ethanol. This may result in the detection of significant concentrations in postmortem samples. Forensic pathologists and toxicologists must be aware of and consider this possibility in postmortem cases, especially if there are signs of decomposition during autopsy. The probability of postmortem ethanol synthesis increases as storage temperature and the interval between death and autopsy increase. Some analytical methods used for screening alcohols have the ability to test for other volatiles that arise during putrefaction, for example n-propanol, and can be useful for assessing whether neoformation has occurred [15].

Benzodiazepines

Nitrobenzodiazepines (e.g. clonazepam, nitrazepam and flunitrazepam) have been shown to be unstable in blood as a result of anaerobic bacterial action [16]. The use of preservatives, e.g. sodium fluoride, and storage of samples at −20 °C can help reduce the loss of nitrobenzodiazepines during storage.

Tetrahydrocannabinol (THC)

It is well established that THC is susceptible to degradation during certain storage conditions. For example, loss of THC in blood samples can be up to 90% over a 6-month time period when stored at room temperature [17] and up to 100% loss can occur over 4 weeks when stored in plastic vs. glass tubes [18].

Gamma-Hydroxybutyric Acid (GHB)

Increases in GHB concentrations have been observed in unpreserved postmortem blood samples, but this can be minimized with the use of sodium fluoride preservative and storage of samples below 5 °C. Urine, antemortem blood and vitreous samples are less susceptible to increased GHB concentrations so testing of additional sample types may be helpful to determine if GHB was consumed prior to death.

Tolerance

The history of drug use by the deceased can be an important consideration in the interpretation of toxicology results. Drug tolerance can be described as a reduced response to the same dose of a drug after repeated exposure. Higher doses of a drug are required to elicit the same response compared with a naïve drug user; therefore, history of drug use is useful in determining the role of the toxicology results. A classic example of the importance of tolerance would be cases involving alcohol consumption. Ethanol fatalities have been associated with blood average ethanol concentrations of 355 mg/100 mL; however, some people with high levels of tolerance show no outward signs of intoxication at comparable concentrations [19, 20].

Cross tolerance can also occur for drugs in the same category, for example opioid users will develop tolerance to other opioids and their history should be considered when assessing toxicology results. A drug concentration in an individual who is on the methadone maintenance program may be an incidental finding, but the same concentration could be potentially fatal in an opioid-naïve individual.

Tolerance acquired due to repeated drug exposure occurs over time, and there are situations that will influence drug toxicity even in an experienced user. Despite previously established tolerance, if there is a period of abstinence (e.g. during incarceration), a loss of tolerance will occur making the individual vulnerable to a drug overdose. Fatalities shortly after release from custody may result due to this type of loss of tolerance. In addition, if their dose is increased or they use a higher potency drug, then they may not be protected. For example, if an experienced heroin user consumes fentanyl, due to its increased potency in comparison with heroin, the individual may experience serious toxicity.

Pharmacogenomics

Pharmacogenomics is the study of an individual's genotype and the disposition of drugs in the body. When studying the role of drugs in individuals, pharmacokinetics is an important consideration in the area of pharmacogenomics. Pharmacokinetics is the study of drug absorption, distribution, metabolism and elimination in the body. Absorption occurs after drugs enter the body and travel from the site of administration into the body's circulation. Distribution is the process by which the drug is distributed throughout the body. Metabolism describes the process of how the drug gets broken down in the body, e.g. via enzyme action, and excretion describes how drugs leave the body, e.g. in urine, bile or exhalation.

Individual genetic variations may influence drug metabolism in a number of ways including genetic polymorphism of CYP P450 enzymes, drug transport proteins and drug targets [21, 22]. Cytochrome P450 enzymes are essential for the metabolism of many drugs and genetic variability (polymorphism) in the cytochrome P450 (CYP) genes can lead to either increased or decreased enzyme activity, and this may result in significant effects on drug concentrations in the body. Examples of enzymes where genetic polymorphism has been documented are CYP2D6, CYP2C19 and CYP3A [23]. The CYP2D6 enzyme was the first human polymorphic enzyme to be investigated, and four categories of metabolizers have been identified: poor metabolizer, intermediate metabolizer, extensive metabolizer and ultra-rapid metabolizer. An example of a drug where genetic polymorphism is important is codeine. Codeine can be classified as a prodrug, and it is metabolized via CYP2D6 to its active metabolite, morphine. If an individual is an ultra-rapid metabolizer, it is possible to experience serious toxicity due to elevated morphine concentrations even when taking therapeutic concentrations of codeine [24].

In medicolegal investigations, postmortem genotyping may provide assistance in the interpretation of toxicological results and provide valuable information that could help in determining not only the cause but also the manner of death. If pharmacogenomic testing is not available, the knowledge that individual genetic differences may result in changes to drug concentrations can still be valuable to the bereaved family members who may wish to be investigated.

Drug Interactions

Interactions between drugs frequently occur and can cause either an increase or decrease in blood concentrations and/or drug effects; therefore, it is important to consider the potential for adverse drug interactions which may result in increased toxicity and even a potential cause of death. Information about specific drug interactions is available in many pharmaceutical reference textbooks and can be a useful resource when the medication history is available, and the toxicological analysis has detected the presence of multiple drugs.

The combination of several drugs belonging to the same pharmacological class may increase the risk of adverse effects, even if multiple drugs are present at therapeutic concentrations. In addition, ethanol, which is frequently detected in death investigations, can increase the central nervous system depressant effects of many other drugs, for example, opioids and benzodiazepines.

Combinations of some drugs can increase the risk of abnormal heart rhythms, e.g. prolonged QT interval. Drugs that have been associated with a risk of QT prolongation belong to many different drug categories including antibiotics (e.g. clarithromycin), antipsychotics (e.g. haloperidol) and opioids (e.g. methadone). This provides an example of when thorough knowledge of the case history is important as forensic toxicology laboratories may routinely test for antipsychotics and opioids but may not have methods for the testing of antibiotics. Prescription history may provide evidence of a potential drug interaction and explain an unexpectedly elevated drug concentration.

Another important factor to consider when interpreting toxicology results is drug-induced interactions involving cytochrome P450 enzymes. Many drugs act as potent enzyme inducers, whereas other drugs act as inhibitors. Drugs that induce enzyme inhibition reduce metabolism, whereas drugs that cause enzyme induction can increase metabolism. These changes in drug metabolism may lead to unexpected and serious adverse effects.

An example of this is the following case study: A 46-year-old woman had a history of prescriptions for transdermal fentanyl and hydromorphone for the treatment of headaches. She arrived at a friend's home and was observed to be drowsy and required frequent wakening while engaged in conversation. She went to lie down and was found sometime later without vital signs. Resuscitation attempts at the hospital were unsuccessful. Postmortem examination revealed acute congestion and oedema of the lungs with patchy bronchopneumonia. Toxicology testing reported a femoral blood fentanyl concentration of 12 ng/L and a therapeutic concentration of venlafaxine (<0.4 mg/L), and there were no other major toxicology findings despite comprehensive drug screening. Additional case history revealed that the deceased was taking Kaletra®, an anti-retroviral formulation containing lopinavir and ritonavir in combination; however, toxicology methods to confirm the presence of these two drugs were not available to the forensic laboratory. The possibility of simultaneous use of lopinavir, ritonavir and fentanyl was considered significant as the protease inhibitors, particularly ritonavir, are potent inhibitors of the cytochrome P450 (CYP) 3A4 enzyme system. Because fentanyl metabolism occurs mainly by CYP3A4, inhibition of this enzyme system may result in decreased clearance and prolonged fentanyl half-life, and concomitant use of these drugs is contraindicated. In the present case, the cause of death was classified as an accidental fentanyl overdose as a consequence of drug interaction with Kaletra® [25].

Postmortem Alcohol Interpretation

Ethanol (colloquially referred to as alcohol) is the most frequently detected drug in death investigations. The blood alcohol concentration (BAC) can be used to interpret whether an individual has consumed alcohol, a general time frame of when alcohol was consumed, possible impairing effects of alcohol and any toxic effects either due to alcohol alone or in combination with other substances. Testing for ethanol is a relatively accurate and reliable way of determining alcohol concentration, but the interpretation of results depends on a number of factors including type of specimen, presence of putrefaction and storage conditions.

When alcohol is consumed, the BAC rapidly increases (absorption phase) and the peak blood concentration is usually reached within 30 min after completion of the last drink. In the post-absorptive phase, alcohol is eliminated from the body at a faster rate than it is being absorbed and the BAC will gradually decline. The elimination rate for alcohol most often used for forensic purposes is 10–20 mg/100 mL/h, but higher elimination rates (up to 35 mg/100 mL/h) may be observed in chronic heavy drinkers.

Concentration of Alcohol in Different Biological Fluids/Tissues

Alcohol is distributed around the body according to the water content of the biological sample, so body fluids containing more water than blood will also have a higher concentration of alcohol when equilibration is reached (see Table 5.1).

Two samples that are the most frequently available for alcohol analysis in death investigations are blood and urine, and the results from both samples can provide an indication of whether a person has recently consumed alcohol. Urine has a higher water content than blood, so a urine alcohol concentration (UAC) will naturally have a higher alcohol concentration compared with blood (see Fig. 5.11) and a low UAC:BAC ratio indicates recent drinking and the individual is still in the absorptive stage, whereas a higher UAC:BAC implies the person in the postabsorptive stage and there was no recent drinking (Fig. 5.11).

Table 5.1 Average ratios of ethanol concentration in biological specimens/ethanol concentration in blood during a state of equilibrium

Serum	1.16
Vitreous fluid	1.27
Urine	1.30
Liver	0.60
Brain	0.80

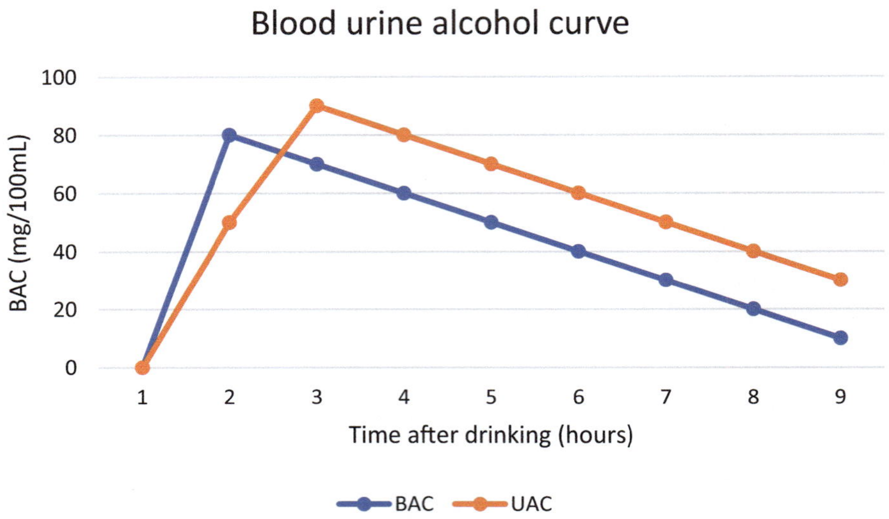

Fig. 5.11 Concentration–time curves of alcohol in blood (BAC) and urine (UAC)

Hospital vs. Forensic Alcohol Testing

It is important for investigators to be aware of differences between clinical alcohol test results compared to postmortem alcohol testing. Hospital alcohol analysis is frequently performed using serum samples and is reported using SI units, so the conversion of test results is required to change the units of measurement and also the different sample types. As an example, a serum ethanol concentration of 25 mmol/L can be converted to the typical units used in forensic laboratories (mg/100 mL) by multiplying the result by 4.61 to convert the units of measurement followed by dividing by 1.16 to correct for differences in water content. This means that the equivalent blood alcohol concentration is 99 mg/100 mL.

In addition, hospital analysis is usually based on an enzymatic alcohol method of analysis (based on the conversion of alcohol to acetaldehyde by alcohol dehydrogenase) and is validated for use in serum or plasma but may not be suitable for postmortem alcohol testing. It is advisable to ensure that any postmortem alcohol results used for a criminal investigation are confirmed using headspace gas chromatography in a forensic laboratory.

Analysis of Subdural or Epidural Hematomas

If an injury produces a subdural or epidural hematoma, it can be submitted for toxicological testing and may provide useful information for investigators.

A hematoma is a relatively protected sample due to reduced circulation in the damaged area of the brain and metabolism of alcohol will not occur at the same rate compared with a peripheral blood sample. A comparison of the peripheral blood concentration with the concentration detected in the hematoma may provide additional information about (at the time the trauma occurred).

Effect of Trauma and Blood Transfusion

Alcohol is a factor in many death investigations involving traumatic injuries. The possibility of significant blood loss or blood transfusion affecting an individual's BAC is something both toxicologists and pathologists should be aware of. Although some dilution of a person's BAC can occur, due to the physicochemical properties of ethanol, any trauma and significant blood loss or blood transfusion cause a minimal reduction in postmortem BAC by less than 10% [26]. This is primarily due to the distribution of alcohol into the total body water (approximately 40 L) and not just the blood volume (approximately 5 L).

Another important factor to consider is when a traumatic injury causes the stomach to rupture. If there is a high concentration of alcohol in the stomach due to recent drinking, then the risk of diffusion into pericardial fluid is significant. A peripheral blood sample would be the preferable sample to test in this situation.

Novel Psychoactive Substances

One of the biggest challenges currently facing forensic toxicology laboratories is the proliferation of novel psychoactive substances (NPS) that has occurred over the last decade with new substances appearing on a regular basis. NPS refer to different categories of drugs that have been designed to imitate the effects of established illicit drugs.

NPS can be categorized into four main groups:

- Cannabinoids
- Depressants
- Hallucinogens
- Stimulants

The use of the term "novel" or "new" refers to the fact that these substances are newly misused, but many NPS are older drugs that were synthesized many years ago and never marketed or approved for use in humans.

NPS have been detected in 133 countries and territories from all regions of the world, and data from UNODC have reported that 1079 substances have currently been identified [27]. The appearance of these drugs in death investigations creates many challenges. To assist in the determination of cause and manner of death, a toxicology laboratory has to be able to quickly develop methods that can detect and quantitate compounds at toxicologically significant concentrations. Sometimes, reference materials (including deuterated internal standards) that are critical for method development are not readily available due to the rapid emergence of drugs into the illicit market. Another major challenge is that many NPS drugs are transient, and by the time a laboratory has developed a method, the drug disappears from casework and a newer drug appears. This creates a situation where a forensic pathologist may not be able to obtain toxicological confirmation of a suspected overdose. In many cases, even if a quantitative result can be provided, there is a paucity of research into factors required for appropriate interpretation. Information about drug stability during storage and postmortem redistribution is rarely available, and pharmacological data from clinical studies may be difficult to obtain due to ethical considerations and concerns of toxicity.

Death investigations involve collaboration between many individuals, and the problem of NPS is an example of how information obtained from a thorough case history can be invaluable. Information from a seized drug sample from a scene, knowledge of testing capabilities of the toxicology laboratory and autopsy findings can provide useful information that can be used to determine the cause and manner of death.

The Opioid Crisis

The increasing use of prescription and non-medical prescription opioids has created a significant public health crisis. Opioid-related deaths have increased significantly since the early 2000s beginning with prescription opioid use followed by illicit heroin and then fentanyl and other synthetic opioids. The rising rate of opioid-related deaths across North America has led to a proliferation of opioids in forensic casework and had a significant impact on the workload of forensic pathologists and toxicology laboratories.

Forensic pathologists, medical examiners and coroners working in conjunction with forensic toxicologists can play a crucial role in identifying trends in the opioid crisis and provide important information for the public health community. Due to the severity of the problem, it is important that the investigation of opioid-related deaths is comprehensive.

Information that can assist in the interpretation of suspected opioid death includes:

- Multiple prescriptions of opioids from different physicians and pharmacies

- Altered transdermal patches, e.g. patches that are cut up or placed next to a heat source for increased absorption
- Multiple transdermal patches on many different body areas or in unusual areas, e.g. mouth and rectum
- The presence of lung oedema and froth in the airways
- Needle tracks or "skin popping" scars
- Indication of naloxone use

A common feature of opioid toxicity is respiratory depression, but it should be noted that some opioids are associated with cardiac toxicity. Methadone has been associated with sudden death due to its cardiac effects, even therapeutic doses of methadone may trigger ventricular arrhythmias such as torsade de pointes tachycardia. In recent years, abuse of the non-prescription opioid loperamide has been reported. Loperamide is used for the treatment of acute diarrhoea, is readily available and has been described as "poor man's methadone" [28]. If a death occurs in an individual with a history of opioid use with a clinical history of unexplained syncope or ventricular dysthymias, then it may be important to ensure that toxicology testing includes loperamide.

Bias in Forensic Toxicology

This chapter has discussed the importance of collaboration between people working in the field of death investigations. Testing decisions and interpretation of results cannot be done effectively in isolation, but it is also important to guard against cognitive bias. There have been three key aspects identified as potential sources of cognitive bias for a case that may require toxicology testing [29]:

1. Selection of tests/case strategy
2. Identification of a substance during drug screening
3. Interpretation of results

Existing frameworks within an organization are frequently used to guide the choice of analysis. This could help avoid different tests being performed based on assumptions about drug use in people of different ages, ethnicities or gender. Examples of testing frameworks can include protocols for sudden unexpected deaths in infancy or standardized drug screening for all homicide investigations. If a laboratory has a standardized testing protocol based on case type and not just specific case history, then full toxicology testing will be done no matter what the case history or background of the deceased is. Protocols can often be established in collaboration with a pathologist, medical examiner or coroner to ensure that relevant testing will be performed in various case types.

If toxicological testing is done in an accredited laboratory, then quality assurance procedures can help prevent bias influencing the identification of a substance during screening. If set values for the identification of a positive or negative result are clearly identified in laboratory operating procedures, then it removes subjectivity in decision-making based on irrelevant case information.

In terms of interpretation, the case history can be critically important in making an informed opinion on an appropriate cause of death (see Box 5.1); however, questioning of established knowledge is also important. An example of this is the diagnosis of cocaine-induced excited delirium. Since the mid-1980s, the role of cocaine in excited delirium has been reported and used as the primary cause of death in many police-involved fatalities [30]. Recent evaluations of this diagnosis have highlighted a lack of scientific scrutiny of this diagnosis and suggest that it has racist and unscientific origins [31]. This highlights the need for all individuals involved in death investigations to be aware of bias and ensure they are aware of the scientific basis of their opinions.

It is not feasible (or appropriate) for toxicology testing to be done in isolation, but if forensic toxicology laboratories use standard frameworks for performing appropriate testing and if scientists are able to provide scientific support for their interpretations (e.g. use of peer-reviewed scientific literature), then this can help mitigate cognitive bias and provide objective toxicological testing and interpretations to assist in death investigations.

References

1. Pounder DJ, Jones GR. Post-mortem drug redistribution—a toxicological nightmare. Forensic Sci Int. 1990;45(3):253–63.
2. Morley SR, Bolton J. Variation in postmortem liver sampling: implications for postmortem toxicology interpretation. J Clin Pathol. 2012;65(12):1136–7.
3. Anderson DT, Fritz KL, Muto JJ. Oxycontin®: the concept of a "ghost pill" and the postmortem tissue distribution of oxycodone in 36 cases. J Anal Toxicol. 2002;26(7):448–59.
4. Savini F, Tartaglia A, Coccia L, Palestini D, D'Ovidio C, De Grazia U, Merone GM, Bassotti E, Locatelli M. Ethanol determination in post-mortem samples: correlation between blood and vitreous humor concentration. Molecules. 2020;25(12):2724.
5. Allen DR, McWhinney BC. Quadrupole time-of-flight mass spectrometry: a paradigm shift in toxicology screening applications. Clin Biochem Rev. 2019;40(3):135.
6. Remane D, Wissenbach DK, Peters FT. Recent advances of liquid chromatography–(tandem) mass spectrometry in clinical and forensic toxicology—an update. Clin Biochem. 2016;49(13–14):1051–71.
7. Pélissier-Alicot AL, Gaulier JM, Champsaur P, Marquet P. Mechanisms underlying postmortem redistribution of drugs: a review. J Anal Toxicol. 2003;27(8):533–44.
8. Yarema MC, Becker CE. Key concepts in postmortem drug redistribution. Clin Toxicol. 2005;43(4):235–41.
9. Cook DS, Braithwaite RA, Hale KA. Estimating antemortem drug concentrations from postmortem blood samples: the influence of postmortem redistribution. J Clin Pathol. 2000;53(4):282–5.
10. Ferner RE. Post-mortem clinical pharmacology. Br J Clin Pharmacol. 2008;66(4):430–43.
11. Hargrove VM, McCutcheon JR. Comparison of drug concentrations taken from clamped and unclamped femoral vessels. J Anal Toxicol. 2008;32(8):621–5.
12. Baselt RC. Disposition of toxic drugs and chemicals in man. 12th ed. Biomedical Publications; 2020.

13. Isenschmid DS, Levine BS, Caplan YH. A comprehensive study of the stability of cocaine and its metabolites. J Anal Toxicol. 1989;13(5):250–6.
14. O'Neal CL, Poklis A. Postmortem production of ethanol and factors that influence interpretation: a critical review. Am J Forensic Med Pathol. 1996;17(1):8–20.
15. Wigmore JG, Chow BL. Case report: detection of neo-formation of ethanol in a postmortem blood sample using n-propanol and a urine sample. J Can Soc Forensic Sci. 2000;33(3):145–9.
16. Robertson MD, Drummer OH. Stability of nitrobenzodiazepines in postmortem blood. J Forensic Sci. 1998;43(1):5–8.
17. Johnson JR, Jennison TA, Peat MA, Foltz RL. Stability of Δ9-tetrahydrocannabinol (THC), 11-hydroxy-THC, and 11-nor-9-carboxy-THC in blood and plasma. J Anal Toxicol. 1984;8(5):202–4.
18. Christophersen AS. Tetrahydrocannabinol stability in whole blood: plastic versus glass containers. J Anal Toxicol. 1986;10(4):129–31.
19. Heatley MK, Crane J. The blood alcohol concentration at post-mortem in 175 fatal cases of alcohol intoxication. Med Sci Law. 1990;30(2):101–5.
20. Perper JA, Twerski A, Wienand JW. Tolerance at high blood alcohol concentrations: a study of 110 cases and review of the literature. J Forensic Sci. 1986;31(1):212–21.
21. Kupiec TC, Raj V, Vu N. Pharmacogenomics for the forensic toxicologist. J Anal Toxicol. 2006;30(2):65–72.
22. Musshoff F, Stamer UM, Madea B. Pharmacogenetics and forensic toxicology. Forensic Sci Int. 2010;203(1–3):53–62.
23. Di Nunno N, Esposito M, Argo A, Salerno M, Sessa F. Pharmacogenetics and forensic toxicology: a new step towards a multidisciplinary approach. Toxics. 2021;9(11):292.
24. Kirchheiner J, Schmidt H, Tzvetkov M, Keulen JT, Lötsch J, Roots I, Brockmöller J. Pharmacokinetics of codeine and its metabolite morphine in ultra-rapid metabolizers due to CYP2D6 duplication. Pharmacogenomics J. 2007;7(4):257–65.
25. Martin TL, Woodall KL, McLellan BA. Fentanyl-related deaths in Ontario, Canada: toxicological findings and circumstances of death in 112 cases (2002–2004). J Anal Toxicol. 2006;30(8):603–10.
26. Kintz P. Influence of antemortem perfusion on autopsy blood ethanol concentration. Forensic Toxicol. 2012;30(1):76–9.
27. United Nations Office of Drugs and Crime. Data from the UNODC early warning advisory on new psychoactive substances [cited Jan 17, 2022]. Available from: https://www.unodc.org/unodc/en/scientists/ewa/data.html.
28. Wu PE, Juurlink DN. Clinical review: loperamide toxicity. Ann Emerg Med. 2017;70(2):245–52.
29. Hamnett HJ, Jack RE. The use of contextual information in forensic toxicology: an international survey of toxicologists' experiences. Sci Justice. 2019;59(4):380–9.
30. Wetli CV, Mash D, Karch SB. Cocaine-associated agitated delirium and the neuroleptic malignant syndrome. Am J Emerg Med. 1996;14(4):425–8.
31. da Silva Bhatia B, et al. "Excited delirium" and deaths in police custody: the deadly impact of a baseless diagnosis. Physicians for Human Rights. phr.org. Mar 2022. https://phr.org/our-work/resources/excited-delirium/.

Chapter 6
Physics 101 and Classification of Injury

Rebekah Jacques

Trauma is the transfer of energy from an external moving object to tissues. Physical injuries may arise in the transference of kinetic energy that exceed the resilience of tissues. Kinetic energy is expressed as a mathematical equation, where kinetic energy is the product of half the mass and squared velocity (i.e. kinetic energy = 1/2 m x v2). The nature of the kinetic energy and the vessel by which the kinetic energy is transferred can convey. The human body has a limited number of ways to respond to injury. Studying trauma, in particular, the biomechanics of trauma in humans comes from a range of study types including cadaveric and human skull studies, animal models, computational models and magnetic resonance imaging. There are inherent limitations to each study type and inherent ethical limitations in the study of living humans. For example, animal models may give some insight into traumatic biomechanics, but the animal brain and skulls are vastly different compared with humans in anatomy and complexity.

A wound is a disruption of the continuity of tissues produced by external mechanical force. Although 'injury' is used synonymously with wound, injury typically has a wider meaning and encompasses not only damage produced by physical force but also damage produced by heat, cold, chemicals, electricity and radiation. The term injury derives from the Latin word 'injuria' which translates to not lawful. This concept has expanded to include an area of injury, disease or local degeneration in a tissue causing change in its function or structure. Therefore, the use of the term injury or wound implies damage from unnatural causes, while the term lesion is non-committal on whether the cause of the damage was natural disease. An example of this is the difference between a bruise and a purpura. Using the term bruise denotes that the cause of this pathological finding was from physical injury, such as blunt force trauma, whilst purpura denotes that there is bleeding under the epidermis but is non-specific and non-committal as to the cause.

R. Jacques (✉)
London Health Sciences Centre, London, ON, Canada
e-mail: rebekah.jacques@lhsc.on.ca

R. Jacques (ed.), *Forensic Pathology*,
https://doi.org/10.1007/978-3-031-42038-2_6

The human body has the ability to absorb forces by the resilience and elasticity of its tissues until the intensity of the applied force exceeds the capability of the tissues to adapt. Consequently, once this happens, an injury occurs. Force is not the only factor but also is the distribution on the body. For example, in sharp force injuries, the force is typically distributed over a small area and a blunt force injury, the force is distributed over a broad area. Overall, the amount of force is dependent on the intrinsic properties of the tissue and the extrinsic properties of the object/implement used to generate the force (Fig. 6.1). The intrinsic properties of the tissue are dependent on the viscoelasticity that allows tissues to deform under a force but able to return to their original form once the force is removed. This can also be dependent on age-related factors that alter the resilience of tissues when identical forces are applied. For example, bones have a higher elastic component in young individuals than adults in advanced age with more brittle bones. Consequently the differences can lead to the presence or absence of a fracture but also differences in fracture patterns, if a fracture were to occur. This affects the quantity and extent of fractures, the anisotropic properties and the fact that the physical properties of the tissue are not constant depending on where and how the force is applied. For example, special skins of the hands, axillae and genitals may have different appearances of injury followed by similar forces and nature of that force.

Extrinsic factors of injury follow Newton's three laws of motion and conservation of momentum.

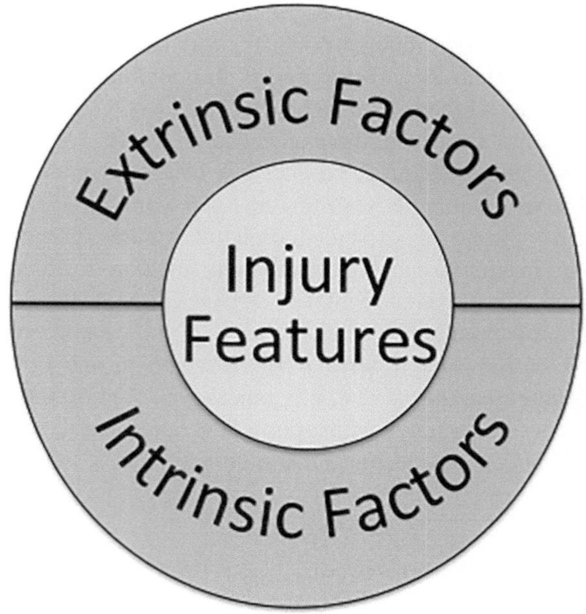

Fig. 6.1 Injury assessment triad. In the forensic setting, often the extrinsic factors, such as the amount of force, the directionality of force and the weapon used, are not known. The forensic pathologist can assess the features of the injury (i.e. laceration versus incision) and the intrinsic factors of the tissues (i.e. bone versus cartilage) to make deductions about the extrinsic factors (i.e. force, nature of the weapon, sharpness of knife, etc.)

Table 6.1 Summary of Newton's law of motion

1. Law of inertia
2. $F = ma$ ($\frac{1}{2} mv^2$)
3. Action–Reaction

Newton's **first law** of motion indicates that an object at rest will stay at rest and an object in motion will stay in motion at a constant velocity unless acted upon by an unbalanced force. In other words, inertia is the resistance to change in motion and is the tendency of an object to resist changes in its velocity (in motion/motionless). For example, if a vehicle descends down a hill, the vehicle will stay at the velocity unless gas, braking or the impact of friction alters the motion of the vehicle. In addition, if the vehicle stops abruptly, the body will temporarily continue to move forward due to inertia.

The **second law** is that force is the product of mass and acceleration. In other words, the greater the acceleration, the greater the force. Therefore, the higher the velocity and therefore acceleration of a vehicle, the more the braking force required to overcome the velocity. This law is particularly important for linear force. Rotational force (torque) is the product of moment of inertia and angular acceleration.

The **third law** is that, for every action, there is an equal and opposite reaction. For example, as the vehicle suddenly stops and the driver is wearing a seatbelt, the seatbelt catches the body, and as the body pushes onto the seatbelt, the seatbelt also pushes against the body (Table 6.1).

The **conservation of momentum** principle states that the total momentum of an isolated system stays constant. For example, the total momentum before a collision equals the total momentum after a collision. At high speed, a vehicle and passengers possess a great deal of momentum. A sudden head-on collision exerts tremendous force on the passengers in an extremely short period of time. There is less time spent stopping such that the force is much greater than if the stopping time was greater (i.e. slowing down). Outside of the vehicle, during a collision, the momentum of each object adds to the final momentum. The law of conservation states the momentum of any closed, isolated system does not change. For example, if a car collides into a tree at 50 km/h (31 mph), the force of hitting a tree at this speed 50 km/h (31 mph), but if the car collides with an oncoming car at 50 km/h (31 mph), collides with another vehicle at the same speed, the force of the collision is the sum of the two at 100 km/h (63 mph).

Classification of Injury

Injuries are generally classified according to their cause as blunt force injuries, sharp force injuries, gunshot injuries, 'asphyxia' and miscellany of others, such as environmental injuries. This is the classification followed in this text, and each group of injuries is discussed in successive chapters (Fig. 6.2). Using standard generally accepted descriptive terms for classifying wounds conveys the mechanism of

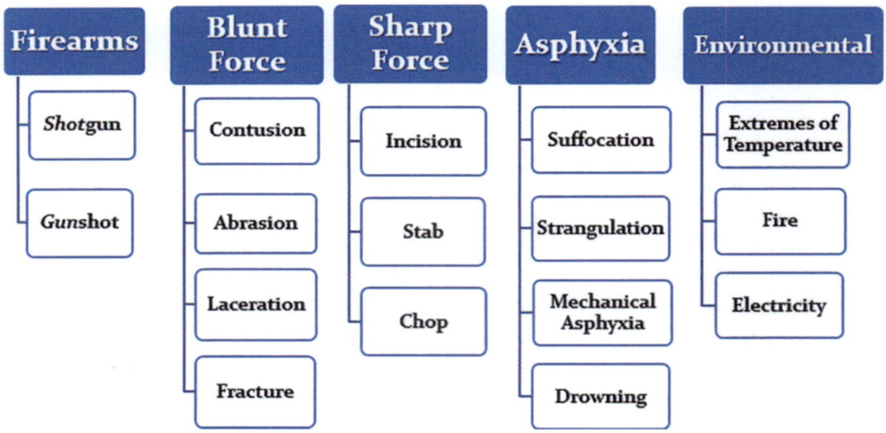

Fig. 6.2 Trauma can be classified based on their mechanism of injury

injury and force required. Blunt force trauma is typically classified as contusions (colloquially referred to as bruises), abrasions (colloquially referred to as scarpes), lacerations (colloquially referred to as tears) and fractures. Sharp force injuries include incised wounds, stab wounds and chop wounds. 'Asphyxial' deaths have a contentious classification.

Chapter 7
Blunt Trauma

Michael J. Shkrum

Introduction

In medicolegal autopsy practice, there are common scenarios that result in blunt trauma injuries. Similar trauma can be seen under different circumstances, but typical injuries do occur in certain scenarios that assist in differentiating how a person died.

As the external examination and dissection of the body unfolds systematically, observations occur sequentially which, in some cases, are supplemented by additional examinations that address issues arising from the circumstances described to the pathologist during the initial death investigation. Progression at each step during the autopsy reveals trauma that requires documentation and interpretation.

During the external examination, skin wounds from blunt trauma (contusions, abrasions, and lacerations) may or may not be readily evident (see section "Scalp"). At this stage, the pathologist needs to be mindful of deformities due to fractures (Fig. 7.1). External examination is followed by incisions along the torso to expose the chest wall and abdominal cavity which can be examined in situ. After the sternum is removed, the thoracic viscera can be inspected in situ. The viscera from the chest, abdomen, retroperitoneum, and pelvis are removed allowing examination of the internal rib cage, thoracic and lumbosacral spine, and pelvis. This is followed by opening the head by reflection of the scalp and removing the calvarium to examine the brain and skull. To minimize the presence of artifactual hemorrhages due to postmortem seepage of blood, the last step in a "routine" autopsy is the removal of the anterior neck structures. This step exposes the cervical spine. In certain cases, e.g., a beating death, additional examinations (i.e., incisions of the extremities and back) can reveal deep soft tissue hemorrhage not evident externally as bruising.

M. J. Shkrum (✉)
London Health Sciences Centre, London, ON, Canada

R. Jacques (ed.), *Forensic Pathology*,
https://doi.org/10.1007/978-3-031-42038-2_7

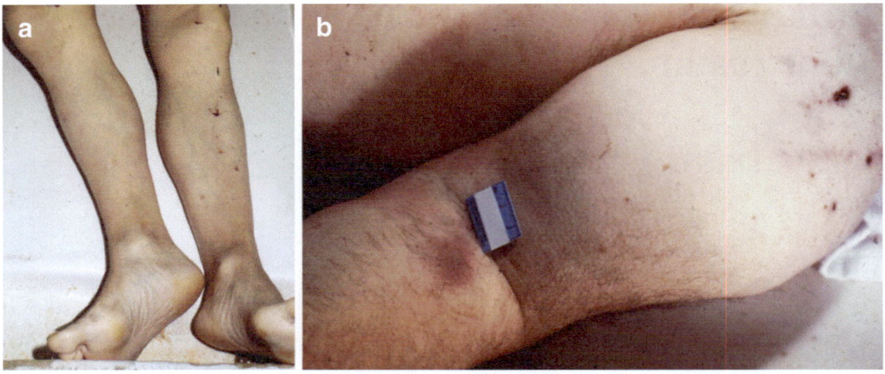

Fig. 7.1 Fracture deformities. (**a**) Fracture of the right hip. Note shortened and externally rotated right leg. (**b**) Fracture of the right humerus (upper arm bone). Note deformity of the arm due to swelling from hemorrhage at the fracture site

Injuries are documented by the pathologist in working notes and diagrams which form the basis of the final narrative report. Features such as location, type, size, and color, if applicable, of a wound are recorded. Photographs of not only the presence but also the absence of findings are equally relevant to the issues of a case. Photographs are complementary records that ensure a case is reviewable by another expert and can be used as exhibits to inform a legal proceeding. A diagram prepared by the pathologist showing the distribution of injuries on the body is an alternative to graphic photographs in a criminal proceeding if there is concern about upsetting jurors. A diagram is effective in conveying the totality of the trauma sustained by a victim. Radiographic findings observed either during the clinical course or at the postmortem examination can confirm or add to the autopsy record of trauma particularly if there are subtle findings that are inapparent during a conventional autopsy.

Injury interpretation requires a systematic approach by the pathologist before, during, and after the autopsy. Integration of information about the circumstances, scene, and relevant medical history forms the basis for the questions to be addressed during the postmortem examination. The contribution of blunt trauma to not only the determination of the cause of death but also its significance regarding other specific issues of the case is built on the foundation of the evolving medicolegal death investigation, the pathologist's knowledge of injury patterns and their origins, and relevant supplementary testing. How injuries lead to death ("mechanism") and whether they "fit" the timeline and the circumstances of the death ("manner") are important in medicolegal death investigations and legal proceedings.

Objectivity in injury interpretation is a must for a pathologist particularly when a police investigation is focused on a "criminally suspicious" death. By engaging in "tunnel vision" and assuming the death is suspicious, a pathologist can fall into the trap of "confirmation bias" in interpreting postmortem findings to support the initial investigative hypothesis and ignoring exculpatory evidence that could lead to a different conclusion about how those injuries arose.

Scene and Medical Information

As in any medical practice, where the physician is guided by the patient's history to reach a diagnosis, a pathologist does not function in an information vacuum. Information from investigators to the pathologist regarding the circumstances, the scene, and relevant medical history guides the steps the pathologist will need to take during the postmortem examination to address the issues raised by a specific case.

Scene

Scene visitation or review of digital images of a scene taken by police provides context prior to the autopsy. Body location and position, observable injuries, state of clothing, evidence of purposeful activity, the nature and state of the surrounding environment including potential sources of injury, the presence of alcohol or drug paraphernalia, and resuscitative efforts at the scene are some details that can assist in the documentation and interpretation of trauma observed at autopsy.

Past Medical History

Review of the past clinical history of a blunt trauma victim can reveal prior medical conditions that can predispose an individual to injury, e.g., falling due to a neurological disorder, exacerbate the consequences of a wound, e.g., increased bleeding from impaired clotting due to cirrhosis, or diminish the physiological response to trauma, e.g., heart disease. Certain trauma seen at the time of autopsy may have been documented in a medical record of a prior incident unrelated to the fatal event.

Acute Injuries: External

There may be information from the clinical record or investigation prior to the autopsy that an impact (e.g., blow) occurred at a specific site on the body, but that injury is not visible at autopsy. The possibilities include the following:

- The impact force was insufficient to cause a visible wound.
- The impact caused transient erythema which disappeared by the time of the autopsy.
- The impact was dissipated over a wide surface area. There may be underlying soft tissue bruising revealed by dissection (e.g., subscalp injury).
- Clothing or hair absorbed the impact.
- The information was inaccurate.

As cutaneous (skin) and soft tissue injuries are usually not life-threatening, clinical management is focused on the diagnosis and treatment of serious and potentially life-threatening internal injuries. Consequently, there may be little information about external injuries when the hospital chart is reviewed prior to the autopsy. Clinical documentation may be in the narrative of the chart. There may be a diagram showing the approximate location, type, and measurements of the external injuries. In some criminal investigations, photographs will be taken by police either by consent or under a criminal warrant while the victim is hospitalized. Clinical data can assist in confirming certain postmortem observations of wounds that have been either altered by resuscitation and treatment, e.g., sutured lacerations, or changed due to healing. These data may be absent in the chart and will require clarification by discussion with the clinician.

Acute Injuries: Internal

The clinical record informs the pathologist about the therapeutic and diagnostic procedures performed during resuscitation, radiologic imaging findings, and the injuries that were observed and treated including surgical intervention. Information from radiologic imaging showing injuries in an organ can be correlated with trauma found during the postmortem examination. An injured organ (e.g., spleen) that has been surgically resected can be examined by the autopsy case pathologist, photographed, and documented in a surgical pathology report. In other situations, a carniectomy specimen from surgery may need to be reunited with the skull at the time of postmortem examination to assess for skull fractures.

If there was resuscitation at the scene or in the hospital, then iatrogenic trauma can occur which may or may not be distinguishable from injuries that happened prior to resuscitation particularly if they are associated with hemorrhage from artificial circulation created by chest compressions (see section "Cardiopulmonary Resuscitation (CPR)").

External Examination

In contrast to the clinical situation, the pathologist has more time to inspect, record, and interpret cutaneous trauma.

Antemortem, Perimortem, or Postmortem?

Generally, the presence of hemorrhage distinguishes an antemortem injury from postmortem trauma. A visible contusion alone or associated with an abrasion or a laceration indicates a survival period during which blood circulated to the injured site. Incision of a skin wound to demonstrate soft tissue hemorrhage can confirm an injury is antemortem.

An antemortem injury can be perimortem if the injury occurs around the time of death. The amount of associated hemorrhage in the surrounding soft tissue can vary from minimal to considerable and depends on how rapidly death ensued. Injuries can be considered perimortem when the trauma or disease or both causing death was "immediate" or "near instantaneous" leading to a rapid decrease in cardiac output. For example, a terminal fall from a cardiac arrhythmia can result in perimortem facial injuries. Head trauma from any type of assault can cause rapid brainstem dysfunction leading to cardiorespiratory arrest and be manifest as perimortem facial and scalp injuries (see section "Commotio Medullaris (Brainstem Concussion)").

Postmortem changes can mimic antemortem injuries. Extravasation of blood can occur into postmortem lacerations in areas of lividity particularly when there is progression to decomposition. Typical postmortem yellow or orange abrasions can turn red or brown from lividity (Fig. 7.2).

Antemortem Injuries: Survival Interval

The gross and histological features of a skin wound can only estimate its age.

The color of a contusion progresses with the survival interval, but when a certain color occurs and its order in the temporal sequence is debatable [1, 2]. Colour changes in bruises of different ages have been described in various historical textbooks. Based on these observations, a red or purple contusion could occur in seconds to about 24 h before death which means that in the case of a victim who has succumbed quickly from injuries, a red or purple contusion could have occurred either during the fatal incident or at some time before and been unrelated to the terminal event. Brown, blue, or dark purple bruises have been described as ranging from 24 to 72 h old. A yellow bruise can be at least 1 week old [3]. But one study of photographic assessment of bruises found that yellow was present in bruise that was more than 18 hours old whereas red did not alter significantly with time [1, 2]. Studies have shown that photographic and clinical assessment of the age of a bruise based on its color is highly inaccurate and subject to inter- and intra-observer variation in color perception and description [3]. Many variables can affect the appearance of bruises such as site on body (e.g. loose tissue around the eye), age of the individual, i.e. an increased tendency to bruise in children and the elderly, underlying medical conditions associated with a bleeding tendency (e.g. cirrhosis) and the rapidity of death [2]. At autopsy, the pathologist must also consider that there can be a gradation of color in a bruise. For example, the central area of a large healing bruise can appear more recent compared with its periphery where healing has commenced. Aging of multiple contusions of different colours can be expressed in relative terms (i.e. a yellow bruise appears older than bruises of other colours) (Fig. 7.3).

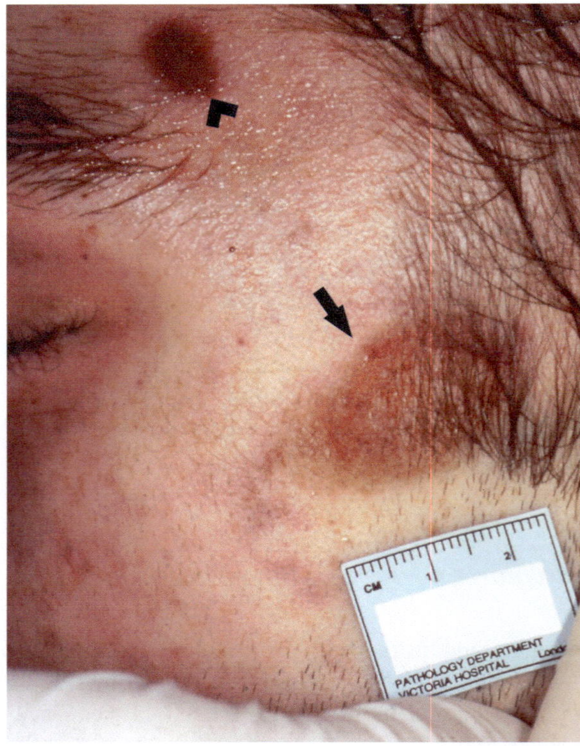

Fig. 7.2 Postmortem abrasions. The deceased was found lying on her left side after a fall. Lividity was absent on the left side of the face where it impacted the floor. Typical postmortem yellow abrasion on the prominence of the left cheek (arrow). Another abrasion on the ridge of the lateral eyebrow (arrowhead) in an area of lividity was also likely yellow, i.e., postmortem but appeared dark red suggesting an antemortem injury

Histology can narrow the estimation of a survival interval, but it only allows an opinion which is "in the ballpark" and not specifically "in the seats." Neutrophils appear outside of areas of hemorrhage in about 1–24 h after the injury [1]. Macrophages follow and ingest red blood cells. Histochemical stains (e.g., Perl's Prussian Blue) highlight hemosiderin-laden macrophages (siderophages) and indicate a survival interval of about 2–3 days or more. Histological sections of a healing abrasion or laceration show certain features (scab formation, granulation tissue, and re-epithelialization of wound edges) indicative of survival [1].

When issues arise about either trauma occurring at different times or during a survival interval or both, sampling of representative cutaneous wounds to determine the histological stage of inflammation can estimate their relative ages. Estimation of survival interval can be bolstered by correlating the histology of an external wound with that of an internal injury, e.g., the stage of inflammation in a scalp wound with the finding of diffuse axonal injury (see section "Diffuse Axonal Injury (DAI) and Diffuse Vascular Injury (DVI)").

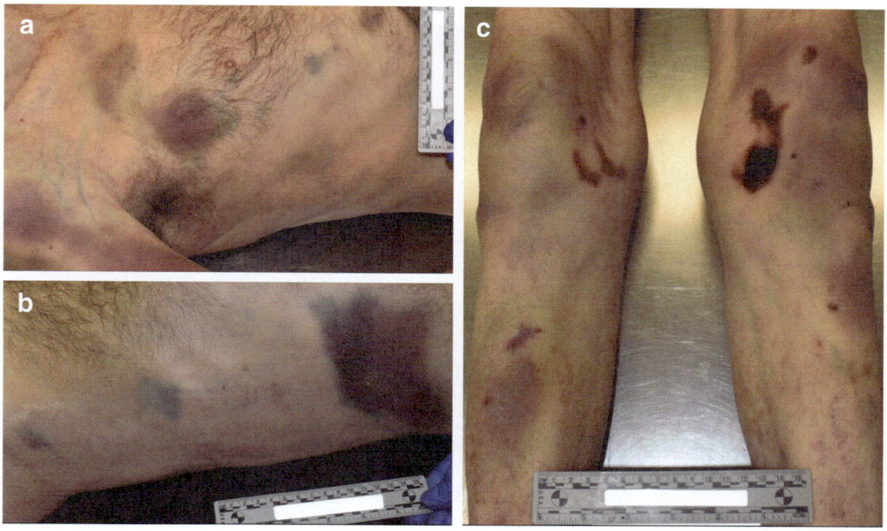

Fig. 7.3 Chronic alcoholic. Contusions showing a range of colors on the torso (**a/b**) indicative of different stages of healing were supportive of repeated episodes of falling due to intoxication. Abrasions and contusions on the knees and shins (**c**) reflect a typical injury pattern from stumbling and falling

Degree and Direction of Force

A common question posed to the pathologist is how much force caused an injury. The nature of the cutaneous wound, i.e., open (abrasion, laceration), compared with a contusion suggests greater force. The size of the wound can be influenced by various factors that include not only the degree of force but also the impact surface area and anatomic site. An impact to a site with a thin layer of skin covering bone (e.g., scalp) can cause wide splitting (Fig. 7.4). A stellate laceration can suggest equal dispersion of energy around the impact site due to a perpendicular impact. Eccentric undermining of a laceration suggests a tangential impact.

A contusion can enlarge as blood spreads from its original impact site, e.g., from the supraorbital ridge into loose periorbital tissues, and create the false impression of its origin from the larger surface (Fig. 7.5). Medications (e.g., anticoagulants), bleeding diatheses (e.g., leukemia), and decreased skin strength from aging can enhance bleeding. A small, seemingly innocuous, skin wound at an impact site can be a sign of considerable internal trauma.

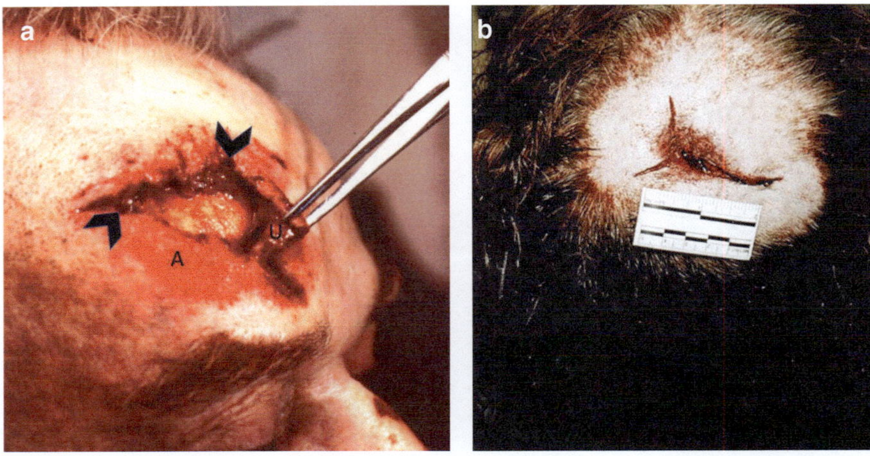

Fig. 7.4 (**a**) Laceration on forehead. Note features characteristic of a laceration: irregular wound edges; undermining (U); and tissue bridging (arrowheads). The presence of undermining supports that the force had a tangential impact. Associated abrasion (A) under the inferior edge of the wound. (**b**) Haircut and shave reveal a stellate laceration on vertex of scalp Indicative of a possible perpendicular impact

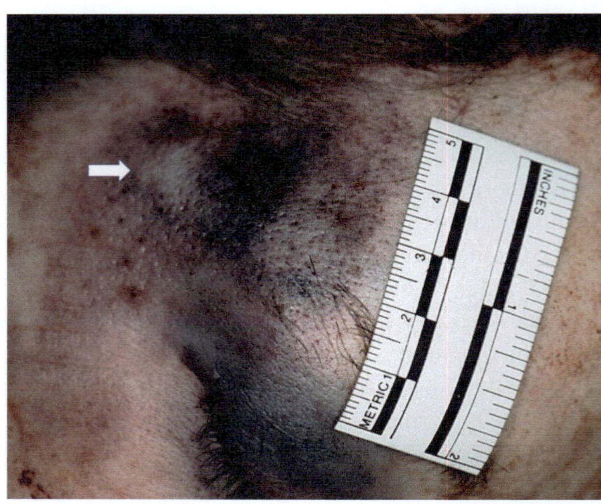

Fig. 7.5 Contusion right temple. Central area of pallor (arrow) in the contusion suggests a forceful impact with blood dispersed around the impact site. Note blood tracking into the right periorbital area

Patterned Injuries

Pattern recognition is a fundamental skill in pathology practice. The determination by a pathologist of a common injury pattern based on the distribution of wounds on the body requires an accurate examination and documentation of all cutaneous injuries. Less commonly, the pathologist's expertise is needed to determine whether a cutaneous injury is patterned and reflects the design of the surface that caused it (Figs. 7.6 and 7.7).

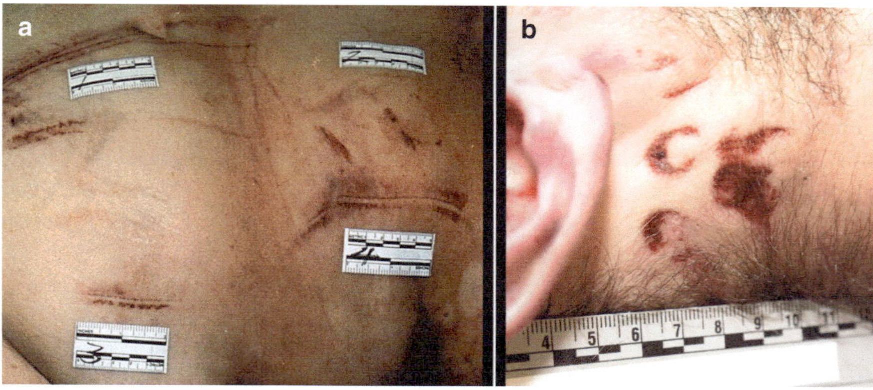

Fig. 7.6 (**a**) Multiple sets of parallel linear abrasions on the anterior torso. The assailant, who was a right-front passenger, was said to have used a snow/ice scraper to repeatedly press the floor pedals while he was driving the vehicle in which he had wedged his murdered wife on the driver's side. (**b**) Semicircular/circular abrasions on the side of the neck from blows due to a narrow circular object

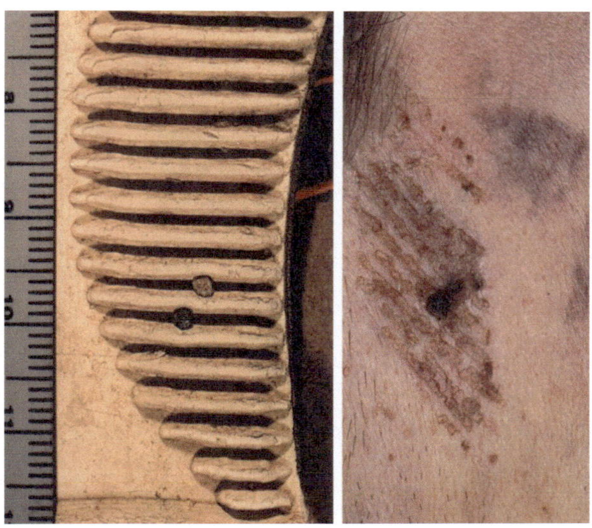

Fig. 7.7 Victim kicked in head. Patterned abrasion. The pattern of the treads on the sole of the assailant's running shoe (left photograph) matches linear abrasions on the right side of the victim's face below the temple (right photograph). Two small round abrasions within the linear abrasions correspond to small stones caught in the grooves of the sole. (Reprinted by permission from Wolters Kluwer Health, Inc. Ramsay DA, Shkrum MJ. Homicidal blunt head trauma, diffuse axonal injury, alcoholic intoxication, and cardiorespiratory arrest: a case report of a forensic syndrome of acute brainstem dysfunction. Am J Forensic Med Pathol. 1995 Jun;16(2):107–14. https://pubmed.ncbi.nlm.nih.gov/7572861/)

Motor Vehicle Collisions

Motor vehicle collisions (MVCs) are the most common cause of deaths from blunt trauma. Fatal injuries can be either isolated in one body region or involve multiple sites. MVC-related trauma is the archetype of death from "multiple blunt trauma injuries." Although there may be a myriad of injuries that are not necessarily unique to MVCs, certain injury patterns can be present which can assist in collision reconstruction.

Injury Patterns

"The Fatal Triad" of skull-pelvic-lower extremity fractures was an injury pattern described in a clinical study by Farley of upright adult pedestrians struck by motor vehicles [4]. In their clinical study of pedestrians, Waddell and Drucker described an injury triad involving the knee, hip (femur) or pelvis, and the head [5].

Weisz et al. classified injuries sustained by unrestrained drivers into levels [6]. Craniocerebral and cervical spine (Level 1) injuries were due to contact with the windshield, A-pillar, or front header. Loading of the steering wheel caused trauma in the chest and abdomen (Level 2). Contact with the dashboard caused loading of the knee leading to fractures of the femur and pelvis (Level 3).

These injury patterns in pedestrians and drivers were described about a one-half century ago. Although features in the current motor vehicle fleet such as vehicle type and exterior design and occupant safety features have evolved and may modify the trauma patterns currently seen in pedestrians and occupants, respectively, the historic descriptions of injury patterns continue to be applied to present-day autopsy practice.

Lower Extremity Injuries in Pedestrians

The finding of lower extremity injury can support the scenario that a pedestrian was upright when struck by a motor vehicle. Trauma from initial impact with a vehicle bumper can be limited to cutaneous and soft injuries, or it can cause "bumper" fractures which typically involve the tibia or fibula or both [7–9]. A femur fracture can occur in a short pedestrian or from a high bumper [4, 10]. Proximal femur fractures can be due to impact with the vehicle hood and be associated with pelvic fractures [5, 11]. A lower extremity fracture may be obvious as a compound fracture or a visible deformity; however, radiography or dissection or both may be necessary to show a closed or isolated fracture (Fig. 7.8). Radiographs are evidentiary and reviewable records that not only supplement the pathologist's documentation of

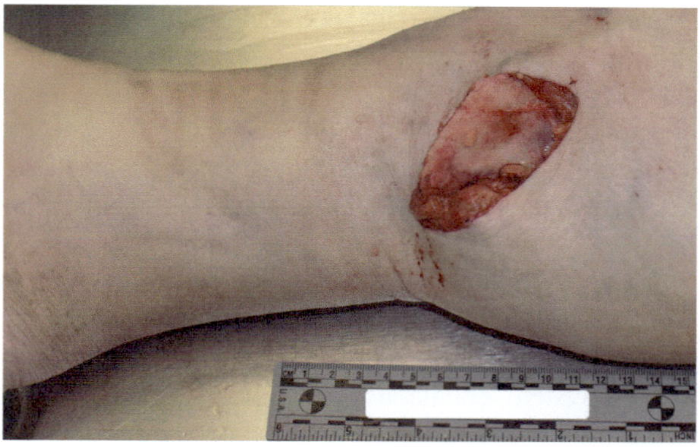

Fig. 7.8 Upright pedestrian struck by motor vehicle. Compound fracture, right tibia ("bumper" fracture)

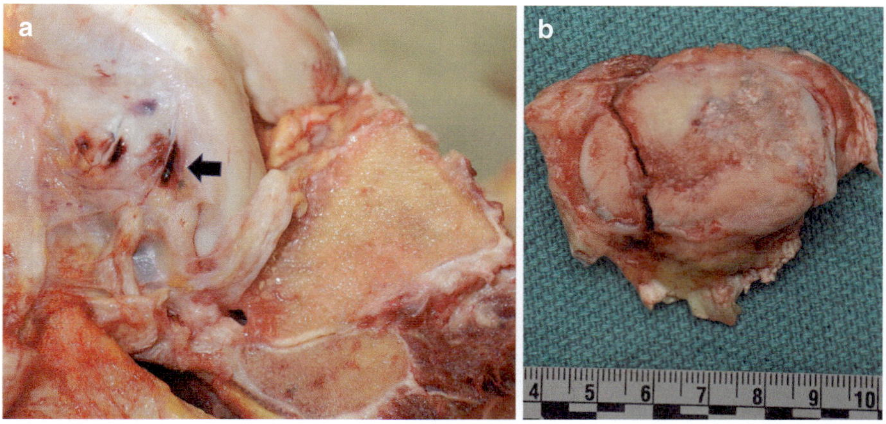

Fig. 7.9 Upright pedestrians struck by motor vehicles. "Typical" bumper fractures of tibia/fibula/femur absent. Knees were examined in both cases. (**a**) Hemorrhage at the insertion of the lateral collateral ligament (arrow). Proximal tibia and fibula shaved—no evidence of hemorrhage ("bone bruise"). (**b**) Patellar fracture

injuries and assist the medicolegal death investigation but can also be used to inform a legal proceeding.

Radiographs may miss knee injuries which may be the only evidence of lower extremity trauma. They can be demonstrated by dissection of the knee joint. After removal of the patella (knee cap) and shaving of the proximal tibia and distal femur, certain injuries can be revealed. They include hemoarthrosis, ligamentous laceration and dislocation, and fractures of the tibial plateau, high tibia, supracondylar femur, and patella (Fig. 7.9) [5, 12]. Tearing of the collateral and cruciate ligaments can result in hemorrhage localized to their bony attachment sites and avulsion fractures [5, 13]. Compression between the femur and tibia due to movement around the knee joint from impact can lead to bleeding in the corresponding cancellous bone resulting in "bone bruises" [13]. In one study, bone bruises were seen only in upright pedestrians (77% frequency versus 0% in run-over cases) [13].

Measurement of the distance of the bumper injury site (fracture site, skin wound) from the sole of the foot is a traditional autopsy practice. Whether this measurement can be correlated with the distance of the bumper height to the ground has been questioned [8]. This uncertainty could be due to where to measure the height of a lower extremity fracture because of either displacement of the fracture end resulting in shortening of the leg or the complexity of the fracture. Another factor could be the bumper width (Fig. 7.10). A broad bumper can cause fractures at different levels.

Lower extremity injuries including fractures can occur in a recumbent pedestrian who is run over [13, 14]. External evidence of being dragged under an automobile (e.g., tire tread marks, grease marks from the vehicle undercarriage, burns from the exhaust system, cutaneous brush abrasions, skin and soft tissue avulsions, abrasions of exposed bone, and limb amputations) can occur (Fig. 7.11). These injuries can also be observed in an upright pedestrian who is run over after being struck [13, 14].

Chest

MVCs are a common cause of blunt chest trauma [15, 16].

Contact of the torso and upper body with the hood or front of the impacting vehicle occurs when the center of gravity of a pedestrian is above the hood edge height of the impacting vehicle.

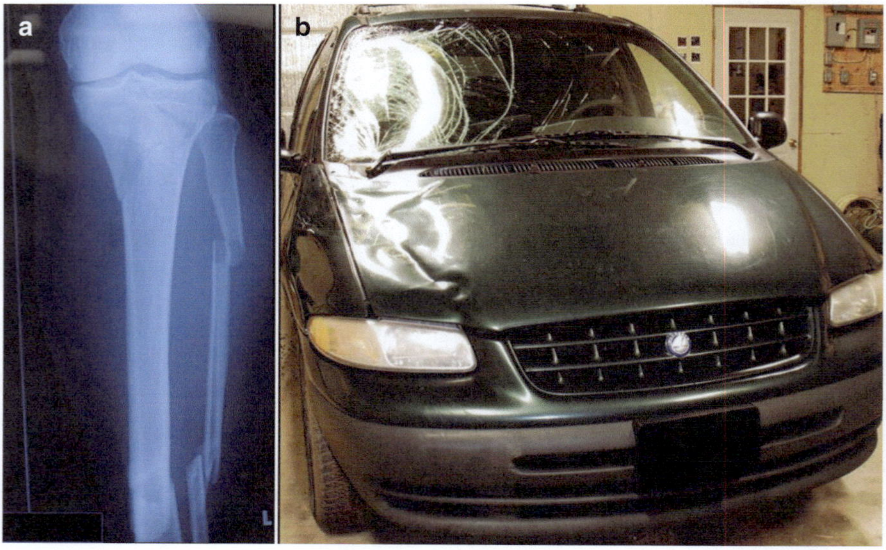

Fig. 7.10 (**a**) Fractures of proximal and distal tibia and fibula in an upright pedestrian struck by a van shown in (**b**). Damage to the hood and windshield was caused by the deceased wrapping onto the vehicle. The distribution of the fractures may reflect the width of the bumper

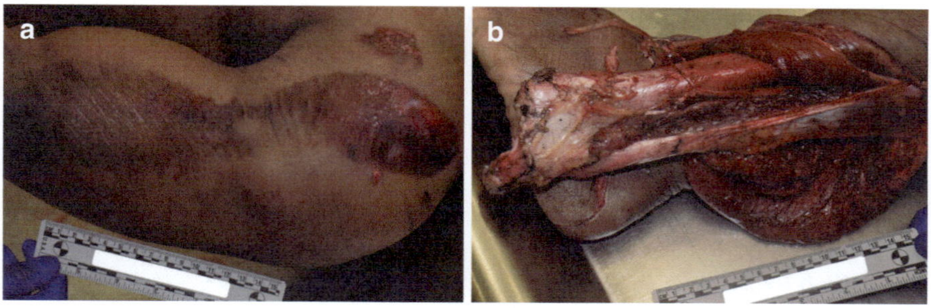

Fig. 7.11 Pedestrian run-over and dragged. (**a**) Extensive brush-type abrasions on arm. (**b**) Extensive avulsion injury of leg with dislocation of ankle

In the case of a driver fatality, there will be investigative information about airbag deployment, and the question may arise whether it had any role in injury causation because of historical data when "first-generation" ("aggressive") air bags were introduced [17, 18]. In a study of motor vehicle driver fatalities occurring in frontal impacts, the injury pattern with the deployment of "less aggressive" third-generation air bags installed in the current motor vehicle fleet trended to a greater incidence of intra-thoracic trauma compared with first-generation air bags suggesting increased loading of the chest through the airbag. No deaths were attributed to third-generation airbag deployment in this study. Collision severity rather than airbag deployment was a major factor in causing fatal injuries [19].

Traumatic Pneumothorax

Pneumothorax, pneumomediastinum, and subcutaneous emphysema can be caused by air leaks either from the respiratory tract (e.g., lacerated bronchus) or lungs (e.g., lung laceration by a displaced rib fracture). Mechanical ventilation can result in pulmonary barotrauma, particularly in a patient with lung disease (e.g., emphysema). Esophageal rupture can also lead to pneumomediastinum and subcutaneous emphysema.

Clinical or postmortem radiographic imaging prior to the autopsy can demonstrate a pneumothorax.

Decompression of a pneumothorax by insertion of intravenous catheters (needle thoracostomy) through the upper chest wall may have been attempted during resuscitation. Whether the catheters entered the pleural cavities can be assessed when the chest flap is reflected at autopsy. One study found that a 5-mm catheter inserted at the level of the second intercostal space failed to enter the pleural cavity in 42.5% of cases [15]. A chest tube (tube thoracostomy) is typically introduced unilaterally or bilaterally through the fourth or fifth intercostal spaces. In situ inspection of the chest cavities can determine whether the tips of the tubes are free or penetrate a lung. An Asherman Chest Seal is used to treat open chest wounds.

At autopsy, crepitus in the neck and chest is a sign that a pneumothorax may have occurred. If the pneumothorax has not been decompressed during resuscitation, then it can be demonstrated by the insertion of a 60 cc syringe filled with a few cc of water into the anterolateral fourth or fifth intercostal space. Air expelled from a tension pneumothorax can be seen as air bubbles in the water inside the syringe, and the volume of air can be quantified in the syringe.

Chest Wall Fractures

Up to 50% of rib fractures are missed in plain film chest radiographs [15, 20, 21]. In one study, 86% of the fractures found at autopsy had been missed by chest radiographs [22]. Antemortem or postmortem CT imaging is more sensitive in detecting rib fractures [23]. CT imaging showing axial (inward/outward) displacement of rib fractures is a potential marker for hemothorax, hemopneumothorax, flail chest, and visceral injury [20, 24].

Sternal and rib fractures with or without displacement and associated soft tissue hemorrhage may be visible on the anterior and anterolateral chest wall when the first autopsy incision is made. Complete documentation of the extent and distribution of rib fractures is done after the viscera are removed. Costosternal and anterior rib fractures can be seen or palpated on the sternal plate. Anterolateral, lateral (at maximum curvature of rib), posterolateral, posterior (at the level of a horizontal line drawn through the anterior border of the thoracic vertebrae), or costovertebral fractures can be found on inspection of the pleural cavities [20]. Because anterolateral fractures are adjacent to ribs that have been cut when the sternum is removed, the pathologist may need clarification from the assistant on whether they could be dissection artifact. Rib fractures represent sites of direct impact, but they can occur indirectly from an impacted area at the posterolateral angle, the structurally weakest area of the rib cage [15].

Complete fractures, particularly if they are displaced and associated with pleural lacerations, are usually obvious, but rib fractures that are incomplete ("buckle fracture") can be less apparent. Biomechanical studies have shown that chest impact resulting in compression of the outer cortex of the rib is less likely to cause a fracture compared to the consequent tension on the inner cortex; therefore, a buckle fracture may only be evident inside the chest [20, 25, 26]. Focal subpleural areas of hemorrhage can help localize "buckle" and complete fractures.

Age-related changes decrease bone elasticity and increase the likelihood of a complete fracture and displacement [21, 26, 27].

Flail chest is a common injury in MVCs [28]. A flail chest occurs when there are fractures of:

- three or more continuous ribs in two or more locations, or
- three or more bilateral consecutive ribs, or
- three or more ribs associated with a sternal fracture [29].

Flail chest is a cause of death. Hospitalized patients need mechanical ventilation which increases the risk of pulmonary barotrauma, pneumonia, sepsis, and adult respiratory distress syndrome (ARDS) [29].

Traumatic Hemothorax

The volume of blood drained from a chest tube may be recorded in the clinical chart. At autopsy, blood in a chest tube drainage container can be quantified. Sources of traumatic hemothorax are outlined in Table 7.1.

Traumatic Hemoperitoneum

A Focused Assessment with Sonography for Trauma (FAST) scan is a point-of-care ultrasound examination done during the initial trauma management to determine whether bleeding has occurred, but its origin cannot be localized by FAST. CT imaging can identify possible sources of bleeding, but a patient who is hemodynamically unstable may be taken directly to laparotomy. In some cases, bleeding from intra-abdominal organs can be delayed, and catastrophic hemorrhage occurs later in the clinical course (e.g., spleen, liver, and mesentery) (Figs. 7.13 and 7.14) [1, 35, 36]. Histology showing an inflammatory reaction and healing changes can confirm that delayed rupture has occurred [37].

Table 7.1 Sources of traumatic hemothorax

Rib fracture
– Pulmonary laceration
– Laceration of intercostal vessel[a] [30]
Sternum fracture (laceration of the internal mammary vessel)[b]
Clavicle fracture (laceration of the subclavian vessel) [31]
Thoracic spine fracture [32]
Intrapericardial trauma (hemopericardium) with pericardial tear
– Cardiac laceration[a] [33]
– Inferior vena cava
– Ascending aorta
Transmural laceration of descending thoracic aorta (isthmus) (Fig. 7.12) with pleural laceration (left hemothorax) ± mid-thoracic spine fracture
Azygos vein laceration with pleural tear and mid-thoracic vertebral fracture (right hemothorax) [34]
Diaphragm rupture with
– Herniation of lacerated spleen (left hemothorax)
– Herniation of lacerated liver (right hemothorax)

[a] Delayed presentation possible
[b] Hemomediastinum also

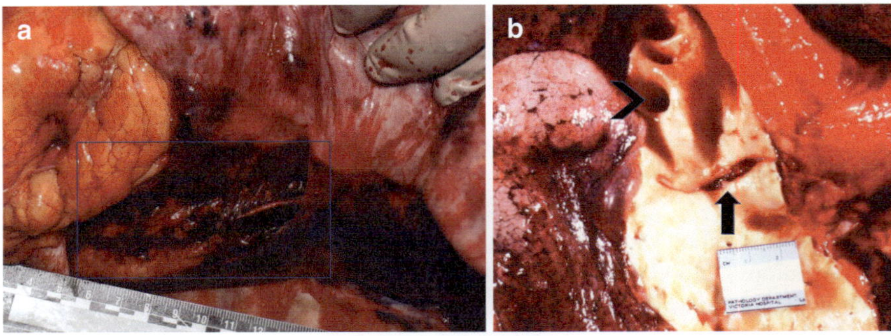

Fig. 7.12 Fatal motor vehicle collisions. (**a**) Left lung retracted to allow in situ examination of the left pleural cavity. Subpleural hemorrhage along the length of the thoracic aorta is a sign of an aortic laceration. An associated pleural tear results in a left hemothorax. (**b**) Posterior view of en bloc dissection of heart and lungs. Opening along the length of the descending thoracic aorta toward the arch reveals a horizontal transmural laceration (arrow) in the isthmic area just below the subclavian artery ostium (arrowhead) which is the most common site of aortic injury from sudden deceleration. Note that aortic lacerations can have defined edges mimicking a cut that could be misinterpreted as due to postmortem dissection

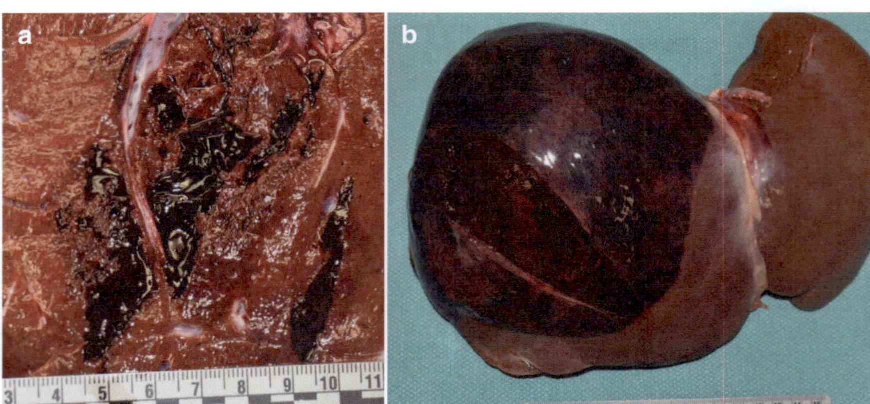

Fig. 7.13 Thin fibrous capsules cover the liver and spleen which have soft parenchyma. The more resistant capsule may not tear, but an intraparenchymal laceration can occur. An expansile hematoma can form which can lead to rupture. (**a**) Intraparenchymal hepatic laceration. (**b**) Expansile subcapsular hepatic hematoma, unruptured

In the case of a motor vehicle occupant fatality, there may be loading evidence from a seatbelt that was positioned on the abdomen instead of the pelvis. The "seatbelt sign" is a sign of potential intra-abdominal trauma (Fig. 7.15) [1].

To determine the origin of the hemoperitoneum, the abdominal cavity can be examined in situ for lacerations of major organs and structures (liver, spleen, mesentery, and gastrointestinal tract).

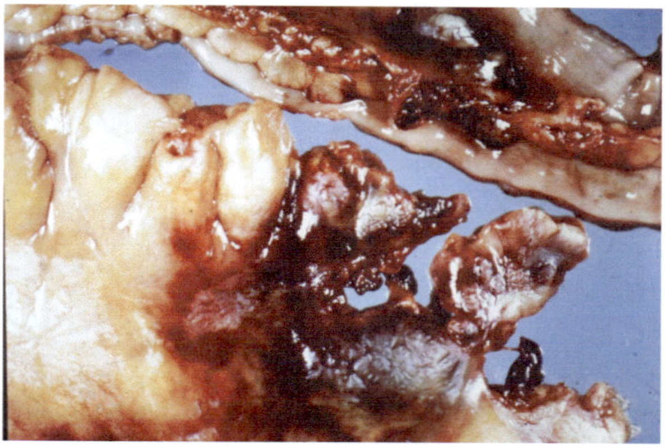

Fig. 7.14 Victim stomped on abdomen. Small bowel mesenteric laceration. In any case of hemoperitoneum, in situ examination of the peritoneal cavity to determine the origin of the hemorrhage should include inspection of the mesentery in addition to the more common sites, i.e., spleen and liver

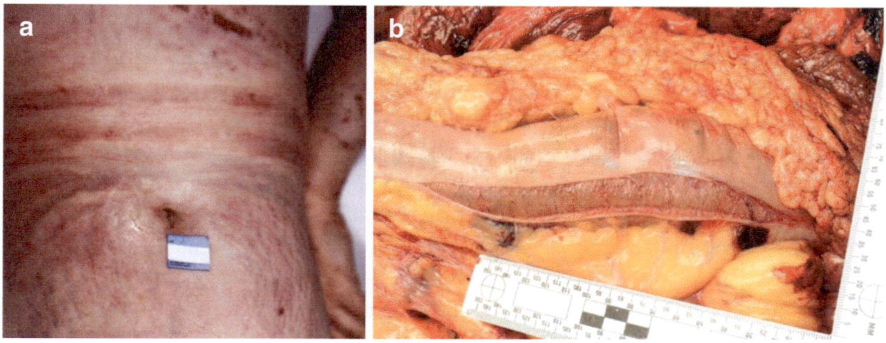

Fig. 7.15 Motor vehicle occupant—"Seat Belt Sign." (**a**) Parallel horizontal linear bruises extending across the upper abdomen indicative of an improperly positioned lap belt. (**b**) Seromuscular tear, bowel, due to seatbelt loading. (Courtesy of Dr. R. Jacques)

Hemoperitoneum can be retroperitoneal in origin (see sections "Retroperitoneal Hemorrhage" and "Pelvis").

Retroperitoneal Hemorrhage

During the in situ examination of the abdominal cavity, retroperitoneal hemorrhage may be seen. Once the abdominal viscera have been removed, it will be more evident.

Although the total volume of hemorrhage cannot be quantitated because of blood tracking around organs and in tissue planes, the extent and expansion of the retroperitoneal space by hemorrhage are evidence of the severity of the bleeding (see section "Pelvis").

Sources of traumatic retroperitoneal hemorrhage include:

- Zone I—central (pancreas, duodenum, abdominal aorta and branches, inferior vena cava and branches)
- Zone II—flank (kidney, adrenal gland; duodenum and pancreas also)
- Zone III—pelvis (fractures, intrapelvic veins or arteries, urinary bladder)
- Zone IV—combinations of the above [38]

Hemorrhagic Shock

The average adult blood volume is 70 mL/kg (7% of body weight) or about 5 L [39]. Blood volume varies with age and is decreased in older individuals. The estimated blood volume in children is 8–9% of body weight and up to 9–10% in infants [39]. The Nadler or Lemmens–Bernstein–Brodsky equations can give a more accurate determination of blood volume based on sex, height, and weight [40, 41].

Blood loss greater than 750 cc in the average person (blood volume > 15%) can result in early hemorrhagic shock (Class IV) [39]. Continued bleeding resulting in more than a 40% loss of blood volume (>2000 cc) is preterminal (Class IV hemorrhagic shock) requiring immediate treatment [39].

Although the volume of blood lost at a scene from trauma cannot be quantified, its extent can be correlated with the severity of the injuries seen at autopsy. During the autopsy, blood in the pleural and peritoneal cavities can be measured and correlated to the decedent's body weight to estimate the percentage of blood volume lost. Observations seen during the autopsy such as diminished lividity, subendocardial hemorrhages ("shock hemorrhages"), and pallor of kidneys are signs that have been associated with hemorrhagic shock.

Thoracolumbar Spine

MVCs are a common cause of thoracic and lumbar fractures.

In one study of motor vehicle occupants who presented to a trauma center, most fractures occurred at the thoracolumbar junction (T11–L2) followed by the thoracic (T1–T10) and lumbar (L3–L5) regions [42]. Although fracture-dislocation was more likely in unbelted occupants, the authors found that three-point appropriately belted occupants were not more protected from thoracic and lumbar spine injury compared with unbelted occupants. Other factors such as increased stiffness of the occupant's seat combined with its upward contour may introduce additional compressive forces on the spine and increase the likelihood of compression and burst fractures. Airbag deployment in three-point belted occupants appeared to have a protective effect against thoracolumbar spinal injury. Chest injuries were the most common associated injuries. The stability that the bony chest wall provides to the thoracic spine and the partial protection by the lower ribs of the lumbar spine may be responsible for the association of chest injuries with thoracolumbar spine trauma.

Pelvis

A pelvic binder may be applied during resuscitation to control internal bleeding from a pelvic fracture. Linear ("stretch") abrasions on the anterior pelvic brim may be a sign of a pelvic fracture (Fig. 7.16). Antemortem or postmortem radiographic imaging, particularly a CT scan, can confirm and document fracture-dislocations. Separation of the symphysis pubis is easily palpable at autopsy. Fractures of the pubic rami and sacroiliac joint disruption can also be carefully felt to avoid prosector injury.

Anterior–posterior compression of the torso can separate the symphysis pubis and cause posterior ligamentous injury and separation of the sacroiliac joints [43, 44]. Widening of the symphysis pubis by more than 2.5 cm is associated with a significant degree of separation of one or both sacroiliac joints [44, 45]. Sacroiliac joint widening is a sign of serious soft tissue and visceral injury because considerable force is needed to tear the interosseous sacroiliac ligaments, the strongest ligaments [41, 43]. Vertical shear from axial loading resulting in unstable pelvic fractures can occur not only in MVCs (e.g., ejection from a motorcycle and submarining under a restraint system) but also from falls from heights (see section

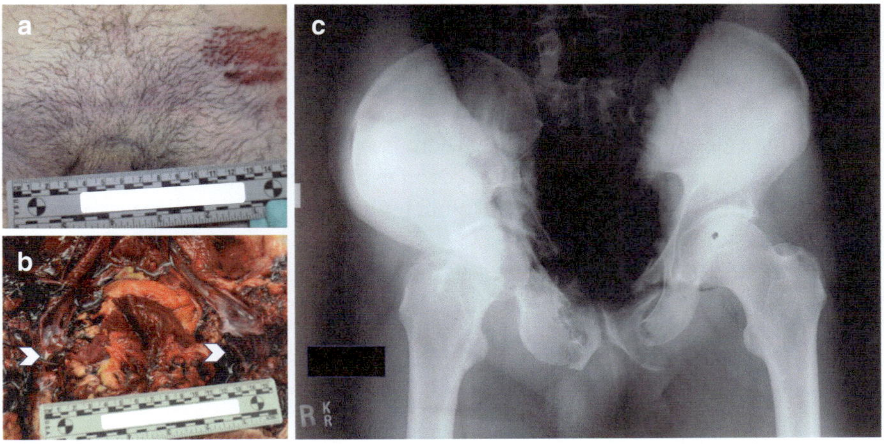

Fig. 7.16 Pelvic trauma. (**a**) "Stretch" abrasions on the left lower abdominal quadrant and bruising extending across the lower abdomen/suprapubic area are visible signs of underlying pelvic fractures and intrapelvic injuries. (**b**) Disruption of bilateral iliofemoral veins (arrowheads) with associated intrapelvic hemorrhage. (**c**) Postmortem plain film anterior-posterior radiograph of pelvis. Fractures of pubic rami

"Descent from Heights") and impact by a heavy load on the head, shoulders, or back (e.g., logging/mining accidents) [43, 44, 46].

An initially conscious person with any type of pelvic fracture regardless of its stability can become hemodynamically unstable [47–50]. Older individuals can be predisposed to severe pelvic hemorrhage because of the increased fragility of arteriosclerotic (plaques) arteries and loss of intrapelvic support tissue [51]. Venous bleeding is more common and accounts for a less rapid decline into shock compared to arterial bleeding [47, 49, 50]. Hemorrhage from intrapelvic vascular injury can spread into the abdominal retroperitoneal space, thighs, and gluteal areas [48]. Up to 4 L of blood can accumulate in the retroperitoneal space before more widespread bleeding occurs [49].

Craniocerebral Trauma

Scalp

Accurate documentation of a scalp wound requires washing away blood and cutting/shaving of hair around the injury (Fig. 7.4). Occult subscalp contusions are revealed when the scalp is incised and reflected.

A cutaneous scalp injury may be the impact site for a skull fracture. Subscalp hemorrhage can be diffuse if head impact is on or from a surface with a large area. Neurosurgical incisions can alter skin injuries and cause diffuse subscalp hemorrhage.

Skull Fracture

A calvarium fracture may be palpable. There may be external signs of a basal skull fracture such as periorbital bruises ("raccoon eyes"), scleral hemorrhage, bleeding with or without expulsion of blood and brain tissue from the ear and nose, and bruising in the mastoid area.

Stripping the dura reveals fractures in the inner table of the calvarium and base that, in the case of the calvarium fractures, may not be evident on the outer skull.

Brain Retention

In general, the need to retain the brain will depend on the circumstances of the case and the statutory regulations regarding organ retention in the jurisdiction where the autopsy is done. Death from major head trauma in the context of a homicide investigation will necessitate brain retention after the body is released to ensure adequate formalin fixation to allow an optimum neuropathological examination (see section "Diffuse Axonal Injury (DAI) and Diffuse Vascular Injury (DVI)").

Diffuse Axonal Injury (DAI) and Diffuse Vascular Injury (DVI)

Classical acute DAI (severe traumatic axonal injury) and diffuse vascular injury (DVI) commonly occur in MVCs from shear stress on the brain due to sudden acceleration–deceleration (inertia), but they can occur when there is rapid movement of the head from other causes [52]. Evidence of scalp and skull contact injuries may not be present. DAI also occurs in assaults and falls from heights.

Unconsciousness from classical acute DAI happens immediately and persists until death [1]. Traumatic axonal injury is applied to cases in which there is a lucid interval before death. Victims of DVI are either dead at the scene or unconscious a few hours before dying.

Minimal subarachnoid hemorrhage may be seen. Brain sections may be unremarkable or show focal hemorrhagic foci [i.e., gliding (parasagittal) contusions at the dorsal angle of the frontal and parietal lobes, hemorrhagic laceration of the corpus callosum, and hematomas in the dorsolateral quadrants of the upper brainstem] [1]. Petechiae in DVI may be seen grossly in the deep gray matter, the frontal and temporal lobe white matter, corpus callosum, midline of the hypothalamus, dorsal and lateral pons, midbrain, and around the third and fourth ventricles and cerebral aqueduct (Fig. 7.17) [1, 52]. Because the diagnosis of DAI and DVI rests on histology, formalin fixation ensures optimum cutting and sampling. Generally, in MVC-related deaths, a non-fixed brain can be cut at autopsy, and representative brain slices required for histology are kept and fixed in formalin, and the remainder of the brain can be released with the body (see section "Cerebral Edema and Herniation").

Histological sections taken from the frontal subcortical white matter and adjacent corpus callosum, deep gray matter including posterior limb of the internal capsule, splenium of the corpus callosum, cerebellar white matter, caudal midbrain (level of decussation of the superior cerebellar peduncle), and rostral pons (basis pontis and superior and middle cerebellar peduncles) can determine whether classical DAI is present [1]. Numerous axonal swellings detected by immunohistochemical staining for beta-amyloid precursor protein (BAPP) in the corpus callosum, subcortical white matter, and basis pontis support the diagnosis of classical DAI (Fig. 7.18) [1]. Axonal swellings are less extensive and numerous in traumatic axonal injury [1]. The older medical literature has documented that BAPP-labeled axonal swellings can occur within 2 h of survival time; [53, 54] however, BAPP-labeled axonal swellings can be seen after about 35 minutes of survival [55].

Hypoxic Ischemic Encephalopathy (HIE)

A transient cardiorespiratory arrest can occur at the time of the head injury and cause HIE. In certain cases (see section "Commotio Medullaris (Brainstem Concussion)"), removal of the spinal cord to show histological evidence of neuronal necrosis supports global ischemia arising from a transient cardiorespiratory arrest. The microscopic features of ischemic neuronal necrosis are not apparent until

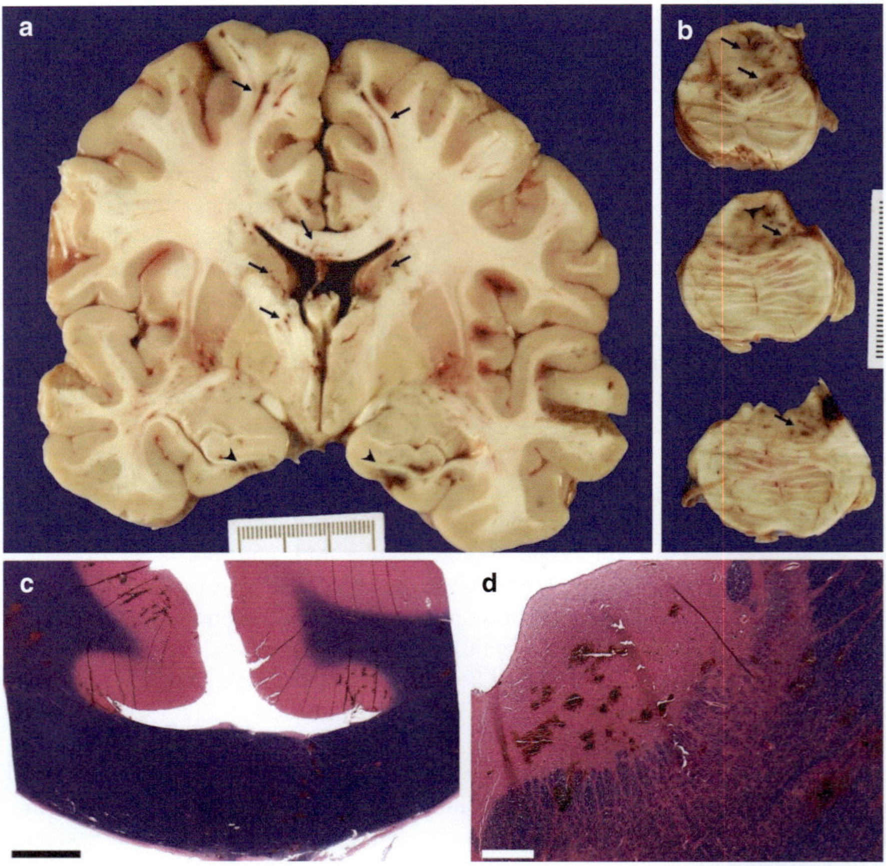

Fig. 7.17 (**a**) Coronal sections of the cerebral hemispheres at the level of mammillary bodies. There are scattered petechial hemorrhages in the parasagittal white matter, corpus callosum, internal capsule, and basal ganglia (arrow). Also presented are the small cortical hemorrhages in bilateral parahippocampal gyri, secondary to uncal herniation due to brain swelling (arrowhead). (**b**) Horizontal sections of the brainstem. Extensive petechial hemorrhages are seen in the dorsal pons, more prominent at the dorsolateral aspect (arrow). (**c**, **d**) Microscopic images of hematoxylin-eosin and Luxol fast blue stained sections from (**a**) and (**b**). Note the perivascular hemorrhages in the parasagittal white matter, corpus callosum (**c**), and dorsal pons (**d**) are more extensive than shown in the gross images (**a**, **b**). Scale bars represent 3 mm in (**c**) and 600 µm in (**d**). (Reprinted by permission from Oxford University Press. Stewart MKG, Shkrum MJ, McClafferty KJ, Mao H, Zhang Q. A Neuropathological Study of Diffuse Vascular Injury in Fatal Motor Vehicle Collisions. J Neuropathol Exp Neurol. 2022 Jan 29;81(2):88–96)

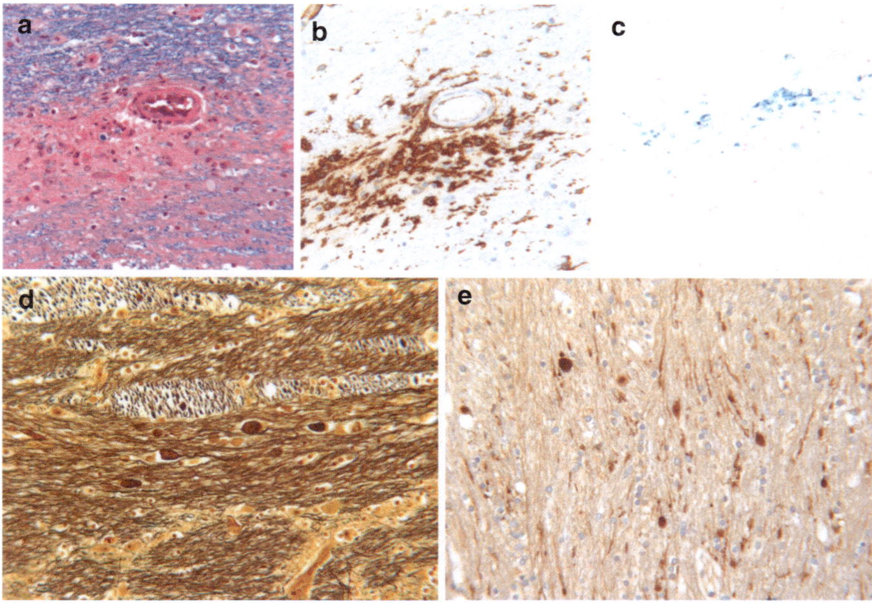

Fig. 7.18 Photomicroscopy of diffuse axonal injury in a 49-year-old man who remained unconscious until death, 18 days following an assault. (**a**) Basis pontis, HE/LFB, 25×. Perivascular petechial hemorrhage in pontine white matter. (**b**) Basis pontis, HLA-DR1 immunohistochemistry, 25×. Marked activation of microglia/macrophages at the site of petechia. (**c**) Basis pontis, Perls' Prussian blue, 25×. Perivascular siderophages. (**d**) Basis pontis, Bielschowsky's method, 25×. Argyrophilic axonal swellings (with tadpole-like morphology). Swellings are most prominent in the crossing fiber (elsewhere they were more prominent in the vertical tracts)—i.e., "tract dysjunction." (**e**) Internal capsule, amyloid precursor protein immunohistochemistry, 25×. Note immunopositive axonal swellings and strands. (Courtesy: David A. Ramsay. Emeritus Professor and Neuropathologist, Western University and London Health Sciences Centre)

6–12 h after a head injury, and they may not be evident if, during this interval, cerebral blood flow has stopped because of cerebral edema [1].

Cerebral Edema and Herniation

Traumatic brain swelling can be either diffuse and associated with HIE or localized and adjacent to contusions, intracerebral hematomas, or peridural hemorrhage.

Gyral flattening and narrowing of sulci creating a smooth cerebral outline are external signs of diffuse cerebral edema. Cerebral ventricles narrow. Various types of herniation can occur: uncal/transtentorial herniation (unci, parahippocampal gyri, and basilar temporal and occipital lobes) with occipital lobe infarction if the posterior cerebral arteries are compressed; central herniation of the thalamus; secondary brainstem or "Duret" hemorrhages (midline rostral pons, tegmentum of pons, and midbrain) (Fig. 7.19); and cerebellar tonsillar herniation resulting in necrotic tissue in the spinal subarachnoid space. Localized cerebral edema can lead to subfalcine herniation of the cingulate gyrus under the falx cerebri. Large cerebellar hematomas can lead to upward herniation.

The removal and sectioning of swollen brains at autopsy can be challenging. If retention of the whole brain is not possible, then delaying the release of the body up to 48 h to allow partial formalin fixation of the brain and representative sectioning with the return of non-retained brain to the body is another option.

Cervical Spine

Neck hyperextension (e.g., pedestrian struck by a car) or hyperflexion (e.g., motor vehicle occupant in frontal collision) are common injury mechanisms. Head impact may or may not be present [1].

Hypermobility of the neck felt during the external examination raises the possibility of cervical spine trauma. After the larynx is removed, soft tissue hemorrhage, either tracking down or localized on the anterior cervical spine, is a sign that a fracture or dislocation or both may be present (Fig. 7.20). Hemorrhage indicates an antemortem or perimortem trauma and distinguishes it from a postmortem fracture due to manipulation of an osteoporotic neck. Dissection of hemorrhagic tissue can

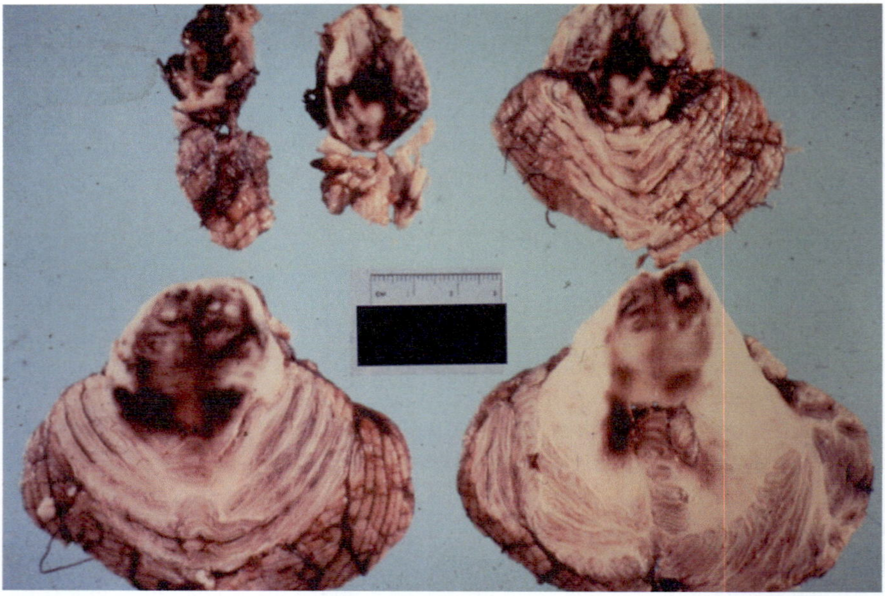

Fig. 7.19 Secondary brainstem ("Duret") hemorrhages due to cerebral edema. Duret hemorrhages are typically prominent in the pontine midline or throughout the pontine and midbrain tegmentum. Note the contrast to the more subtle and smaller petechial hemorrhages seen in the pons in diffuse vascular injury (see Fig. 7.16)

reveal mid- and lower cervical spine vertebral body/intervertebral disc fractures and dislocations. Inspection of the base of the skull and rotation of the head can show a visibly displaced spine in the foramen magnum from an atlanto-occipital dislocation. An atlas fracture and gaps created by ligamentous tears can be palpated through the foramen. Palpation of the cervical spine from below can detect an atlanto-axial junction fracture-dislocation and odontoid peg fracture. Plain film radiography can confirm and document fracture-dislocation. CT imaging can assist in demonstrating a cervical spine injury particularly if it is subtle.

Trauma involving the atlanto-occipital (AO) junction and upper cervical vertebrae can cause fatal brainstem or upper spinal cord injury. Mid-cervical spinal trauma can injure the spinal cord (C3, C4, C5) that controls diaphragmatic movement. Lower cervical spine injury can result in paralysis and lead to eventual death from pulmonary thromboembolism or sepsis (e.g., urinary tract infection).

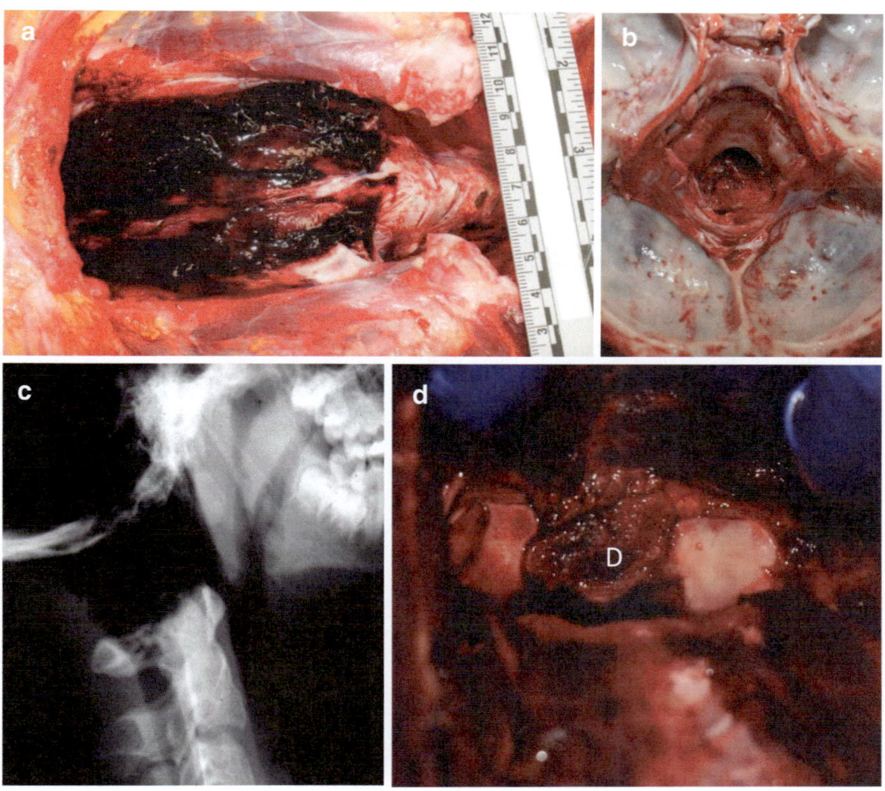

Fig. 7.20 Upper cervical spine trauma. (**a**) Larynx removed. Hemorrhage tracking down the cervical spine. (**b**) Base of skull. Cervical spine visible in foramen magnum due to atlanto-occipital dislocation. (**c**) Lateral skull radiograph. Atlanto-occipital dislocation. (**d**) View from below after neck dissection. Atlas reflected to show inferior articular surfaces for the axis and fractured odontoid process (**d**). (Courtesy of Dr. E. Tweedie)

Partial tearing or transection at one or more levels of the brainstem (ponto-medullary junction, cervico-medullary junction, or midbrain) can occur with AO-dislocation (Fig. 7.21). Subarachnoid hemorrhage may be seen at the base of the brain. The basilar artery may or may not be torn. Care is required when removing the brain because forceful tugging can result in an artifactual ponto-medullary junction tear. Partial lacerations of the pons-medulla junction can be subtle particularly when sectioning an unfixed brain at autopsy. Longitudinal sections of the junction for histology will show hemorrhagic foci around the lacerated site confirming a perimortem injury. Because the cervico-medullary junction is cut to remove the brain, the determination that transection has actually occurred at this level is better appreciated by examining it through the foramen magnum while the brain is in situ and gently reflecting it posteriorly. Exposure of the spinal cord by either an anterior or posterior approach and sampling for histology can demonstrate trauma (contusion, contusion–laceration, and transection) at other levels.

Spinal cord injury can occur in adults and children without radiological evidence (SCIWORA) of a fracture or soft tissue injury. MRI (magnetic resonance imaging) has shown trauma of non-bony supporting tissues of the vertebral column [56, 57].

Falls from Standing Height

Victims of falls can be either found dead at the scene or active for a period of time before dying.

Falls from a standing height can result in a pattern of cutaneous injuries on the face and head. Chronic alcoholics who stumble and fall repeatedly while

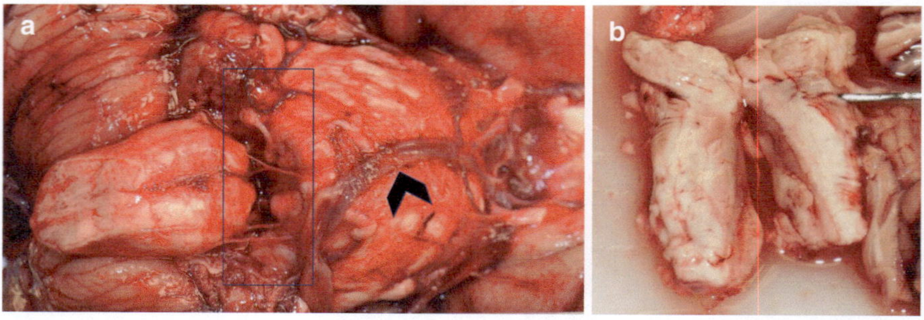

Fig. 7.21 (**a**) Pontomedullary laceration (rectangle). Basilar artery intact (arrowhead). (**b**) Longitudinal cut through caudal pons and medulla during the examination of brain at autopsy. Probe pointing to tear at pons-medulla junction. Histological sections showing parenchymal hemorrhages will confirm that the laceration happened while the victim was alive in contrast to a "tug" artifact caused when the brain is removed at autopsy

intoxicated can sustain multiple injuries that appear suspicious for assault (see section "Assaults"). Injuries can occur not only on the bony prominences of the face (forehead, supraorbital ridge, tip of nose, zygoma, and chin) but also on the chest, posterior elbows, ulnar aspect of the forearms, knees, shins, and dorsal surface of the toes (Fig. 7.3). One or more facial or scalp lacerations can bleed extensively and cause hemorrhagic shock [58, 59]. In these cases, there may be signs of extensive bleeding at the scene where trauma occurred. Other than cutaneous lacerations, no other source of bleeding is found at autopsy [58]. Clinically, the significance of a facial or scalp laceration may not be appreciated until blood pressure and volume are restored during resuscitation, and profuse bleeding follows [58]. Compensatory physiological response to blood loss can be compromised by ischemic heart disease [58].

A major focus at autopsy is to determine whether fatal craniocerebral trauma has occurred. Subdural hemorrhage (SDH) occurs when there is short-duration acceleration of the brain relative to the skull following head impact and is typically associated with falls but can occur in assaults [55, 60, 61]. A skull fracture may or may not be present. Linear or radial fractures are typical [61]. SDH is situated over the convexity of the cerebral hemispheres and can extend onto the skull base. The location of SDH may be unrelated to the site of impact. At autopsy, SDH can be a thin film of blood or a space-occupying mass. The volume of an acute SDH is a guide to whether it caused death: >120 cc, invariably fatal; 50–120 cc, likely fatal if subfalcine and uncal herniation; and <50 cc, unlikely fatal [1].

SDH can evolve over time before death ensues, and purposeful activity by the victim is possible. A review of death scene images may show the effects on increased intracranial pressure such as vomiting, incontinence, and stumbling and falling. The nature of the blood in the SDH seen can give an estimate of its age: acute, blood clotted (time of injury to about 48 h old); subacute, blood partly clotted, and liquid (2 days to 3 weeks old); chronic, blood completely liquified (>3 weeks old) (Fig. 7.22) [1]. A chronic SDH has a thick outer membrane and thin inner membrane enclosing a variably sized cavity containing liquid blood or bloody fluid. The determination of the age of SDH can be supplemented by histology [61, 62]. Yellow staining of the dura indicates significant hemosiderin deposition. Siderophages indicate that the SDH is at least several days old.

Although contrecoup contusions can be seen in sites that are not necessarily diagonally opposite the point of impact, involvement of the frontal and temporal lobes due to an occipital skull impact from a fall backward is a classical and frequent observation (Fig. 7.23) [63, 64]. Cerebellar coup contusions can also occur from an impact to the back of the head as a result of a fall. A coup contusion can result from a fall against a protruding object [61].

Cervical spine and cord injury can occur (see section "Cervical Spine").

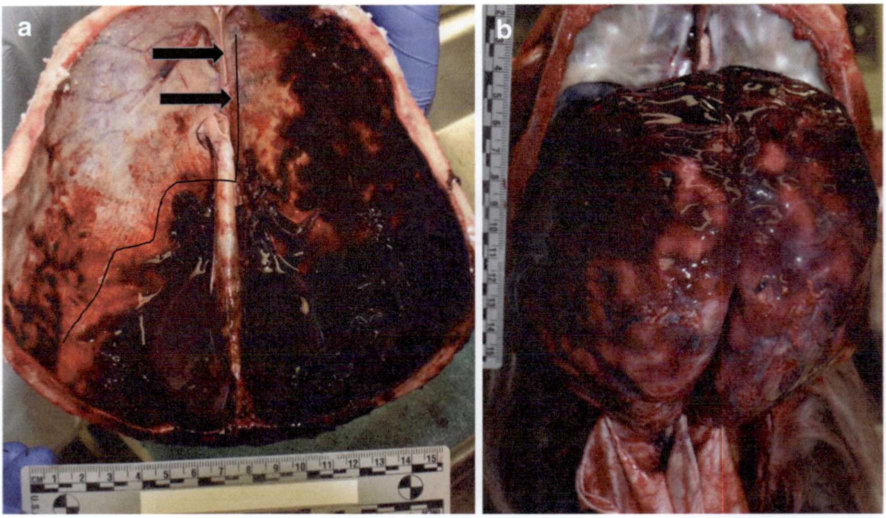

Fig. 7.22 (**a**) Undersurface of calvarium showing subdural hemorrhage. Outline of recent and healing subdural hemorrhage (SDH). At the edges of the SDH particularly in the frontal area (arrows), yellow discoloration from hemosiderin deposition indicates healing. Blood from the recent SDH has pooled on the posterior calvarium. An acute SDH will have blood caked under the dura which can be measured in three dimensions to determine its volume. If the victim survives, SDH will liquefy. A pan positioned under the head can be used to collect blood that will inevitably seep when the skull is being opened. Subdural blood has been used for toxicological analysis. The rationale is that this blood is sequestered from the circulation and not subject to metabolism that normally occurs during a survival period. (**b**) Subarachnoid hemorrhage. In contrast to a SDH, wiping the surface of the brain at autopsy will not remove subarachnoid blood

Fig. 7.23 Contrecoup contusions: inferior frontal lobes (rectangular outlines) and temporal poles (oval outlines). Yellow subarachnoid staining adjacent to contusions indicates the formation of hemosiderin as part of the healing process

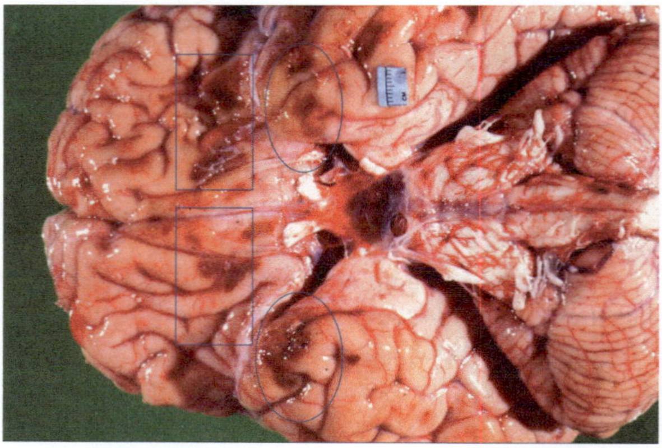

Assaults

Victims of fatal assaults frequently sustain head injuries. The pathologist's interpretation of all postmortem observations including the pattern of craniocerebral trauma

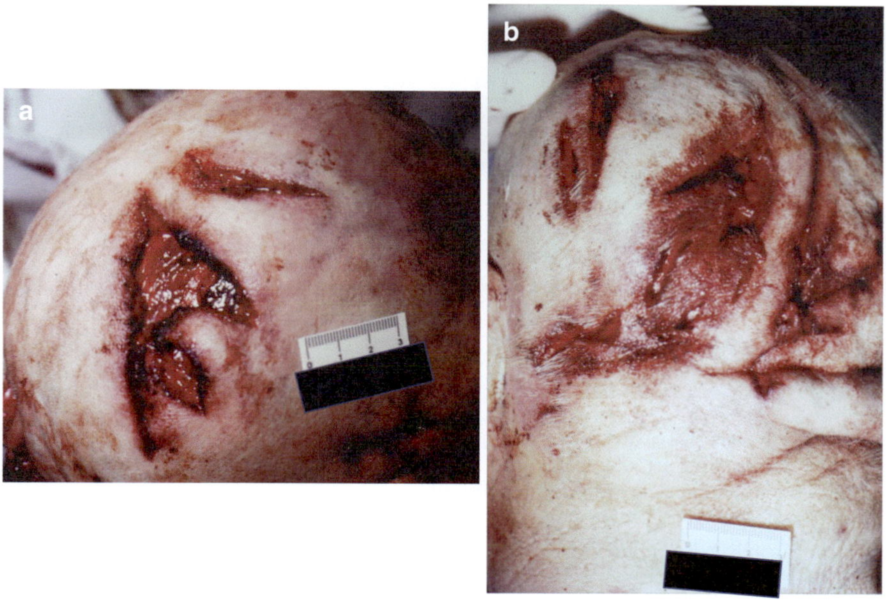

Fig. 7.24 Homicide. Hair has been cut and scalp shaved to show multiple lacerations on the right parietal (**a**) and posterior (**b**) scalp. Cutaneous injuries on different aspects of the scalp and above the level of the ears are indicative of multidirectional blows. In general, blows can be from punches, kicks, or strikes from an object

with the circumstances of the death and scene and other investigative information supports that a homicide has occurred.

Head Trauma: External Examination

Cutaneous injuries on different aspects of the face and the curvature of the scalp indicate multi-directional impacts (Fig. 7.24). The pattern is supportive of repeated trauma, from either blows due to punches, kicks, impacts from blunt objects, or falls on projecting surfaces. One study found that scalp lacerations were on average longer from blows (7 cm) compared with falls (3 cm), a reflection of the greater application of force in an assault [65]. Other blunt trauma injuries suggesting an altercation (e.g., contusions on the metacarpophalangeal joints from punching) or different modes of trauma (e.g., sharp-force injuries) may be present.

The hat brim rule has been proposed as a method of distinguishing falls from assaults. The hat brim line zone is an approximately 3-cm-wide area of the skull between a lower horizontal line at the level of the ear canal and an upper horizontal line at the level of the eyebrow ridges, the latter approximating the saw cut made at autopsy to remove the calvarium [65–67]. The hat brim rule states that injuries from

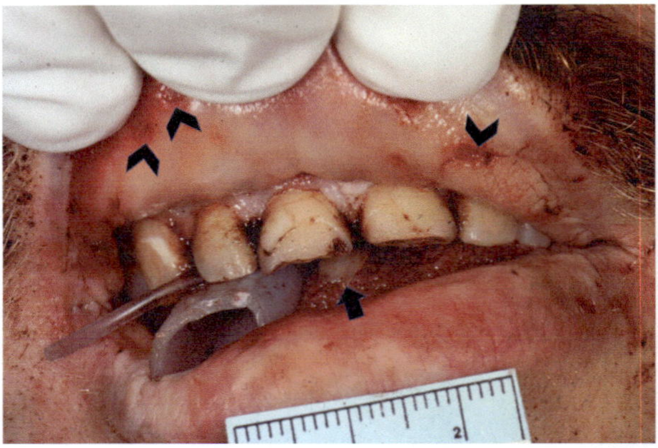

Fig. 7.25 Homicide. The victim was struck in the mouth. Superficial lacerations on the upper lip (arrowheads) from impact with lower teeth. Chipped upper central incisor teeth. Tooth fragment (arrow) on tongue. Note the endotracheal tube left in situ to confirm its position in the trachea. Its end has been cut to visualize the intraoral injuries. Clarification from the resuscitation team about preexisting injuries prior to intubation may be needed

a fall from a standing height in the absence of intermediary blows to the head do not occur above the hat brim line [65]. Several criteria have been described that favor blows over falls: a fracture and a laceration above the hat brim line; and a greater number of lacerations (average of five for blows vs. three or less for falls) [67, 68]. Victims of falls tended to have right-sided skull fractures. Because most people are right-handed, this fracture location could be due to the extension of the right arm by falling individuals to protect themselves from head impact [67]. Fractures in the hat brim line zone did not distinguish between falls and blows [67].

During resuscitation, injuries on the nose, lower jaw, and mouth (e.g., lip lacerations) can occur and mimic trauma from an assault (Fig. 7.25) [69, 70]. Poor dentition can predispose teeth to fracture or dislodge during the insertion of an airway. A fresh injury will have blood in the tooth socket. Information from the clinical record, clinical team, or a reliable person familiar with the deceased can clarify whether a broken tooth was iatrogenic or antedated resuscitation.

Craniocerebral Trauma: Internal Examination

Blows to the face are more likely than falls to cause facial fractures [65]. They may be palpable at autopsy. Radiography or facial dissection or both can accurately document fractures.

One study showed that there was a greater risk of dying from "neurologic injury" when fractures occurred in the upper or mid-face compared with isolated mandibular fractures [71]. The ability to cushion the energy of an impact by the upper and mid-facial bones can be overcome increasing the risk of brain injury (see section

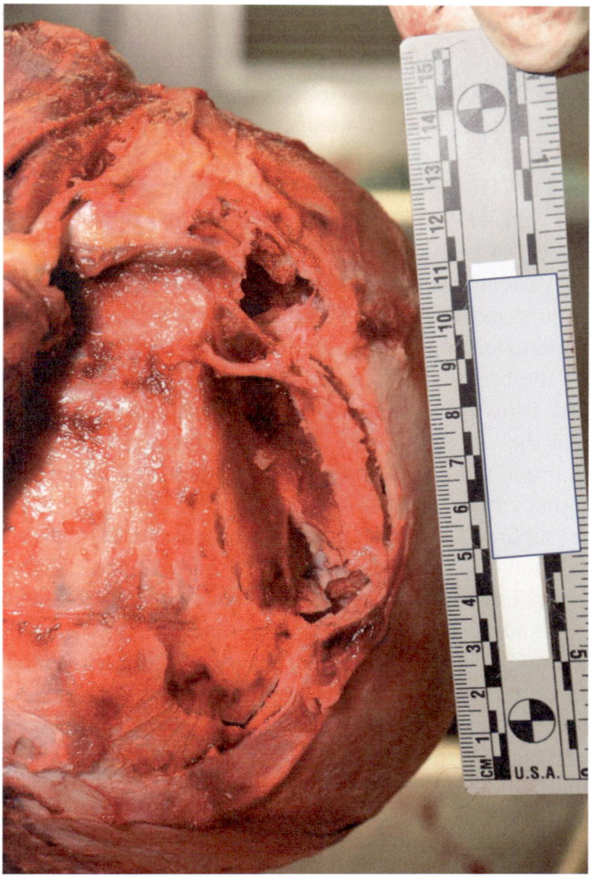

Fig. 7.26 Depressed skull fracture. The extent of the fracture suggests the nature and size of the object or surface that caused it

"Diffuse Axonal Injury (DAI) and Diffuse Vascular Injury (DVI)"); however, even a blow to the mandible resulting in hyperextension of the neck can result in fatal upper cervical spine injury (see sections "Cervical Spine" and "Traumatic Basal Subarachnoid Hemorrhage (TBSAH)") [72–74].

Comminuted and depressed fractures tend to be more common from blows than falls consistent with a greater application of force [65]. The extent of these fractures can approximate the size of the blunt object that caused it (Fig. 7.26). The sequence of multiple fractures may be determined by Puppe's rule, i.e., the line of a pre-existing fracture will arrest all the fracture lines caused by subsequent impacts) [75].

A coup contusion can be typically seen when a stationary head is struck by a blow from a relatively narrow surface [61]. Contrecoup contusions can also be seen after a blow, but, usually, a larger coup contusion is present [61, 76]. A blow to the top of the head can force the unci and cerebellar tonsils onto the edges of the tentorium and foramen magnum, respectively, causing herniation contusions.

Traumatic Basal Subarachnoid Hemorrhage (TBSAH)

Spontaneous rupture of a berry aneurysm is a common cause of basal subarachnoid hemorrhage. Rarely, aneurysmal rupture can be due to head trauma such as an assault [77].

TBSAH typically occurs after impacts (blows, kicks) to the head, face, or neck [78, 79]. TBSAH presents with rapid loss of consciousness and death either immediately or within a few hours (ibid.).

Various mechanisms have been proposed to explain how vertebral artery injury occurs and results in TBSAH: direct impact to the artery; vascular tension from hyperextension or rotation of the neck such as from a blow to the face; shear stress on the brain; and increased intravascular pressure due to vessel compression [78, 79]. Blows to the occiput or near the ear can fracture the C1 transverse process and tear the vertebral artery causing an intracranial dissection [79]. The force may be indirect and occur during the avoidance of an impact (ibid.). Co-existing axonal injury can occur (ibid.).

Victims of TBSAH are frequently intoxicated with alcohol and consequent vasodilation may predispose to vessel rupture. Intoxication can decrease reaction time to blows leading to more vigorous head or neck movements [79].

Examination of the site of vertebral injury has focused on its intracranial segment [78, 79] (Fig. 7.27). The vertebral artery is divided into four segments: V1 (pre-foraminal segment) arising from the subclavian arteries; V2 (foraminal segment) coursing through the foramina in the transverse processes from sixth to third cervical vertebrae (C6 to C2); V3 (extradural or atlantic segment) passing vertically through the transverse foramen of C1 (atlas), coursing medially in a groove on the upper surface of the posterior arch of C1 and entering the vertebral canal through the dura; and V4 (intradural or intracranial segment) passing on either side of the medulla joining to form the basilar artery.

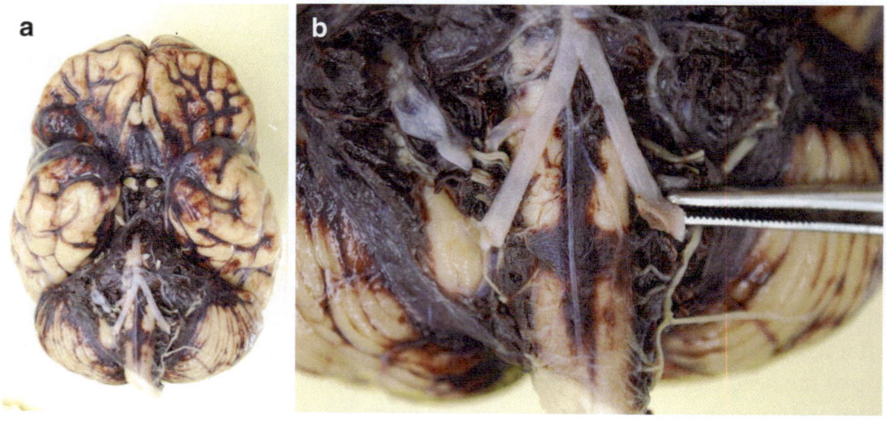

Fig. 7.27 Vertebral artery tear with associated subarachnoid hemorrhage. (**a**) Base of brain with a basal subarachnoid hemorrhage. (**b**) Close-up view of the torn intracranial segment (V4) of the left vertebral artery. (Courtesy Dr. M. Pollanen)

An intracranial vertebral injury can be subtle. A longitudinal fissure in the midpart of the vessel may be seen [78]. Injection of water into the artery during the autopsy may show a leak (ibid.). Histology can demonstrate the injury [78, 79]. Histology can also assess whether a pre-existing vasculopathy could have predisposed to rupture and the need for further investigation for a heritable connective tissue disease [79, 80].

As the intracranial segments of the vertebral arteries are routinely cut during brain removal, posterior neck dissection is the preferred method to find vessel injury [78, 81].

Cause of Death from Blunt Trauma Not Obvious at Autopsy

The cause of death in some assault cases may not be obvious particularly if the extent and severity of the blunt trauma injuries appears to be minimal. Other mechanisms may come into play.

Oculocardiac Reflex

The oculocardiac reflex is a rare cause of severe hypotension or bradycardia/asystole that occurs from facial trauma including blows [82]. Pressure on the orbit or periorbital area results in stimulation of the trigeminal-vagus nerve reflex. Orbital fractures and other facial fractures (zygoma) may or may not be present.

"Homicide by Heart Attack"

In rare cases, apparently minor external injuries or non-fatal internal trauma inflicted during an assault arouses an emotional response causing a terminal collapse of the decedent either during or shortly after ("emotional response period") the interaction with the perpetrator [83]. Death may be delayed if there is medical intervention. The postmortem examination may reveal cardiac disease that could predispose to a lethal cardiac arrhythmia. In the absence of a gross or microscopic cardiac disease, a functional cardiac disorder (e.g., channelopathy) with possible hereditary implications may have predisposed a person to an arrhythmia and may be detected by molecular diagnostic techniques.

Commotio Cordis (Cardiac Concussion)

A precordial impact can cause sudden death [84]. Ventricular arrhythmia can arise when an impact happens during the repolarization (T-wave) of the cardiac electrical cycle. Commotio cordis can occur from the impact of a projectile (e.g., ball) striking the chest such as during a sports event or from a blow from an assault. Minimal, if any signs, of external chest wall trauma may be seen. There are criteria to determine that an assault caused death from commotio cordis: witnessed occurrence of a blunt, nonpenetrating chest blow preceding cardiovascular collapse; absence of structural damage to the sternum, ribs, or heart; and absence of any underlying cardiovascular abnormalities (such as other causes of sudden death) [85].

Commotio Medullaris (Brainstem Concussion)

A person who is beaten about the face while acutely intoxicated can collapse at the scene and be found dead [86]. The determination of death from commotio medullaris is by the exclusion of other causes. The mechanism may be brainstem (medullary) dysfunction resulting in prolonged apnea from stretching of the lower brainstem by rapid movements of the head and exacerbated by ethanol which diminishes the corrective reflex attempts by the cardiorespiratory centers in the brainstem. Associated traumatic axonal injury can be seen if there is a period of survival [87].

Descent from Heights

Injury patterns seen in adults who fall 3 m or more may not distinguish accidents and suicides due to multiple factors such as the height of the fall, the initial body impact site, secondary impacts after bouncing from the initial impact, the surface impacted, and the victim's age (Fig. 7.28) [88]. In one study, victims of accidental

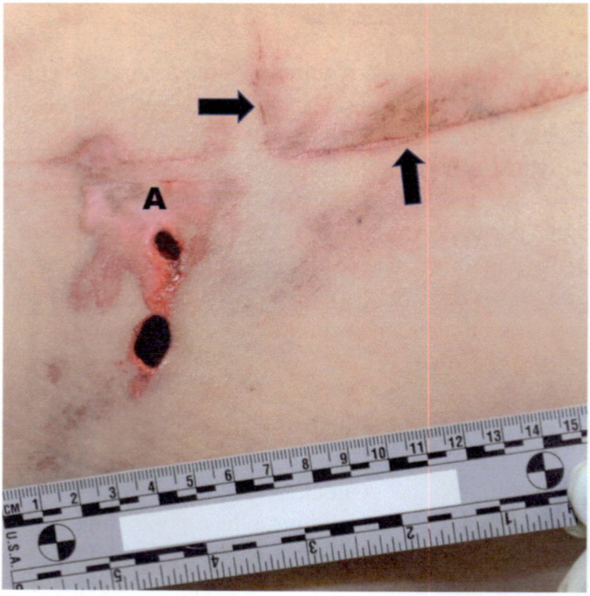

Fig. 7.28 Descent from apartment building. Imprint of paving stone on torso (arrows). Note two lacerations mimicking stab wounds caused by rib fractures displaced at the time of impact. Lacerations associated with abrasion (A) supporting blunt trauma rather than sharp-force causation

falls had spinal and upper extremities fractures likely reflecting attempts to protect themselves, whereas individuals who intentionally fell sustained fractures mostly of the lower limb, pelvis and spine, and head injuries (ibid.). Infants (≤2 years of age) have a predilection to head injury because their larger head size relative to their bodies results in a more cephalad center of gravity and less tendency to right themselves to a feet-first position like adolescents and adults [89–91]. Consequently, fractures of the pelvis, spine, and lower extremities due to axial loading are less frequent compared with older age groups [90]. Children between 3 and 10 years of age may incompletely right themselves and sustain extremity fractures [91].

Cardiopulmonary Resuscitation (CPR)

Abrasions or contusions on the mid-sternum are common. In one review, based on autopsy data, they were seen in about 60% of cases, and defibrillator burns occurred in about 30% [70].

A systematic literature review of autopsy and clinical studies found that the cardiovascular and thoracic injury rate following standard CPR ranged from 32% to 45% [92]. It rose to 58–75% with active compression-decompression (ACD) devices, and up to 100% when standard CPR was followed by ACD-CPR. Major injuries occurred in up to 3% and 7% of CPR-treated pediatric and adult patients, respectively. One study found no difference in the adverse effects of CPR administered by lay and trained individuals [22].

The incidence of rib fractures based on autopsy data was 12.9–96.6% following conventional CPR [22]. Rib fractures tend to be left-sided, but fracture distribution can vary due to hand placement [22]. The average number of fractures can usually range from six to eight [22]. Sternal fractures in one review ranged from 1.3% to 31% (ibid.). The sternum is typically fractured at the level of the fourth rib [22, 92]. Bilateral fractures of the second to seventh ribs along the mid-clavicular line are a common pattern (Fig. 7.29) [25]. Costochondral junction separation is less frequent [92]. Posterior rib fractures are uncommon [93]. Clavicle and vertebral fractures are rare [92].

The risk of fractures and CPR-related injuries increases in older individuals and during long CPR [94]. CPR in infants and children seldom results in fractures [95–97]. In a review of four autopsy studies of CPR in children (0–240 months of age), rib fractures were found in 0–2.1% [22]. Posterior rib fractures have been observed in infants when two-handed CPR has been applied [97–99]. Birth-related posterior rib fractures are uncommon and are associated with macrosomia and shoulder dystocia [100, 101].

Intrathoracic and intra-abdominal trauma can occur in the absence of chest wall fractures [92]. Epicardial, intramural, or subendocardial hemorrhage can be seen [92]. The posteroseptal myocardium is a typical site for hemorrhage due to compression of the heart against the spine. The right atrium and right and left ventricles can rupture creating a hemopericardium [22, 92]. Papillary muscle laceration and

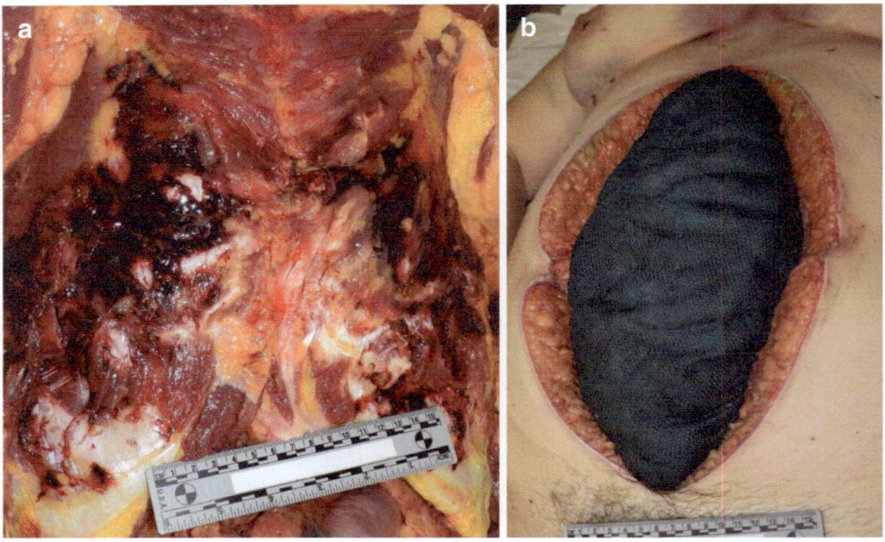

Fig. 7.29 Cause of death: complications of treatment for pulmonary thromboembolism. Resuscitation with active compression-decompression device (ACD) for 2 h before return of spontaneous circulation. (**a**) Multiple bilateral rib fractures. (**b**) Extensive liver lacerations resulted in hemoperitoneum (1½ L) requiring laparotomy, and surgical repair and packing

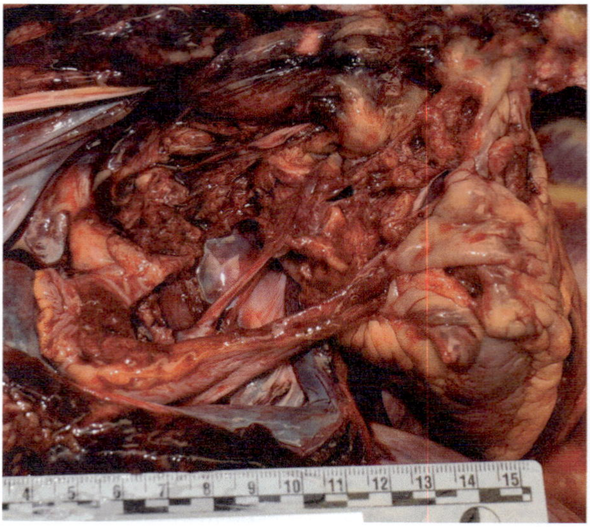

Fig. 7.30 Prolonged cardiopulmonary resuscitation. Massive laceration of the right atrium. (Courtesy of Dr. E. Tweedie)

prosthetic valve dehiscence have been observed [92]. Disruption of coronary arteries or bypass grafts, aorta, subclavian artery and vein, and the vena cava has been described following manual and ACD-CPR (Fig. 7.30) [92]. Aortic dissection can occur with ACD-CPR. Pulmonary contusions do not usually happen with standard CPR but can be caused by ACD-CPR [70, 92]. Lacerations of the esophagus, stomach, liver, and spleen have been observed [22, 92].

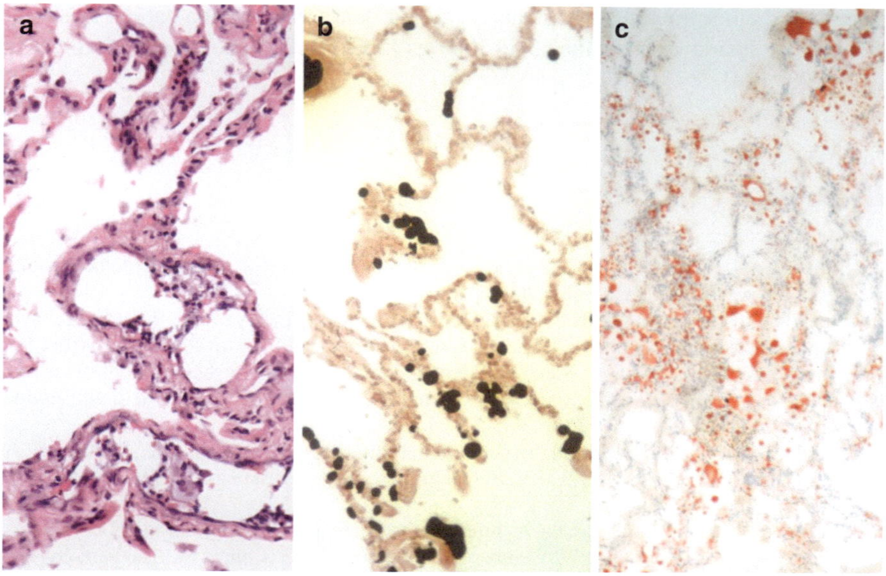

Fig. 7.31 Pulmonary fat embolism, microscopic examination. (**a**) Intravascular vacuoles (formalin-fixed tissue H&E; original magnification 200×). (**b**) Multiple fat emboli (formalin-fixed tissue, postfixation with osmium tetroxide; original magnification 100×). (**c**) Multiple fat emboli (fresh frozen tissue, oil-red-O stain; original magnification 100×). (Reprinted by permission from Springer Nature Customer Service Centre GmbH: Springer Nature, Forensic Pathology of Trauma by Michael J. Shkrum, David A. Ramsay, 2007)

Histology of the lungs showing bone marrow and fat emboli is indirect evidence that fractures have occurred (Fig. 7.31). They could be from CPR-related chest wall fractures, but origin from other fractures or soft tissue injury alone (fat emboli) occurring prior to resuscitation cannot be excluded.

Fat Embolism Syndrome

FES typically develops after a latent period of 12–48 h after the traumatic incident [102]. Major and minor clinical criteria, e.g., Gurd and Wilson, have been used to define FES and can assist in the pathologist's assessment if the person has been hospitalized [102]. Although a petechial rash, a major criterion, is considered a pathognomonic sign, it is transient and can disappear in 24 h. Petechiae are typically seen on the upper chest and can also be found on the oral mucosa, conjunctiva, neck, and axilla [102]. The symptoms and signs of other major criteria—respiratory insufficiency, and cerebral involvement—and minor criteria (e.g., fever and tachycardia) are relatively non-specific [102].

The determination that the histological observation of fat embolism could be a significant factor in causing the sudden death of a trauma victim from fat embolism syndrome (FES) rather than an incidental finding from CPR-related chest wall fractures or other fractures, particularly of long bones, in a trauma patient is a diagnosis of exclusion of any other fatal injuries [102]. Soft tissue alone can result in FES [103, 104].

References

1. Shkrum MJ, Ramsay DA. Forensic pathology of trauma—common problems for the pathologist. Totowa, NJ: Humana Press; 2007. p. 646.
2. Langlois NE, Gresham GA. The ageing of bruises: a review and study of the colour changes with time. Forensic Sci Int. 1991;50(2):227–38. https://doi.org/10.1016/0379-0738(91)90154-b.
3. Grossman SE, Johnston A, Vanezis P, Perrett D. Can we assess the age of bruises? An attempt to develop an objective technique. Med Sci Law. 2011 Jul;51(3):170–6. https://doi.org/10.1258/msl.2011.010135.
4. Farley HH. The fatal triad-skull, pelvis, extremity fractures. Minn Med. 1965;48:905–7.
5. Waddell JP, Drucker WR. Occult injuries in pedestrian accidents. J Trauma. 1971;11(10):844–52.
6. Weisz GM, Schramek A, Barzilai A. Injury to the driver. J Trauma. 1974;14(3):212–5.
7. McCarroll JR, Braunstein PW, Weinberg SB, Seremetis MG, Copper W. The pathology of pedestrian automotive accident victims. J Trauma. 1965;5:421–6.
8. Otte D, Haasper C. Characteristics on fractures of tibia and fibula in car impacts to pedestrians and bicyclists—influences of car bumper height and shape. Annu Proc Assoc Adv Automot Med. 2007;51:63–79.
9. Brainard BJ, Slauterbeck J, Benjamin JB. Fracture patterns and mechanisms in pedestrian motor-vehicle trauma: the ipsilateral dyad. J Orthop Trauma. 1992;6(3):279–82.
10. Matsui Y. Effects of vehicle bumper height and impact velocity on type of lower extremity injury in vehicle—pedestrian accidents. Accid Anal Prev. 2005;37(4):633–40.
11. Iwadate K, Ono K, Ohashi N, Zhang S, Misawa S, Takatori T. Analysis of pedestrian injuries in traffic accidents (2)—especially on leg injury. Nihon Hoigaku Zasshi. 1995;49(3):187–92.
12. Halari MM, Shkrum MJ. Fatal motor vehicle-pedestrian collision injury patterns—a systematic literature review. Acad Forensic Pathol. 2020;10(3–4):144–57.
13. Teresinski G, Madro R. Evidential value of injuries useful for reconstruction of the pedestrian-vehicle location at the moment of collision. Forensic Sci Int. 2002;128(3):127–35.
14. Karger B, Teige K, Fuchs M, Brinkmann B. Was the pedestrian hit in an erect position before being run over? Forensic Sci Int. 2001;119(2):217–20.
15. Morley EJ, Johnson S, Leibner E, Shahid J. Emergency department evaluation and management of blunt chest and lung trauma (Trauma CME). Emerg Med Pract. 2016;18(6):1–20.
16. Pumarejo Gomez L, Tran VH. Hemothorax. In: StatPearls. Treasure Island, FL: StatPearls Publishing; 2021. p. 2022.
17. Shkrum MJ, McClafferty KJ, Nowak ES, German A. Driver and front seat passenger fatalities associated with air bag deployment. Part 1: a Canadian study. J Forensic Sci. 2002;47(5):1028–34.
18. Shkrum MJ, McClafferty KJ, Nowak ES, German A. Driver and front seat passenger fatalities associated with air bag deployment. Part 2: a review of injury patterns and investigative issues. J Forensic Sci. 2002;47(5):1035–40.
19. Kuk M, Shkrum MJ. Injury patterns sustained in fatal motor vehicle collisions with driver's third-generation airbag deployment. J Forensic Sci. 2018;63(3):728–34.
20. Talbot BS, Gange CP Jr, Chaturvedi A, Klionsky N, Hobbs SK, Chaturvedi A. Traumatic rib injury: patterns, imaging pitfalls, complications, and treatment. Radiographics. 2017;37(2):628–51.

21. Sharma OP, Oswanski MF, Jolly S, Lauer SK, Dressel R, Stombaugh HA. Perils of rib fractures. Am Surg. 2008;74(4):310–4.
22. Hoke RS, Chamberlain D. Skeletal chest injuries secondary to cardiopulmonary resuscitation. Resuscitation. 2004;63(3):327–38.
23. Whitson BA, McGonigal MD, Anderson CP, Dries DJ. Increasing numbers of rib fractures do not worsen outcome: an analysis of the national trauma data bank. Am Surg. 2013;79(2):140–50.
24. Bugaev N, Breeze JL, Alhazmi M, Anbari HS, Arabian SS, Rabinovici R. Displacement patterns of blunt rib fractures and their relationship to thoracic coinjuries: minimal displacements count. Am Surg. 2016;82(3):199–206.
25. Yang KM, Lynch M, O'Donnell C. "Buckle" rib fracture: an artifact following cardio-pulmonary resuscitation detected on postmortem CT. Leg Med (Tokyo). 2011;13(5):233–9.
26. Love JC, Symes SA. Understanding rib fracture patterns: incomplete and buckle fractures. J Forensic Sci. 2004;49(6):1153–8.
27. Flagel BT, Luchette FA, Reed RL, Esposito TJ, Davis KA, Santaniello JM, et al. Half-a-dozen ribs: the breakpoint for mortality. Surgery. 2005;138(4):717–23; discussion 723–5.
28. Sirmali M, Türüt H, Topçu S, Gülhan E, Yazici U, Kaya S, et al. A comprehensive analysis of traumatic rib fractures: morbidity, mortality and management. Eur J Cardiothorac Surg. 2003;24(1):133–8.
29. Dehghan N, de Mestral C, McKee MD, Schemitsch EH, Nathens A. Flail chest injuries: a review of outcomes and treatment practices from the National Trauma Data Bank. J Trauma Acute Care Surg. 2014;76(2):462–8.
30. Choi J, Anand A, Sborov KD, Walton W, Chow L, Guillamondegui O, et al. Complication to consider: delayed traumatic hemothorax in older adults. Trauma Surg Acute Care Open. 2021;6(1):e000626 [cited 2022 Apr 28]. https://doi.org/10.1136/tsaco-2020-000626.
31. Faisham WI, Mohammad P, Juhara H, Munirah NM, Shamsulkamaruljan H, Ziyadi GM. Clavicle fracture and subclavian vessels disruption with massive haemothorax mimic intrathoracic injury. Malays J Med Sci. 2011;18(2):74–7.
32. Ninomiya K, Kuriyama A, Uchino H. Massive hemothorax due to bleeding from thoracic spinal fractures: a case series and systematic review. Scand J Trauma Resusc Emerg Med. 2020;28(1):92.
33. Tsugu T, Nagatomo Y, Tanigawa T, Endo J, Itabashi Y, Murata M, et al. Delayed hemopericardium due to non-penetrating chest trauma: a report of new case and literature review. J Med Ultrason (2001). 2019;46(1):159–62 [cited 2022 Apr 28]. https://doi.org/10.1007/s10396-018-0895-9. Epub 2018 Aug 9.
34. Endara SA, Davalos GA, Nuñez MF, Manzano JE. Azygous vein laceration secondary to blunt thoraco-abdominal trauma. Interact Cardiovasc Thorac Surg. 2010;11(3):342–4.
35. Henry L, Fischer N. Delayed haemorrhage and pseudoaneurysms following liver trauma. Eur J Trauma Emerg Surg. 2022 [cited 2022 Apr 28]. https://doi.org/10.1007/s00068-022-01889-z. Epub ahead of print.
36. Shkrum MJ. Delayed fatal hemorrhage due to small bowel mesenteric laceration. Am J Forensic Med Pathol. 2015;36(4):236–8.
37. Riezzo I, Di Battista B, De Salvia A, Cantatore S, Neri M, Pomara C, et al. Delayed splenic rupture: dating the sub-capsular hemorrhage as a useful task to evaluate causal relationships with trauma. Forensic Sci Int. 2014;234:64–71.
38. Goins WA, Rodriguez A, Lewis J, Brathwaite CE, James E. Retroperitoneal hematoma after blunt trauma. Surg Gynecol Obstet. 1992;174(4):281–90.
39. Gutierrez G, Reines HD, Wulf-Gutierrez ME. Clinical review: hemorrhagic shock. Crit Care. 2004;8(5):373–81.
40. Nadler SB, Hidalgo JH, Bloch T. Prediction of blood volume in normal human adults. Surgery. 1962;51(2):224–32.
41. Lemmens HJ, Bernstein DP, Brodsky JB. Estimating blood volume in obese and morbidly obese patients. Obes Surg. 2006;16(6):773–6.

42. Rao RD, Berry CA, Yoganandan N, Agarwal A. Occupant and crash characteristics in thoracic and lumbar spine injuries resulting from motor vehicle collisions. Spine J. 2014;14(10):2355–65.
43. Burgess AR, Eastridge BJ, Young JW, Ellison TS, Ellison PS Jr, Poka A, et al. Pelvic ring disruptions: effective classification system and treatment protocols. J Trauma. 1990;30(7):848–56.
44. Pennal GF, Tile M, Waddell JP, Garside H. Pelvic disruption: assessment and classification. Clin Orthop Relat Res. 1980;151:12–21.
45. Tile M. Acute pelvic fractures: I. causation and classification. J Am Acad Orthop Surg. 1996;4(3):143–51.
46. Young JW, Burgess AR, Brumback RJ, Poka A. Pelvic fractures: value of plain radiography in early assessment and management. Radiology. 1986;160(2):445–51.
47. Coccolini F, Stahel PF, Montori G, Biffl W, Horer TM, Catena F, et al. Pelvic trauma: WSES classification and guidelines. World J Emerg Surg. 2017;12:5 [cited 2022 Apr 29]. https://doi.org/10.1186/s13017-017-0117-6.].
48. Uludag N, Tötterman A, Beckman MO, Sundin A. Anatomic distribution of hematoma following pelvic fracture. Br J Radiol. 2018;91(1085):20170840 [cited 2022 Apr 29]. https://doi.org/10.1259/bjr.20170840. Epub 2018 Feb 22.
49. Geeraerts T, Chhor V, Cheisson G, Martin L, Bessoud B, Ozanne A, et al. Clinical review: initial management of blunt pelvic trauma patients with haemodynamic instability. Crit Care. 2007;11(1):204 [cited 2022 Apr 29]. https://doi.org/10.1186/cc5157.
50. Pascarella R, Del Torto M, Politano R, Commessatti M, Fantasia R, Maresca A. Critical review of pelvic fractures associated with external iliac artery lesion: a series of six cases. Injury. 2014;45(2):374–8.
51. Krappinger D, Zegg M, Jeske C, El Attal R, Blauth M, Rieger M. Hemorrhage after low-energy pelvic trauma. J Trauma Acute Care Surg. 2012;72(2):437–42.
52. Stewart MK, Shkrum MJ, McClafferty KJ, Mao H, Zhang Q. A neuropathological study of diffuse vascular injury in fatal motor vehicle collisions. J Neuropathol Exp Neurol. 2022;81(2):88–96.
53. Johnson VE, Stewart W, Smith DH. Axonal pathology in traumatic brain injury. Exp Neurol. 2013;246:35–43.
54. Bruggeman GF, Haitsma IK, Dirven CMF, Volovici V. Traumatic axonal injury (TAI): definitions, pathophysiology and imaging-a narrative review. Acta Neurochir (Wien). 2021;163(1):31–44.
55. Smith C, Margulies SS, Duhaime A-C. Trauma. In: Love S, Perry A, Ironside J, Budka H, editors. Greenfield's neuropathology, vol. 1. 9th ed. Boca Raton, FL: CRC Press; 2015. p. 637–82.
56. Pang D. Spinal cord injury without radiographic abnormality in children, 2 decades later. Neurosurgery. 2004;55(6):1325–42; discussion 1342–3.
57. Bonfanti L, Donelli V, Lunian M, Cerasti D, Cobianchi F, Cervellin G. Adult spinal cord injury without radiographic abnormality (SCIWORA). Two case reports and a narrative review. Acta Biomed. 2019;89(4):593–8.
58. Hamilton JR, Sunter JP, Cooper PN. Fatal hemorrhage from simple lacerations of the scalp. Forensic Sci Med Pathol. 2005;1(4):267–71.
59. Yumoto T, Kosaki Y, Yamakawa Y, Iida A, Yamamoto H, Yamada T, et al. Occult sources of bleeding in blunt trauma: a narrative review. Acta Med Okayama. 2017;71(5):363–8.
60. Gennarelli TA. Head injury in man and experimental animals: clinical aspects. Acta Neurochir Suppl (Wien). 1983;32:1–13.
61. Leetsma JE, Thibault KL. Physical injury to the nervous system. In: Leetsma JE, editor. Forensic neuropathology. 2nd ed. Boca Raton, FL: CRC Press; 2009. p. 399–559.
62. Rao MG, Singh D, Vashista RK, Sharma SK. Dating of acute and subacute subdural haemorrhage: a histopathological study. J Clin Diagn Res. 2016;10(7):HC01–7 [cited 2022 Apr 29].

63. Adams JH, Scott G, Parker LS, Graham DI, Doyle D. The contusion index: a quantitative approach to cerebral contusions in head injury. Neuropathol Appl Neurobiol. 1980;6(4):319–24.
64. Ryan GA, McLean AJ, Vilenius AT, Kloeden CN, Simpson DA, Blumbergs PC, et al. Brain injury patterns in fatally injured pedestrians. J Trauma. 1994;36(4):469–76.
65. Guyomarc'h P, Campagna-Vaillancourt M, Kremer C, Sauvageau A. Discrimination of falls and blows in blunt head trauma: a multi-criteria approach. J Forensic Sci. 2010;55(2):423–7.
66. Geserick G, Krocker K, Wirth I. Über die Walcher'sche Hutkrempenregel—eine Literaturstudie (Walcher's hat brim line rule—a literature review). Arch Kriminol. 2014;234(3–4):73–90. German.
67. Kremer C, Racette S, Dionne CA, Sauvageau A. Discrimination of falls and blows in blunt head trauma: systematic study of the hat brim line rule in relation to skull fractures. J Forensic Sci. 2008;53(3):716–9.
68. Kremer C, Sauvageau A. Discrimination of falls and blows in blunt head trauma: assessment of predictability through combined criteria. J Forensic Sci. 2009;54(4):923–6 [cited 2022 May 1]. https://doi.org/10.1111/j.1556-4029.2009.01072.x. Epub 2009 May 26.
69. Härm T, Rajs J. Face and neck injuries due to resuscitation versus throttling. Forensic Sci Int. 1983;23(2–3):109–16.
70. Krischer JP, Fine EG, Davis JH, Nagel EL. Complications of cardiac resuscitation. Chest. 1987;92(2):287–91.
71. Plaisier BR, Punjabi AP, Super DM, Haug RH. The relationship between facial fractures and death from neurologic injury. J Oral Maxillofac Surg. 2000;58(7):708–12; discussion 712–3.
72. Imaizumi T, Sohma T, Hotta H, Teto I, Imaizumi H, Kaneko M. Associated injuries and mechanism of atlanto-occipital dislocation caused by trauma. Neurol Med Chir (Tokyo). 1995;35(6):385–91.
73. Ardekian L, Gaspar R, Peled M, Manor R, Laufer D. Incidence and type of cervical spine injuries associated with mandibular fractures. J Craniomaxillofac Trauma. 1997;3(2):18–21.
74. Lewis VL Jr, Manson PN, Morgan RF, Cerullo LJ, Meyer PR Jr. Facial injuries associated with cervical fractures: recognition, patterns, and management. J Trauma. 1985;25(1):90–3.
75. Viel G, Gehl A, Sperhake JP. Intersecting fractures of the skull and gunshot wounds. Case report and literature review. Forensic Sci Med Pathol. 2009;5(1):22–7.
76. Lindenberg R, Freytag E. The mechanism of cerebral contusions. A pathologic-anatomic study. Arch Pathol. 1960;69:440–69.
77. Steinmann J, Hartung B, Bostelmann R, Kaschner M, Karadag C, Muhammad S, et al. Rupture of intracranial aneurysms in patients with blunt head trauma: review of the literature. Clin Neurol Neurosurg. 2020;199:106208 [cited 2022 May 1]. https://doi.org/10.1016/j.clineuro.2020.106208. Epub 2020 Sep 9.
78. Kim S. Inconspicuous longitudinal tears of the intracranial vertebral artery in traumatic basal subarachnoid hemorrhage. J Pathol Transl Med. 2020;54(2):179–83.
79. Wong B, Ong BB, Milne N. The source of haemorrhage in traumatic basal subarachnoid haemorrhage. J Forensic Legal Med. 2015;29:18–23.
80. Pickup MJ, Pollanen MS. Traumatic subarachnoid hemorrhage and the COL3A1 gene: emergence of a potential causal link. Forensic Sci Med Pathol. 2011;7(2):192–7. Epub 2010 Nov 19.
81. Galtés I, Rodríguez-Baeza A, Subirana M, Barbería E, Castellà J, Medallo J. A proposed dissection procedure for vertebral arteries in forensic pathology. J Forensic Sci. 2012;57(1):212–4.
82. Yoo JJ, Gishen KE, Thaller SR. The oculocardiac reflex: its evolution and management. J Craniofac Surg. 2021;32(1):e80–83 [cited 2022 May 1]. https://doi.org/10.1097/SCS.0000000000006995.
83. Turner SA, Barnard JJ, Spotswood SD, Prahlow JA. "Homicide by heart attack" revisited. J Forensic Sci. 2004;49(3):598–600.

84. Menezes RG, Fatima H, Hussain SA, Ahmed S, Singh PK, Kharoshah MA, et al. Commotio cordis: a review. Med Sci Law. 2017;57(3):146–51.
85. Lupariello F, Curti SM, Di Vella G. Diagnostic criteria for commotio cordis caused by violent attack: review of the literature. Am J Forensic Med Pathol. 2018;39(4):330–6.
86. Milovanovic AV, DiMaio VJ. Death due to concussion and alcohol. Am J Forensic Med Pathol. 1999;20(1):6–9.
87. Ramsay DA, Shkrum MJ. Homicidal blunt head trauma, diffuse axonal injury, alcoholic intoxication, and cardiorespiratory arrest: a case report of a forensic syndrome of acute brainstem dysfunction. Am J Forensic Med Pathol. 1995;16(2):107–14.
88. Papadakis SA, Pallis D, Galanakos S, Georgiou DF, Kateros K, Macheras G, et al. Falls from height due to accident and suicide attempt in Greece. A comparison of the injury patterns. Injury. 2020;51(2):230–4.
89. Lallier M, Bouchard S, St-Vil D, Dupont J, Tucci M. Falls from heights among children: a retrospective review. J Pediatr Surg. 1999;34(7):1060–3.
90. Roshkow JE, Haller JO, Hotson GC, Sclafani SJ, Mezzacappa PM, Rachlin S. Imaging evaluation of children after falls from a height: review of 45 cases. Radiology. 1990;175(2):359–63.
91. Sawyer JR, Flynn JM, Dormans JP, Catalano J, Drummond DS. Fracture patterns in children and young adults who fall from significant heights. J Pediatr Orthop. 2000;20(2):197–202.
92. Miller AC, Rosati SF, Suffredini AF, Schrump DS. A systematic review and pooled analysis of CPR-associated cardiovascular and thoracic injuries. Resuscitation. 2014;85(6):724–31.
93. Sperry K. Anterior thoracic wall trauma in elderly homicide victims. The "CPR defense". Am J Forensic Med Pathol. 1990;11(1):50–5.
94. Ram P, Menezes RG, Sirinvaravong N, Luis SA, Hussain SA, Madadin M, et al. Breaking your heart—a review on CPR-related injuries. Am J Emerg Med. 2018;36(5):838–842 [cited 2022 May 1]. https://doi.org/10.1016/j.ajem.2017.12.063. Epub 2017 Dec 28.
95. Maguire S, Mann M, John N, Ellaway B, Sibert JR, Kemp AM, Welsh Child Protection Systematic Review Group. Does cardiopulmonary resuscitation cause rib fractures in children? A systematic review. Child Abuse Negl. 2006;30(7):739–51.
96. Weber MA, Risdon RA, Offiah AC, Malone M, Sebire NJ. Rib fractures identified at postmortem examination in sudden unexpected deaths in infancy (SUDI). Forensic Sci Int. 2009;189(1–3):75–81.
97. Matshes EW, Lew EO. Two-handed cardiopulmonary resuscitation can cause rib fractures in infants. Am J Forensic Med Pathol. 2010;31(4):303–7.
98. Duval JV, Andrew TA. Two thumb method of infant CPR: is there an increased risk for posterior rib fractures? Paper presented at National Association of Medical Examiners 41st annual meeting. Georgia: Savannah; 2007.
99. Clouse JR, Lantz PE. Posterior rib fractures in infants associated with cardiopulmonary resuscitation. In: Paper presented at American Academy of Forensic Sciences annual meeting. Washington, DC; 2008.
100. Lonergan GJ, Baker AM, Morey MK, Boos SC. From the archives of the AFIP. Child abuse: radiologic-pathologic correlation. Radiographics. 2003;23(4):811–45.
101. van Rijn RR, Bilo RA, Robben SG. Birth-related mid-posterior rib fractures in neonates: a report of three cases (and a possible fourth case) and a review of the literature. Pediatr Radiol. 2009;39(1):30–4.
102. Akhtar S. Fat embolism. Anesthesiol Clin. 2009;27(3):533–50.
103. Lee KA, Opeskin K. Death due to superficial soft tissue injuries. Am J Forensic Med Pathol. 1992;13(3):179–85.
104. Nichols GR 2nd, Corey TS, Davis GJ. Nonfracture-associated fatal fat embolism in a case of child abuse. J Forensic Sci. 1990;35(2):493–9.

Further Reading

Acres MJ, Morris JA. The pathogenesis of retinal and subdural haemorrhage in non-accidental head injury in infancy: assessment using Bradford Hill criteria. Med Hypotheses. 2014;82(1):1–5.

American Academy of Pediatrics Committee on child abuse and neglect: shaken baby syndrome: inflicted cerebral trauma. Pediatrics. 1993;92(6):872–5.

Bruce DA, Zimmerman RA. Shaken impact syndrome. Pediatr Ann. 1989;18(8):482–94.

Caffey J. Multiple fractures in the long bones of infants suffering from chronic subdural hematoma. Am J Roentgenol Radium Ther. 1946;56(2):163–73.

Caffey J. On the theory and practice of shaking infants. Its potential residual effects of permanent brain damage and mental retardation. Am J Dis Child. 1972;124(2):161–9.

Caffey J. The whiplash shaken infant syndrome: manual shaking by the extremities with whiplash-induced intracranial and intraocular bleedings, linked with residual permanent brain damage and mental retardation. Pediatrics. 1974;54(4):396–403.

Case ME, Graham MA, Handy TC, Jentzen JM, Monteleone JA, National Association of Medical Examiners Ad Hoc Committee on Shaken Baby Syndrome. Position paper on fatal abusive head injuries in infants and young children. Am J Forensic Med Pathol. 2001;22(2):112–22.

Choudhary AK, et al. Endorsements of consensus statement on abusive head injury. Pediatr Radiol. 2019;49:421.

Choudhary AK, Servaes S, Slovis TL, et al. Consensus statement on abusive head trauma in infants and young children. Pediatr Radiol. 2018;48(8):1048–65.

Christian CW, Block R, Committee on Child Abuse and Neglect, American Academy of Pediatrics. Abusive head trauma in infants and children. Pediatrics. 2009;123(5):1409–11.

Cory CZ, Jones BM. Can shaking alone cause fatal brain injury? A biomechanical assessment of the Duhaime shaken baby syndrome model. Med Sci Law. 2003;43(4):317–33.

Duhaime AC, Gennarelli TA, Thibault LE, Bruce DA, Margulies SS, Wiser R. The shaken baby syndrome. A clinical, pathological, and biomechanical study. J Neurosurg. 1987;66(3):409–15.

Elinder G, Eriksson A, Hallberg B, Lynøe N, Sundgren PM, Rosén M, Engström I, Erlandsson BE. Traumatic shaking: the role of the triad in medical investigations of suspected traumatic shaking. Acta Paediatr. 2018;107(Suppl 472):3–23.

Geddes JF, Tasker RC, Hackshaw AK, et al. Dural haemorrhage in non-traumatic infant deaths: does it explain the bleeding in 'shaken baby syndrome'? [published correction appears in Neuropathol Appl Neurobiol. 2003 Jun;29(3):322]. Neuropathol Appl Neurobiol. 2003;29(1):14–22.

Geddes JF, Whitwell HL. Inflicted head injury in infants. Forensic Sci Int. 2004;146(2–3):83–8.

Gilliland MG, Folberg R. Shaken babies—some have no impact injuries. J Forensic Sci. 1996;41(1):114–6.

Gilliland MG. Interval duration between injury and severe symptoms in nonaccidental head trauma in infants and young children. J Forensic Sci. 1998;43(3):723–5.

Guthkelch AN. Infantile subdural haematoma and its relationship to whiplash injuries. Br Med J. 1971;2:430–1.

Kempe CH, Silverman FN, Steele BF, et al. The Battered-Child syndrome. JAMA. 1962;181(1): 17–24.

Lynøe N, Elinder G, Hallberg B, et al. Insufficient evidence for 'shaken baby syndrome'—a systematic review. Acta Paediatr. 2017;106(7):1021–7.

Lynøe N, Eriksson A. Is there a common denominator for brief resolved unexplained events, sudden infant death syndrome, and alleged shaken baby syndrome? Med Hypotheses. 2020; https://doi.org/10.1016/j.mehy.2020.10993.

Matschke J, Büttner A, Bergmann M, et al. Encephalopathy and death in infants with abusive head trauma is due to hypoxic-ischemic injury following local brain trauma to vital brainstem centers. Int J Legal Med. 2015;129(1):105–14.

Scheimberg I, Cohen MC, Zapata Vazquez RE, et al. Nontraumatic intradural and subdural hemorrhage and hypoxic ischemic encephalopathy in fetuses, infants, and children up to three years of age: analysis of two audits of 636 cases from two referral centers in the United Kingdom. Pediatr Dev Pathol. 2013;16(3):149–59.

Wolfson DR, McNally DS, Clifford MJ, Vloeberghs M. Rigid-body modelling of shaken baby syndrome. Proc Inst Mech Eng H. 2005;219(1):63–70.

Chapter 8
Sharp Force Injuries

Rebekah Jacques

History and Scene Findings

The availability of information on the circumstances surrounding a death by sharp force injuries is quite variable and sometimes can be misleading. Ideally, before performing the autopsy, the pathologist should have all the information available regarding the deceased's background, the circumstances of death, involvement of resuscitation efforts, and the scene findings, including photographs.

The amount of blood at the scene can be variable and may reflect attempts at cleaning but also may reflect the anatomical position of the body relative to injuries. Blood observed at the scene may be from the decedent and, where relevant, the assailant. The quantity of blood observed at the scene may speak to the mechanism of death, such as exsanguination.

Knives are often used as an implement of opportunity. The presence of a knife or other related object with a point or sharp-edge may be present at the scene (Fig. 8.1). Some scenes may be more challenging to isolate which knife may have been used because of large number of knives at the scene (e.g., kitchen) or the knife has been removed from the death scene. However, observations of the knives at the scene may be assessed for intactness of blade, dimensions of the blade (e.g., length, width, thickness of the blade), face of the guard ('hilt') of the knife's handle adjacent to the blade, presence/absence of blood, double or single edged and presence/absence of serrations (teeth), and any other peculiarities. If the knife remains in the body of the decedent at the scene, discussion with investigating law enforcement about assessing this evidence prior to safe transportation of the body to the morgue maybe necessary. This may include photodocumenting the knife in situ, collecting fingerprints on the knife handle and careful removal of the knife. Keeping the knife in situ has

R. Jacques (✉)
London, ON, Canada
e-mail: rebekah.jacques@lhsc.on.ca

R. Jacques (ed.), *Forensic Pathology*,
https://doi.org/10.1007/978-3-031-42038-2_8

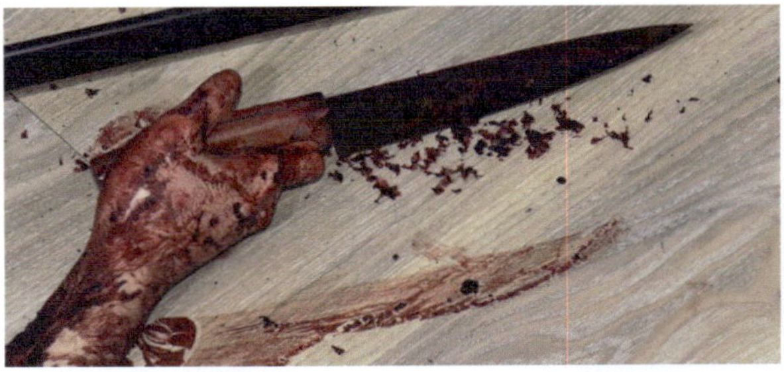

Fig. 8.1 The implement used, such as a knife, may be present at the scene and the quantity of blood may be noted

safety risks for body removal services and mortuary staff. In addition, if the knife is located in the back of the decedent and not removed, this may prevent transporting the decedent on their back and to development of postmortem hypostatic hemorrhages on the ventral (front) surfaces of the body, such as the face. Further, the pathologist may be called upon to examine a knife that may have been used to cause sharp force injuries. Unless the knife, or a portion of the knife (e.g. blade or broken tip of the blade), often a pathologist can only provide general opinion about the object used to cause an injury, such as an object with an edge, and/or point. A pathologist cannot definitively link a knife to a wound unless the knife remains in the body. If the tip of the blade or the blade remains in the body, this should be collected following photodocumentation and transferred into the custody of law enforcement. The tip of the knife can then be sent to an expert to physically re-unite the tip of the knife to the remaining blade.

Knives are the weapons most frequently involved, and their physical characteristics are important in shaping the wound. The common physical characteristics of the knife that a pathologist may be asked about as they are important in shaping the wound include the length, width, and thickness of the blade; however, whether a serrated cutting edge was used may also be important in shaping the wound. These features relate to the anatomy of the knife, specifically the handle and blade (Fig. 8.2). A knife is an object that has an edge and a point but has different shape wounding functions, as follows:

- A pointed instrument lacking an edge (i.e., pin) can stab but does not readily incise
- A sharp-edged surface lacking a point (i.e. paper) incises but does not readily stab

Individuals that have been transferred to a health care facility prior to autopsy may have undergone a variety of resuscitation efforts, including surgical treatment that can hinder assessment of findings on the body. In these circumstances, review of the medical records is paramount since the resuscitation procedures carried out may alter the characteristics of the original injury or cause confusion with findings that are not real injuries. Further confusion can be minimized, or avoided, when the body is sent with all medical devices in place; however, there are centers where this is not a common practice. Preferably, medical intervention would not alter injuries, such as

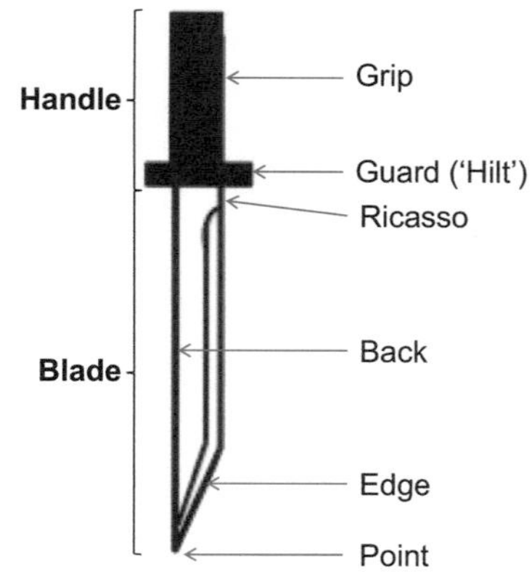

Fig. 8.2 Forensic anatomy of a single-edged, non-serrated, knife

extending the original injury with surgical incisions to access injured internal organs and other structures. A separate surgical incision, that is documented and does not alter the original injury, is preferable. Any surgical incisions and the nature of these surgical incisions should be documented in the medical record. Otherwise, a discussion with the medical team by the pathologist could clarify any confusion. The autopsy should describe evidence of medical and surgical intervention in addition to the presence of medical devices, if still present. It will be recorded if the injury has sutured or manipulated in any other way. These findings can correlate with the medical record. Sometimes surgically excised tissues may have to be directly evaluated by the forensic pathologist. Common resuscitation-related efforts that may be misconstrued as sharp force injuries include thoracostomy incisions that may be misinterpreted as a stab wound. Traditional thoracostomy incisions are typically 1–2 cm in length and are located of the lateral (side) of the mid chest to allow for the placement of a chest tube. The chest tube can be a life saving measure to evacuate fluid, such as blood, and air in the chest cavity. The approximate amount of blood removed from the chest cavity may be documented in the medical record. In the absence of a in situ chest tube, this finding can be misinterpreted as a stab wound (Fig. 8.3). The needle thoracostomy incision, also referred to as needle decompression, is the insertion of a needle into the chest cavity. Anatomically, this is landmarked in the anterior (front) second intercostal space of the midclavicular line of the chest. A thoracotomy incision is a larger chest incision that sometimes can be bilateral. The purpose of this incision is for the treating physician to gain access to the chest organs. A chest retractor is used to open the chest wall. These are often associated with an irregular injury in the axilla (armpit) and sometimes false starts. The injury of the axilla can be misconstrued as a stab wound because areas of the body with loose skin, such as the axilla, can appear irregular due to puckering of skin at the time of cutting the tissue. It is the association of the retractor that makes this finding supportive of a resuscitation-related artifact rather than a true injury.

Also, the medical records can indicate whether relevant radiographs such as X-rays or computed tomography scans have been performed. If the relevant area of

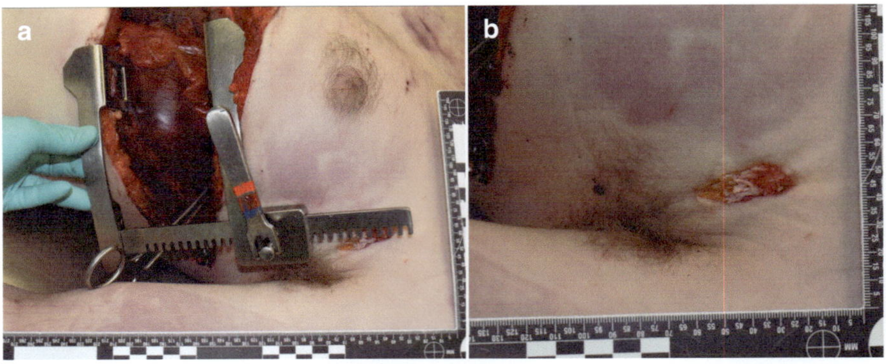

Fig. 8.3 The Finochietto rib spreader can cause an injury of the axilla (armpit) that may be confused as a sharp force or blunt force injury. (**a**) Rib spreader in situ of the left chest. (**b**) Associated injury of the anterior axilla

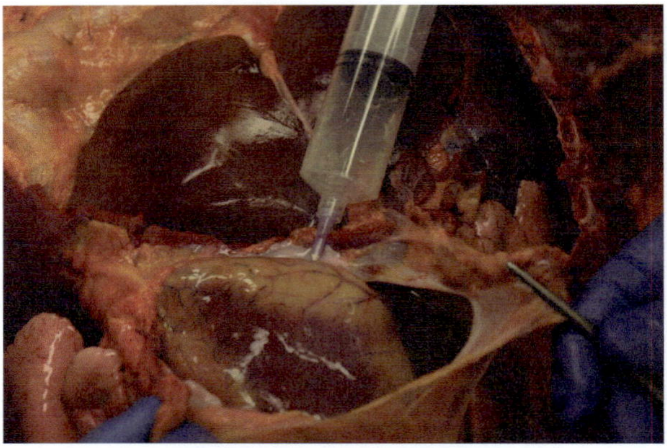

Fig. 8.4 Sharp force injuries to the neck may result in injuries to the jugular vein thereby permitting air into the circulation and causing an air embolous. Assessing for an air embolus by filling the pericardium with water and partially filling a syringe with water prior to insertion of the syringe in the right ventricle. This method can also quantify the amount of air in the heart, if present. X-rays of the chest can also be examined for air embolous

the body has been radiographed and is accessible to the pathologist, this ancillary investigation may not have to be repeated at the time of the autopsy. This can give an indication of internal injuries are present, including the presence of retained foreign objects, such as the tip of a blade, entire blade or air. The presence of air can be in the heart, such as an air embolism (Fig. 8.4) in the setting of neck injuries, pneumothorax (air in the chest cavity), or pneumoperitoneum (air in the abdomen in the setting of a viscus injury).

Morphology

Sharp force injury classification is dependent on the appearance on the skin surface but also the internal appearance. The features of an incised wound (incision) and stab wound show well-demarcated edges that can be easily approximated. A chop wound will also show well-demarcated edges but the edges exhibit bruises and/or abrasions. The difference between an incised wound and a stab wound is the depth of the wound track relative to the length of the skin injury (Fig. 8.5).

Stab Wounds

Stab wounds are injuries produced by the application of mechanical force of a pointed object whose main characteristic is that their depth is greater than their length. This arises because the force is more perpendicular to the skin surface as opposed to tangential or parallel. Stab wounds have a linear or oval shape, sharp margins, and two corners/angles (Fig. 8.6). The edges of a stab wound are clearly demarcated and the adjacent skin is often unremarkable with the exception of 'hilt' marks that may be observed. The corners or angles can blunt or pointed to indicate whether that blade is double- or single-edged. This is problematic because a blade that has entered the body to the level of ricasso of the blade may appear blunt at each corner. Further, a corner can split, giving a "fishtail"

INCISED WOUND	STAB WOUND
Depth (D) < Length (L)	Depth (D) > Length (L)

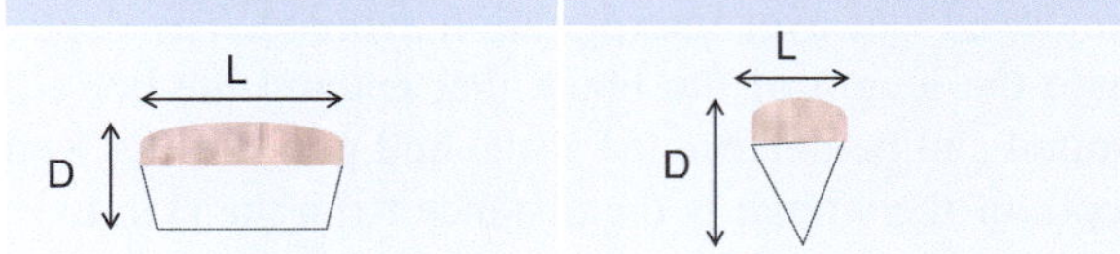

Fig. 8.5 Depth of the wound track, relative to the length of the skin wound, distinguishes a stab wound from an incised wound

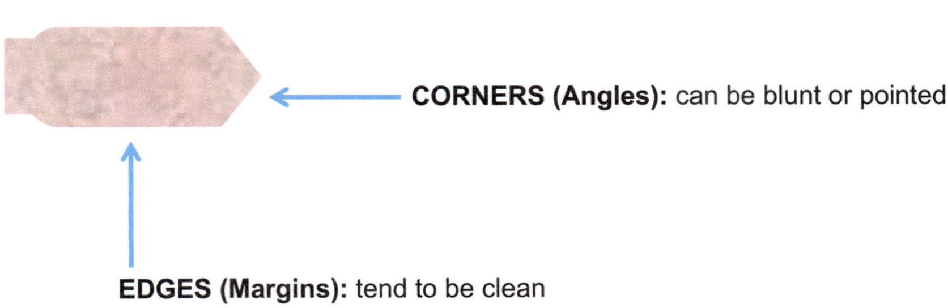

Fig. 8.6 Skin features of a stab wound

appearance from the spine of the blade. A superficial penetration may also give an appearance of a double-edge blade because of the pointed corners. The shape and length of a stab wound are related to the orientation of the wound in the body surface and are determined by the distribution of tension lines of the skin (Langer's lines) [1]. These tension lines, also referred as skin cleavage lines, are the result of parallel bundles or rows of fibroconnective tissue in the reticular dermis (deeper layer of skin) of the skin. In general, the direction of these tension lines in the skin tends to be horizontal and circumferential in the trunk and neck but longitudinal in the limbs. This is because they are generally parallel to the orientation of muscle fibers under the skin. Wounds that are oriented parallel to tension lines have a narrow and linear shape; however, wounds that are perpendicular to tension lines appear short and wide. In this way, wounds perpendicular to tension lines are oval and have a gaping appearance. Consequently, to have an accurate length in gaping stab wounds and assessment of corners/angles of the stab wound, the margins need to be re-approximated by digital pressure or tape. The length and width can also be measured if the stab wound involves the skull. The length of the wound is then measured from one corner/angle to the other along the longitudinal axis of the wound when the margins are apposed and gaping. The length of the wound in the skin can approximate the width of the knife but can also be smaller or larger. The inherent elasticity or laxness of the skin can decrease or increase the dimensions of the wound relative to the width of the blade of the knife. When there is relative movement between the knife and the decedent's body either by the individual holding the knife or by the victim's movement, the wound may be L or V shaped.

The dimensions of the object used may be a vital part of the investigation of a homicide, especially if the weapon has been removed from the scene. The features of the stab wound can speak to the implement used but caution has to be used to not over interpret findings. A common tenet in forensic work that caution must be employed and over interpretation avoided. The depth of the wound can approximate the length of the blade that entered the body (Fig. 8.7). The depth of the wound can be determined if the end point of the wound can be ascertained. The depth of the wound is the distance from the skin to the deepest point of penetration. In practice, this can be challenging to ascertain as the end point can sometimes only be confirmed only after evisceration. The depth of the wound can approximate the length of the blade that entered the body, therefore giving a minimal length (Fig. 8.8). However, the length of the wound does not necessarily mean that the entire blade of the knife entered the body. The presence of a 'hilt' mark around the stab wound indicates that the entire length of the blade entered the body and the knife has a guard or hilt. A 'hilt' mark is a patterned abrasion or bruise on the skin surrounding the stab wound. The absence of a 'hilt' mark does not mean the entire length of the blade entered the body. A common misconception is that the presence of a 'hilt' mark indicates that significant force was used. The quantity of force required to cause a stab wound is based primarily on the tissues involved and the sharpness of the object used. The presence of a 'hilt' mark on its own is not an indicator of forces. In addition, caution must be taken in

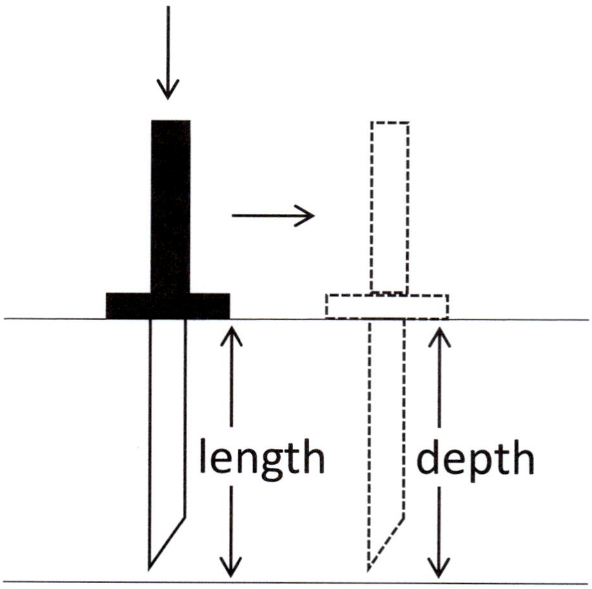

Fig. 8.7 The length of the wound can approximate the length of the blade. However, forcible compression of the body can make the depth of the wound exceed the length of the blade

Stab Wound	Blade	Possible Over-interpretations
Depth (D)	≈ Length (L)	Forcible compression: D>L
Length	≈ Width	Effect length: - Skin elasticity - Langer's Lines - Muscle fibers
Width	≈ Thickness	Re-approximation is subjective
Striations	Serrated	Striations not always present with serrated knives

Fig. 8.8 Summary of stab wound observations that may speak to class characteristics of the blade used to cause the injury

ascertaining the length of the blade via the depth of the wound in the body in areas that can be compressed, such as the chest and abdomen, during the stab wound and then recoil. This compression and subsequent recoil can make the estimation of the length of the blade longer than actuality. The length of the wound can approximate the width of the blade unless there has continued extension of the wound at one end. The cautionary inference is that relative movement of the weapon and the decedent may be due to 1) the knife actively moving or 2) the decedent moving or 3) both can lengthen the wound. An indicator to this relative movement due to leverage or angulation in the plane of the wound is the skin defect which is enlarged and maybe notched or "L-shaped." This finding supports that these events are often dynamic situations. The width of the wound can approximate the thickness of the blade but is of least value because the thickness of the blade of knife is generally only a few millimeters. The width of the wound is the widest measurement between the two opposing margins. Also, the re-approximation of the margins can be subjective.

Other features of the stab wound that can indicate class characteristics of the knife include the presence of striations (i.e., lands and grooves). The presence of striations in the wound is helpful and can indicate that the knife has a serrated cutting edge (i.e., has teeth); however, the absence of striations in the wound can be either from serrated or non-serrated blades (Fig. 8.9). The presence of striations can be observed in the cartilage, typically in stab wounds involving the anterior (front) chest and the costochondral junction of the anterior aspect of the ribs, but has also been observed in the skin of a stab wound [2]. The striations need to be photodocumented and consideration of retaining the cut surface for possible tool mark examination, especially in criminally suspicious cases, should be considered. Further, serrated blades can also cause a patterned wound on the skin as the blade grazes along the dermis resulting in a cluster of superficial parallel periodic wounds at regular intervals.

Internally, the path in the body may be observed by noting which organs and structures are injured. In the torso, this is facilitated by layered musculocutaneous dissection and careful inspection in the body cavities. When there are multiple stab wounds, these can overlap internally precluding definitive assessment of each stab wound path. These may be better described collectively and identified the limitations of determining each pathway.

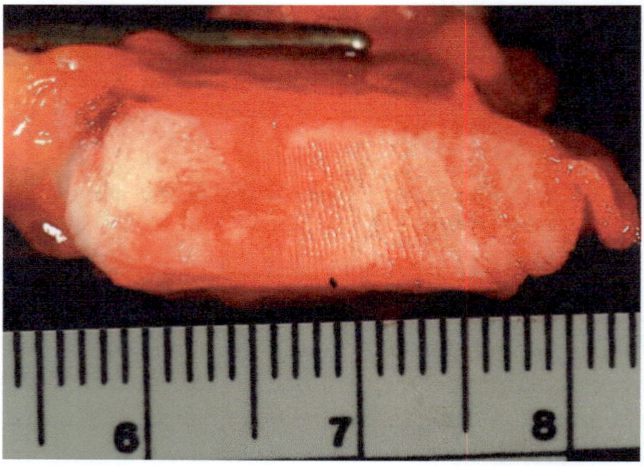

Fig. 8.9 Striations on the cartilage of the rib in a stab wound indicated that the knife/implement used was serrated (Courtesy Dr. Tweedie Department of Pathology and Laboratory Medicine, Schulich School of Medicine and Dentistry, Western University)

Stab Wounds by Objects Other than a Knife

Although knives are the most commonly used object to cause a stab wound, other objects with a point may be used. These can include pens, pencils, pool cues, broken glass, broken porcelain, etc. It can be challenging to determine the nature of the stab wound when there is only one injury. The nature of the stab wound may indicate the nature of the object used. An ice pick tends to result in small, round, or slit-like injuries. These injuries may mimic a gunshot wound. A linear cluster of three to four wounds can indicate a fork. The pattern of injury from a screwdriver depends on the type of screwdriver. A Phillips screwdriver has an X-shape at its tip which can lead to a patterned X-shape injury with a central round defect. A standard, or slotted, screwdriver may produce a slit-like appearance with squared corners. Stab wounds with scissors are variable in appearance depending on the positioning of the blades. If the two blades of the scissors are open and both injure the body, this will result in paired stab wounds or a zig-zag appearance, if partially opened. If only 1 blade enters, it can have a similar appeareance as a knife-related injury. If the blades are closed, this may result in a slit-like appearance. Arrows produce stab wounds that take on the appearance of the shape of the stab wound (Fig. 8.10).

Incised Wounds

Incised wounds are injuries produced by sharp-edged objects whose length is greater than their depth. Like stab wounds, the most common objects that cause incised wounds are knives; however, scissors, barbed wire, and box cutters may also be used.

The mechanism of injury involves a sliding movement of the edge of the instrument on the body surface. Most incised wounds (cuts) occur when the sharp edge of the object is pressed and slid over the skin. This can be a slashing motion as well.

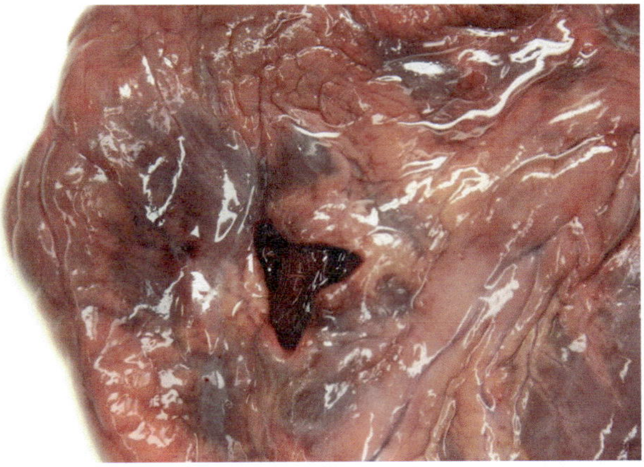

Fig. 8.10 Perforating injury of the heart that exhibits the features of the arrow used

Depending on their depth and location, incised wounds can injure skin as well as subcutaneous tissue, muscles, bone and other structures (tendons, blood vessels, airway).

While incised injuries are very common in emergency services, fatalities are less common. In the postmortem context, they are often observed in suicidal attempts by cutting the wrists and other parts of the body or homicidal maneuvers with deep cuts in the neck of defensive injuries. Cases that become fatal usually involve major blood vessels, often in the neck.

Morphology of Wounds

Incised wounds have clean-cut edges with no macroscopic abrasion or contusion. In most cases, the differential diagnosis with lacerations is straightforward (Fig. 8.11). A laceration is a blunt force injury that tears the tissue, typically the skin. A laceration has irregular margins, tissue bridging (e.g. visible strands of tissue from one margin to another margin of the wound), and bruised and/or abraded margins. These features are not observed in incised wounds. A laceration is a blunt force injury that tears the tissue, typically the skin. However, differentiation could be difficult if the laceration is linear with non-abraded margins more. On the other hand, when the edge of the object used is not very sharp and/or irregular, a cut could

FEATURES	LACERATION	INCISED WOUND
Cause	Blunt force injury	Sharp force injury
Edges	Ragged/irregular	Cleanly divided
Bruising/abraded margins	+	-
Tissue Bridging	+	-
Location	Bony Prominences	Any location
Image	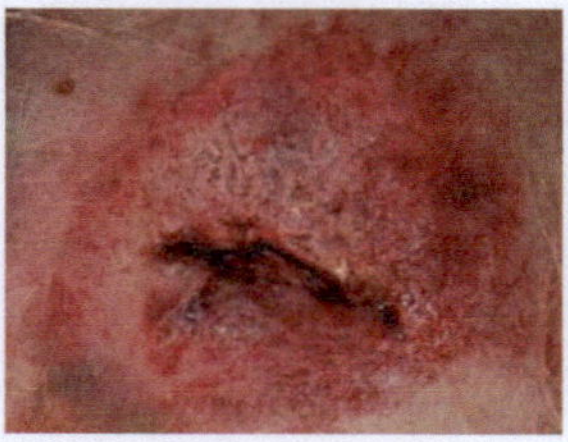	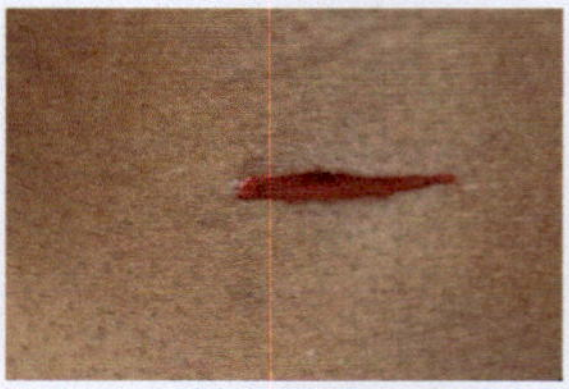

Fig. 8.11 Features to distinguish a laceration from an incised wound

show abraded or irregular margins. In those cases, the absence of tissue bridges in the depth of the incised wound allows the definite differential diagnosis with lacerations.

Depending on the orientation of the cut in the body surface, as already discussed for stab wounds, could have linear or gaped appearance. In both cases, the depth is often maximum in the center of the wound.

The incised wound(s) should be described in terms of its anatomical region, precise location in relation to anatomical landmarks and its orientation in relation to the body segment where it is located. Total length of the wound should be measured facing its edges. Any irregularities in its edges and/or its angles as well as presence of abrasions and bruises in its vicinity should be described. Each wound should be photographed, showing its location, and with a suitable scale.

For incised wounds in upper or lower extremities, the internal examination may require dissection of deep planes at the level of the wound to document injuries to muscles, blood vessels, nerves, and tendons as well the extent of bleeding. Respective photographs may be considered.

In case of neck incised injuries, internal examination depends on the size and depth of wounds present. Small and shallow injuries, usually located in one or more of the anterolateral regions of the neck, can be approached by performing an anterior musculocutaneous dissection, following the removal of the brain and viscera, to document for the presence and absence of injuries to muscles, blood vessel(s) and other structures involvement and extent of hemorrhage in soft tissues.

Incised-Stab Wounds

These are sharp force injuries that have features of both a stab and incised wound. This is to account for some of the semantics of trying to classify injuries and the overlap of features related to length and depth of a stab and incised wounds. It is suggested that the injury starts as a stab wound with the knife entering the body but the length is extended as the blade pulls across the body.

Chop Wounds

Chop wounds have attributes of both sharp force and blunt force injuries due to the object that caused the injury as being both heavy and having a sharp cutting edge. Examples of objects that may cause chop wounds include axes, hatchets, boat propellers, lawn mower blades, and airplane propellers. On the skin, the defect has sharp margins but the margins are also bruised or abraded due to the combination of cutting and crushing forces. The defect tends to be wider and deeper than an incised wound. There is typically an underlying fracture if a bone is present under the impact site. This is because the weight of the object acts as a force to penetrate the tissues.

Ancillary Investigations

Before proceeding with the autopsy, the possibility of an air embolism should be considered, especially in cases of deep incised wounds of the neck. The presence of air in the right heart chambers can be demonstrated by performing a chest radiograph or other imaging studies such as CT scan or MR when available. Radiographs are also useful in identifying the tip of a blade and even whole blades.

Manner in Which Sharp Force Injuries Occurred

The autopsy is an essential tool to help establishing whether the fatal sharp force injuries can be classified as an accident, suicide, or homicide. The pattern, quantity, anatomical location, and types of wounds may indicate the manner of death. Accidental and suicides often have the object used at the scene, but the same can be true for homicides. The absence of the object used requires explanation. Sharp force injuries as a means to complete suicide is less common than hangings, firearms, and drug toxicity methods. In suicides, clusters of parallel, horizontal (and sometimes vertical), incised wounds may be present in accessible sites of the body, such as on the anterolateral (side and front) neck (Fig. 8.12) and anterior (front) wrist or forearm (Fig. 8.13). The injury to wrist is rarely fatal, largely in part due to the lack of knowledge related to the anatomy, including blood vessels, of the wrist. Also, cluster of superficial stab wounds of the left chest may also be observed in suicides. These patterns of injuries are referred to as "hesitation marks" (also referred to as tentative injuries) as they are thought to represent previous

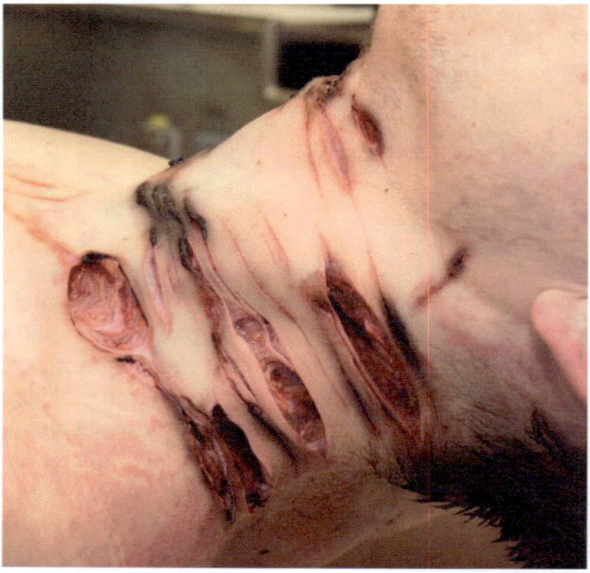

Fig. 8.12 Cluster of multiple parallel incised wounds to the neck some of which are gaping to the loss of skin tension from adjacent incised wounds

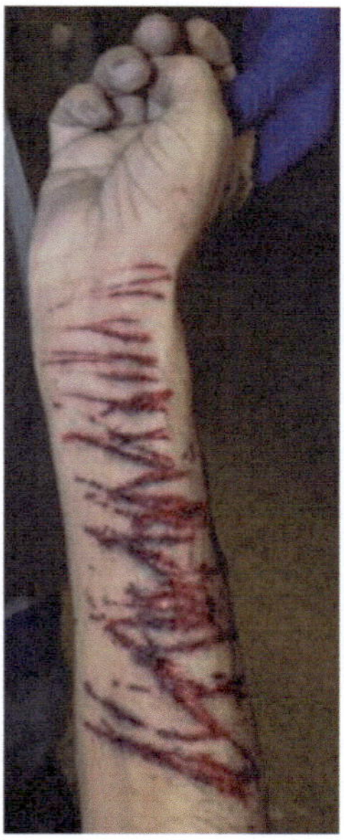

Fig. 8.13 Cluster of parallel, predominantly horizontal, incised wounds of the forearm. These are sometimes referred to as 'hesitation' marks and indicate a form of self-harm

unsuccessful attempts to injure an organ, such as the heart, or a major blood vessel, such as the jugular vein [3]. These are often superficial incised wounds adjacent or continuous with the fatal injury. The impression is that the individual attempts to cut the skin and stops because of pain or hesitancy. The cluster of incised wounds can also be observed in homicidal cases highlighting the overlap and avoid being dogmatic related to a single injury. Determination of an injured radial or ulnar artery can be challenging due to their depth and elasticity. Dissection and exploration of the adjacent proximal (closer to trunk of body) forearm maybe facilitated identifying the artery and the injury.

In contrast, defensive injuries are sharp force injuries that commonly arise on the hands and arms, and less rarely on the soles of feet and inner thighs in homicides [3]. These occur as the individual tries to protect themselves from injuries of vital structures located in the head, neck, and torso (trunk). In general, incised wounds in homicides are multiple and in different planes. In homicides, the number of stab wounds can vary to a single stab wound to multiple stab wounds. Defensive injuries often arise on the palms of the hands and fingers and extensor side of the forearms. The palm injuries may arise as an attempt to grasp the sharp-edged object. These injuries can also arise in the web between the thumb and fingers. The presence of defensive injuries are not required to make a determination that the manner of death is a homicide. In homicides, the number of stab wounds can vary to a single stab wound to multiple stab wounds. In attacks with knives, it is very common to find incised wounds located in the upper extremities, especially on forearms and hands, due to attempts by the victim to avoid the weapon, these are called defense injuries. Sometimes, the cluster of incised wounds of the neck has overlapping features of suicides and homicides. In homicides, a common question put to the pathologist is the handedness of the assailant or the relative positions of the decedent and assailant. This cannot be determined by the pathological findings and these questions are better answered by non-medical evidence.

Sharp force injuries may also be used to dismember a body. Examination of the amputations can indicate the nature of the object used to cause amputations. These amputations are often postmortem injuries and are not what caused an individual's death.

Accidental sharp force injuries are rare and can involve a variety of sharp items, including knives. A careful evaluation of the history, scene, and circumstances, in addition to evaluation of the wounds can facilitate discovery of the manner of death.

Mechanism of Death

The mechanism of death from sharp force injuries is variable and can include blood loss such as exsanguination (bleeding to the point of death), hypovolemic shock, and hemorrhage being the most common. The mechanism of blood loss is supported by quantifying blood in the body cavities in addition to blood collected during resuscitation and death scene observations. Other findings supportive of blood loss include subendocardial (inner surface of the heart) hemorrhage of the left ventricle and diminished livor mortis in the absence of blood transfusion. The subendocardial hemorrhage is bleeding on the inner surface of the left ventricle, typically arising in the outflow tract. Subendocardial hemorrhages are non-specific and can arise in other settings outside of sharp force injuries and trauma. The pathophysiology is thought to be due to a non-cardiac cause but due to the effects of stress hormones, such as catecholamines. Other mechanisms of death include air embolus and pneumothoraces. An air embolus arises when there is injury of the jugular vein in the neck. This injury allows air from the surrounding environment to enter the vascular system and travel into the right side of the heart due to the negative intra-thoracic pressure from respiration, which causes negative pressure in the veins [4]. This can be identified using a chest radiograph and by aspirating the right ventricle in situ with a syringe once the chest plate is removed and pericardium is opened. The radiograph of the chest is not sensitive in detecting smaller volumes of air in the heart. Filling the pericardium and partially filling the syringe with water ensures accuracy and better means to document the presence of air (i.e., bubbles) in the right ventricle. The amount of air that can cause death in a venous air embolus is 10–280 mL [5]. A pneumothorax is the accumulation of air in the chest cavity. This is best assessed with a radiograph but can also be demonstrated at autopsy with dissection. Following careful Y-incision of the torso and reflection of the skin and subcutaneous tissue, a pocket in the supraclavicular space or lateral chest is filled with water. The ribcage is punctured in the intercostal space or supraclavicular fossa with a partially filled water syringe. The detection of air to determine the presence of an air embolism and/or pneumothorax is limited by decompositional changes. At autopsy, the atelectatic lung may be observed in a large pneumothorax. Other mechanisms include cardiac tamponade with a stab wound involving the heart, proximal thoracic aorta, and/or other major vessel adjacent to the heart, arrythmias, and hemoaspiration due to injuries related to the neck, lungs, and tracheobronchial tree.

The survival ability and opportunity for volitional activity are dependent on the circumstances, organs and vessels injured, and mechanism of death.

In legal proceedings, the amount of force is often asked. This can be answered using broad categories of force that are based on common sense notions of force such as minimal pressure to significant force in the setting of bone fractures [6, 7]. This is largely unsatisfactory for the courts. There are two main drivers of force that are at play: (1) The sharpness of the edge and (2) the tissues injured in the stab wound path. The sharper the cutting of the object the more easily it can enter the body. The sharpness of the object is not typically known by the pathologist. However, a pathologist can offer opinions on the force needed to overcome the rigidity and elasticity of tissues. After the teeth, bone, and cartilage, skin is the next most resistant tissue. Once the skin is breeched, comparatively little force is required to injure major blood vessels and organs. So even if there is pathological evidence to indicate the entire length of blade of the knife has completely entered the body, this does not mean that significant force was inflicted.

Sharp Force Trauma in Decomposed and Embalmed Bodies

Sharp force injuries can be obscured by the process of decomposition. Depending on the degree of decomposition, there may not be sufficient skin, soft tissues, or organs to assess. Careful examination of the tissue, bones, and cartilage present needs to be assessed. However, not all sharp force injuries will have skeletal trauma. This may require consultation with an anthropologist.

In addition, prior surgical interventions or procedures may dehisce due to the breakdown of tissues and development of putrefactive gases (Fig. 8.14). The locations need to correlate with the medical record.

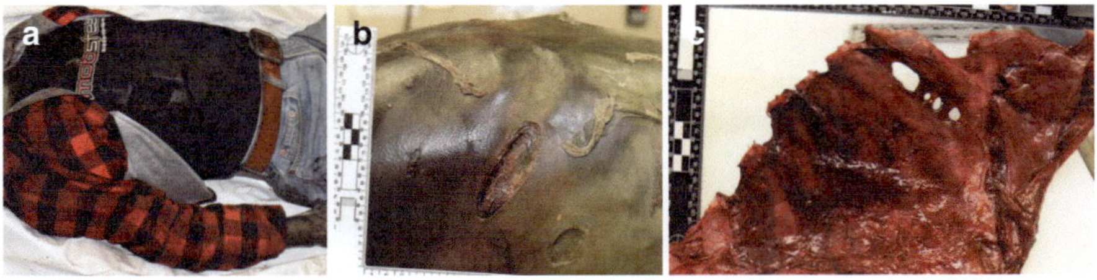

Fig. 8.14 A previous video-assisted thoracoscopic surgery (VATS) that was performed many months before death appeared as stab wounds at autopsy. The margins of the previous incisions had separated due to decompositional changes. There were no fatal internal injuries and evidence of a lobectomy was present. (**a**) Clothing without defects. (**b**) Multiple VATS sites in the same locations as described in the medical record. (**c**) Evidence of healing in the intercostal space associated with the VATS sites

Embalmed bodies will also have multiple internal trocar injuries; however, the circumstances and formalin fixation will distinguish these from true injuries.

Summary

Sharp force injuries are commonly encountered in a medico-legal practice and represent suicides, accidents, and homicides. The pattern and distribution of injuries speak to the manner of death. In addition, the features of the stab wounds can be used to provide class characteristics of the implement used.

References

1. Langer K. ON the anatomy and physiology of the skin. I. the cleavability of the cutis. Br J Plast Surg. 1978;31(1):3–8.
2. Jacques R, et al. An experimental model of tool mark striations by a serrated blade in human soft tissues. Am J Forensic Med Pathol. 2014;35(91):59–61.
3. Racette S, et al. A suicidal and homicidal sharp force injury: a 5-year retrospective comparative study of hesitation marks and defense wounds. Forensic Sci Med Pathol. 2008;4:221–7.
4. Gordy S, Rowell S. Vascular air embolism. Int J Crit Illn Inj Sci. 2016;5(11):93.
5. Prichard PD. A suicide by self-decapitation. J Forensic Sci. 1993;38:981–4.
6. Hainsworth SV, et al. How sharp is sharp? Towards quantification of the sharpness and penetration ability of kitchen knives used in stabbings. Int J Legal Med. 2008;122(4):281–91.
7. Parmar K, et al. Quantification of forces required for stabbing with screwdrivers and other blunter instruments. Int J Legal Med. 2012;126(1):43–53.

Chapter 9
Asphyxia & Anogenital Injuries

Rebekah Jacques

Asphyxia

There are no pathognomonic signs for asphyxial deaths. Historical attempts to look for signs of asphyxia include cyanosis, petechiae, congestion, edema, engorgement of the right heart, and fluidity of the blood. These observations are non-specific, which further adds to the difficulty in classification of causes of asphyxial deaths. There are many different classifications of asphyxia [1] that make attempts in differentiating asphyxial deaths. A summary of common asphyxial deaths that includes both a chemical and mechanical approach to asphyxia based on the circumstances and the autopsy findings is shown (Fig. 9.1). Alternatively, a classification on asphxyial deaths could be based on pathophysiological approach that that examines the failure in (a) supply, (b) transfer, (c) transport, or (d) uptake and utilization of oxygen [2]. Recognizing that a consensus on standardization terminology is still evolving, just like other areas of medicine.

Chemical asphyxia

Chemical asphyxia is the inhalation of gaseous compounds, or the ingestion of toxic substances prevents the utilization of oxygen at the cellular level and causes death. The most common substances are carbon monoxide, cyanide, and hydrogen sulfide. More recently, the ingestion of nitrites has led to a rise in acquired fatal methemoglobinemia.

R. Jacques (✉)
London, Canada

R. Jacques (ed.), *Forensic Pathology*,
https://doi.org/10.1007/978-3-031-42038-2_9

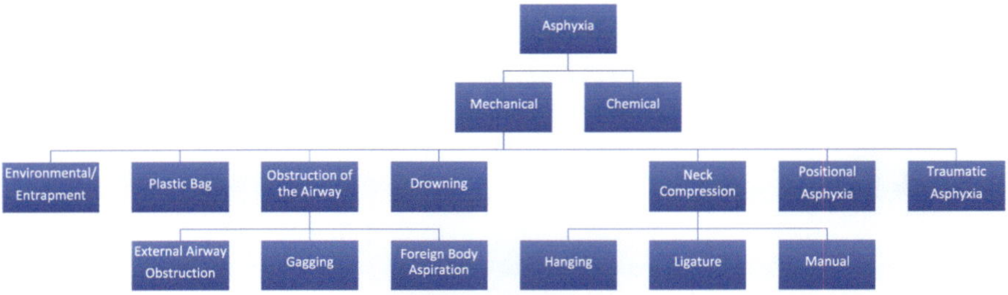

Fig. 9.1 Proposal of asphyxial classification that includes both mechanical and chemical asphyxia

Fig. 9.2 Ventral 'cherry-red' lividity in a fatal carbon monoxide death

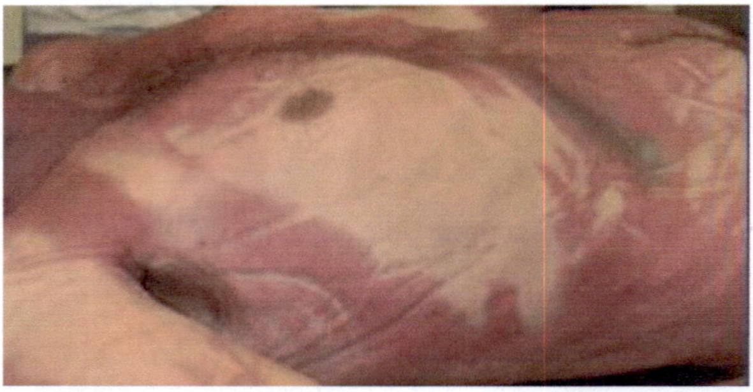

Carbon monoxide is a gas that is produced during incomplete combustion of carbon-based fuels. It is commonly produced with the burning of organic materials and the use of internal combustion motors. It has a higher affinity for the hemoglobin (a protein) in red blood cells than oxygen. Once carbon monoxide is breathed in, it will diffuse into the bloodstream and bind to hemoglobin. The bond between carbon monoxide and hemoglobin is called carboxyhemoglobin. This bond displaces oxygen because carbon monoxide has a higher affinity that is hundreds of times stronger than oxygen. This displacement causes death because hemoglobin is the major transporter of oxygen in the body and when oxygen is displaced it cannot be efficiently be transported to cells. At autopsy, the clue to carbon monoxide toxicity includes the circumstances and the bright "cherry" red appearance of lividity and blood. This red appearance is maintained even in formalin-fixed tissues, which normally tissues become pale over time (Fig. 9.2). The color of the lividity can be difficult to ascertain depending on the lighting of the mortuary, and also red lividity can arise in colder temperatures, such as mortuary refrigeration. The circumstances can be variable and can include a pipe connected between a vehicles' exhaust pipe and placed in the car window, fire-related deaths, dysfunctional furnace, multiple deaths in one residence, evidence of tampering with a gas line, etc. Further, carbon monoxide levels can be measured at the scene for the safety of first responders and death investigators. In suspected deaths, toxicological analysis is used to determine the carboxyhemoglobin saturation to confirm carbon monoxide exposure. Smokers can have a carboxyhemoglobin level of 12%.

Fatal levels are usually over 50% but lower levels can also cause death in individuals with cardiac or respiratory diseases.

Cyanide is formed from the combination of cyanide salts with acid. It can be used commercially for the production of synthetic products, mining, and fumigation. At autopsy bright "cherry" red lividity, hemorrhagic gastritis, and the odor of bitter almonds, of which a large minority of individuals are unable to detect, may be observed. The absorption of cyanide from the skin is rapid. Cyanide impairs oxidative phosphorylation by binding to cytochrome oxidase and impairing its ability to function. Specifically, cyanide reversibly binds to ferric ions in cytochrome oxidase within the mitochondria (an organelle in the cell). This stops cellular respiration by preventing the reduction of oxygen to water. Essentially, the oxygen molecules can be brought to the cell but the cell itself cannot use it in its metabolism. Toxicological analysis is necessary to confirm cyanide exposure.

Hydrogen sulfide is much more toxic than carbon monoxide and gives a rotten egg smell. It arises in the breakdown of organic matter in an anaerobic environment, such as sewers, poorly ventilated basements, and manure pits. It can also be made using a combination of household cleaning products and pesticides. Like cyanide, this causes death by impairing oxidative phosphorylation and blocking oxygen utilization at the cellular level. At autopsy, there is green discoloration of the lividity and internal organs. There may also be discoloration of metal objects, such as belt buckles and coins.

Another increasing observed cause of chemical asphyxia is **secondary methemoglobinemia** [3]**.** This is most commonly due to ingestion to nitrite or nitrate containing salts such as sodium nitrite ($NaNO_2$) or nitrate ($NaNO_3$) ingestion but there are a variety of other causes. Primary methemoglobinemia is a genetic disorder and will not be discussed here. In methemoglobinemia, the hemoglobin protein is converted such that its ability to release oxygen to tissues is reduced. This results in hypoxia. The blood can have a chocolate brown appearance (Fig. 9.3) and purple/blue-gray appearance of the skin and mucous membranes. Testing for methemoglobin saturation in the blood needs to be undertaken to confirm exposure.

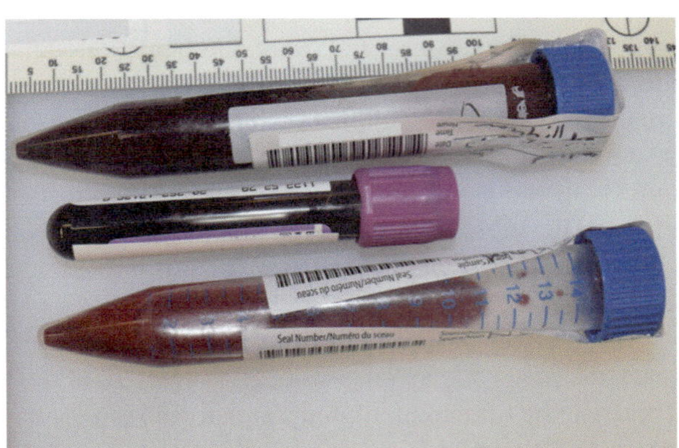

Fig. 9.3 Brown blood in a methoglobinemia due to nitrate ingestion. The upper tube is postmortem blood following a short hospital admission. The middle tube shows the admission blood. The lower tube is an example of postmortem blood from an unrelated case to function as a control for colour

Mechanical Asphyxia

Mechanical asphyxia includes deaths that impair the utilization of oxygen usually due to physical forces rather than chemicals. These can include displacement of oxygen in the local environment, a foreign object that obstructs the airway or compression of the neck or chest. Death scene examination is paramount in cases of possible asphyxia because in the absence of acute pathological abnormality, the circumstances can point to a particular form of asphyxia including helium devices, impermeable plastic bags secured over the head, entrapment in airtight containers, exposure to gases in silos or sewers. In these latter cases, gas analyses at the scene can be performed.

Environmental/entrapment: These are deaths that arise due to decreased levels or no atmospheric oxygen. These can include airtight spaces that are initially sufficient to breath oxygen but the supply is limited or when an individual enters an area that is oxygen deficient. To be clear, these deaths are due to lack of oxygen, not the presence of a poison. This cause of death is rare because of safety regulations have been implemented in many regions as a means to prevent death. Common circumstances include deaths in shipholds, underground chambers, surgical anesthesia, and children getting trapped in household appliances. Given that the scene findings can be variable, first responders and death investigators may have to use caution when extricating the body in some of these environments. Consideration of measuring oxygen levels at the scene may be warranted. Autopsy findings have no acute pathology that readily explains death and conjunctival petechiae are typically not observed. Ancillary investigations include routine microscopic examination and toxicology to rule out competing causes of death.

Plastic bag asphyxia: This is a death due to a plastic bag that has been placed over the head. These are often suicides but can also include homicides and accidents. Often, family, friends, or first responders have removed the plastic bag at the death scene. Consequently, this cause of death can be missed if the pathologist is not informed about this finding.

Asphyxiating gases: An asphyxiant gas is non-toxic, or minimally toxic, and reduces or displaces oxygen. Once all of the remaining oxygen is utilized, this will lead to unconsciousness and death. Common gases include methane, carbon dioxide, and inert gases such as helium, nitrogen, and argon. Consequently, these deaths are due to lack of oxygen, not the presence of a poison. Often a plastic bag is used in combination with asphyxiating gas such that oxygen can be displaced more quickly. If there are concerns related to the circumstances or the pathological findings and the presence of helium needs to be tested in postmortem samples, the toxicologist must be aware of this as helium is commonly added in toxicologically analysis.

Smothering (External Airway Obstruction): This is the inability of oxygen to reach the lungs due to a mechanical obstruction at the level of the mouth and nose. There can be little to no findings at autopsy, especially if the decedent cannot offer much resistance such as individuals that are intoxicated, or incapacitated from non-toxicological causes or at the extremes of age. A variety of manners of death including accident, suicide, and homicide can be ascribed. Autopsy findings are variable and can include a range from nothing to subtle findings including

- Blunt force injuries, typically bruises and abrasions around the nose, mouth, inner lips, masseter muscles, tongue, and inner cheeks
- Petechial hemorrhages of the conjunctivae are usually absent

Drowning: Drowning is defined as the process of respiratory impairment from submersion or immersion in a liquid medium (Fig. 9.4). Drowning is a common cause of death and represents a specialized form of asphyxia in which environmental oxygen is displaced by a liquid. Drowning can occur at all swimming skill levels but risk factors for drowning include cold water, strong current, young age, intoxication, and seizure disorder.

Pathophysiologically, drownings in water can be divided into fresh water and saltwater drownings. The mechanism of drowning in freshwater is that some of the water that enters the lungs enters the vascular system. Water entry causes hemodilution (dilution of blood) and hemolysis (ruptures the red blood cells). Hemolysis occurs due to excess water entering the red blood cells beyond the capacity of the cell. This can ultimately lead to a cardiac arrhythmia. In saltwater drownings, the high concentration of dissolved salt has the opposite effect on the red blood cells and draws water molecules from the red blood cells and the vascular system into the alveoli. This further fills up the alveoli, which are the functional units of air exchange in the lungs, with water and prevents gas exchange. At autopsy, both these types of drownings result in pulmonary edema and heavy lungs. However, in some individuals that have drowned, the lungs are not particularly heavy with water and pulmonary edema. In these "dry" drownings, it is hypothesized that the mechanism of death is due to laryngospasm in which the upper airway, namely the larynx (voicebox) restricts the entry of water into the lungs. The presence or absence of a laryngospasm cannot be determined from the pathological findings. Those that have been rescued from bodies of water are still at risk of complications of drowning. These include hypoxic-ischemic injury to the brain (Fig. 9.5) and diffuse alveolar disease of the lungs.

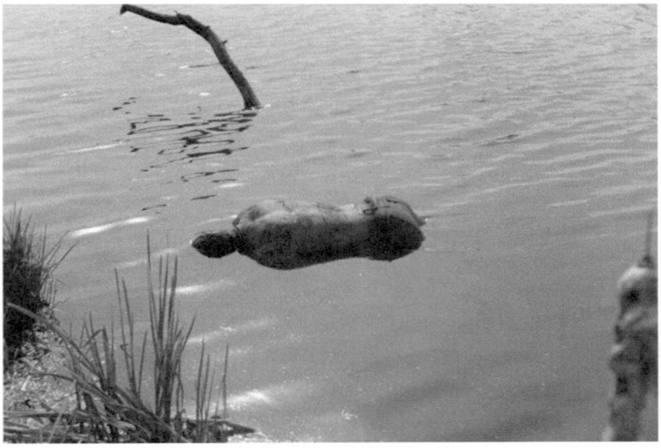

Fig. 9.4 Bodies recovered in water present challenges to the pathologist to determine if the decedent entered the water alive or dead as there are no pathognomonic findings of drowning

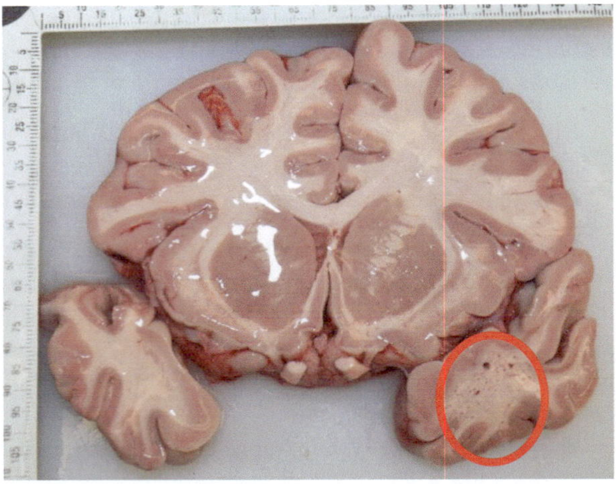

Fig. 9.5 Early changes of hypoxic-ischemic encephalopathy that can be observed following rapid anoxial injuries to the brain following a period of successful resuscitation. The changes are best noted in vacuolation of the subcortical white matter of the right temporal lobe of the brain (see circle)

The scene findings can be variable when a body is recovered from water. If the body of water is shallow, confirmation that the nose and mouth were submerged needs to be sought as drowning can still occur in a few centimeters of water. If the body is recovered from a bathtub with water, there is usually an underlying reasoning for the drowning and the cause needs to be sought at the time of the autopsy. Possible eyewitness statements of individual drowning can be helpful and other findings that would indicate the individual were alive before they entered the water. It is also a good opportunity to look for and photodocument for the presence of a foam cone on the mouth at the scene. A foam cone represents pulmonary edema that has developed from the lungs and emanated through the airway orifices. This foam cone may be fleeting with transportation of the body from the scene to the morgue. A subcategory of bodies recovered from water includes SCUBA (self-contained underwater breathing apparatus) divers. SCUBA divers recovered from water can die from a variety of causes including drowning, barotrauma, environmental asphyxia due to running out of oxygen or other equipment failures. In these deaths, the equipment needs to be assessed in addition the postmortem examination to assess for the presence or absence of barotrauma (i.e., arterial gas embolism).

There are no pathognomonic findings at autopsy to make the determination of drowning. Drowning is based on inclusionary and exclusionary data. This also includes consideration that not all bodies recovered from water had entered the water while alive. Generally the determination of drowning is made in a recently dead body in order to exclude other competing causes of death. The exclusionary data that the autopsy can provide is to assess for the absence of acute competing causes of death (i.e., gunshot wound to head). Findings support that the body has been recovered from water include wet body and clothing, immersion changes (wrinkling of skin) primarily of hands and feet. Pathological findings of drowning are variable and non-specific. These include pulmonary edema, hyperinflated lungs, water in the sphenoid sinus, foam in the upper airway and mouth, and congestion in the temporal bones of the skull. The congestion in the temporal bones may result from the prolonged head down position that occurs after drowning. Muscle hemorrhage in the strap muscles and platysma may occur in drowning [4]. Hemorrhages of the strap muscle are typically symmetrical and are along the longitudinal muscle bundles and can be quite extensive [4]. It is suggested that the mechanism of hemorrhage in the anterior muscles to the neck may be due to forceful muscle contractions during drowning [4]. Petechial hemorrhages are usually not present in adults. However, in children, petechial hemorrhages in the conjunctiva and periorbital area may be observed [5]. This may be due to an increase in cephalic intravascular pressure due to events associated with drowning including laryngospasm, vomiting, aspiration of water, muscle contraction, and venous congestion [5]. In particular, children have an increased microvascular density, increased elastin fibers, and decreased collagen in the dermis compared to adults, which may explain the differences between adults and children [5].

Other findings that may be observed on a body that is recovered from an open body of water include postmortem predation of aquatic animals and abrasions of the protuberant areas of the back of the hands. The abrasions of the hands arise because after drowning, the body often initially descends to the bottom of the water and may be carried in the water by a current. During this time period, the upper extremities hang down from the rest of the body and drag along the ground. If putrefactive decomposition occurs, the gas formation can be sufficient for the body to come to the surface of the water.

There are a few ancillary investigations that have been used as an attempt to support that drowning occurred. These investigations are controversial and may be variably utilised depending on local practice.

Diatom: (microscopic algae) Studies that compare the diatoms of the water collected at the site of drowning and a body tissue sample (i.e., intact femur) by identifying and quantifying these silica organisms. The principle of the diatom test in drowning is based on the inference that diatoms are present in the water where the drowning took place and the inhaled water enters the alveolar space of the lungs, penetrates the circulation and become deposited in different organs of the body. The diatoms in the sampled water may serve as evidence of drowning and the location of drowning.

Gettler chloride test: Examines the difference in chloride levels between blood samples and between the right and left ventricles of the heart. In seawater drownings, there is less chloride on the right side than the left. The opposite finding is found in freshwater drownings.

Strontium: In seawater drownings, the level of strontium, a trace element, is compared in samples of blood taken from the right and left ventricles.

Other ancillary investigations include microscopic examination of the lungs. This may show emphysematous aquosum changes to the airspaces but these changes can be related to other disease processes that have to be excluded.

Further, microscopic examination of tissues may show natural causes, such as myocarditis, that may have an underlying cause to the drowning. Toxicology may show the presence of substances and is an important investigation to request since intoxication is a risk factor for drowning

Foreign body aspiration (Internal airway obstruction): This is the inability for oxygen to reach the lungs due to a foreign body occlusion in the conducting airways. The level of obstruction may be at any level between the oropharynx (back of the mouth) to the principal bronchi (branches of conducting airways to lungs). If the foreign body is removed from the conducting airways by first responders, and the pathologist is not informed, this cause of death may be missed. Risk factors for internal airway obstruction include young children, edentulous/markedly incomplete natural dentition, intoxication, and dementia. A variant of this is gagging, which is when a cloth, or other foreign object, is placed in the oral cavity. The presence of gastric contents in the conducting airways may also be a consideration of internal airway obstruction. However, the presence of gastric contents in the airways can be due to antemortem aspiration in addition to agonal (perimortem) aspiration, or postmortem displacement into the airways by handling of the body in death. Agonal aspiration or postmortem displacement usually results in a small amount of gastric contents in the airway, and there may be a readily explainable cause of death. The colloquial term "choking" may be used to denote internal airway obstruction due to foreign body aspiration but this is a "loose" term and can also denote manual strangulation. Therefore, the term choking is best avoided as a cause of death in order to avoid confusion.

Traumatic asphyxia: This is impairment of expansion of the chest for respiration due to external compression of the chest and/or abdomen (Fig. 9.6). Consequently, air and its accompanying oxygen cannot enter the lungs and reach the bloodstream. In adults, this can include being crushed by the land in a collapsing dugout, avalanche, or a vehicle. There is often florid petechial hemorrhage and congestion above the point of restriction. In the pediatric population, this can occur in the setting of a larger person lying on top of the small child. This is sometimes referred to as overlay. Petechial hemorrhages are not usually observed in cases of overlay.

Positional asphyxia: Occurs when the body is in a breathing-restricted position that an individual cannot extricate themself from. This inability to remove one's self from this compromised position may be due to intoxication, obesity, seizure disorder, dementia, neuromuscular disease, and young age. At the death scene, the body is observed to be in a position where the neck is hyperflexed (bent forward with chin toward chest) and torso is positioned above the head. If the decedent's terminal

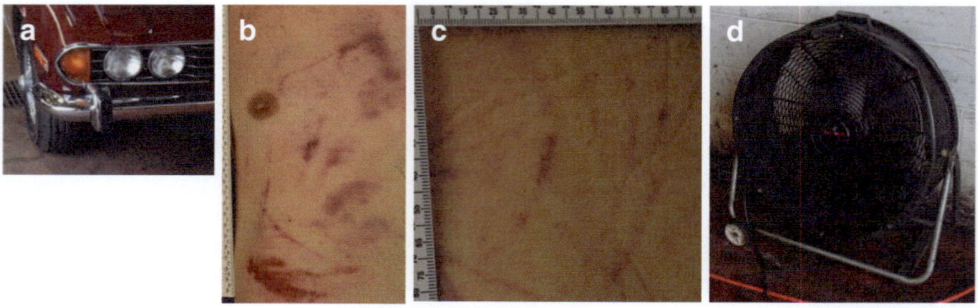

Fig. 9.6 Traumatic asphyxia: The chest was crushed between a car and a fan that was against a wall. (**a**) Car bumper that impacted the front of the chest. (**b**) Chest showing bruising that aligns with features of car bumper. (**c**) Back shows curvilinear bruises that aligns with features of the fan. (**d**) Fan that impacted the back

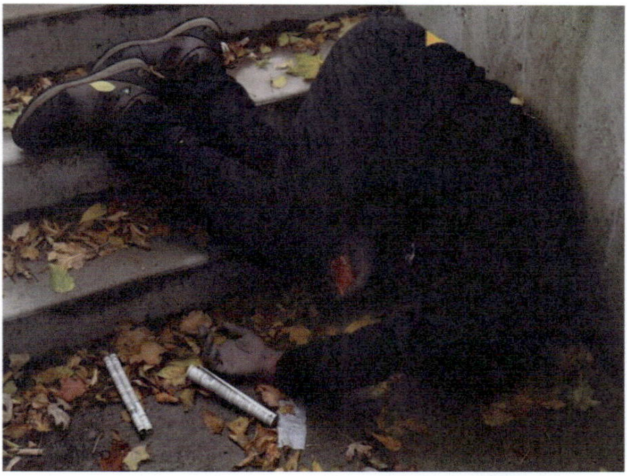

Fig. 9.7 Positional asphyxia with a hyper flexed neck

position was changed at the scene or this was not recognized as a possible positional asphyxia at the death scene and photodocumented, a clue at autopsy that this may be the cause of death is ventral lividity of the head, face, and upper chest and sparing of the anterior neck. This can be associated with petechial and hypostatic hemorrhages (hemorrhages in areas of lividity). There are variations on the position of the body including a head positioned declined below their feet such that the weight of the abdominal contents pushes up on the thoracic cavity impairing chest expansion for breathing (Fig. 9.7). There is some overlap with traumatic asphyxia.

Neck Compression

External neck compression, also referred to as strangulation, represents impaired transportation of blood between the heart and brain and may include compression of the airway. Reduced blood flow of the brain due to neck compression includes hanging and strangulation. The lack of postmortem diagnostic criteria for asphyxial deaths leads to challenges for the forensic pathologist. Forensic pathologist can make this determination based on observations that collectively in the appropriate context can have diagnostic value but individually do not. These observations include conjunctival petechial hemorrhages, evidence of external and internal blunt force injury of the anterior (front) of the neck (Fig. 9.8). However, the spectrum of findings in strangulation can be widespread, and the minimal acceptable criteria for homicidal strangulation have not been determined.

Forensic Anatomy of the Anterior Neck Structures

The internal structures of the anterior neck are complex and include muscles, the hyoid bone, the upper airway, and major blood vessels. Below the skin of the anterior neck lie two muscle groups. Superficially there is a thin, sheet-like muscle that covers most of the anterolateral (front and sides) aspect of the neck and spans from the clavicles (collar

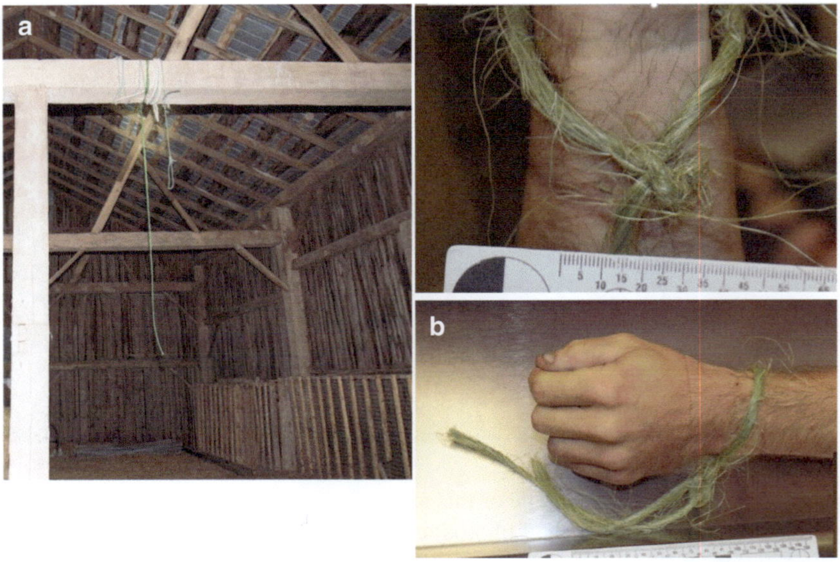

Fig. 9.8 Atypical hanging with ligatures around the wrists. (**a**) Scene images showing multiple ligatures. (**b**) Autopsy images of the loose ligatures around the wrists. Not indicative of homicide as these could be self-applied and removed

bones) to the lower face and is called the platysma muscle. Behind the platysma muscle are paired strap muscles that lie just in front of the bony and cartilaginous structures of the anterior neck. These paired muscles are referred to as strap muscles because of their long and flat shape that is similar to a belt or strap. From anterior to posterior (front to back), the strap muscles include the sternocleidomastoid, omohyoid, sternohyoid, sternothyroid, and thyrohyoid muscles. The origin and insertion sites are indicated by their names with the etymology of "omo" meaning shoulder in Greek.

The structures behind the strap muscles include the hyoid bone and the cartilaginous larynx. The **hyoid bone** is a solitary horseshoe-shaped bone located centrally at the base of the tongue. The hyoid bone develops in a segmented fashion, whereby the continuous nature of the hyoid bone identified in adults may not be observed in infants and youth [4]. The hyoid bone is composed of a central body, paired greater horns, and lesser horns. The body is located anteriorly in the neck. The lesser horns project up, and the greater horns extend posteriorly. There is a synchondrosis joint between the articulation of the body and the greater horns. Overtime the synchondrosis joints ossify making the segments of the hyoid bone as one continuous bone. This ossification usually begins in the third decade of life and finishes in the fourth or fifth decade [6]. The developmental progression is variable and may lead to asymmetrical mobility and flexibility. Once the bones are fused, the hyoid bone is more vulnerable to fractures. Below the hyoid bone sits the **larynx** (voice box). There is marked sexual dimorphism of the larynx resulting in a greater size in post pubertal males than females. The larynx is composed of two cartilages: thyroid cartilage and cricoid cartilage that are adjacent to the esophagus and the vertebral bodies that make up the spine. The thyroid cartilage is a shield of cartilage that opens at the back and sits above the cricoid cartilage. The shield of cartilage consists of two laminae united anteriorly in an acute angle in adults and forms the laryngeal prominence (Adam's apple). A V-shaped notch separates the laminae superiorly. Posteriorly the laminae diverge into two long slender processes called the superior and inferior horns. The superior horns are long and narrow. They extend upwards and medially toward the vertebral bodies located in the back of the neck. The superior horns attach laterally to the thyrohyoid ligament, which frequently house the triticeous cartilages. The triticeous cartilages are small pieces of fibrocartilage that lie superior and in close association to the superior horns. The inferior horn is short, thick and directed downwards. The cricoid cartilage sits below the thyroid cartilage and that fully encircles the trachea. The cricoid cartilage is a smaller but thicker than the thyroid cartilage. The cricoid cartilage has a signet ring shape that forms a narrow arch anteriorly and has a broad plate posteriorly. The pathologist must be aware of the anatomical variants of the thyroid cartilage in order to avoid overinterpret these differences as fractures [7]. Paired jugular veins and carotid arteries run vertically and sit on either side of the hyoid bone and larynx.

Mechanism of Death

The anatomical and physiological effects need to be considered when sustained pressure is applied to the front of the neck. Occlusion of the blood vessels in the neck impairs proper oxygenation of the brain. The occlusion of the jugular veins results in congestion, petechiae, and edema above the point of constriction due to the rapid rise in venous pressure in the head in the setting of arterial perfusion. Occlusion of the carotid arteries causes rapid unconsciousness because the arterial supply to the brain by the paired vertebral arteries in the posterior neck is insufficient for brain perfusion. Occlusion of the carotid arteries for 4–5 min can cause irreversible hypoxic-ischemic brain injury. If there has been resuscitation and a period of survival, hypoxic-ischemic injury to the brain can be observed at the time of autopsy. Given the higher blood pressure within the carotid arteries than the jugular veins, it takes more force to occlude the arteries than the veins. Another hypothesized mechanism of death is the effects of pressure on the baroreceptors in the carotid arteries that can cause bradycardia (slow the heart rate). This mechanism is not without controversy and if this mechanism in fact occurred cannot be determined at autopsy. Airway occlusion may also have a role in the mechanism of death and can occur in two ways: First, the external pressure on the neck lifts the larynx and/or the hyoid such that the base of the tongue is pressed up against the roof of the mouth and occludes at the oropharynx (back of the mouth). Second, direct compression of the larynx or trachea. Given that cartilage has more resistance than blood vessels, occlusion of the larynx will require more force than occlusion of the blood vessels. Fractured hyoid and larynx usually speak to the force applied to the neck, rather than the mechanism of injury. It is the occlusion of the blood vessels that has the predominant role in causing hypoxia (low oxygen) and anoxia (lack of oxygen).

Hanging

Hanging is a distinct form of neck compression in which the constricting force applied to the neck is from the gravitational weight of the body or body part, such as the head. The head is a body part that is sufficiently heavy to cause hanging in the seated or recumbent positions. Hanging deaths are most commonly due to suicide followed by accident. Homicidal hangings are rare.

Hangings are typically initially identified by scene findings (Fig. 9.8). The decedent may be discovered partially or completely suspended from a ligature. Incomplete body suspension indicates that part of the weight of the body is supported, usually from the lower extremities. The examination of the body may exhibit a constellation of injuries and is dependent on the nature of the ligature material, weight of the body, length of descent, complete versus incomplete suspension, and length of the time of suspension [8]. When the ligature is tied to high point of suspension, such as a rafter, there often is a ladder or similar aid to assist the decedent to tie the ligature. These aids may be moved by families or first responders and may require further inquiry. A wide variety of ligatures may be used but should correspond to the ligature mark (Fig. 9.9). The features of ligatures are that they have some length and are flexible (e.g., belts, ropes, cords). There is often an upslanted, abraded, and indented ligature furrow that corresponds to the ligature. If a broad soft ligature was used or padding was placed between the neck and ligature, a ligature furrow may not be present (Fig. 9.10). The ligature furrow on the neck is often more proximal than in ligature strangulations. The ligature furrow sometimes can be horizontal rather than upslanting. A horizontal ligature mark can arise in

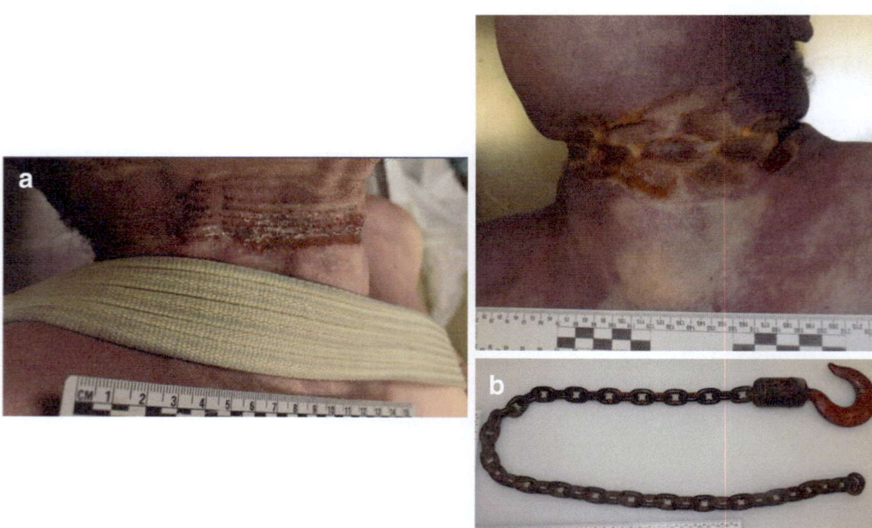

Fig. 9.9 Ligature marks that corresponds to ligature. (**a**) Ligature mark due to belt. (**b**) Ligature mark due to a chain

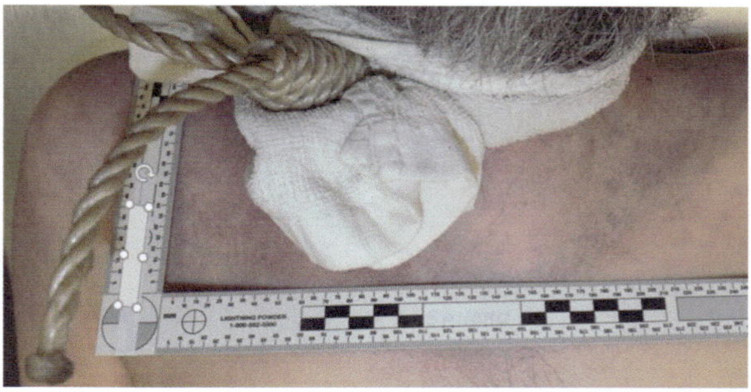

Fig. 9.10 An intervening item between the neck and ligature may be used as an attempt to minimize pain associated with constriction of the neck. This can lead to the absence of a ligature mark

hangings when the suspension point is low and decedent leans away from the point of suspension. Correlation with the death scene can facilitate understanding of ligature furrow. The tip of the tongue is often protruding and often shows postmortem drying of the tip of the tongue if the body remains hanging. The tip of the tongue protrudes due to sustained external pressure from the ligature that lifts the larynx and/or the hyoid such that the tongue is pressed up and forward. A saliva stain may be present on the lower face, anterior torso or clothing. Petechial hemorrhages are not always observed when a body has been completely suspended because both veins and arteries are occluded. Arterial pressure and the occlusion of the veins are required to increase the intravascular pressure in the head. This is why petechial hemorrhages above the point of constriction can be observed in incomplete suspensions because support of the body alleviated constriction and occlusion of the carotid arteries. If the body remains vertical after death, the distribution of lividity that develops is circumferentially around the lower extremities and distal upper extremities. The lividity is more pronounced in the distal lower extremities. Internally, there may be no to some hemorrhage, fractures of the hyoid bone and larynx, unless there is a long drop there may also be damage to the cervical (neck) vertebrae and spinal cord (spine). More extensive injuries of the neck, including decapitation may be observed with the combination of a long drop and elevated body weight.

Hangings are usually suicides but there are variations on the scene and circumstances that do not change the cause of death but can speak to the manner of death. A variant of hanging is "autoerotic asphxyia" and the "choking game." In autoerotic asphyxia, the scene findings are variable but can include pornographic materials, exposure of the decedent's genitals, features of cross dressing, fetishism, and sadomasochism [9] (Fig. 9.11). Autoerotic asphyxia is commonly described in young adult males but also has been reported in adolescents, women, and the elderly [10]. The autoerotic asphyxiation occurs by inducing cerebral hypoxia and concurrent masturbation. The decreased oxygen supply to the brain, or cerebral hypoxia, is often due to hanging, neck ligatures, plastic bags over the head, and oxygen replacement with gas or chemicals [10]. This hypoxic state is reportedly believed to heighten sexual pleasure [10]. The risk is that the hypoxic euphoria can lead to unconsciousness and death. Death is usually accidental due to failure of self-rescue. Since this may be a habitual act, there are typically methods to minimize trauma

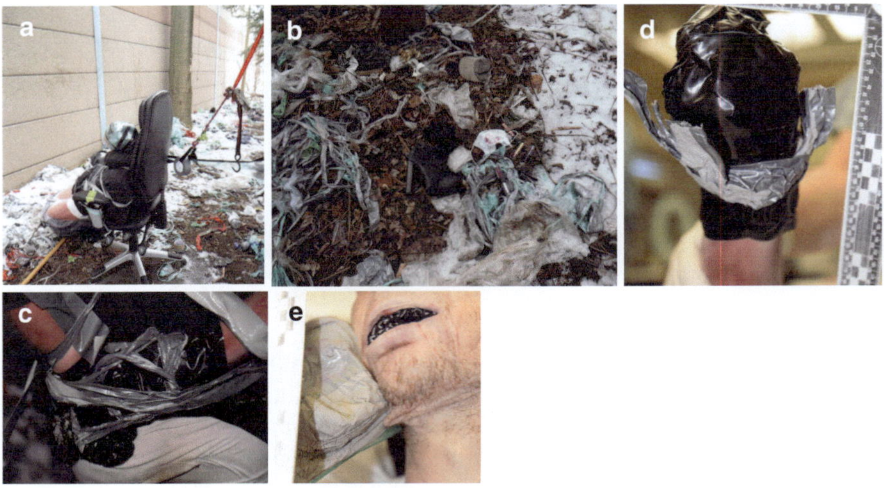

Fig. 9.11 Autoerotic asphyxia. (**a**) Scene images show complex mechanism for bonadge. (**b**) Scene images showing habitual use of various bondage materials, women's clothing and makeup. (**c**) The use of tape in bondage to hold wrists around back. (**d**) The use of tape to create a mitten. (**e**) Handkerchief in the oral cavity that was covered with tape (tape reflected)

related to causing the asphyxia (i.e., ligature mark) as not to draw attention to these injuries. These methods can include the placement of an intervening cloth between the neck and ligature or utilizing a soft broad ligature. There may be evidence of self-rescue at the scene and this can be as simple as standing up to remove the neck compression. In the choking game, the decedent is often a child or young adolescent. The intent is to produce the feeling of light-headedness or other neurological symptoms related to occluding the blood vessels of the neck. This is often performed in groups or pairs with the other person applying pressure on the neck but may be performed in isolation.

Manual and Ligature Neck Compression

Manual and ligature neck compression, also referred to as manual and ligature strangulation is a form of neck compression that is due to external physical force(s) on the front of the neck. The external findings of sustained neck compression include petechial hemorrhages of the conjunctivae, injuries of the skin of the neck, and injuries of the internal anterior neck structures (Fig. 9.12). In the absence of conjunctival petechial hemorrhages, the presence of laryngohyoid fractures need to be cautiously interpreted.

Manual strangulation indicates that hands were used to compress the neck. Manual neck compression indicates that the manner of death is homicide. Ligature neck compression indicates that a ligature was used to constrict the neck by an

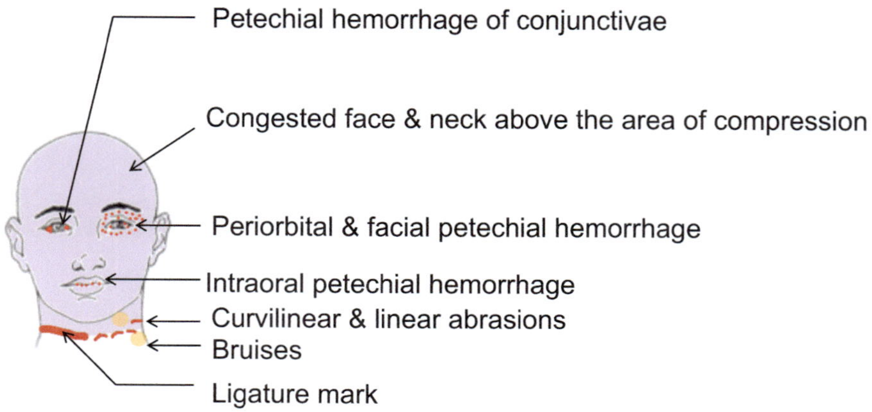

Fig. 9.12 External findings that may be observed in neck compression

external force rather than the weight of the decedents' body (i.e., as observed in hangings). Ligature neck compression is often homicidal but some are suicidal or accidental. The determination between manual and ligature strangulation depends on the external findings of the neck. Manual strangulation is free of a ligature mark but may have discoid bruises and abrasions. Ligature strangulation has a horizontal ligature mark. Variants of external neck compression includes compression of the neck by a limb, baton, flashlight, cane, etc. The "bar arm" typically occurs with an arm, baton, or similar object compressing the neck, squeezing the larynx against the cervical spine and occludes the airway. The "carotid sleeper" occurs when a flexed arm compresses the anterior neck and occludes the carotid arteries bilaterally.

Petechial Hemorrhages

Petechial hemorrhages (petechiae) are small, pinpoint, hemorrhages that arise from ruptured postcapillary venules. In sustained neck compression, petechiae can be observed in conjunctivae, sclera, periorbital skin, facial skin, mucosa of oral cavity, and airway (Fig. 9.13). Although, petechiae first appear in the conjunctivae, the time taken for petechiae to appear is unknown. Recognizing and documenting petechiae are important because of their evidentiary value to support the currently understood mechanical pathogenesis of sustained neck compression. Petechiae are not pathognomonic of asphyxia because they are not typically present in other forms of asphyxia such as entrapment, obstruction of the airway, internal airway obstruction, and plastic bag asphyxia. This is because in those asphyxial deaths, there is no mechanism that results in an increase in vascular pressure in the postcapillary venules of the eyes, face, and head. The hypothesized mechanism of petechiae hemorrhage formation is a sustained increase intravascular pressure rather than endothelial damage from hypoxia [11, 12]. Unless there has been sustained pressure on the neck, the presence of petechiae supports a mechanical rather than hypoxic cause.

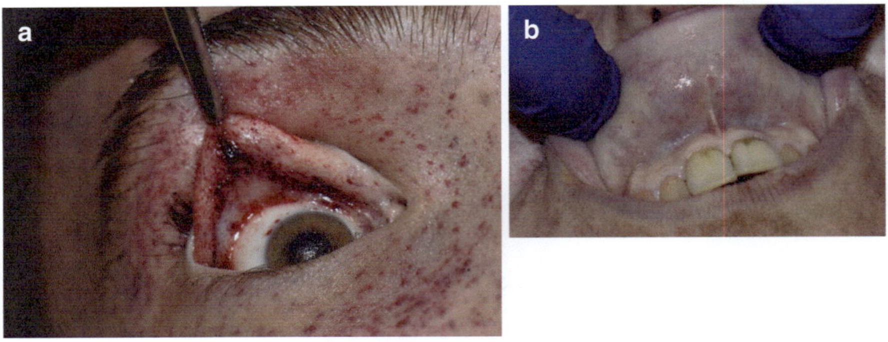

Fig. 9.13 Multiple petechial (pinpoint) hemorrhages of the conjunctivae (inner surface of eyelid) and periorbital (around the eye) skin and oral (mouth) mucosa in sustained neck compression. (**a**) Petechiae of the eye. (**b**) Petechia of the upper inner labial mucosa of the mouth

Care must be taken in interpreting petechial hemorrhages. Petechial hemorrhages can be observed in other circumstances such as heart failure, electrocution, status epileptic, head trauma, cardiopulmonary, paroxysms of sneezing and coughing, sepsis, gravity inversion, childbirth, drowning in children, and vomiting or other valsalva maneuvers [5]. Rare or isolated petechial hemorrhages in the setting of benign circumstances and the absence of traumatic findings must be considered. Further, petechial hemorrhages of the eyes and face may arise as a postmortem change when the decedent's body is in prone position resulting in hypostatic hemorrhages due to lividity rather than petechial hemorrhages from neck compression. However, when petechial hemorrhages of the eyes are observed, external neck compression needs to be assessed for at the time of the postmortem examination. Therefore, although petechiae may be indicative of external neck compression, conjunctival and facial petechiae alone are not diagnostic per se of external neck or chest compression. In addition, deaths due to neck compression sometimes may not have external neck injury, especially among females [13]. Therefore, in the setting of conjunctival petechial hemorrhages, especially if multiple or florid, and in the absence of external neck injuries, assessment for the presence or absence of internal neck injuries can assist in ascertaining the significance, if any, the petechiae. Like many things in forensic pathology, the observation of petechiae must be interpreted in the greater context of the investigation and autopsy findings.

External Neck Injuries

The injuries associated with pressure applied to the neck can be variable [4]. The injuries can also extend to the lower face, usually along the jawline, the posterolateral sides of the neck, along the clavicle(s) (collar bones) and upper chest. The findings on the skin of the neck in **manual neck compression** can include evidence of blunt force injury:

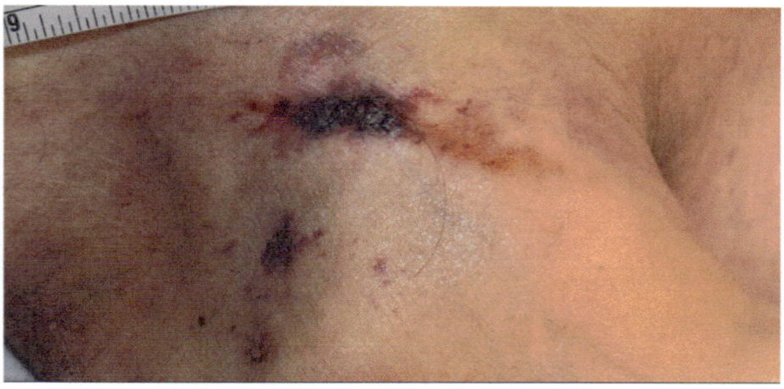

Fig. 9.14 Blunt force injuries in the form of abrasions and bruises at the anterior (front) neck. The significance of these injuries requires incorporation of the scene and remaining pathological findings

1. Bruises:
   (a) Usually discoid
   (b) Usually red or purple but not always
   (c) May be isolated, cluster, or become confluent
   (d) May represent injuries from the fingertips of the hands of the assailant
2. Abrasions: A wide variety of shapes may be observed on the skin. Fingernails may produce linear and curvilinear abrasions. Some of these abrasions may be from the assailant or from the decedent as they attempt to free themself from external neck compression.

The findings on the skin of the neck in **ligature strangulation** can include evidence of blunt force injury (Fig. 9.14):

1. Ligature mark:
   (a) Appearance depends on the nature of the ligature & may be patterned
   (b) Ligature mark has a nearly horizontal appearance
2. Ligature:
   (a) Ligature may be present on the body or at the death scene
   (b) Often an implement of opportunity so can be variable
   (c) Ligatures with a pattern may imprint this pattern onto the skin. Recognizing the pattern is invaluable in tracing a potential implement
3. Abrasions:
   (a) Fingernails may produce linear and curvilinear abrasions
   (b) These injuries may reflect the decedent attempts to free themself from the compressive effects from the ligature.

Internal Neck Injuries

The internal neck injuries can be divided predominantly into hemorrhages and fractures.

Hemorrhages: The hemorrhages of the anterior neck can be variable in its distribution but can involve the neck subcutis, soft tissues of the neck, thyroid gland, and muscles. Hemorrhages may involve the superficial platysma muscle but also the deeper strap muscles. The deeper intramuscular hemorrhages may not correspond with the cutaneous injuries. A layered musculocutaneous dissection of the anterior neck following the removal of the brain and viscera can avoid artifactual hemorrhage by allowing blood in blood vessels of the neck be drain into the chest cavity and/or intracranial cavity. In addition, intercartilaginous laryngeal hemorrhages can be associated with subepithelial laryngeal hemorrhages and intralaryngeal muscular hemorrhages [14].

Artifactual hemorrhages of the posterior surface of the esophagus are referred to as Prinsloo-Gordon artifact [15]. Further caution needs to be taken in artifactual postmortem hypostatic hemorrhages (Tardieu spots) in areas of lividity due to prone position (face down) of the body at the scene (Table 9.1) [16]. This is because lividity can mimic soft tissue bruising (pseudo-bruising) related to external neck compression. In an experimental study that induced hemorrhagic lividity of the neck, gross and microscopic examination was unable to distinguish hypostatic hemorrhages from acute bruises [16].

Fractures: Fractures of the laryngohyoid are relatively common findings at postmortem examination in deaths due to external neck compression but are not always present. The presence of fractures indicates the degree of force that was applied to the neck rather than a significant contribution to death. More force is required to fracture bone and cartilage than to occlude blood vessels. Not all individuals that have died from external neck compression will exhibit fractures as there is a variety of factors that have to be considered. For example, differences in shape and rigidity of the hyoid bone may explain the differences in the presence or absence of fractures [17]. Hyoid fractures are usually observed in the posterior third of the greater horns. They may be unilateral or bilateral, and local hemorrhage is observed at the site of discontinuity. Experimental studies involving blunt impacts of the thyroid cartilage demonstrated that the thyroid fractures are commonly located near the base of the superior horns due to biomechanical reasons [18]. Fractures of the cricoid cartilage and laminae of the thyroid cartilage are less common. Fractures of the cricoid cartilage traverse the ring structure typically in a vertical or oblique manner (Fig. 9.15). Given the ring structure of the cricoid cartilage may exhibit more than 1 fracture, requiring careful exam-

Table 9.1 The main pitfalls in diagnosing external neck compression as a cause of death

Hyoid bone development misinterpreted as a fracture
Triticeous cartilage misinterpreted as a fracture
Prinsloo-Gordon artifactual hemorrhage
Postmortem hypostatic hemorrhage
Resuscitation-related artifacts

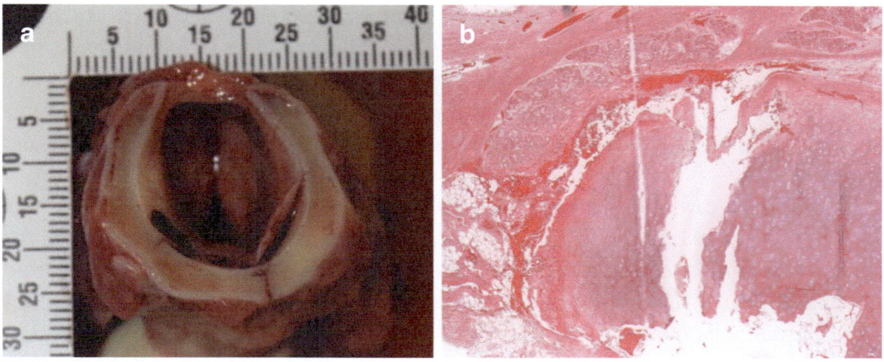

Fig. 9.15 Transverse section of the cricoid cartilage showing an acute hemorrhagic fracture without an associated inflammatory reaction. (**a**) Macroscopic view of the cricoid cartilage fractures. (**b**) Microscopic view of cricoid cartilage fracture showing discontinuity of the cartilage in the center of the image

ination for the presence or absence of another fracture. The fractures of the laminae are usually oblique. Histologically, there may be hemorrhagic microscopic fractures of the thyroid cartilage [14].

Blunt Impact Trauma to the Neck

Blunt impact trauma can cause injuries to the anterior neck that are similar to strangulation. The distinguishing feature between external neck compression and blunt impact trauma is the presence of petechiae in the conjunctivae that arise in sustained neck compression. Blunt impact trauma that is not sustained does not cause an increased intravenous pressure. It is thus increased intravenous pressure that is necessary to cause rupture of blood vessels that appear as petechial hemorrhages. Causes of blunt impact trauma include a punch or kick to the throat but also falls onto the neck.

Tissue Management of Suspected Laryngohyoid Injuries

Artifactual hemorrhaged can be avoided by performing a musculocutaneous dissection following the removal of the brain and viscera to extravasation of blood into soft tissues of the neck due to dissection. Photodocumentation of the internal structures in situ and/or once removed can allow for reviewability. This can include photographs of the anterior and sides of the neck once the skin with the platysma muscle is reflected. Taking photographs after each paired muscle is reflected can also highlight hemorrhage that may be on the anterior and posterior surfaces of the strap muscles. Macroscopic evidence of hemorrhage in areas of fractures supports the notion that the fracture is antemortem. The fracture site will have sharp edges and be crepitant on palpation. Exposing the greater hyoid horns and thyroid superior horns in situ can minimize the risk of misinterpreting artifactual fractures, especially in areas of soft tissue hemorrhage. The presence of hemorrhage in a mobile area of the hyoid bone may be supportive of a fracture, while the absence of hemorrhage is supportive of a natural joint. To maximize detection of fractures in the cricoid cartilage by making a transverse section to divide the superior and inferior half.

Histological examination can be variable [19]. Microscopy can differentiate that an area of abnormal mobility as either a fracture or a natural joint, especially in the presence of hemorrhage at a site of interest [6, 14, 19]. The hyoid bone and thyroid cartilage typically require formalin fixation and then decalcification prior to sectioning. Alternatively, methacrylate can be used to decalcify the tissues [6]. Removal of large soft tissues, such as the thyroid gland will speed up the fixation process, but leave a small amount of the soft tissues attached to the areas of interest prior to fixation. Following decalcification, sectioning of the horns and submitting the horn from the fracture to the tip into the histology cassette. Alternatively, the hyoid bone is cut through the body and the two halves are bisected along their length [6]. Similarly, histology of the cricoid cartilage can differentiate an area of hemorrhage from bone marrow (Fig. 9.16). Transverse section of the cricoid cartilage can reveal fractures that usually traverse the cricoid cartilage. Histology can distinguish between fractures and triticeous cartilage. Triticeous cartilage are characterized by an island of fibrocartilaginous completely surrounded by perichondrium where a fracture line will pass through the cartilage and the perichondrium overlying the fracture line will be breeched. Awareness of the triticeous cartilage is important because fracture of the superior horn of the thyroid cartilage is the most commonly observed in strangulation [4]. In addition, the syndronchotic joints of the hyoid bone may also be misinterpreted as a fracture. Radiographs and histology can facilitate distinguishing a fracture from a joint.

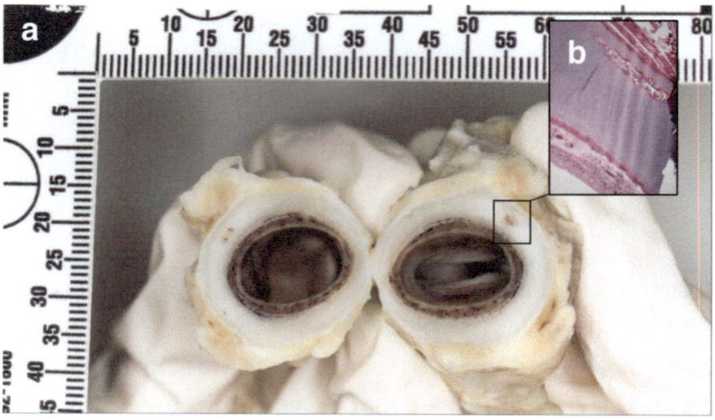

Fig. 9.16 Macroscopic focus of hemorrhage in the cricoid cartilage that may be due to an injury or bone marrow. (**a**) Macroscopic view of cricoid cartilage that was cut transversely to reveal an area of hemorrhage. (**b**) Inset: microscopic examination of the area of hemorrhage determines the etiology as bone marrow rather than injury

Anogenital Injuries

There is little written in the medical literature concerning anogenital injuries. In part because of the circumstances may result in withholding information and attempts to conceal the facts [20]. Most sex-related acts would not have signs of anogenital injury [21]. In addition, anogenital injuries are not commonly observed at autopsies resulting in variable experience among forensic pathologists when confronted with this uncommon entity. However, when injury is present, the distinction between consensual and non-consensual sex-related injuries cannot be determined by the pathological findings alone [22]. Both consensual and non-consensual sexual activity can result in anogenital injury. There is an overlap between physical findings between consensual and non-consensual activity such that the pathological findings are often insufficient to differentiate between the two groups. In both consenting and non-consenting sexual intercourse, a wide range of genital injuries can be observed including rapidly healing microscopic lacerations to major vaginal vault lacerations [23]. Most are minor injuries, which either do not require medical treatment or at most minimal treatment [20]. In addition, superficial injuries such as mucosal disruption may disappear over hours to days [24]. This occurs because the tissues in this area are capable of rapid and usually complete regeneration. More extensive injuries are rare and can result in death. Consequently, many forensic pathologists may have only rarely encounter anogenital injuries that have resulted in death. Although consent cannot be determined by the postmortem examination, consent to sex is irrelevant in the case of young children and infants, who are unable to legally consent [24]. After complete assessment, a report to Child Protective Services might be indicated in some cases of pediatric anogenital injury.

The occurrence of extra-anogenital injuries is variable depending on the research methodology and ranges from 20 to 64% [25–27]. Clinical studies on alleged non-consensual sex-related acts indicate that 5–8% have detectable genital trauma and 11–29% have trauma in extra-genital areas [28]. However, the reported ranges is also age and hormone status dependent as genital trauma is more common in young children and postmenopausal females [28]. The higher incidence of trauma in children is due to the disproportionate anatomy and being estrogen deficient [29]. In postmenopausal females, increased rate of injury was attributed to atrophy of connective tissue and vaginal epithelium, loss of soft tissue elasticity due to decreased estrogen levels.

The prevalence of anogenital injuries after a non-consensual sexual act is estimated between 9% and 87% depending on the ages of the survivors studied, method of examination, and the type of injuries included [30–32]. A national epidemiological study of suspected rape homicides in females over 13 years found the most common genital injuries in females over 13 years included in descending order: vaginal, posterior fourchette, urethral, hymenal, and introital [22]. However, another study found that trauma most commonly involves the fossa navicularis, labia minora, posterior fourchette, vagina, cervix, anus, and perineum [33]. Among sexual assault survivors, genital injuries in women of color may be more frequently missed up to four times more [34–37]. In females over 13 years, commonly injured locations of the extra-anogenital included injuries to the head, face, neck, pelvis, buttocks, and lower limbs [22]. Evidence of human bites and external neck compression were strongly associated with sex-related homicides in women [22].

Outside of injuries, there are other indicators of sexual activity which can include pregnancy, presence of semen, or a sexually transmitted disease. However, like injury, a determination of consent cannot always be determined.

Causation of Anogenital Injury

Causation of anogenital injuries is also not well studied. This is in part because the information provided in reported in non-consensual sexual acts may lack sufficient detail [38]. Further scientific research of genital injury is limited, in part to the risk of objectifying patients or unjustifiably serving research interests rather than the care of the patient [24]. In addition, many genital injury studies in non-consensual sexual acts do not make attempts to correlate physical findings with the nature of the act [38]. Specifically, it is unclear if there was vaginal or anal penetration and if so, what was the nature of the object [38]. The paucity of this information is limited given the range of possible non-consensual sexual acts that exist [38]. The mechanism of injury can vary, and little research is present on mechanism of injury in the anogenital injuries. Clinical research has been hindered by poor systematized research methodology due to contradiction in findings, lack of standardized terms, different examination techniques, mixed children and adult patient populations, lack of controls and non-blinded design, paucity of peer review variations in examiner training and experience [24].

Anogenital Anatomy

The forensic pathologist's knowledge in range of variations of normal anatomy and disease states is necessary for the reliable documentation and interpretation of any injuries of the anogenital area. Age, parity, abuse history, hormonal milestones all have associated anatomical variations that are normal [24]. Further, exclusion of recent birth and anal fissures related to inflammatory bowel disease or chronic constipation is warranted. Also the recognition of the cultural practice of female cutting (formerly referred to as female genital mutilation) can alter the appearance of the external genitalia in females.

Biological Female Anatomy

Vulva

The vulva, or the female external genitalia, is demarcated by the mons pubis anteriorly, the anus posteriorly and laterally to the inguinal-gluteal folds. The vulva is composed of multiple structures including the mons pubis, clitoris, labia minora, labia majora, vulval vestibule, vestibular bulbs, urethral meatus, hymen, and vaginal introitus. The prepuce of the clitoris represents the anterior fusion of the labia minora. A bilateral frenulum of the clitoris attaches posteriorly to labia minora. The vestibular bulbs are two long masses of erectile tissue that within and adjacent to the clitoris and introitus. The labia minora fuse anteriorly to form a prepuce of the clitoris and end posteriorly as the fourchette. The labia minora are folds of skin lying medial to the labia majora. The labia minora contains sweat glands and sebaceous glands but no hair follicles and there is no underlying adipose tissue. The area where the labia *majora* meet posteriorly is called the posterior *commissure*. The posterior *fourchette* is where the labia *minora* meets posteriorly. The labia minora is located lateral to the vulvar vestibule and medial to the labia majora and is bounded by the sulcus interlabialis. The labia majora are lateral to the intralabial sulcus and medial to the inguinal-gluteal fold. The hymen is the most distal extent of the vagina, which is an internal structure. The hymen is a thin membrane composed of connective tissue that overlies the introitus, which is the vaginal opening. The hymen may be imperforate, round, annular, septate, cribriform, or porous. Coitus or the use of intravaginal tampons results in tears in the hymen, which can be observed as hymenal tags, called caruncle hymenales. On the vaginal surface, the hymen has a non-keratinized stratified squamous epithelium that becomes glycogenated with exposure to estrogen.

The anatomy of the female genitalia differs in prepubertal children and adult females due to estrogen exposure. In children up to 2 years of age, when maternal estrogen is present, the hymen may appear thick and have a convoluted, waxy appearance. The waxy appearance is typically seen in infants and children that are breast-fed. Once the maternal estrogen disappears, the hymen becomes thin and vascular.

During the prepubertal period, the labia majora have a flat appearance and the labia minora is thin. The clitoris is usually hidden by the labia majora, and the mucosal redundancy in the lower vagina may appear near the hymen as a fold. The posterior fourchette (the area where the labia minora meet posteriorly) does not exist in prepubertal children because the labia minora do not reach the midpoint posteriorly. However, in both pre-pubescent and adult females, the posterior commissure is present. The mucous membranes of the vagina in pre-pubescent children are thin, pink, and atrophic.

In later childhood, the external genitalia show signs of early estrogen exposure including thickened mons pubis, the labia majora and labia minora fill out, the labia minora extends toward the posterior fourchette, the hymen thickens, the introitus enlarges, the vagina elongates, and vaginal mucosa thickens.

Anatomical variations of normal vulva include (Table 9.2) [39]:

1. **Intravaginal longitudinal ridges:** Narrow ridge of mucosa covered connective tissue tissue on the vaginal wall that may attach to the inner lining of the hymen
2. **Linea vestibularis:** Pale vertical line across the posterior fourchette and/or fossa navicularis
3. **Failure of midline fusion:** Congenital anomaly that may extend from the fossa navicularis to the anus

Table 9.2 Some variations of normal in the pre-pubescent hymen

Variation	Appearance
Imperforate hymen	No opening in the hymen, rare
Fimbriated	Redundant tissue that folds over itself
Cribriform	Multiple small opening
Crescentic	Half-moon shape hymenal tissue at the posterior introitus
Annular	Hymenal tissue that surrounds the introitus and that spares the center or may be displaced from the center
Septate	Multiple larger openings in the hymen tissue

4. **Labial adhesions:** Fusion of the adjacent mucosal surfaces of the posterior portion of the vestibular walls (Fig. 9.17)
5. **Periurethral/peri-hymenal bands:** Small bands of connective tissue connecting to opposing surfaces

During puberty, the external genitalia gradually assumes an adult appearance including formation of the posterior fourchette, pubic hair on the mons pubis, thickened, elastic hymen with folds, mucous production of the vagina increase length of the vagina, and thickened vagina mucosa.

In adults, there may be variation in the size, pigmentation, and shape of the labia, size, and visibility of the clitoris and the location of the urethral orifices and introitus (vaginal opening). During pregnancy, there are marked physiological and anatomical changes in female bodies depending on the gestation of the fetus. In the first trimester, the uterus is enlarging but is still protected by the pelvis. There is increased vascularity of the vulva and vaginal tract in addition to increased physiological discharge that may be misinterpreted as seminal fluid. In the third trimester, the cervix comes into the vaginal axis and direct contact to the cervix can cause bleeding. At delivery, there can be trauma to the genital area. A history of the use of forceps, episiotomies, and degree of anogenital lacerations, if present, should be in the medical record. Following delivery, vaginal lubrication and distention can occur and the vagina can become thinned and the fugal (folded) pattern can be lost.

During menopause, estrogen levels drop and menstruation ceases. This can be reflected in anatomical and structural changes including thinning of the pubic hair, decrease in subcutaneous adipose tissue, drying of the mucosa, fragility of tissues, smaller or a gaping introitus, the presence of rectoceles, cystoceles or uterine prolapse, thin, loss of elasticity of the vaginal walls.

Vagina

The vagina extends from the introitus of the vulva to the uterus. Internally, lies posterior to the urinary bladder and anterior to the rectum. The vagina is a muscular tube lined by a mucous membrane that surrounds the exocervix, forming vault like fornices between the cervical attachments anteriorly, laterally and posteriorly. The vaginal

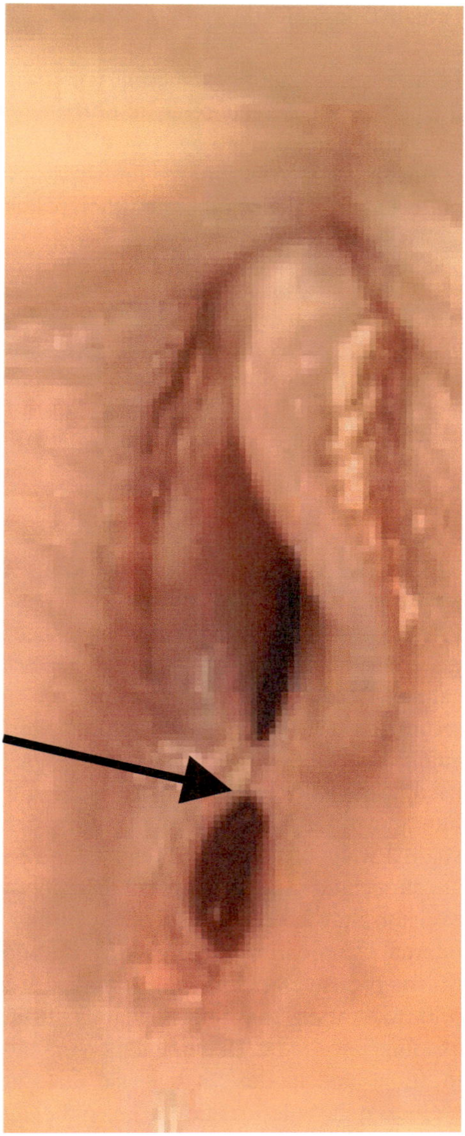

Fig. 9.17 Labial adhesions indicated by arrow is a normal anatomical variation of the vulva

musculature is continuous with the uterus. The middle half of the vagina is closely opposed to the rectum, separated by a fibrofatty adventitia and the rectovaginal septum. The lower one-fourth of the vagina is separated from the anal canal and anorectal sphincters and perineal body. The urethra lies anterior to the vagina and courses approximately about 1/3 of its length on the vagina and enters the vaginal wall and terminates with its external meatus in the vulvar vestibule. The ureters course along bilaterally the upper third of the vagina before entering the urinary bladder.

Female Genital Cutting

Female genital cutting, sometimes referred to as female genital mutilation, which is the partial or complete removal of the external female genitalia. This will result in an altered genital anatomy. The WHO defines this as: all procedures involving the partial or total removal of the female external genitalia or other injury to the genital organs for cultural or other non-therapeutic reasons [40].

There are four distinct types:

- Type 1: Excision of the prepuce +/− all or part of the clitoris
- Type 2: Excision of the clitoris & all or partial excision of the labia minora
- Type 3: Excision of part or all of the external genitalia and stitching/narrowing the vaginal opening (also known as infibulation)
- Type 4: Unclassified and can include all other procedures to the female genitalia for non-medical purposes (i.e., pricking, piercing, incising, scraping, and cauterizing the genital area)

Tissue Management of Injured Female Anatomy

Prior to obtaining biological swabs inspection and photodocumentation for foreign materials, blood and injuries can be performed. Following the collection of biological swabs and other exhibits a more comprehensive in situ external and internal examination of the vagina, cervix, and uterus can occur. Internal examination of the vagina can be aided with labial traction/separation. In addition, a speculum can be used, if the pathologist is comfortable in using this aid. The assistance of a speculum allows for direct inspection of the cervix and vaginal walls. Alternatively, the vaginal walls can be examined once the pelvic organs have been removed. If there are anogenital injuries, a formal dissection of the pelvic organs with trans-anal disc excision may be performed. Prior to this special dissection being performed, an internal examination of the pelvic and abdominal cavity can be performed to assess for the presence or absence of injuries. It is easier to examine the vaginal fornices prior to fixation, as formalin fixation stiffens the tissues making it more difficult to examine once fixed. Documentation of vaginal and vulvar injuries using anatomical locations and landmarks but also utilising the face of an analog clock with 12 o'clock at the anterior midline and 6 o'clock located at the posterior midline may be helpful.

Findings due to other conditions, which can be mistaken for injury

1. Urethral prolapse
2. Lichen sclerosus et atrophicus
3. Vulvar ulcer(s), such as aphthous ulcers or those seen in Behcet disease

4. Inflammation, and fissuring of the perianal or vulvar tissues due to infection with bacteria, fungus, viruses, parasites, or other infections that are not sexually transmitted
5. Rectal prolapse
6. Rectocele and cystocele
7. Red/purple discoloration of the genital structures (including the hymen) from lividity (Fig. 9.18)

External Male Genitalia

The external male genitalia is composed of the penis and scrotum. The penis is composed of a base, shaft, and distally of a glans (head) that contains the urethral meatus (opening) with or without a prepuce (foreskin). The prepuce is a prolongation of the skin of the shaft and normally covers most of the glans. The prepuce can reflect

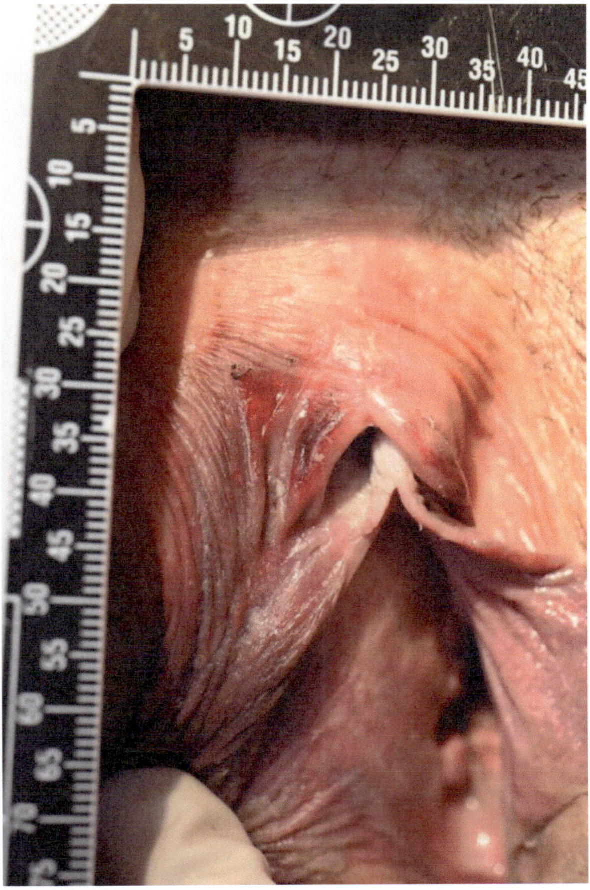

Fig. 9.18 Vulva showing lividity that was suspicious for a bruise. Histoloigcal evaluation showed congested blood vessels and no hemorrhage

beyond itself, showing its mucosal inner surface, which is continuous with the epithelium of the coronal sulcus of the glans penis. The removal of the prepuce via male circumcision is commonly practiced in some communities and may be absent. The prepuce will not retract in the majority of infants because the narrow tip will not pass over the glans penis and the inner mucosal surface of the prepuce is fused to the glans penis. However, by 5 or 6 years old, the prepuce can be completely retracted beyond the level of the glans corona. The testes may be descended into the scrotum at birth but can remain intra-abdominal. During puberty, the testes enlarge, the scrotum becomes thickened, and pubic hair begins to cover the mons pubis.

Injury

Sex-related injuries of male children and adults are poorly studied resulting in little knowledge and experience [41]. The lack of information available about genital injury among males may reflect smaller numbers of males reporting non-consensual sexual acts. Those studies available focus on anal injuries but penile or scrotal injuries have not garnered a body of literature [38].

External examination includes the scrotum, testicles, penis, periurethral meatus and requires reflection of the prepuce, if present. Given that the mucosa of the glans and inner surface of the prepuce is initially fused, the ability to reflect the foreskin depends on the age of the decedent. Documentation of injuries uses anatomical location such as dorsal penis, ventral glans, etc.

Perineum

The perineum comprises the surface area of the torso between the thighs and the buttocks, extending from the coccyx to the symphysis pubis. It functions as the external pelvic floor that supports and surrounds the urogenital and gastrointestinal tracts. The perineal body is the central tendon of the perineum, a fibromuscular structure located in the midline of the perineum at the junction of the anus and urogenital triangle in both males and females.

Injury

Perineal lacerations are not common but when exist are typically classified into 4 categories [42]:

- 1st degree: superficial lacerations limited to the epithelial layer
- 2nd degree: lacerations that extend into the perineal body but not the external anal sphincter
- 3rd degree: involving the superficial or deep injuries to the external anal sphincter
- 4th degree: extending throughout the rectal mucosa

Anus

The anus, or anal canal, is the opening of the lower gastrointestinal tract and connects the colon via the rectum to the outside world. The anal canal is composed of internal and external sphincter muscles that are formed by the puborectalis muscle. There is normal variation between individuals of the anus that include: degree of pigmentation, rugal patterns, symmetry, and prominence and distribution of vascular structures. Pubic hair can develop and surround the external anal tissues.

The surgical anal canal is approximately 5 cm long [43] and based on functional criteria, which cannot be determined at autopsy due to the loss of tone. Similarly, the term anal verge, that is used in the clinical setting, is defined as the point where the walls of the anal canal come in contact in their normal resting state [44, 45], which also cannot be determined postmortem.

The anus may become lax postmortem. The "funnel anus" appearance should be interpreted as an anatomical variant rather than evidence of sexual act involving the anus.

The histological anal canal is composed of different types of epithelium that in formalin-fixed specimens, the average length of the anal canal has a length of 3 cm [43].

There are structures observed in the surfaces of the anal canal that can be identified with naked eye examination in formalin-fixed tissue. Microscopically there is a sequence of epithelium that can be identified in longitudinal sections:

1. Colorectal zone: complete ring of colorectal type mucosa. There is no line line of demarcation that marks the transition to the anal canal; however, some shortening and irregularity of the crypts may be observed in the area closest to the anal transitional zone [46]. Macroscopic staining, such as Alcian blue or green, wherein the mucin of the colorectal zone has a dark stain, the anal transition stains lighter due to the sparse mucin production and paucity of staining in the squamous zone [47].
2. Anal transition zone: Macroscopically, this has a smoother, gray-blue more glistening appearance. Histologically composed of epithelial variants, including sparse mucin production in the surface epithelium and scattered crypts. This is defined as the zone between the uninterrupted colorectal mucosa and uninterrupted squamous epithelium [47]. The epithelium is 4–9 cell layers with the basal cells being small with perpendicular nuclei to the basement membrane. The surface cells may be columnar, cuboidal, flat, or polygonal [48–50]. In addition, other epithelial type cells include small areas of mature squamous epithelium, occasional goblet cells, colorectal type, and simple columnar epithelium. Anal glands can be observed in the submucosal. This may not always be present.
3. Squamous zone: non-keratinizing squamous epithelium with short or no papillae. This uninterrupted squamous epithelium typically occurs at the level of the dentate line. The most important macroscopic landmark is the dentate line that divides the anal transitional zone from the squamous zone line, which is com-

posed of anal valves, sinuses, and the bases of anal columns. These are not always readily apparent. At a minimum, the dentate line should be defined by the lowest sinuses visible.

4. Perianal skin (This is not part of the anal canal but included for completion): dull and wrinkled with or without hair. Microscopically, this is keratinized squamous epithelium with or without hair and skin appendages and anogenital mammary-like glands.

Injury & Artifacts

Many of foreign body insertions may cause mucosal injury only [20]. Injuries observed of the anus include lacerations, which tend to radiate from the orifice (Fig. 9.19). These may be best sampled for histological assessment by taking cross sections perpendicular to the laceration. If there is an injury to the anus, careful

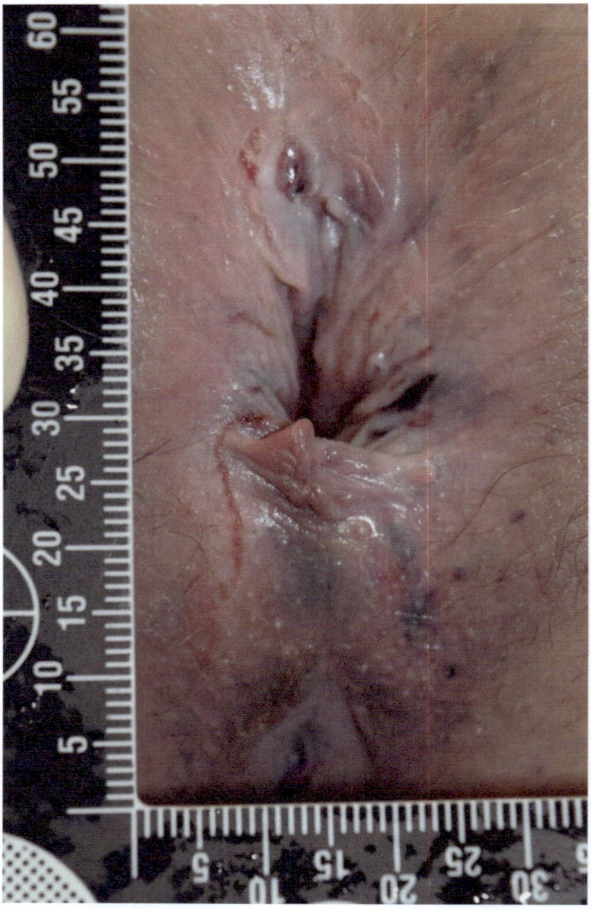

Fig. 9.19 Anus showing multiple radiating injuries

inspection and opening of the intestines, in particular the rectum, as there may be intestinal injuries associated with anal injuries. Careful consideration of natural causes of what could be considered as anal injuries such as anal fissures related to inflammatory bowel disease or defecation of hard stool. Similarly to vaginal/vulvar injuries anal injuries may be documented using the face of an analog clock. Further, hemorrhoids can sometimes passively bleed postmortem depending on the position of the body. For example, in a case report of hanging, the decedent's hemorrhoids bled postmortem due to positioning of the body [51]. Further, the presence of lividity in the area of anal injury may lead to some passive bleeding. This can challenge the forensic pathologist in determining if the injuries are antemortem, postmortem, or perimortem.

Biological Samples

Collection of biological samples can be used to determine the occurrence of recent sexual act. This evidence can include saliva, seminal fluid, pulled head hair, fingernail clippings or scraping, swabs of suspected bite marks or suction bruises (i.e., hickeys), pubic hair, blood, urine, fiber, debris, and soil. Some law enforcement agencies have access to alternate light source or forensic light source, which is an instrument containing ultraviolet light from a black light source that can illuminate trace biological materials such as blood, semen, and saliva on skin causing visible fluorescence. Biological samples can be collected following photodocumentation. DNA analysis is the test choice for most samples. This can be a means to exclude or include suspects. Testing for sexually transmitted infections may also be warranted. In addition, the presence of tampons, sanitary napkins, condoms, etc. may be transferred into the custody of the police as exhibits.

Swabs can be dampened with sterile normal saline when collecting from dry surfaces (i.e., skin) but all swabs need to be dried either in a drying container or before being placed in a container to avoid the destruction of the material from bacterial and fungal overgrowth. Exhibits need to be sealed and a chain of custody established.

References

1. Sauvegeau A. Classification of asphyxia: the need for standardization. J Forensic Sci. 2010;55(5):1259–67.
2. Byard R. Issues in the classification and pathological diagnosis of asphyxia. Aust J Forensic Science. 2011;43(1):27–38.
3. Hickey, et al. Fatal metheglobinemia: a case series highlighting new trend in intentional sodium nitrite or sodium nitrate ingestion as a method of suicide. Forensic Sci Int. 2021;326:110,907.
4. Pollanen MS. Pitfalls and artifacts in the neck at autopsy. Acad Forensic Pathol. 2016;6(1):45–62.
5. Somers et al. Presence of periorbital and conjunctival petechial hemorrhages in accidental pediatric drowning. Forensic Sci Int 2008;175:198-201.

6. Davison AM, Williams EJ. Microscopic evidence of previous trauma to the hyoid bone in a homicide involving pressure to the neck. Forensic Sci Med Pathol. 2012;8:307–11.
7. Pinheiro J, et al. Laryngeal anatomical variants and their impact on the diagnosis of mechanical asphyxias by neck pressure. Forensic Sci Int. 2018;290:1–10.
8. Kumar P, Rayamane AP. Pattern of neck injuries in hanging deaths and its correlation with recent concepts and theories. J-SIMLA. 2015;7(1):20–5.
9. Byard RW, Branwell NH. Autoerotic death. a definition. Amj Forensic Med Pathol. 1991;12:74–6.
10. Myers WC, et al. The relationship between serial sexual murder and autoerotic asphyxiation. Forensic Sci Int. 2008;176:187–95.
11. Rao VJ, Wetli CV. Asphxyial deaths and petechiae: a review. Am J Forensic Med Pathol. 1988;9:32–4.
12. Ely SF, Hirsch CS. Asphxyial deaths and petechiae: a review. J Forensic Sci. 2000;45:1274–7.
13. James R, et al. Homicidal neck compression of females: autopsy and sexual assault findings. Acad Forensic Pathol. 2013;3(4):454–7.
14. Pollanen MS. A triad of laryngeal hemorrhages in strangulation: a report of eight cases. J Forensic Sci. 2000;45(3):614–8.
15. Prinsloo I, Gordon I. Postmortem dissection artifacts of the neck: their differentiation from antemortem bruises. S Afr Med J. 1951;25(2):358–61.
16. Pollanen MS, et al. Hemorrhagic lividity of the neck: controlled induction of postmortem hypostatic hemorrhages. Am J Forensic Med Pathol. 2009;30(4):322–6.
17. Pollanen M, Chiasson D. Fracture of the hyoid bone in strangulation: comparison of fractured and unfractured hyoids from victims of strangulation. J Forensic Sci. 1996;41:110–3.
18. Bockholdt et al. Experimental investigations of fractures of the upper thyroid horns. Led Med. (Tokyo). 2003:5:S252-S255.
19. Rajs J, Thiblin I. Histologic appearance of fractured thyroid cartilage and surrounding tissues. Forensic Sci. Int. 2000;114:155–66.
20. Syllabi M, et al. Rectal perforation following fist fornication. Clin Res Hepatol Gastroenterol. 2020;44:e216–8.
21. Adams JA, et al. Interpretation of medical findings in suspected child sexual abuse: an update for 2018. J Pediatr Adolesc Gynecol. 2018;31:255–31.
22. Abrahams N, et al. The epidemiology and the pathology of suspected homicide in South Africa. Forensic Sci Int. 2008;178:132–8.
23. Biggs M, et al. Genital injuries following sexual assault of women with and without prior sexual intercourse experience. CMAJ. 1998;159:33–7.
24. Brennan PAW. The medical and ethical aspects of photography in the sexual assault examination: why does it offend? J Clin Forensic Med. 2006;13:194–202.
25. Alempijevic D, et al. Severity of injuries among sexual assault victims. J Forensic Legal Med. 2007;14:266–79.
26. Everett RB, Jimerson GK. The rape victim: a review of 117 consecutive cases. Obstet Gynecol. 1977;50:88–90.
27. Tintinalli JE, Hoelzer M. Clinical findings and legal resolution in sexual assault. Ann Emerg Med. 1985;14:447–53.
28. Ramin SM, et al. Sexual assault in postmenopausal women. Obstet Gynecol. 1992;80:860–4.
29. Cartwright PS. Sexual assault Study Group. Obstet Gynecol. 1987;70:44–6.
30. Jina R, Jewkes R, Vetten L, Christofides N, Sigsworth R, Loots L. Genito-anal injury patterns and associated factors in rape survivors in an urban province of South Africa: a cross-sectional study. BMC Womens Health. 2015;15:29.
31. Astrup BS, Ravn P, Thomsen JL, Lauritsen J. Patterned genital injury in casesof rape—a case-control study. J Forensic Legal Med. 2013;20(5):525–9.
32. Lincoln C, Perera R, Jacobs I, Ward A. Macroscopically detected female genital injury after consensual and non-consensual vaginal penetration: a prospective comparison study. J Forensic Legal Med. 2013;20(7):884–901.

33. Delacroix J, et al. Rectal perforation secondary to rape and fisting in a female adolescent. Pediatr Emerg Care. 2011;27:116–9.
34. Sommers MS, Zink TM, Fargo JD, Baker RB, Buschur C, Shambley-Ebron DZ, et al. Forensic sexual assault examination and genital injury: is skin color a source of health disparity? Am J Emerg Med. 2008;26(8):857–66.
35. Baker RB, Fargo JD, Shambley-Ebron DZ, Sommers MS. Source of healthcare disparity: race, skin color, and injuries after rape among adolescents and young adults. J Forensic Nurs. 2010;6(3):144–50.
36. Cartwright P. Factors that correlate with injury sustained by survivors of sexual assault. Obstet Gynecol. 1987;70(1):44–6.
37. Sommers MS, Zink TM, Baker RB, Fargo JD, Porter J, Weybright D, et al. Effects of age and ethnicity on physical injury from rape. J Obstet Gynecol Neonatal Nurs. 2006;35(2):199–207.
38. Lincoln C. Genital Injury: Is it significant? A review of the literature. Med Sci Law. 2001;41(3):206–16.
39. Heger A, et al. Apperance of the genitalia in girls selected for nonabuse: review of hymenal morphology and nonspecific findings. J Pediatr Adolesc Gynecol. 2020;15:27–35.
40. https://www.who.int/news-room/fact-sheets/detail/female-genital-mutilation. Accessed: July 29, 2021.
41. Ernst AA, et al. The utility of anoscopy and colposcopy in the evaluation of male sexual assault victims. Ann Emerg Med. 2000;36:432–7.
42. Cappelletti S, et al. J Forensic Medicine and Legal Medicine. 2016;44:58–62.
43. Fenger C. The anal transitional zone. Location and extent. Acta Pathol Microbiol Scand A. 1979;87:379–86.
44. Symington J. The rectum and anus. J Anat Physiol. 1888;23:106–15.
45. Buie LA. Practical proctology. Philadelphia: WB Saunders; 1937. p. 40–50.
46. Fritsch H, Aigner F, Ludwikowski B, et al. Epithelial and muscular regionalization of the human developing anorectum. Anat Rec. 2007;290:1449–58.
47. Fenger C. The anal transitional zone. A method for macroscopic demonstration. Acta Pathol Microbiol Scand A. 1978;86:225–30.
48. Wendell-Smith CP. Anorectal nomenclature: fundamental terminology. Dis Colon Rectum. 2000;43:1349–58.
49. Federative Committee on Anatomical Terminology. Terminologia anatomica: international anatomical terminology. Stuttgart, New York: Thieme; 1998.
50. Fenger C, Knoth M. The anal transitional zone: a scanning and transmission electron microscopic investigation of the surface epithelium. Ultrastruct Pathol. 1981;2:163–73.
51. Bhardwaj DN, Sharma SK, Gupta S. Haemorrhoids leading to post-mortem artefact: a case report. Med Sci Law. 2005;45:265–6.

Chapter 10
Firearm-Related Injuries

Rebekah Jacques

Firearm injuries are a form of penetrating and perforating trauma. The nature of the firearm, its associated ammunition, and distance from the body can result in a variety of different injuries.

The Anatomy and Function of Firearms

An understanding of the nature of firearms is helpful to understand the injuries that can be observed when a firearm discharges a projectile that impacts a body.

The basic anatomy of a firearm is composed of the following:

- **Grip:** handle of the gun
- **Trigger:** small projecting lever that activates the firing pin
- **Firing pin:** an internal structure that transfers the pull of the trigger into firing the projectile
- **Barrel:** a metal cylinder where the projectile (bullet) travels and exits out the muzzle
- **Bore:** the inside of the barrel
- **Muzzle:** the end of the barrel
- **Choke:** constriction of the shotgun bore at the muzzle
- **Chamber:** contains the ammunition

When the trigger of a firearm is pulled, in a loaded firearm, this sets into motion, a rapid chain of events. This chain of events starts when the firing pin strikes the primer at the base of the ammunition. The firing pin ignites the primer composition, which in turn ignites the (smokeless) gunpowder (Table 10.1). The

R. Jacques (✉)
London, Canada
e-mail: rebekah.jacques@lhsc.on.ca

R. Jacques (ed.), *Forensic Pathology*,
https://doi.org/10.1007/978-3-031-42038-2_10

Table 10.1 Firearm and ammunition terms

Term	Definition
Shotgun	Type of long barreled firearm that uses a shotgun shell for ammunition and does not have a rifled barrel resulting in a thin-walled barrel
Rifle	Type of long barreled firearm that has a thick rifled barrel, which is composed of clockwise or counterclockwise spiraled lands and grooves that provides gyroscopic stability during the trajectory of the fired projectile
Revolver	Type of short barreled handgun that has a rotating cylinder that houses the ammunition
Caliber	Internal diameter of the barrel of a gun (handgun or rifle) or external diameter of a bullet. Typically measured in millimeters (i.e., 9 mm) or hundredths/thousandths of an inch (i.e., 0.22 or 0.357)
Gauge	Internal diameter of a shotgun barrel. Initially based on the diameter of spheres of the pellets that could be made from a pound of lead. For example, a 12-gauge barrel is the diameter of a sphere of 1/12th of lead. Therefore the largest to smallest gauge is as follows: 10, 12,16, 20, and 28. The exception being the 410-gauge, the smallest, which is actually a caliber that has a 0.410 diameter barrel
Shotgun shell	Ammunition for shotgun that can include pellets of a single projectile called a "slug"
Shot cup	Plastic cup in a shotgun shell that holds the pellets
Wadding	Barrier between the gunshot powder and pellets that is made of paper, felt, or plastic
Primer	Located at the bottom of the ammunition (shotgun shell or bullet casing) that when struck by the firing pin, it ignites the propellant in the bullet casing. It is typically composed of barium, antimony, and lead. SEM can be used to determine gunshot residue from the primer
Gunpowder	Propellant that is composed of nitrocellulose +/− nitroglycerine that is located in the bullet casing above the primer. Once ignited by the primer, it rapidly expands from a solid to a gas sending the projectile down the barrel
Jacketed bullet	A bullet can be fully or semi-encased in copper or similar density material with or without the top of the lead core exposed at the tip. The jacket prevents the lead core from melting. On X-ray the jacket has a lighter radiodensity than the lead core
Choke	A device that constricts the muzzle end of a shotgun that keeps the pellet spread tighter at greater distances. There are four progressively constricted types: cylinder, improved cylinder, modified, and full). This can affect the pathological range
Birdshot	Is a type of shotgun ammunition that has multiple pellets that are designed for small games such as small birds (i.e., partridge). Need to collect a sample of the pellets as an exhibit. Ideally, the pellets with the least damage, if possible.
Buckshot	Is a type of shotgun ammunition that has 8–10 pellets designed for larger game, such as a deer. Given the small number, ideally need to collect all of the pellets that are present in the body at autopsy as an exhibit
Slug	Is a type of shotgun ammunition that has a single "bullet" designed for hunting larger game such as deer

controlled expansion of gases from burning gunpowder generates pressure that forces the bullet down the barrel of the firearm. The combustion of the gunpowder occurs quickly and is mostly complete but can leave unburned gunpowder, soot (smoke), gases, flame, and primer that adhere to the projectile but can also be projected down the barrel out of the muzzle of the gun. The production of the gases from the ignition of the powder pushes the projectiles down the barrel and out the muzzle.

Firearms

Firearms can be broadly classified as shotguns, rifles and, handgun. Each type of firearm has different ammunitions and can cause different wound patterns. Long firearms include shotguns and rifles (Fig. 10.1). These long firearms are shot from the shoulder. Shotguns are designed to fire multiple pellets down a barrel with the exception of the slug. The bore of the shotgun is smooth and contains no rifling resulting in a thinner wall of the barrel. The diameter of the barrel of a shotgun is referred to as a gauge. The gauge is calculated from the weight of a solid lead sphere that fits into the bore of a barrel. The gauge is the multiplicative inverse of a sphere's weight in fractions of a pound. So a 1/12th pound lead sphere fits into a 12-gauge bore. The end of the shotgun can have a choke, which is a device that adds varying levels of constriction to the diameter of the barrel. The level of the constriction determines the diameter of the pattern of spread of pellets. It is the spread of the pellets that determines pathological range. The ammunition used in a shotgun is a shotgun shell.

Handguns and rifles have a series of parallel spiral grooves that have been cut along the length of the bore (internal surface) of the barrel. This is called rifling and results in a thicker bore than in shotguns. The metal of the bore of the barrel that

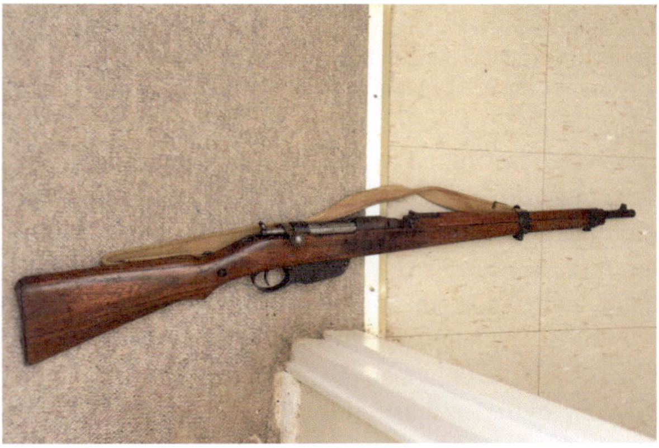

Fig. 10.1 Bolt action rifle. The bolt ejects the spent cartridge case

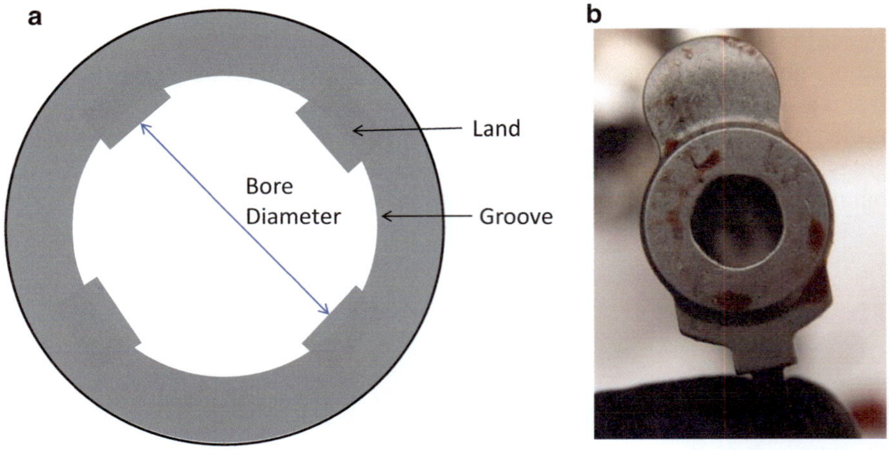

Fig. 10.2 Muzzle end of a rifled gun demonstrating the lands and grooves which provides better accuracy. (**a**) Diagram of the lands and grooves. (**b**) Muzzle end of a rifled gun showing an increased thickness and internal rifling along the length of the barrel

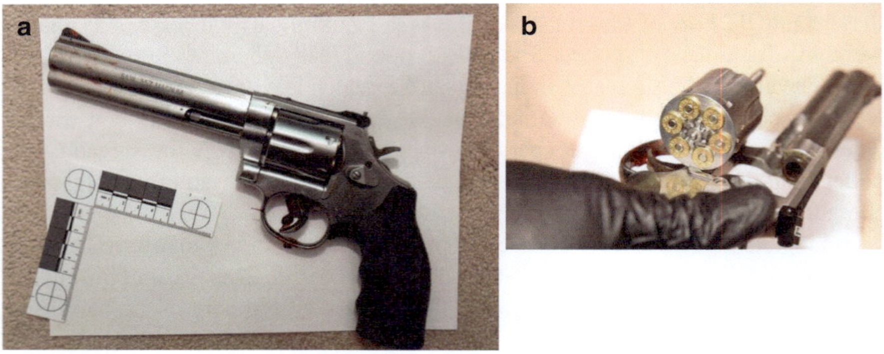

Fig. 10.3 Revolver is a type of handgun. The cylinder just above the trigger can lead to injuries of the hand as products of combustion emanate between the cylinder and the rest of the gun. (**a**) Side view of a revolver. (**b**) View of the cylinder open showing the ammunition within the cylinder

is elevated is referred to as "lands" (Fig. 10.2). The number of grooves can vary and so can the directionality. The function of rifling is that it imparts a gyroscopic spin on the projectile as it moves down the barrel of the gun that stabilize its flight in the air, thereby improving accuracy. Handguns, as the name implies, are shot from the hand, rather than the shoulder. Handguns have the cartridge kept in a magazine (essentially a chamber) which requires the first round of ammunition to be manually loaded into the chamber. A special type of handgun is the revolver. Revolvers have a rotary cylinder that holds the bullet cartridges (Fig. 10.3). Pulling the trigger rotates the cylinder and advances cartridges in-line with the bore prior to each shot.

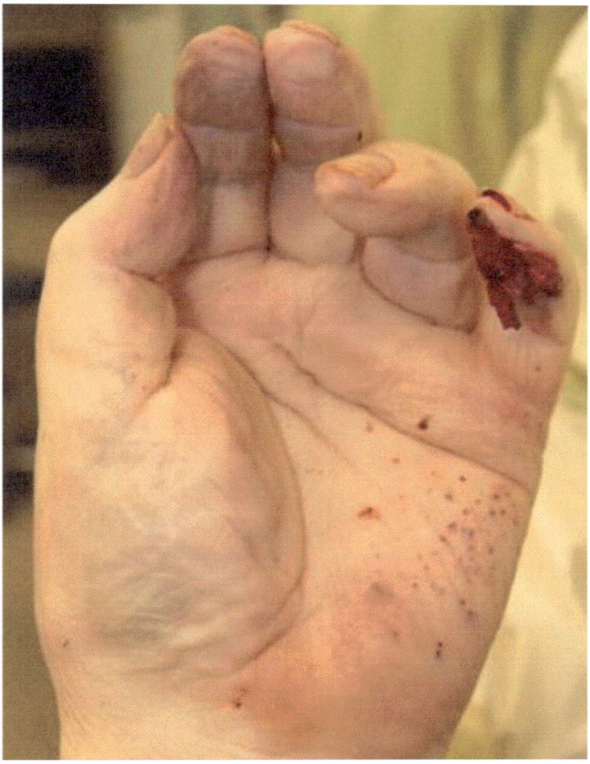

Fig. 10.4 Extensive cylinder gap injuries of the left hand involving the hypothenar eminence (mound of the palm at the base of the pinky finger) and the pinky finger. These injuries may be observed in the decedent when the firearm is a revolver

Revolvers can result in a unique pattern of injury referred to as the cylinder gap (Fig. 10.4).

Ammunition

Shotgun Shells

Shotgun ammunition is most commonly referred to as shotgun shells (Fig. 10.5). A typical shotgun shell is composed of a plastic casing with a metal base and primer, gunpowder, wad, and a crimped end to hold all the components together. The pellets are located at the crimped end. The primer can be centrefire or rimfire depending on the location of the primer cup that lies in the base of the bullet. Rimfire indicates that the primer within the rim casing and centrefire has a primer that is a separate piece held in the center of the casing. The wad functions as a barrier to separate the pellets from the gunpowder so the pellets do not melt from the heat produced during gunpowder combustion but also is a seal to maintain consistent pressure.

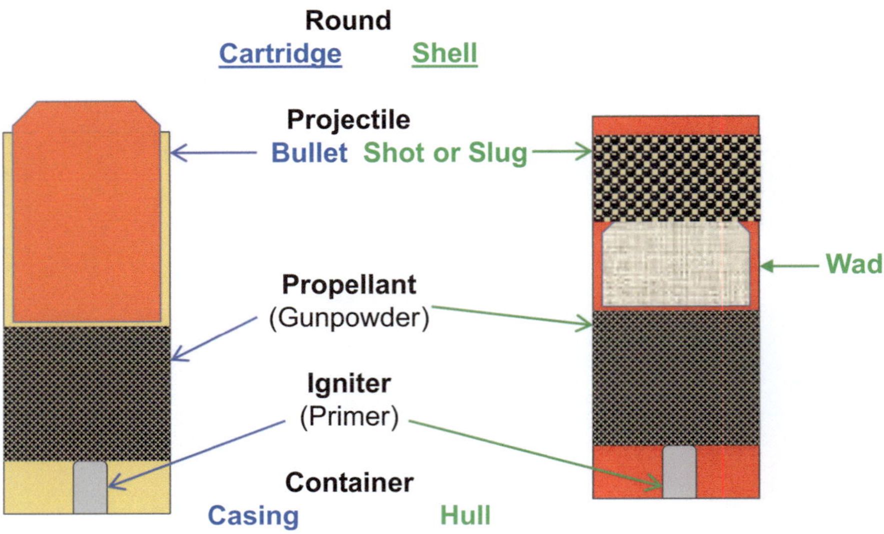

Fig. 10.5 Ammunition anatomy of a cartridge casing and shotgun shell

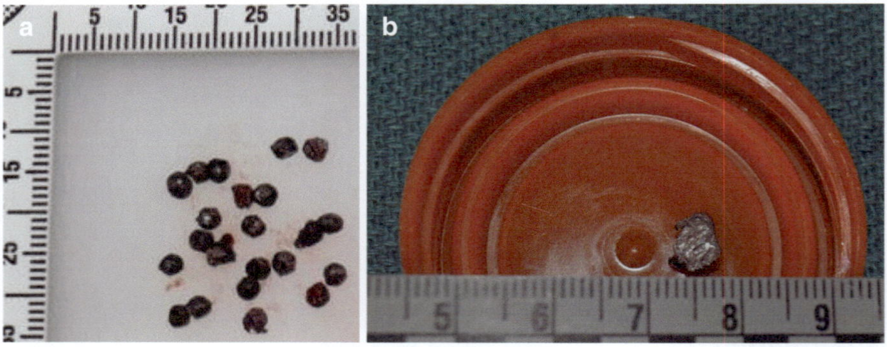

Fig. 10.6 Pellets from a bird shot recovered, some of which are damaged. When there are multiple pellets, collect the undamaged (or least damaged ones) as they carry more significance. (**a**) Sample of pellets. (**b**) Damaged pellet from colliding with other objects, including, other pellets

The shotgun shell contains multiple projectiles, referred to as pellets and collectively called a "shot." The pellets are typically made of lead and sometimes steel. There are wide range of pellets that range in size and quantity from the smallest birdshot to buckshot and single projectile as a slug. **Birdshot** are pellets used for hunting birds or other small animals (Fig. 10.6). A **buckshot** is designed for hunting large game such as deer. A large "000" buckshot pellets measure 0.9 cm each where small no. 9 birdshot pellets measure 0.2 cm each in diameter. The higher the gauge, the smaller the pellets and the more numerous pellets and lower the kinetic energy based on the lower mass (i.e., Kinetic Energy = 1/2 mv^2). Birdshots are often packed in white granulated plastic materials, which will also be expelled in addition to the

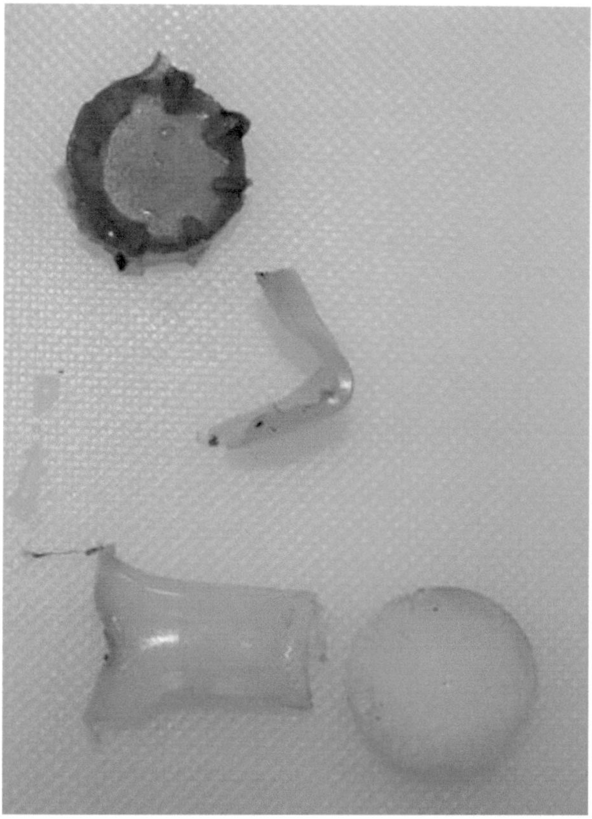

Fig. 10.7 Fragments of a wad from shotgun wound

pellets and wad (Fig. 10.7). An American invention is the **shotgun slug** that is a single large lead projectile.

The wad can be variable and can include a plastic cup with 3–4 petals or a cup and 2 cardboard cushions.

Cartridge Cases

Cartridge cases are often made of brass but aluminum and steel cases are also possible (Fig. 10.8). Like the shotgun shell, there is primer in a primer cup and gunpowder at the base of the cartridge. The bullet sits on top of the gunpowder. The bullet can have a central lead core covered by a full or partial metal jacket typically composed of copper or sometimes steel (Fig. 10.9). A radiographic clue that you are dealing with a partial metal jacket is a "lead snowstorm" whereby as the bullet travels through the body, the jacket peels back exposing the lead core, which breaks into numerous lead fragments. There are a variety of different bullet designs

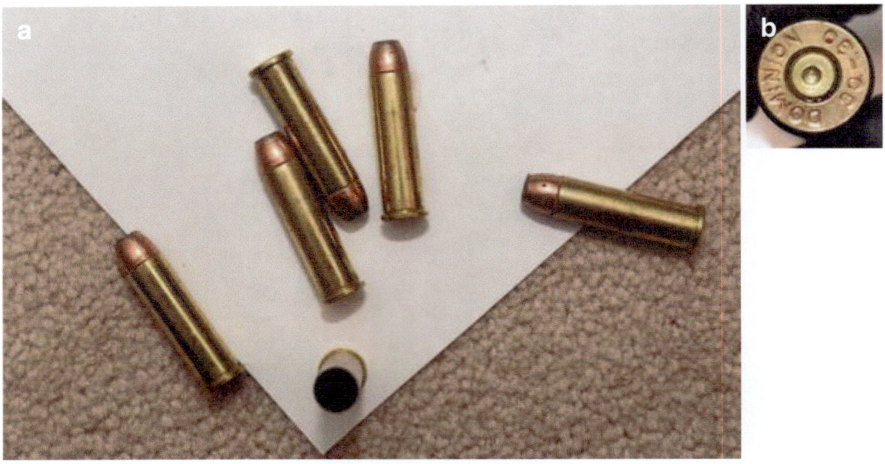

Fig. 10.8 Spent and unspent center fire cartridge cases with copper jacket. (**a**) There are 5 unspent copper jacketed bullet cartridge case and 1 spent cartridge case. (**b**) Base of fired centre-fire cartridge case

Fig. 10.9 Previously fired copper-jacketed bullet with lead core that was removed from a fatal gunshot wound

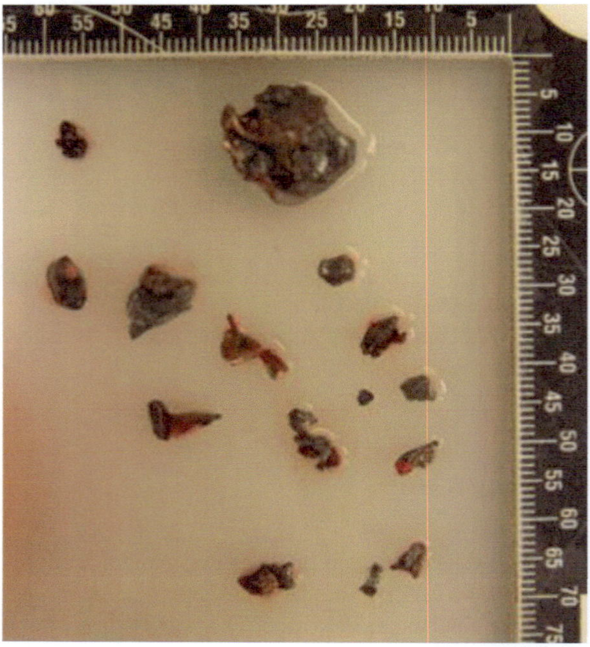

including hollow point, semi-jacketed with or without a hollow point, and total metal jacket. *These are designed to have different tumbling, cavitating, expanding, velocity properties and release energy properties. Jackets are commonly made of a copper alloy* but can also be made of steel *or similar density metal. Other bullet designs include round* tip or hollow point. The size of the cartridge cases is measured by caliber. The caliber is the diameter of the bullet.

Gunshot Residue

Gunshot residue (GSR) is defined as compounds formed during the discharge of a firearm. GSR is the inorganic and metallic residues largely originating from the ammunition that has been discharged but may include contributions from the firearm and previous ammunitions discharged from the firearm." [1]. GSR is expelled from any breached areas of the firearm including the barrel, ejection port, and cylinder gap. GSR is applied to any and all of the materials that are expelled from the discharged firearm. This includes materials from the primer cap, gunpowder grains, burnt and unburnt powder grains, metals associated with the bullet, cartridge casing, or firearm composition. These materials can be used to link a discharged firearm [2]. The nature of GSR can be analyzed by a scanning electron microscopy and energy dispersive X-ray spectrometry. The forensic application has some limitations due to the number of GSR particles deposition can vary significantly with each discharge from a firearm [1].

Kinetic Energy and Wounding

Bullets injure by transferring kinetic energy to tissues. Wound characteristics are the product of the velocity and bullet mass. Once the projectile is in the body, it can tumble and increase its surface area that impacts tissue. The severity of the injury is due to the disruption of the tissue due to:

1. Direct interaction from the projectile (i.e., pellets) and tissue. This creates a permanent path through crushing and laceration.
2. Effects of the **temporary** cavity from the kinetic energy transferred from the bullet. The greater the kinetic energy the projectile possesses, the more energy is transferred to tissues and greater the displacement of tissue. Kinetic energy is half the product of mass (m) and squared velocity (v) that is mathematically written as $\frac{1}{2}mv^2$. The exponential relationship of velocity to kinetic energy makes velocity the main contributor to kinetic energy and thus injury. Consequently, high velocity firearm injuries result in greater injury, which is manifested as cavitation. Cavitation occurs when tissue is thrust away from the bullet path creating a temporary cavity. This temporary cavity has an initial rapid radial expansion and stretching in tissues, which lasts for a few milliseconds, and then collapses onto the permanent track. The size of the temporary cavity is dependent on the rapidity of the kinetic energy transferred and the viscoelasticity of the tissues.

Table 10.2 Firearm-related injuries of the skin

Entrance gunshot wound
– Re-entry gunshot wound
– Atypical
Exit gunshot wound
– Shored exit gunshot wounds
– Atypical
Intermediate wounds
Tangential gunshot wounds
Wad injuries (i.e., petal abrasions)

Firearm Injuries

There are a wide variety of injuries that can arise. The wound pattern depends on the ammunition, firearm, and distance between firearm and injured individual (Table 10.2).

Entrance Versus Exit Gunshot Wounds

Determining whether a gunshot wound is an exit or entry can have challenges but also has implications for the legal system. Sometimes it can be challenging to determine whether a gunshot wound is an entry or exit hole due to alterations by handling, decomposition, healing, removal of clothing at the time of resuscitation and other factors. Still it is an essential task for the forensic pathologist to differentiate the entrance wound from the exit wound, if present, and provide an opinion on pathological range for the entrance wounds (Fig. 10.10). In general, an entrance wound on the skin is circular and has an abraded rim of the wound. The abraded rim or ring abrasion can be eccentric or concentric. This abraded rim occurs because the skin is stretched from the bullet before entering the body. The exit wound tends to be stellate or slit-like and maybe larger than the entrance wound. Exit wounds tend to be larger and more irregular than entrance wounds because during the path in the body the bullet has destabilized, may be deformed, and may be associated with fragments of broken bones that are carried through the body. An abrasion rim is not observed unless the skin is supported as the bullet exits the body. This is referred to as a **"shored" exit wound**. A shored exit wound can arise in a variety of settings including when the skin of the exit wound is supported by a belt, tight clothing, a chair, etc. This highlights the importance of examining the clothing, personal effect, and scene findings. Some gunshot wounds of entry may also have a stellate appearance as well if it is in an area of the body that has underlying bone (i.e., the head) and the muzzle of the gun is in contact with the head at the time of discharge.

In addition, if bone, particularly flat bone such as the skull, is fractured, the fracturing pattern can be useful in distinguishing an entrance wound from an exit wound

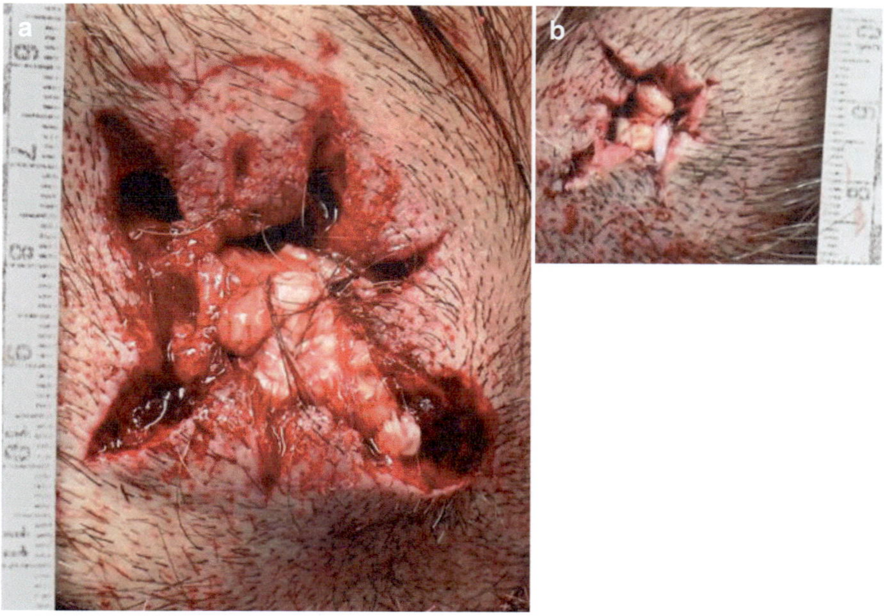

Fig. 10.10 Gunshot wounds of entry of the head can have a stellate appearance do to the pressure buildup between the skull and scalp against the muzzle. (a) Gunshot wound of entry with a stellate appearance but also a muzzle impression shown at the top of the injury. (b) Gunshot wound of exit with a stellate appearance but also smaller in size

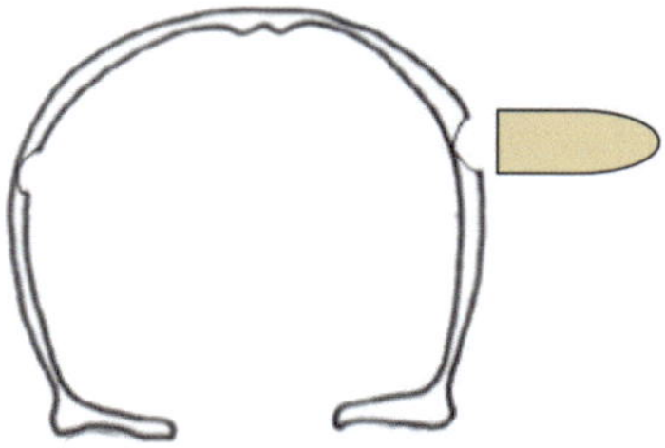

Fig. 10.11 Internal and external beveling can indicate gunshot wound of entry and exit

(Fig. 10.11). In gunshot wounds of entry, the defect on the outer table opens toward the inner table in a cone-like fashion toward the cranial vault. This is called internal beveling. A feature of an exit wound is external beveling, whereby the cone-like defect is on the outer table of the bone. This mechanism of fracture pattern occurs because of the inherent properties of bone. Bone can accommodate compression forces better than tension from the projectile. Consequently, as the forces associated with the bullet cause tension forces on the opposite side of the bone and compression forces on the same side as the bullet. The tension force causes a fracture with a crater-like appearance on the opposite side of the bullet (Fig. 10.12).

Sometimes a "keyhole" defect in the bone may be observed, whereby both internal and external beveling can be observed in a single defect. This defect most

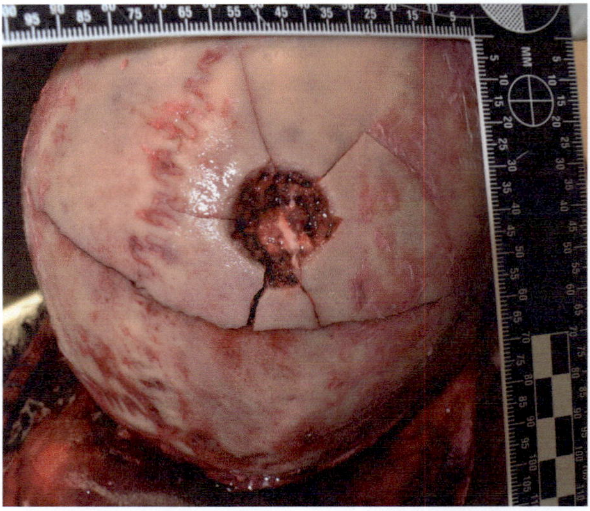

Fig. 10.12 External beveling of the right parietal skull bone indicative of an exit wound. In addition, Puppe's principle, which can speak to the order of injuries, is demonstrated with radiating skull fractures of the exit gunshot wound being interrupted by the linear coronal fracture that extends to the left parietal bone from the gunshot wound of entry

commonly can be observed in entrance wounds, but can also be observed in exit gunshot wounds as well. This pattern occurs when the projectile strikes, a flat bone, at a shallow angle that causes two divergent fractures radiating from the defect in the direction of the projectile.

Microscopic examination of entry gunshot wounds shows coagulative necrosis of the keratinocytes [3]. However, it is unclear if shored exits were also examined histologically. Microscopic examination of exit holes shows no keratinocyte necrosis due to burns, but may show adipose tissue, bone, and muscle tissue [3].

Pathological Range in Gunshot Wounds of Entry

The appearance of the entry gunshot wound can be variable and is dependent on the distance between the muzzle and the body, in addition, to the presence of any intervening objects such as clothing, windows, etc. When a gun is fired, the exiting projectile can be accompanied by the following products: a jet of flame, a cloud of gas, soot, gunpowder, and vaporized metal from the ammunition and primer. As the distance between muzzle and target increases the products that accompany the projectile are able to accompany the projectile at a spectrum of distances. This may influence the appearance on the gunshot wound of entry and speak to the pathological range.

The primary effects of the projectile cause the features of the entrance wound, which is typically a circular hole with an abrasion ring/collar. The secondary effects determine the pathological range depending on the distance of the end of the muzzle and body at the time of discharge. Determination of pathological range is a *qualitative* assessment, rather than a quantitative assessment. To determine a quantitative determination requires that the exact firearm and similar ammunition are fired at known ranges in an attempt to reproduce the same size pattern found on the body.

Pathological range is an opinion on the distance between the end of the muzzle based on the macroscopic appearance of the entrance gunshot wound. The macroscopic appearance is due to secondary effects of the products that accompany the projectile including unburned gunpowder, possible metal fragments from the firearm, gases, flame, and soot that soils the skin. Depending on the distance and the presence of an intermediary target(s) that is between the firearm, this can lead to scorching, soot soiling, and tattooing/stippling on the skin. The flame at the end of combustion can cause thermal effects to the entry gunshot wound. The formation of carbon monoxide due to incomplete combustion can cause the underlying muscle, if present, to have a "cherry" red appearance. Soot deposition is the result of the combustion of gunpowder that soils the entry hole (Fig. 10.13). This soot soiling can be removed with ease and can be observed macroscopically. However, with "smokeless" gunpowder, in which a smokeless chemical powder is employed, the soot deposition can be less intense. Grains of gunpowder that are either burnt, or not, that are projected at the time of discharge can cause "tattooing" around the entry hole. These grains of gunpowder cause punctate abrasions on the skin that cannot be removed by cleaning the surface. They can have a "freckle-like" appearance (Table 10.3).

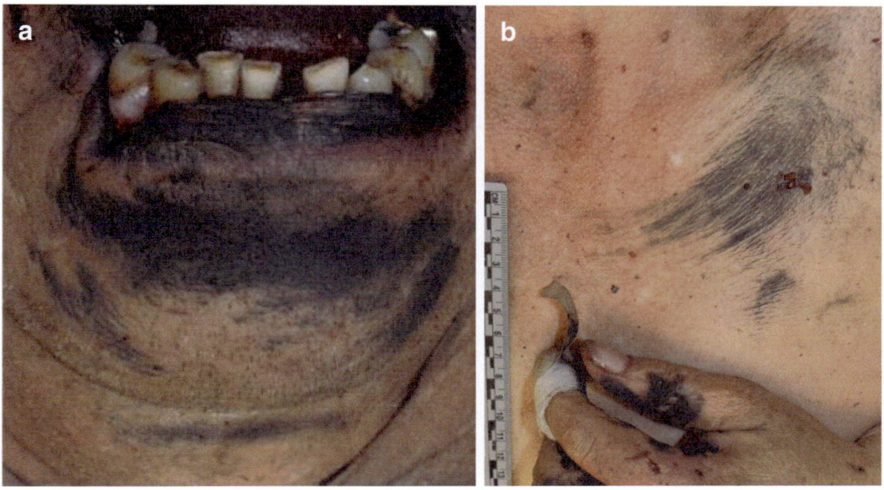

Fig. 10.13 Depending on the nature of the gunpowder and characteristics of the gun a variable amount of soot may be present on the body. Shown is a large amount of soot that is less commonly observed due to the introduction of smokeless gunpowder. (**a**) Soot in the chin and neck. (**b**) Soot on the hand and chest

Table 10.3 Pathological range of the entry gun*shot* wounds can be broadly divided into the four categories but there is a spectrum of appearances due to overlapping densities of soot and gunpowder

1. **Contact:** variable—gases can split skin, blackening, muzzle "impression"
2. **Close:** soot deposition
3. **Intermediate:** powder tattooing/stippling is present
4. **Indeterminate/Distance:** distinctive features are absent. The absence of distinctive features can be due to a distance between the muzzle and target that exceeds the ability of gunpowder and soot to reach the target or that there is an intervening item, such as clothing, in which the soot and/or gunpowder has deposited

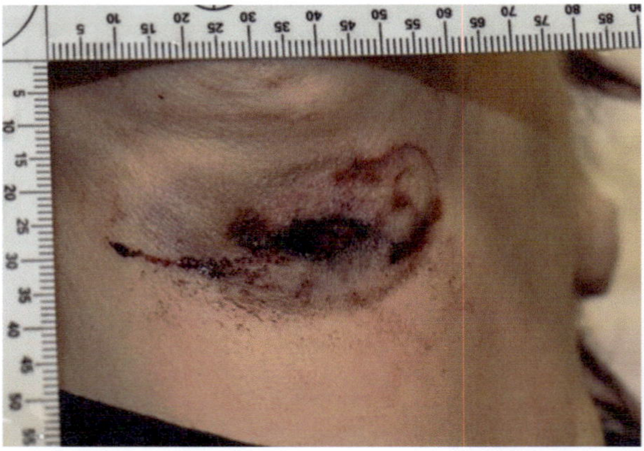

Fig. 10.14 Contact gunshot wound with an abraded muzzle impression and soot. (Courtesy: Dr. Tweedie. Department of Pathology and Laboratory Medicine, Schulich School of Medicine and Dentistry, Western University

Contact Range

In contact gunshot wounds, the muzzle of the gun is against the skin at the time of discharge. All of the material exiting the muzzle of the gun goes beneath the skin. The edges of the wound may be burnt and blackened due to the flame and the impregnation of the soot in this area of burning. The defect can have a circular or stellate appearance. In addition, there may be a patterned abrasion, with or without bruising, due to the muzzle. The stellate appearance and/or muzzle imprint can arise when the muzzle is pressed against skin and bone. This is due to the gas that emanates from the firearm's muzzle and collects between the elastic skin and bone. This gas rapidly expands the skin resulting in a stretching of the skin impacting the muzzle and/or causing stellate lacerations (Fig. 10.14).

Close Range

In close range, the muzzle is short distance away from the skin such that the bullet hole is surrounded by soot. Soot is wipeable. There are overlapping skin appearances between angled contact and close range that the determination between the

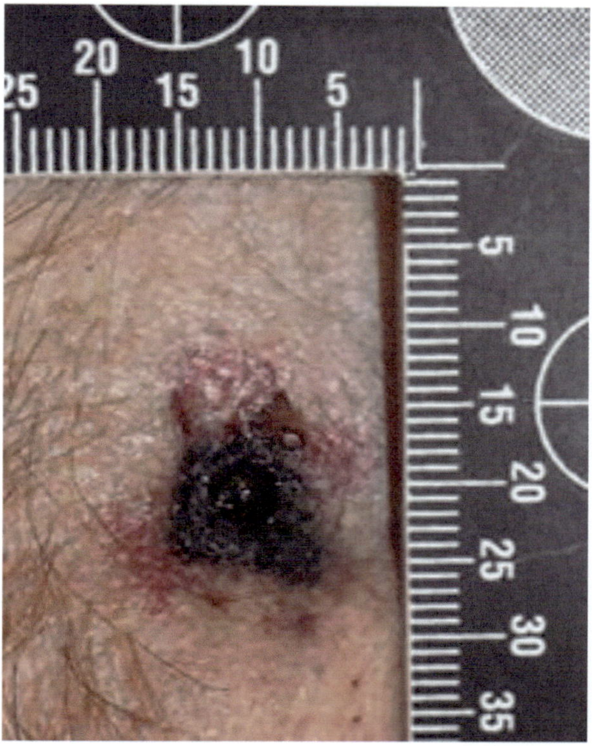

Fig. 10.15 Entry gunshot wound covered in soot

two can be determined by the internal examination. Externally they both have an eccentric soot deposition but in angled contact the bullet and soot in the same direction and angled near-contact, the bullet and soot are in different directions (Fig. 10.15).

Intermediate Range

Intermediate range occurs when the muzzle is held away from the body at a distance where the soot cannot reach the body but close enough that the gunpowder grains strike and abrade the skin. The pathognomonic finding for intermediate range is stippling or tattooing around the gunshot wound of entry. The stippling or tattooing is due to punctate abrasions that have a red to brown appearance due to powder grains and other materials. Unlike soot, stippling cannot be wiped away. The shapes and nature of gunpowder (i.e., disc powder, ball powder, cylindrical powder) are variable and therefore the range in which this observation can be identified is variable.

Indeterminate/Distance Range

Indeterminate and distance range have the same appearance in that the gunshot wound of entry does not exhibit the secondary effects (i.e., soot or stippling) on the skin. Distance range occurs when the distance between the muzzle and body is far enough away that the soot and powder grains do not reach the skin. Indeterminate occurs when there is a secondary object, such as a shirt, that prevents the soot and gun powder grains from depositing on the surface of the skin. Therefore, the distance between the muzzle and the body cannot be ascertained.

Pathological Range for Shotgun Wounds of Entry

The pathological range for shotgun wounds of entry is based on the spread of pellets and injuries related to the wad, if present. The spread of pellets that leave the muzzle determines the overall pattern size (Fig. 10.16). This spread is determined by the present of a choke. As the pellets travel at greater distances from the muzzle, the greater the spread of the pellets. Pellets may also collide with each other altering their individual kinetic energies and deforming their shapes. These intrinsic variables can result in variable penetration into the body [4] (Table 10.4).

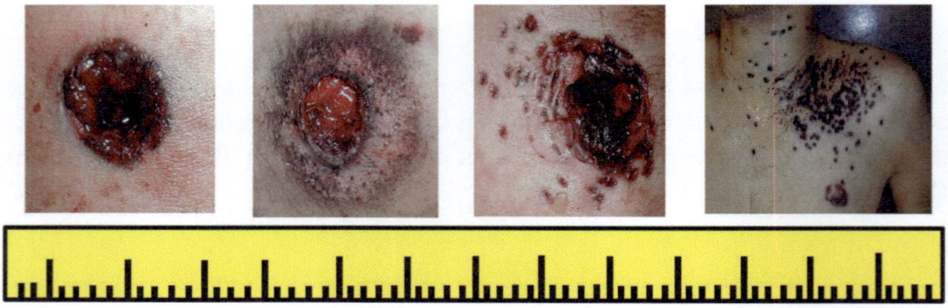

Fig. 10.16 Shotgun wounds of entry at increasing distances between muzzle and human. (Courtesy: Dr. Soledad Martínez, Servicio Médico Legal, Santiago, Chile)

Table 10.4 Pathological range of the entry shot gun wounds can be broadly divided into the four categories

1.	**Contact:** central hole with soot deposition and wad within body (unless fell out later)
2.	**Close:** scalloped hole. May have an abrasion from wad
3.	**Intermediate:** scalloped hole and satellite pellet holes and abrasions
4.	**Distance:** no central hole but individual pellet hole

Shotgun Wounds

Shotguns are a long firearm that fire multiple pellets down a barrel. The size of the pattern of discharged pellets depends on the degree of the choke on the barrel. Unlike gunshot wounds, shotgun wounds have a different type of ammunition that has wadding. A shotgun shell is composed of a plastic shot cup, which holds the pellets. Wadding is a barrier made out of plastic, felt or other materials, that separates the gunpowder from the pellets.

Pathological Range

Contact

The entry shotgun wounds have a circular appearance with blackened and seared margins. A muzzle abrasion may be present. The appearance of contact wounds to the head often has an explosive appearance with numerous associated lacerations due to the development of gas between the skull and scalp.

Close

The entry shotgun wound has a widened, scalloped margins due to the spread of pellets.

Indeterminate

The entry gunshot wound has a dominant hole with scalloped margins and satellite pellet shotgun wounds of entry. As the range increases, the number of surrounding satellite holes increase.

Distant

The entry gunshot wounds is composed entirely of satellite pellet shotgun wounds.

Injury Related to Wadding and Other Materials

In contact shotgun wounds, the wadding will be in the body (unless it falls out) but as the distance increases between the muzzle and body, this allows the wadding to open up due to the air resistance and to have the petals open up. These can cause a Maltese cross patterned abrasion on the body.

The finely granulated white plastic material in the shotgun shell can also cause punctate abrasions similar to powder tattooing.

Intermediate Wounds

The appearance of a shored exit mimics an entry gunshot wound due to the appearance of a ring abrasion. This occurs when the projectile leaves the body, it finds that there is an external object, such as clothing, flooring, wall, etc., that is against the gunshot wound of exit. As the skin is pushed out by the projectile, it slaps against the external object, causing an abrasion.

Graze Wound

A graze gunshot wound occurs when a bullet travels across the skin at a horizontal /parallel or nearly horizontal to surface of the skin resulting in an angled area of abrasion without perforating the skin. If the bullet is deep enough into the tissue, this can result in lacerations along the margins that point in the direction that the bullet was traveling.

Cylinder and Muzzle Gap

In revolvers, there is a gap area between the cylinder, which holds the ammunition, meets the barrel.

Multiple Gunshot Wounds

Multiple gunshot wounds can be a challenge for the forensic pathologist. In general, the number of entry gunshot wounds should equate to the sum of projectiles recovered from the body and exit gunshot wounds. However, there may be exceptions, such as there may be a larger number of exit wounds than entry wounds because of fragmentation of the projectile in the body, typically involving bones. Deviations from this equation can also be observed with keyhole lesions of the skull.

In general, the order of gunshot wounds cannot be determined with the exception of gunshot wounds to the head. Using Puppe's principle, a previous fracture line will terminate a subsequent intersecting fracture line.

Summary

Gunshot wounds have a variety of appearances depending on the type of firearm, ammunition, range, and intervening factors. Sometimes the pattern of injury can be puzzling because there are many exceptions to the rules.

References

1. Blakey L, et al. Fate and behaviour of gunshot residue—a review. J Forensic Sci. 2018;63(1):9–19. https://doi.org/10.1111/1556-4029.13555.
2. Vachon CR, Martinez MV. Understanding gunshot residue evidence and its role in forensic science. Am J Forensic Med Pathol. 2019;40:210–9.
3. Baptista MV, et al. Histopathological detection of entry and exit holes in human skin wounds caused by firearms. J Forensic Legal Med. 2014;25:49–52.
4. Cail K, Klatt E. The effect of intermediate clothing targets on shotgun ballistics. Am J Forensic Med Pathol. 2013, 34:348–51.

Chapter 11
Environmental Injuries

Rebekah Jacques

Temperature-Related Deaths

The average human body temperature is 37 °C with cyclical variations and normal variation ranges. The body temperature is regulated by feedback mechanisms that involve different parts fo the brain including the hypothalamus and brainstem. Heat is produced by the body from metabolism and can be gained or lost to the environment from four mechanisms: (1) **conduction:** direct heat loss from one object to another; (2) **radiation:** heat loss due to emission of infrared rays; (3) **evaporation:** heat loss from the evaporation of liquid such as sweating; (4) **convection:** the loss of heat from air currents on the body, such as wind. When there are environmental temperatures that exceed the body's ability to maintain homeostasis, when prolonged, can result in death. The determination of temperature-related deaths is largely based on scene and circumstances with autopsy findings serving as exclusionary information to rule out competing causes of death.

Hypothermia

Injury caused by cold temperatures is when heat loss exceeds the body's ability to maintain heat production from metabolism. A variety of environmental and individual factors may increase the risk of the development of hypothermia including environments that increase the rate of heat loss from the body such as air movements resulting in convection (Table 11.1). The extremes of age are also at risk for hypothermia. In older persons, there is sarcopenia (loss of skeletal muscle) and elder body

R. Jacques (✉)
London, Canada
e-mail: rebekah.jacques@lhsc.on.ca

R. Jacques (ed.), *Forensic Pathology*,
https://doi.org/10.1007/978-3-031-42038-2_11

Table 11.1 Risk factors for the development of hypothermia

1.	Environment with a low temperature, damp/wet, and windy
2.	Water immersion
3.	Extremes of age
4.	Undernourished
5.	Hypothyroidism
6.	Inadequate clothing and indoor heating
7.	Dementia
8.	Ethanol or other drug use

habitus leads to lower heat production and less insulating subcutaneous fat, respectively. The surface area to mass ratio in infants results in a more rapid heat loss. Undernourished individuals that have low insulating fat stores are at risk of more rapid heat loss. Individuals with dementia can develop wandering behaviors that led them going outside, often inadequately dressed. Ethanol use is an independent risk factor for hypothermia because there is associated impaired judgment, the protective shivering response is impaired, and the effects of vasodilation promote heat loss.

There are no pathognomonic findings for hypothermia at autopsy. Indicators of hypothermia include clinical, scene, and pathological findings. Clinically hypothermia is only a few degrees below the average temperature of the human body and is defined as a core body temperature <35 °C. The person may present with a decreased respiratory rate, decreased heart rate, and decreased consciousness. At the scene, there may be evidence of two behaviors:

1. 'Hide and Die' syndrome:
   (a) This behavioral phenomenon in which the individual is discovered in a location that gives them the impression that they are trying to hide. The decedent may be found in a closet, under a bed or dresser for example. This can also appear burrowing into the ground (Fig. 11.1). Burrowing may result in abrasions and bruises involving the face, hands, and knees (Fig. 11.2).
2. Paradoxical Undressing:
   (a) This behavioral phenomenon occurs in individuals effected by hypothermia who begin removing their clothing. It is thought to be a manifestation of the disruption of the function of the hypothalamus. At the scene, the decedent may be partly, or completely, undressed with clothing strewn about (Fig. 11.3).

Autopsy findings thay may be observed include:

1. Pink-brown areas of discoloration over the extensor surfaces of larger joints such as the knees, elbow, and outer sides of the hips (Fig. 11.4). It can sometimes be observed on the face. The exact reason is unknown.
2. Hemorrhagic gastropathy, often referred to as Wishnewsky spots,: foci of black hemorrhage of the mucosal surface of the stomach (Fig. 11.5).
3. Acute pancreatitis may be hemorrhagic. Histology is needed to differentiate from autolysis, which is more commonly observed postmortem that hemorrhagic pancreatitis.
4. If the hypothermia has been prolonged, areas of frost bite may be observed predominantly of the fingers, toes, nose, and ears.

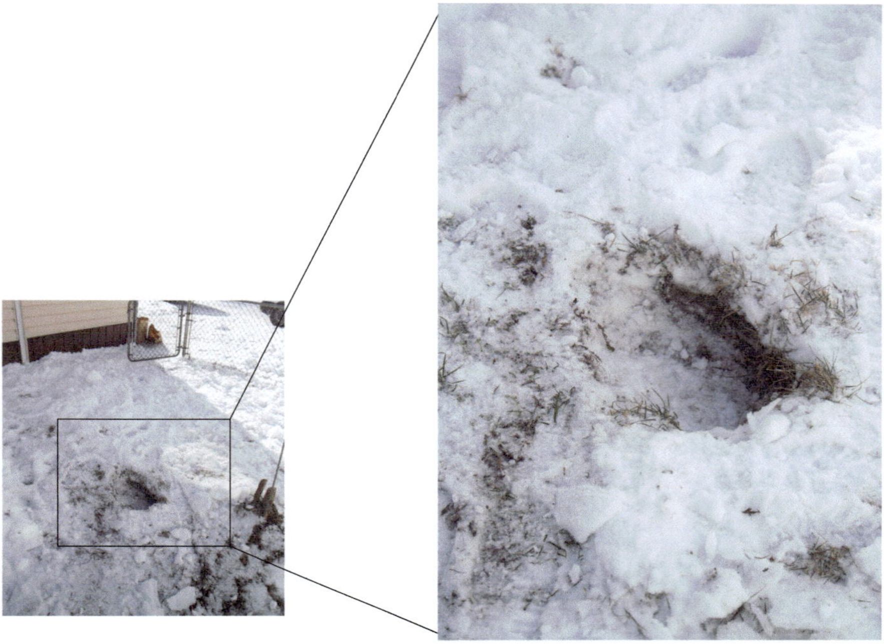

Fig. 11.1 The snow has been dug away by hands as a behavioral change of hypothermia—'hide and die' syndrome. The inset is a closer view of the burrowing

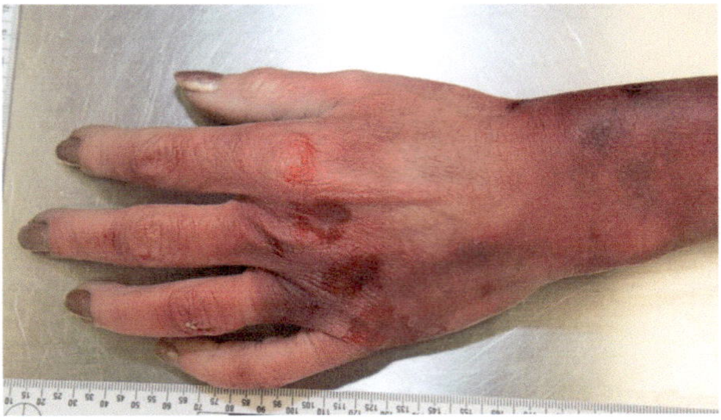

Fig. 11.2 Abrasions of the back of the fingers and hands may be observed at autopsy from attempts at burrowing in 'hide or die, syndrome

Hyperthermia

Hyperthermia arises when the body is unable to compensate for the environmental heat. There is non-environmental hyperthermia, predominantly related to malignant hyperthermia due to genetic vulnerability to anesthetic medicines and drug-induced fever are not described here. Clinically, hyperthermia is defined as a core body temperature ≥40.5 °C. Clinically, persons with hyperthermia may present with a high body temperature, dry skin, nausea, vomiting, dyspnea, and impaired

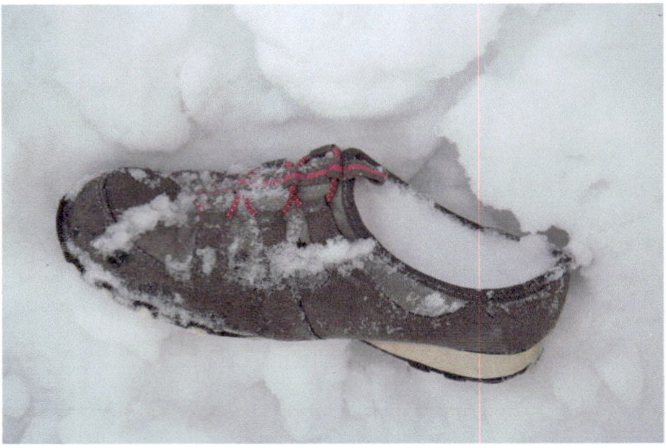

Fig. 11.3 Paradoxical undressing with clothing strewn about at the death scene

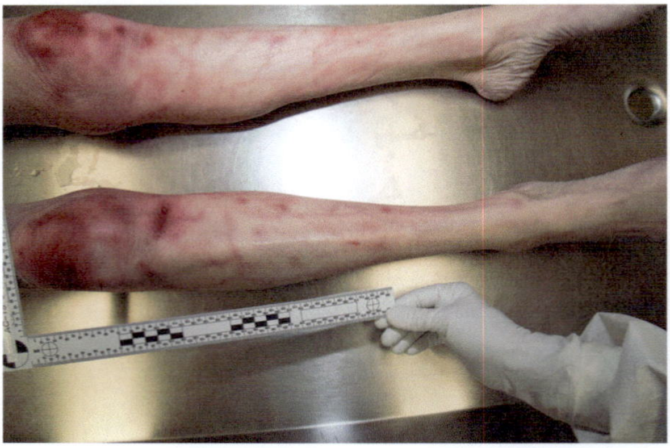

Fig. 11.4 Cold 'erythema' around the larger joints may be observed in hypothermia

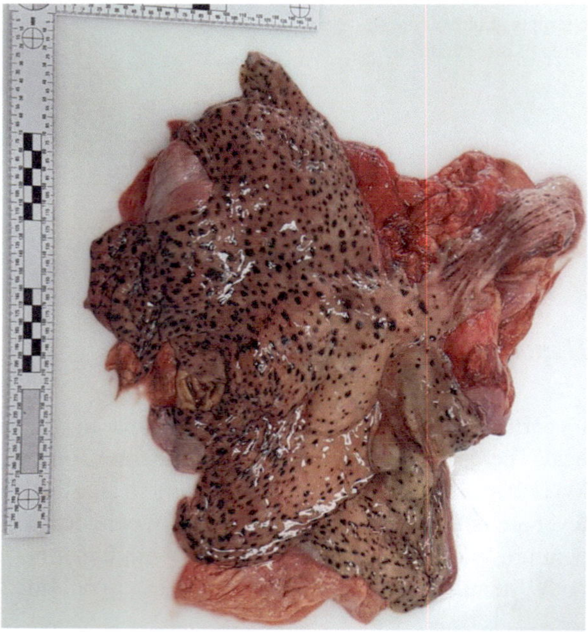

Fig. 11.5 In hypothermia, black hemmorrhagic foci (hemorrhagic gastropathy) may be observed on the mucosal (inner) surface of the stomach

consciousness. At autopsy, the body may still feel warm and have rapid decomposition but the determination relies on warm environment and exclusionary findings at autopsy.

Burns and Fire-Related Deaths

Burns can occur postmortem or antemortem. Burns occur when a heat source comes into contact with the body at a high temperature or a low temperature for a sustained period of time. Common sources of heat include (1) fire/flame, (2) hot liquid/steam, (3) hot objects, (4) electricity, (5) chemical agents. Mortality tends to increase in relation to older adults, area involved, depth, and inhalational injuries. The location, temperature, and duration contribute to the severity of the burn.

Burns are a consequence of elevated temperature in tissue over a threshold value for a period of time. The extent of injury is dependent on both the temperature and duration of exposure. This relationship between temperature of the injurious agent and exposure duration is referred to as the time–temperature relationship [1]. Thermal damage occurs in the skin and most cell types once the temperature reaches approximately 43 °C [1].

Bodies that are recovered from fires may have burns, some of which can be extensive. It is the pathologist's role to determine if the decedent died from the fire or something else (Fig. 11.6). The presence of soot in the airway, in addition to

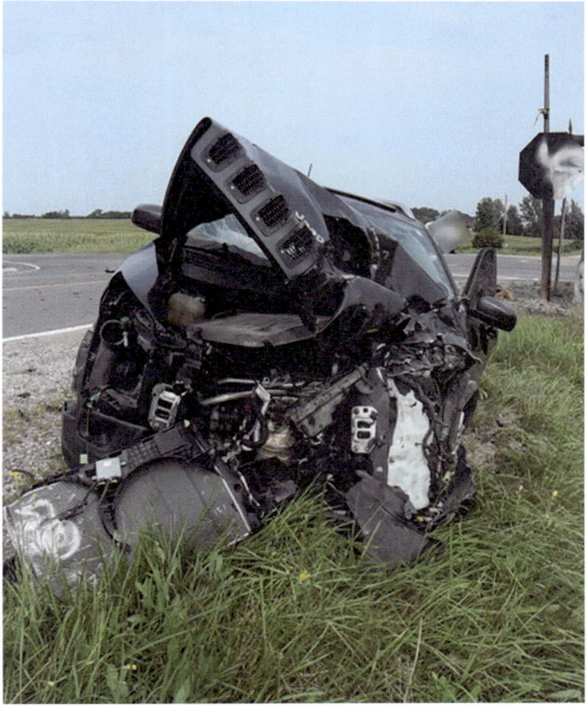

Fig. 11.6 Scene images may show extensive thermal damage. Smoke inhalation is necessary to consider as a competing cause of death to blunt impact trauma in a motor vehicle collision

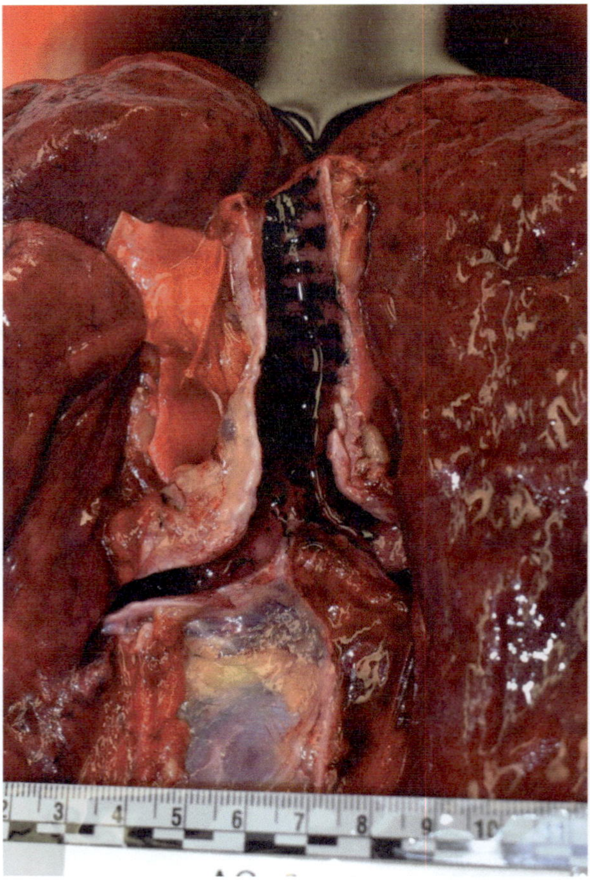

Fig. 11.7 The airway has evidence of smoke inhalation in form of black soot deposited on the trachea and bilateral principal bronchi

elevated levels of carboxyhemoglobin saturation, are supportive that an individual died from a fire (Fig. 11.7). An indicator of fatal level of carboxyhemoglobin saturation may be observed as 'cherry-red' blood and lividity.

Body Surface Area

Burns are quantified using the body surface area, wherein 1% of the body surface is based on the size of the decedent's palm. In addition, the percentage of body surface differs between children and adults. Burn severity is related to the burn depth and the total body surface area but even small burns can become life threatening.

Table 11.2 Summary of burn types based on depth. Severity of burn depends on the temperature and duration of contact. Note: These observations are made on clinical signs. They may be used on decedents; however, the findings do not always correlate with regard to vitality [2].

Types of burn	Description
Superficial	Burn that involves the epidermal layer. Red skin with blanching, dry. There is minimal structural damage, therefore no bullae/blisters (cavities filled with fluid) form. Also referred as a first-degree burn. Example: Minor flash burn, sunburn
Partial thickness	Burn that involves the epidermis and dermis. Structural damage to the dermoepidermal junction results in the formation of bullae/blisters. These are further subdivided in superficial: moist and elastic and will blanch with pressure +/– edema. Deep: more dry & do not blanch with pressure. Also referred to as second degree
Full thickness	Involve the epidermis and dermis. Appear as white and waxy or even charred. Nerve innervation is destroyed so will not be painful
Fourth degree	Burns extend beyond the skin and extend into the muscles & bones.

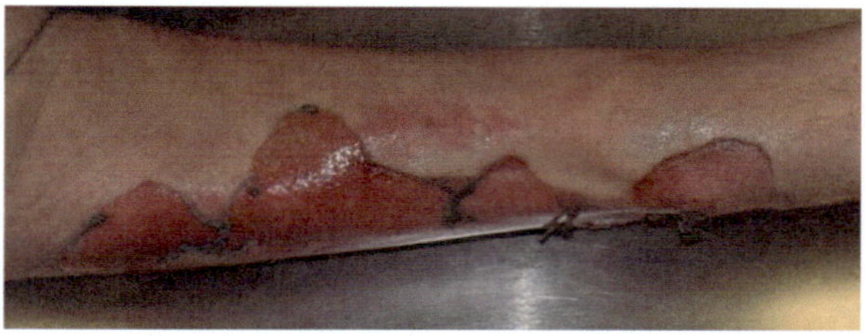

Fig. 11.8 Superficial thickness burns of the left lateral thigh and calf

Depth of Burn

Burns can be classified as partial and full thickness (Table 11.2). A partial burn includes first to second degree. A first-degree burn involves the epidermis of the skin only, such as a sunburn. The skin appears pink to red, lacks blisters, and is dry. Nerve endings are intact and can be painful. These burns heal without scarring. A superficial second-degree burn involves the papillary dermis and therefore results in blisters and thus appears wet (Fig. 11.8). Healing can occur but may be associated with scarring. A third-degree involves the reticular dermis and appears yellow or white. The burn is dry. Healing occurs with scarring. A full thickness burn involves the bone. Charring is typically present. Note that these observations are made on clinical signs. They may be used on decedents; however, the findings do not always correlate with regard to vitality [2]. Clinically, fourth degree burns can be observed in decedents but this is because they usually arise in postmortem period. A red margin may be observed around lesser degree burns but this is not indicative of a burn that arose in the antemortem period. Histologically, this reddened margin can be difficult to detect [2]. However, the presence of leukocyte infiltration and fibrin may indicate an antemortem period in which the burns arose.

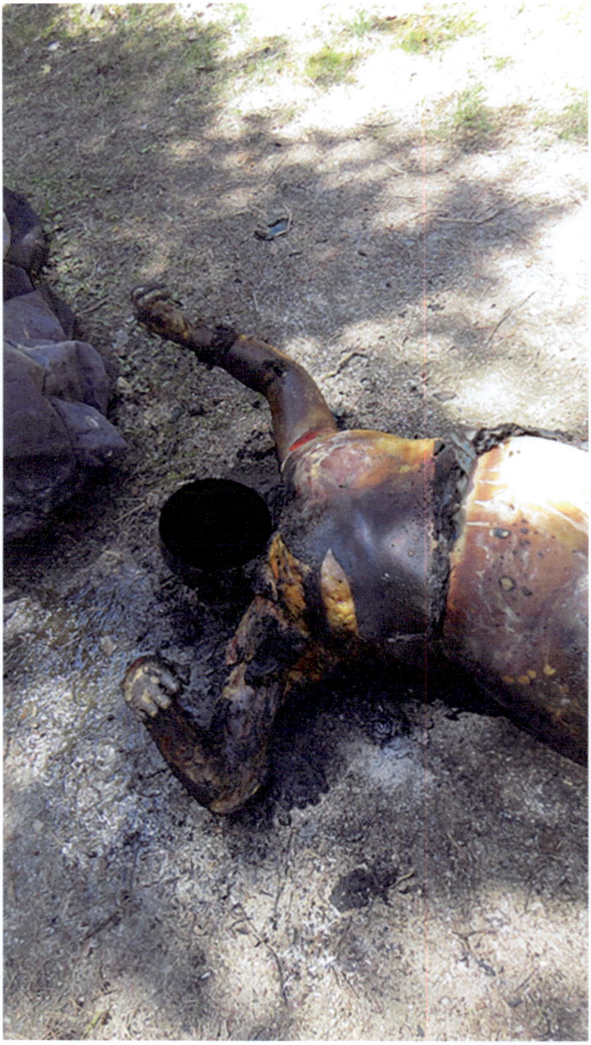

Fig. 11.9 Extensive thermal changes can result in pugilistic posturing and skin splitting. The skin splitting can be observed with the exposure of the yellow underlying fat

Artifacts

Burns are associated with therapeutic and postmortem artifacts. Therapeutic artifacts such as fasciotomies and escharotomies to avoid compartment syndrome appear as deep sharp force trauma. These a medical and sirgical interventions to prevent the development of compartment syndrome. Since muscle bundles are encapsulated in epimysium and perimysium, severe edema response to burns will result in local interstitial hydrostatic pressure resulting in poor perfusion, referred to as compartment syndrome, and lead to muscle necrosis. Fasciotomies and escharotomies can improve perfusion. Postmortem artifacts include (Fig. 11.9):

1. Epidural "heat" hematoma. These occur at the top of the head in the epidural space. Thought to be due to diploe vessels of the skull. Different than antemortem epidural hemorrhage due to its location, which is the lateral head/temporal bone fractures due to the proximity of the middle meningeal arteries at the side of the head
2. Skin splitting
3. Fractures/amputations: No hemorrhage in the area indicates a postmortem thermal change.
4. Embedded metals from structure that was on fire can be from the structure of the residence. Care should be made to ensure that bullets or other fragments of weapons are not represented.
5. "pugilistic posturing": This is to describe the flexion that occurs at the elbows, hips, and knees due to the greater bulk of the flexor muscles around these joints.

Flash burns: The depth of the burn is often proportional to the quantity and type of fuel that explodes [3].

Flame burns: The depth of the burn is typically deep in the dermis. These are often associated with inhalational injuries.

Scalds: Scald is a contact burn with a liquid. The depth of the scald injury depends on the temperature of the liquid, the thickness of the skin, thermal capacity of the liquid, and duration of contact [3, 4]. For example, water at 60 °C in 3 s will cause the simaliar burn in 1 s at 69 °C. Scalds tend to be superficial burns [5]. Child abuse/elder abuse: sparing of skin folds, immersion scalds can give a "doughnut sign" where there is an area of spared skin surrounded by burnt skin. The spared tissue due to direct contact with bottom of the bathtub may also protect the tissue in contact with the bathtub from the water.

Children and older adults have a higher incidence of scalds. In the pediatric population, boys under 2 years of age are susceptible due to increased engagement in their environment and limited motor development to avoid injury [4]. In the geriatric population, their limited mobility to avoid and escape danger puts this cohort at risk of scalds and other burns [6].

Contact burns: Can occur with heated solids such as hot metals, plastics, glass, or hot coals. The object is either extremely hot or there was a prolonged period of contact with the object, such as a heating pad. The latter can be seen in individuals with loss of consciousness (i.e., substance or alcohol use, epilepsy, cerebrovascular accident). These tend to be deep dermal or full thickness burns [5].

Chemical burns: These are burns due to chemicals, most commonly strong alkalis or acids, that damage the skin on contact. The most common chemicals are typically household products such as toilet bowl cleaners, drain cleaners, oven cleaners, detergents, and bleaches. In addition, the lime mineral in cement is an alkali. These substances often include hydrochloric acid, phosphoric acid, sulfuric acid, hydrofluoric acid, sodium hydroxide, and potassium hydroxide. Acid burns tend to create an impermeable "tan" of the skin, which limits further penetration [3]. Chemical burns can cause redness and may appear similar to rash or skin infection, blistering, skin peeling, and edema or can appear darkened due to a hard, dry eschar

[7]. Chemicals cause direct cell injury through a variety of mechanisms including oxidation, reduction, denaturation, and dehydration [7]. Chemical burns are exothermic reaction, thereby releasing energy as heat, which adds a thermal component to the chemical injury [7]. Contact time with a chemical burn is typically longer than a thermal injury because exposure to the chemical is ongoing. The most common categories of chemical burns are alkali and acids. Alkali burns tend to combine with lipids in the body and create soap, which continues to "dissolve" the tissues until neutralized [3]. Therefore alkalis tend to penetrate deeper and cause burns more extensive than acid burns. This causes a coagulative type necrosis in acids and liquefactive necrosis with alkali substances [7].

These substances may also be ingested resulting in chemical burns of the mucosa of the mouth, upper airway, and upper gastrointestinal tract.

Mechanism of Injury

At the cellular level, heat causes protein denaturation of proteins and loss of integrity of plasma membranes [3]. Tissue loss is primarily due to protein denaturation and secondary due to inflammatory mediators, oxidant, and proteases [3]. Following the application of heat, there are three zones of injury [3]:

- **Zone of coagulation:** Center of the wound, irreversible tissue loss and necrosis due to coagulation of proteins
- **Zone of stasis:** Decreased tissue perfusion, mixture of viable and nonviable cells, capillary vasoconstriction, and ischemia. This zone may convert to necrosis due to hypoperfusion, desiccation, edema, and infection

  Zone of hyperemia: Viable cells, vasodilation

Mechanisms of Death

The systemic response of burns in those that initially survive the burn results in a release of cytokines and other inflammatory mediators once the burn reaches a 30% body surface area [5].

1. Fatal dysrhythmia: Capillary permeability is increased resulting in shift of intravascular proteins and fluids to the interstitium. These changes, in addition to fluid loss, lead to peripheral and splanchnic vasoconstriction, and decreased myocardial contractility. This can result in hypotension (low blood pressure) and end organ perfusion.
2. Rhabdomyolysis: Due to massive skeletal muscle tissue necrosis. This can lead to acidosis or myoglobinuria. The myoglobinuria is the accumulation of muscle cells that can also cause renal (kidney) failure.

The next mechanisms are due to loss of the normal skin barrier

1. Infection: Non-specific down regulation of the immune response
2. Hypothermia
3. Hypernatremia
4. Fluid loss: The injury disrupts osmotic and hydrostatic gradients leading to edema and large fluid shifts. Systemically, this results in hemodynamic changes.

Electrocution

Electricity is the flow of electrons across a potential gradient from high to low concentration, typically along a conductor. This difference in potential difference is expressed in voltage (V), which represents the force driving the electrons. The quantity of electrons flowing along this gradient is the current and is measured in amperes (I). The impedance to flow is resistance. The voltage is the unit of force that causes current to flow along a conductor. Voltage is not the sole determinant of injury and death. Fatalities can occur as low as 25 volts [8], and lighting strikes have a high survival rate [9]. The better electrical metric that best describes the ability to cause burns is *power*. Electrical resistance is the quantity of force that opposes the flow of electrical current and is rarely known. However, the skin of adult hand has a resistance of approximately 5000 ohms [8]. This can decrease or increase depending on if the hands are callused or wet. Resistance is an important factor as electricity takes the path of least resistance, and thermal energy is generated when there is greater resistance and is indicative of damage. Different tissue types have different resistance levels, from most to least resistant: bone, fat, tendon, skin, muscle, blood, and nerves [8]. Once the current is beyond the skin, it will find the path of least resistance until it comes to a grounding source. Electrical current in tissues is carried by mobile ions in the extracellular and intracellular fluids, which are highly electrolytic. Within the body, the current carriers change from electrons to ions. This conversion occurs at the surface of the skin through electrochemical reactions [10] of the human body. This current passes from a high potential to a lower potential. The charge in metals is carried by the electrons. The conversion from electrons to mobile ions occurs at the skin surface [9]. Skin is a complex electrical conductor as its resistance depends on the surface hydration [11]. The epidermis has electrical insulator with a high resistivity. High versus low voltage is arbitrarily divided at 1000 V but is often the only variable known with certainty. At low voltages, the sweat glands from the dermis carry the current from the stratum corneum, thereby bypassing the high resistivity of the epidermis [12, 13]. The stratum corneum can be overcome at about 500–600 V but hydration reduces this resistance and the dry stratum corneum is relevant of household voltage (120 or 220 V) [14, 15]. Tissues with higher water content, such as large arteries, nerves, and muscles have low resistance. Resistance is a property of the overall current, while tissue resistivity is a property of a tissue. Tissue resistivities is a property of the tissue, regardless of size. But are defined as the resistance of a centimeter cube of skin and electrodes attached to opposite sides. Tissues in the body have a wide range of resistivities, with the epidermis having the highest resistivity. Blood is the best electrical conductor in the body but given the central location in the body has little clinical relevance as the muscle and dermis carry the current. Bone is the best electrical insulator. Part of the reason for high resistivity of cortical bone and epidermis, compared to other tissues, is due to the lower free-water content. The cell membrane function is an ionic-transport barrier, therefore low frequency currents are shielded. At low electrical frequencies, the plasma membrane appears to determine a diffusion barrier against free ion exchange due to the tightly regulated ion pumps, including the electrochemical potential across the cell membrane [9]. At higher frequencies, the cell membrane is no longer an effective barrier to passage of current, resulting in capacitive coupling across the membrane transferring the current into the cytoplasm [10]. The cell may continue to maintain transmembrane ionic concentrations via adenosine triphosphate (ATP) pumps, which can lead to exhaustion of metabolic energy [10]. The current disrupts these membrane potentials by overcoming the barrier of the plasma membrane and moving ions. The damage includes heat-mediated damage, cell membrane electroporation, electrochemical interactions at the contact points, and blunt impact trauma [9]. Electrical damage to tissues may not be visible on the external and internal examination.

The electric current travels through the body from an entry point to an exit point. The tissues along the path can be damaged. On the skin, a typical electrical or joule burn is typically a well demarcated lesion with a central area with various degrees of thermal injury and sometimes a reddened peripheral margin. As electricity travels through the body, there is resistance of dry skin that permits the electrical energy to convert to heat that is directly proportional to both the current and electrical resistance. The quantity of heat generated and therefore thermal injury to tissue are equivalent to $0.24 \times (\text{Voltage})^2 \times \text{Resistance}$ [5]. Therefore, voltage is the main driver of thermal injury to tissues, and injuries can be classified based on voltage including low voltage and high voltage. [5]. Low voltage injuries (<400 volts) usually do not cause damage beyond a small deep thermal burn at the contact site and can include domestic (i.e. household) current but they can still be fatal by causing cardiac arrhythmias especially due to the alternating nature of the current [3]. High voltage injuries can result in thermal burns, cardiac dysthymias, high tension injuries, and flash injuries. High tension injuries tend to occur a 1 kV or greater and can result extensive tissue damage and limb loss [5]. Low voltage is considered below 1000 volts, but is an arbitrary distinction between high voltage [8].

Rhabdomyolysis and renal failure can also arise in electrocutions due to muscle damage. Muscle necrosis may occur adjacent to bone due to its high resistance [3]. In addition, smaller body parts, such as digits, hands, and limbs may be destroyed, while the trunk remains largely intact. This difference is because smaller body parts have less dissipation of electricity and generate more intense heat than the torso [3].

The exception being, if the entrance or exit is on the chest or abdomen. Voltage greater than 70,000 V is often fatal [3, 5]. Flash injury arises when there is a tangential presence of the body adjacent to a high tension voltage arc. This results in superficial flash burns of exposed body but also clothing can catch fire. No electrical current enters the body.

The diagnosis of fatal electrocution is based on the history and pathological findings. When electrical burns are challenging to determine because the burn may be small or have variable appearances, examination of the burn site should be assessed for metal deposition with scanning electon microscope (SEM). Heat generated in electrocution may cause atomization of metallic electric cable resulting in deposition of minute metal particles from the conducting surface [16]. Additionally, special stains such as Perls Prussian Blue and p-dimethylaminobenzylidene-rhodanine) for iron and copper may enhance diagnostic accuracy [17].

Lightning-related deaths are a special form of natural electrocution source. There are five electrical mechanisms of lightning injury:

1. **Direct strike:** Lightning directly hits individual
2. **Contact:** Lightning strikes an object, such as a metal pole, that the individual is touching
3. **Side flash:** Current extends from a nearby object or another person to the decedent
4. **Ground current:** Lightning strikes the ground and passes from the strike point to the decedent
5. **Blunt force trauma/blast injury:** Decedent is thrown from the blast (thunder)

Lightning strikes are considered to have a high survival rate [9]. The mortality rate ranges from 10–30% [18]. Lightning is a natural form of high voltage electricity. Indicators of a death from lightning can include an outdoor location, cluster/herd of animals that have died, and cutaneous injury pattern on the body. The rapid electrical discharge usually leaves just superficial burns, significant heat generation is not generated because of the rapid discharge; however, there are exceptions [9]. The Lichtenberg pattern is a fern-like pattern of burn injury that is usually confined to the outer layers of skin [10]. The cutaneous manifestation of lightning include [18]:

1. Linear burns: Linear burns occur preferentially in high sweat concentration, under the breasts, arms, & middle of chest. Thought to be due to vaporization of water on the skin's surface.
2. Punctate burns: Multiple, small, closely spaced discoid burns. Includes the "tip-toe sign," which are smaller discoid burns on the tips of toes and sides of soles of feet
3. "Feathering": Includes Lichtenburg figure that is a fern-like, branching, arborizing, serpiginous or fractal extravasation of blood into the subcutaneous tissues
4. Thermal: Occurs if the person is wearing a metal object or clothing ignites

Handheld Conducted Electrical Weapon

Although not considered an environmental injury, handheld conducted electrical weapon is included here for completion. The most common form of handheld conducted electrical weapon (CEW) that a forensic pathologist may be involved in is the TASER but there is a wide array of CEW that includes stun guns, electronic control devices, etc. The TASER is an acronym for Thomas A. Swift's Electric Rifle. TASER is a projectile CEW. Since projectile CEW is a method of force use by law enforcement community, forensic pathologists may be engaged in this type of weapon. Most projectile CEWs deploy two barbed probes or darts. These probes are commonly metal and have a piercing mechanism usually do to a sharpened tip and a latching mechanism, usually a backward-facing barb, to ensure probe remains embedded in the target. They are usually tethered to the source of the electrical current in the device by wires. The probe will call a puncture wound into the skin. Projectile CEWs have two darts that need to enter the individual in order to complete the electrical circuit. The distance between the two darts, or their impact sites, are important to measure as the distance between the two can indicate how far the probes have traveled prior to impact. The spread of the probes becomes greater as the distance from the deployment position to the decedent also increase. In some respects, the distance serves as the pathological range. The length of the probes is variable depending on the expected wardrobe in varying climates to ensure better success. The tissues affected depend on the anatomical location because the current travels down the low resistivity of the metal barbs, there is little thermal damage. The puncture wound may be associated with abrasion and bruising due to cylinder that is attached to the barbed probe. Once the dart is embedded, the pulsating electrical current activates all the muscle fibers in the circuit, thereby overriding voluntary movement. Some of the newer models that law enforcement use also discharges 20–30 small serialized confetti to match the CEW cartridge to the registered owner. This is useful to determine which officer fired which CEW. Most CEW deliver an average of 600 V pulse [19] but delivers only about 2 W of power.

Summary

The commonly considered environmental injuries include temperature-related deaths, burns, and electrocution were explored in this chapter. Temperature-related deaths such as hypothermia and hyperthermia rely on the history, and the autopsy serves as to assess for competing causes of death. Essentially, temperature-related deaths are a diagnosis of exclusion. Burns and electrocutions typically have cutaneous findings to support the cause of death.

References

1. Martin NA, Falder S. A review of the evidence for threshold of burn injury. Burns. 2017;43:1624–39.
2. Bohnert M, Pollak S. Heat-mediated changes to the hands and feet mimicking washerwoman's skin. Int J Legal Med. 2003;117(2):102–5.
3. Keck M, et al. Pathophysiology of burns. Wiener Medizinishe Wochenschrift. 2009;159(13-14):327–36.
4. Lau EYK, et al. Importance of clothing removal in scalds. Hong Kong Med J. 2016;22:152–7.
5. Hettiarach S, Dziewulski P. ABC of burns: pathophysiology and types of burns. BMJ. 2004;328:1427–9.
6. Abu-Sittah GS, et al. Management of burns in the elderly. Annals of burns and fire disasters. 2016;XXIX(4):249–54.
7. Yin S. Chemical and common burns in children. Clin Pediatr. 2017;56(55):8S–12S.
8. Duff K, McCaffrey RJ. Electrical and lightning injury: a review of mechanisms and neuropsychological, psychiatric and neurological sequelae. Neuropscyhol Rev. 2001;11(2):101–16.
9. Bier M, et al. Biophysical injury mechanisms associated with lightning injury. NeuroRehabilitation. 2005;20:53–62.
10. Lee RC, et al. Biophysical Injury mechanisms in electrical shock trauma. Annu Rev Biomed. 2000;02:477–509.
11. Panescu D, Cohen KP, Webster JG, Stratbucker RA. The mosaic electrical characteristics of the skin. IEEE Trans Biomed Eng. 1993;40(5):434–9.
12. Grimnes S. Pathways of ionic flow through human skin in vivo. Acta Derm Venereol. 1984;64(2):93–8.
13. Yamamoto T, et al. Measurement of low-resistance points on the skin by dry roller electrodes. IEEE Trans Biomed Eng. 1988;35(3):203–9.
14. Grimnes S. Dielectric breakdown of human skin in vivo. Med Biol Eng Comput. 1983;21(3):379–81.
15. Blank IH, Finesinger JE. Electrical resistance of the skin; effect of size of electrodes, exercise and cutaneous hydration. Arch Neurol Psychiatry. 1946;56(5):544–57.
16. Nagesh KR, et al. Arcing injuries in a fatal electrocution. Am J Forensic Med Pathol. 2009;30:183–5.
17. Jacobsen H. Electrically induced deposition of metal on the human skin. Forensic Sci Int. 1997;90:85–92.
18. Ritenour AE, et al. Lightning injury: a review. BURNS. 2008;34:585–94.
19. Dawes, et al. Electrical characteristics of an electronic control device under a physiologic load: a brief report. Pacing Clin Electrophysiol. 2010;33(3):330–6.

Chapter 12
The Negative Medicolegal Autopsy

Rebekah Jacques

Concept of the Negative Autopsy

An autopsy is negative if all of the steps of the autopsy fail to demonstrate a cause of death. All of the steps of the autopsy need to be performed to satisfy that a complete postmortem examination has been performed and potential causes of death can be explored and ruled out. This may mean that pathological and historical findings are present but the autopsy is "negative" from a cause and mechanism of death perspective. Essentially, the cause of death is undetermined or unascertained. The negative medicolegal differs from the "false negative" autopsy or the "defective" autopsy. The false negative autopsy arises when the cause of death is actual ascertainable but an essential piece of information was missing from the autopsy. This can include an inadequate history, lapse in external examination, inadequate internal examination, and lack of toxicological analysis. In addition, a lack of training can contribute to a missed cause of death [1].

The incidence of the negative medicolegal autopsy varies. The standard forensic pathology textbooks report an incidence of 5–10% rate of all autopsies [2]. Published articles from large medical centers and forensic pathology departments range from 23.44 to 1.45% [1, 3–8]. There are multiple factors that explain this variation (Table 12.1). The *quality of the death investigation system* is an important factor because this will dictate the types of deaths that will fall under the jurisdiction for a medicolegal autopsy, access to resources to obtain accurate historical and circumstantial information, and training of those participants in the death investigation system. Related to the death investigation system is the *available resources* for the pathologist to perform ancillary investigations and access to scientific articles.

R. Jacques (✉)
London Health Sciences Centre, University Hospital, London, ON, Canada
e-mail: rebekah.jacques@lhsc.on.ca

R. Jacques (ed.), *Forensic Pathology*,
https://doi.org/10.1007/978-3-031-42038-2_12

Table 12.1 Major factors in the incidence of the negative medicolegal autopsy

• Quality of death investigation system
• Pathologist
– Experience
– Training
• Features of the case:
– In-hospital
– Out of hospital
– Donation status (rare)
– Prolonged hospital death
• Completeness of the dissections: consider special dissections
• Available resources
• Postmortem changes
– Decomposition
– Taphonomy
• Features of the decedent:
– Age
– Biological sex

Table 12.2 Ancillary investigations to consider, when appropriate

• Histology:
– Broaden histological assessment of organs
Toxicology:
– Consider vitreous fluid, liver sample, stomach contents when blood is unavailable
• Vitreous biochemistry
• Microbiology & virology studies
• Metabolic studies
• Genetic testing: Collect tissue/blood for DNA
• Radiology
• Consider specialized consultation: Heart, brain
• Ultrastructural studies
• IgE/Tryptase
• Sickle cell disease/trait
• Urine myoglobin

Some types of deaths can only be determined with extensive histological sampling of tissues and organs and specialized high-quality laboratory tests (Table 12.2).

The experience of a pathologist competent in medicolegal autopsies plays a role. It is said that experienced pathologists have a higher rate of negative conclusions compared to their junior colleagues [2]. Reportedly, less experienced pathologists interpret that failing to provide a cause of death reflects upon their ability or are afraid of being viewed as incompetent [2]. Inversely correlated with the incidence of the negative autopsy is experience such that as pathologists reportedly become less inhibited in their admission of ignorance [2]. Further, less experienced pathologists may expect that if extensive effort has been placed to determine the cause of death than this should correlate into a positive outcome.

The characteristics of the decedent have reported to play a role, primarily age and biological sex. The age of the decedent is inversely correlated with age. Although all age-groups have representation of a negative medicolegal autopsy, infants are an overrepresented cohort. In addition, compared to older adults, teenagers and young adults have a higher proportion of negative autopsies. The young adult does not typically have the, almost universal, overlay of degenerative cardiovascular disease that is seen in the older group that live in the Western hemisphere. Thus, it is probable that the same occult disease process (i.e. channelopathies) occurs in that older group as it does among the young population, but the latter do not have a convenient overlay of degenerative disease, which are inevitably found in older adults. Consequently, rare occult disease processes are not sought after when there is a readily identifiable cause of death. In a handful of reported studies, the total number of negative autopsies was higher among males [7, 8]. These sex differences were attributed to a lower autopsy rate for females, possibly due to religious or cultural reasons. In addition, more males were discovered in external environments, compared to females, leading to a larger role for decomposition and taphonomy. This leads to another factor, *case type*, in terms of the postmortem state of the human remains. There is a higher incidence of negative medicolegal autopsies in decomposed and skeletal remains compared to bodies without those changes. These postmortem changes result in a higher incidence of negative medicolegal autopsies because the presence of decomposition indicates a number of observations, wherein data obtained at each step of the autopsy is affected. The data that may be obtained in the first step of the autopsy may not be available because there was nobody present to witness the death and family or friends may not be available to provide information about the decedent. The external and internal findings may be obscured or lost including the loss of organs and tissues from decomposition. Ancillary investigations are hindered because blood and vitreous fluid may not be available to undergo toxicological and biochemical analysis, respectively. In summary, the pathologist has incomplete data set. In addition, the completeness of the autopsy can affect the incidence of negative medicolegal autopsies. In order to have a cause of death, based on history requires relevant negative autopsy findings, which are often not available due to decomposition. Completeness of the autopsy may also relate to the exten of dissections depending on the context. A typical example is a body discovered at the end of the stairs. If anatomical cause of death is not discovered following examination of the major bodies cavities, head, anterior neck, chest, abdomen, and pelvis than consideration of a posterior neck dissection to examine for ligamentous injuries and fractures may be warranted.

Pathologists' Framework

Death is a functional event, not an anatomical one. Therefore, a structural or anatomical cause of death cannot always be the standard to explain death. There are two frameworks a pathologist may use to help them to arrive at a cause of death, these include:

1. Classification of pathological and historical/circumstantial evidence.
2. Step-wise approach to the autopsy & hypothesis testing.

Classification of cause of death was initially outlined in Spitz & Fisher's Medicolegal Investigation of Death [9] as they consider the continuum of types or classes of evidence found during a postmortem examination. This continuum of evidence can be divided into 5 classes that reflect the certainty related to the cause of death based on the pathological and historical/circumstantial evidence [10] (Fig. 12.1). Class 5 is the negative medicolegal autopsy, which represents the minority of cases.

Class 1: *Definitively* fatal acute or perimortem pathological finding(s):

Definitely fatal acute or perimortem pathological findings (Table 12.3) are present in the decedent that indicates the cause of death. These deaths represent a minority (5%) of death investigations wherein the autopsy findings alone provide the necessary foundation for a cause of death opinion [11]. Following the postmortem examination, the autopsy findings alone are sufficient to provide a cause of death with absolute certainty (Fig. 12.2). This is because the autopsy findings of the external and internal examination are completely independent of the history and ancillary investigations due to the pathological findings being

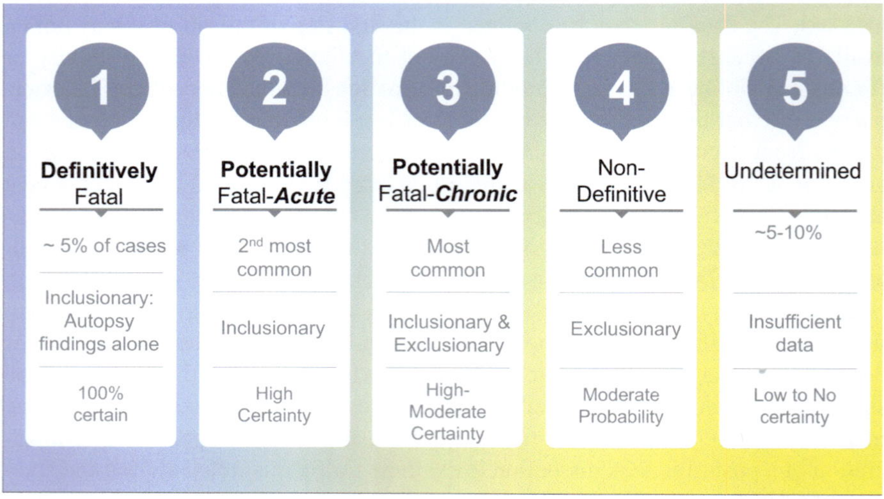

Fig. 12.1 Classification of the cause of death

Table 12.3 Examples of class 1 evidence causes of death

• Intraoral shotgun wound of the head with extrusion of the brain
• Ruptured myocardial infarction
• Ruptured aortic dissection
• High energy multiple trauma (i.e., explosion)
• Decapitation
• Obstructive intracardiac mass
• Massive pulmonary thromboembolism

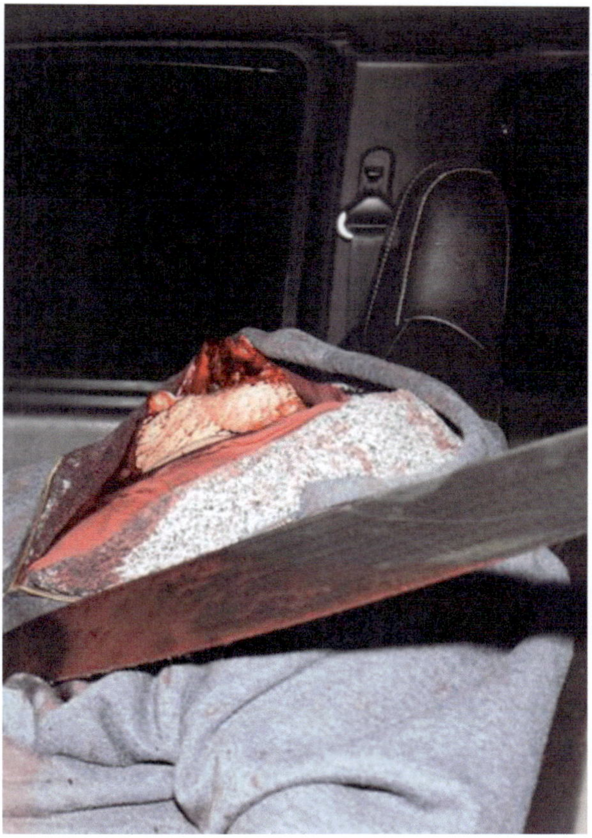

Fig. 12.2 Class 1 cause of death showing a motorised rope assisted decapitation. This is not compatible with continued life

incompatible with continued life (Fig. 12.3). These largely include natural and traumatic causes. In addition, the mechanism of death is structurally demonstrable, such as exsanguination and hemopericardium.

The majority of medicolegal autopsies involve lethal mechanisms that are functional derangements, which are often not structurally demonstrable. The degree of

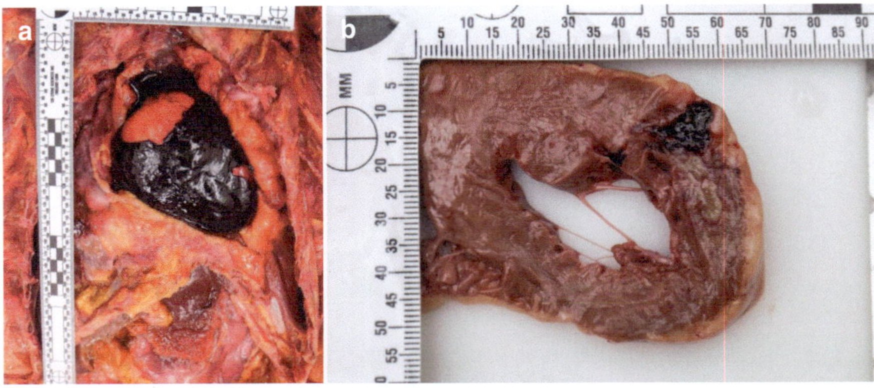

Fig. 12.3 Class 1 evidence showing pathological findings that are incompatible with continued life. This can include a ruptured myocardial infarction that leads to a hemopericardium. (**a**) The mechanism of death is demonstrated as a hemopericardium (blood around the heart) that has come from the rupture site. (**b**) Rupture myocardial infarction was due to coronary artery atherosclerosis and thrombus

certainty with which the pathological findings translate into a cause of death depends on the nature of the available background information. The autopsy findings of the external and internal examination serve to exclude reasonable possible scenarios on fatalities in which opinion rests on circumstantial, historical, or non-autopsy laboratory data.

Class 2: *Potentially* fatal acute or perimortem pathological finding(s):

At autopsy acute or perimortem pathological findings may be identified that imply the cause of death, based on clinicopathologic correlation with the history and exclusionary findings. This class is defined by the presence of a disease or injury with lethal potential, sufficiently advanced that the process is recognized as capable of explaining death (Fig. 12.4, Table 12.4). Although the pathological findings are potentially fatal, some people do survive. These cases represent a slightly larger percentage of cases than class 1. In summary, this is an acute disorder with a ready explanation of death, subject to any other causes of death being excluded. These deaths include diseases, injury, and intoxication. The mechanism of death is not demonstrable. For example, deaths due to hanging or ligature strangulation cannot demonstrate the interference with cerebral circulation of the arteries or neck and airway obstruction (unless there is a period of survival). In addition, carotid stimulation can neither be proven or disproven.

Class 3: *Potentially* fatal *chronic* pathological finding(s):

Class 3 evidence is represented in the majority of medicolegal autopsies. These deaths are characterized by chronic pathological changes (Fig. 12.5, Table 12.5) that are correlated with the history and exclusionary findings including the absence of acute pathology. These deaths imply that the cause of death is based on a clinicopathologic correlation with the history and exclusionary find-

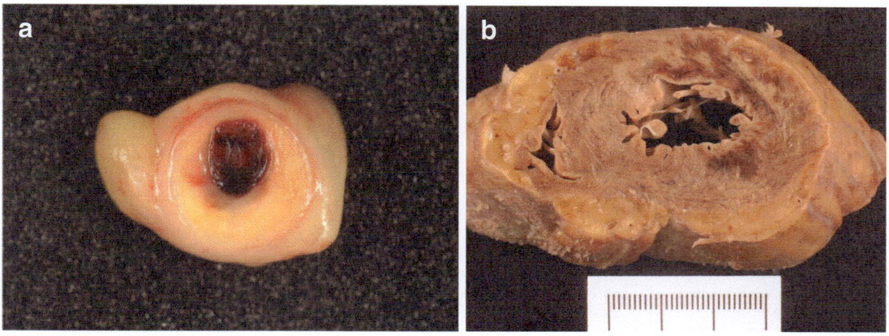

Fig. 12.4 Class 2 evidence example showing an epicardial coronary artery with occlusive thrombus and subendocardial infraction. Acute myocardial infarctions are potentially survivable. The mechanism of death, such as an arrythmia, is not demonstrable at autopsy. (Courtesy: Dr. E. Tweedie Department of Pathology and Laboratory Medicine, Schulich School of Medicine and Dentistry, Western University). (**a**) Coronary artery with occlusive acute thrombus. (**b**) Crosse section of the heart at the left of the ventricles. Reddened area of the left ventricle (shown on right of the image) is an area of an acute myocardial infarction

Table 12.4 Example of class 2 evidence causes of death

• Acute coronary thrombus
• Acute myocardial infraction
• Acute lobar pneumonia
• Hanging
• External neck compression (i.e., strangulation)
• Acute drug/alcohol intoxication

ings. If there is an acute pathology, acute fatal injury, and/or intoxication, this will trump the chronic disease and the decedent is understood to die *with* chronic natural disease, rather than *of* the disease.

Class 4: Non-definitive or non-specific pathologic finding(s):

Class 4 evidence represents a few medicolegal autopsies. At autopsy, there are non-definitive or non-specific pathologic findings (Fig. 12.6, Table 12.6) that can explain death based on inference from clinicopathologic correlation with history and exclusionary findings at autopsy. The pathologist has exhaustively excluded all potential acute and chronic causes of death, and the decedent has a medical condition or in circumstances that may be fatal. There is a lethal lesion that is not structurally demonstrable. The autopsy serves to exclude reasonable possible alternatives. Therefore, the autopsy, by revealing nothing raises the degree of certainty. If the pathologist has not exhaustively excluded alternative causes of death, the death ought to be properly classified as undetermined.

Class 5: No pathologic findings are present that can explain death (Undetermined/Negative Medicolegal autopsy)

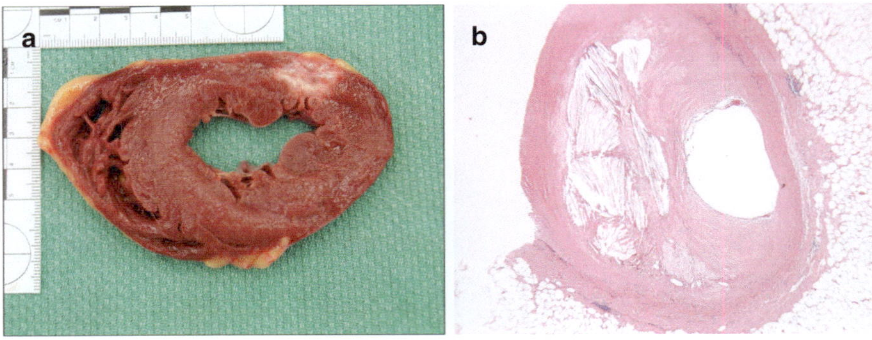

Fig. 12.5 Class 3 evidence to support a cause of death as atherosclerotic heart disease. The cross section of the heart at the level of the ventricle shows a transmural area of fibrosis/scarring of the left ventricle (shown on the upper right hand side of the image). This was due to coronary artery atherosclerotic plaques. (**a**) Cross-section of heart with scarring. (**b**) Severe luminal stenosis with atherosclerotic plaque

Table 12.5 Examples of class 3 evidence causes of death

• Atherosclerotic heart disease
• Hypertensive heart disease
• Cardiomyopathy (i.e., hypertrophic cardiomyopathy)

In class 5 evidence, the autopsy does not reveal pathologic findings that can explain death based on inference, despite clinicopathologic correlation with history and exclusionary findings. The cause of death is undetermined or unascertained following the death investigation into the circumstances, complete autopsy, and relevant ancillary investigations. This is in part due to case selection (i.e., skeletal remains/severely decomposed) (Fig. 12.7), support of toxicology laboratory, and quality of the death investigation system. It also represents a recognition of the limitations of science and the inability of morphologic study to determine functional derangements.

The negative medicolegal autopsy can occur in both natural (i.e., channelopathy) and non-natural (i.e., smothering) deaths. Although the principal aim of the autopsy is to determine the cause of death, a negative autopsy is not a sign of failure. The benefit is that the negative or exclusionary information gained from the autopsy may be of considerable medicolegal value (Table 12.7).

Decision-making on the cause of death is a combination of positive and negative or exclusionary evidence based on interpreting the pathophysiology and circumstances of the death. In a practical sense, this is related to "sliding scale" of evidence that can be classified from 1 to 5. Determining the cause of death is usually straightforward but for some cases the determination can be difficult or controversial due to lower class of

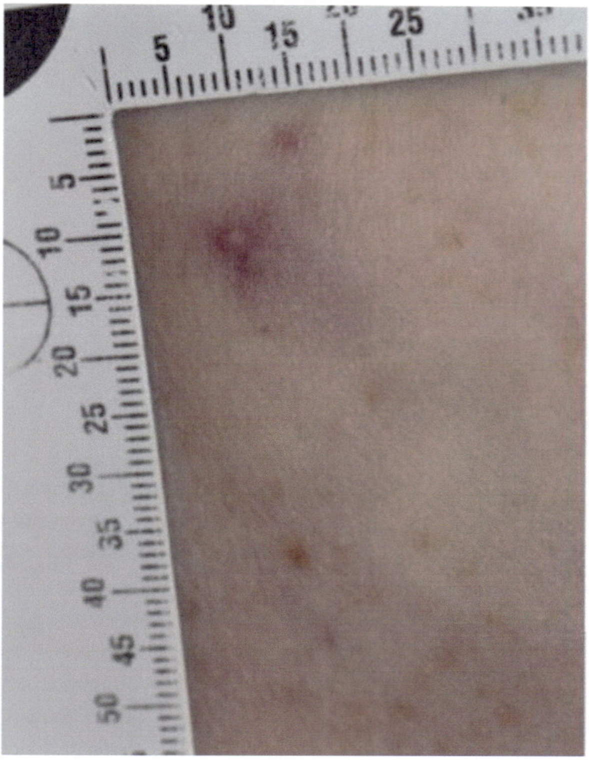

Fig. 12.6 Class 4 evidence to support that this hypersensitivity reaction to a hornet sting resulted in an anaphylactic reaction

Table 12.6 Examples of class 4 evidence causes of death

• SUDEP (Sudden Unexpected Death in Epilepsy)
• Airway obstruction (non-fixed)
• Hypothermia (cold exposure)
• Hyperthermia (heat exposure)
• Anaphylaxis
• Drowning
• Low voltage electrocution

evidence. The majority of medicolegal autopsies are concluded based on class 3 evidence due to the prevalence of chronic heart disease in many countries (Table 12.8).

The precise cause of death may be due to combined effects of co-factors, and knowledge of the relevant factors may limit a reliable conclusion about their significance. This reflects the uncertainty that encompasses some death investigations, as well as the inherent uncertainty that is sometimes an inescapable part of medicine.

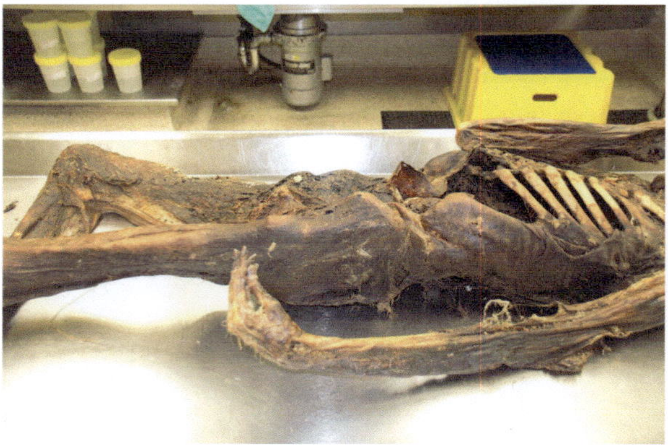

Fig. 12.7 Severely decomposed/skeletal remains often represent a negative medicolegal autopsy as the cause of death cannot be determined due to the absence of organs to evaluate

Table 12.7 Examples of class 5 evidence causes of death

• Negative autopsy findings with no context
• Fresh bodies with no context
• Decomposed bodies
• Skeletonized bodies

Table 12.8 The medicolegal value of a negative medicolegal autopsy

• Detects the absence of heritable diseases
• Eliminates suspicions
• Provide reassurance to families
• Substitute facts for conjecture
• Allows for investigation to remain "open"

Considerations Before Arriving at the Conclusion of a Negative Medicolegal Autopsy—Step-Wise Approach to the Autopsy & Hypothesis Testing

Prior to the completion of the postmortem examination, it is useful to reexamine the steps of the autopsy to ensure that reasonable investigations have been considered.

Scene and Circumstances

The importance of history and circumstances in medical diagnosis is standard training and practice for physicians. History plays a paramount role in decision-making of the cause of death. A study that examined 630 medical case found that history was the most important component in diagnosis in the majority of cases [12]. This finding has been repeated in many studies [13–19]. The history is where a hypothesis is formed about why an individual died. If there is no single hypothesis supported by the background information, more information is probably required. If sufficient information is available, proceed with autopsy. Going through the subsequent steps of the autopsy, the hypothesis (clinically referred to as working diagnoses) may be confirmed or refuted (Fig. 12.8) Additional historical information may be needed to be required following or after the autopsy (Fig. 12.9). There are a variety of sources to review in this step (Table 12.9).

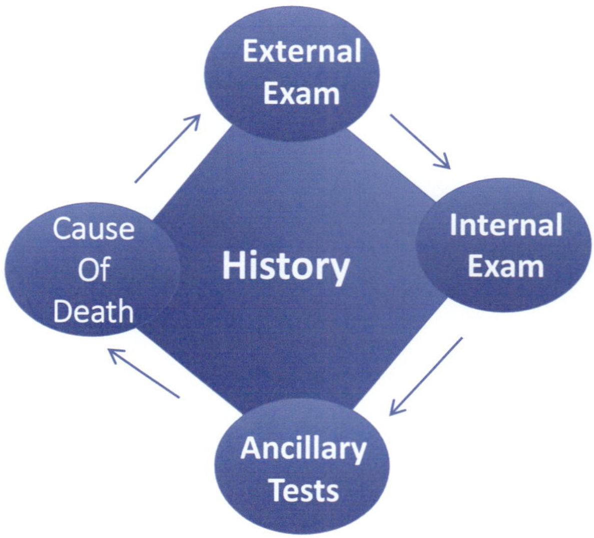

Fig. 12.8 Concept of hypothesis testing in medicine (clinically referred to as a working diagnosis) and medicolegal autopsy. The history and circumstances of the death may form a hypothesis regarding the cause of death but this is tested against the subsequent steps of the autopsy to ascertain a cause of death

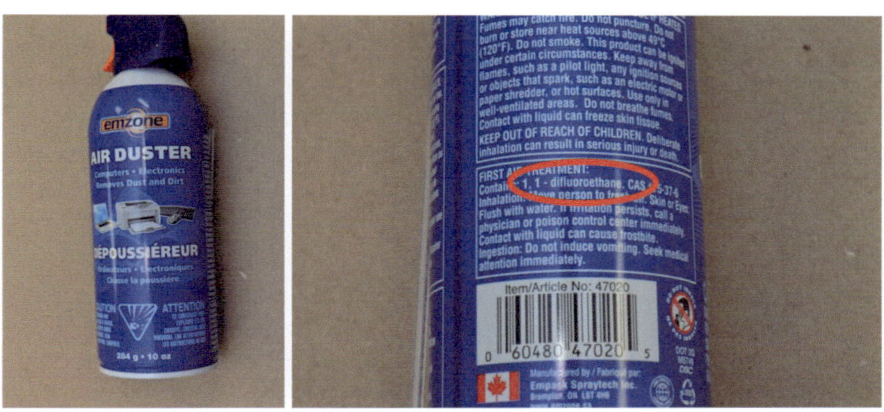

Fig. 12.9 The scene can guide determining ancillary testing for cause of death. The presence of 1,1-diffluourethane at the scene directed toxicological testing for this substance as organic solvents are not routinely tested for. This substance is associated with sudden death due to the cardiotoxic effects on the myocardium

Table 12.9 The evidence that may be collected in the history, scene, and circumstances

• Warrant for postmortem examination/relevant documents
• Scene images:
– Photographs
– Videos
• Scene visit:
– Prospective
– Retrospective
• Medical record
• Paramedic report
• Police:
– Initial police investigation
– Report
• Eyewitness statements
• Position of the body

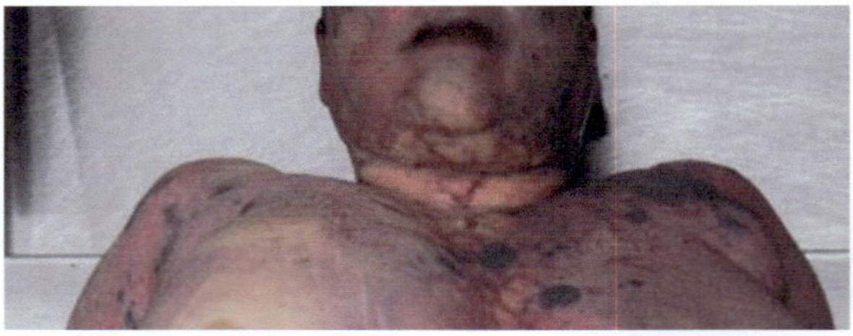

Fig. 12.10 The distribution of lividity could indicate that there was a positional asphyxia at play. Sparing of lividity of the anterior (front) neck in the setting of anterior lividity can indicate a hyperflexed neck

External Examination

The external examination may direct further investigations as this is an opportunity to detect disease and injury but also consider what was among the personal effects (i.e., receipts for over the counter medicines) and postmortem changes (Fig. 12.10, Table 12.10).

Internal Examination

A complete internal examination requires opening the head, consideration of removing the periosteum and reflecting the temporalis muscle to assesses for occult skull fractures. In addition, the dura needs to examine the base of skull (Fig. 12.11, Table 12.11). The neck structures and tongue need to be removed to examine for an internal airway obstruction. Consideration of opening the bowel and any special dissections may be necessary. For example, an individual with an explained acute subarachnoid hemorrhage i.e. no ruptured Berry aneurym) may require a vertebral artery examination to assess for a vertebral artery dissection.

Table 12.10 The evidence that may be collected during the external examination

• Clothing, jewelry & personal effects
• Medical/surgical intervention
• General nutrition & development
• Documentation of identifying features (i.e., tattoos, scars, etc.)
• Postmortem changes
• Body stature & habitus
• Examine all body surfaces
• Injuries, petechiae, etc.
• Natural disease
• Lifestyle
• Congenital anomalies

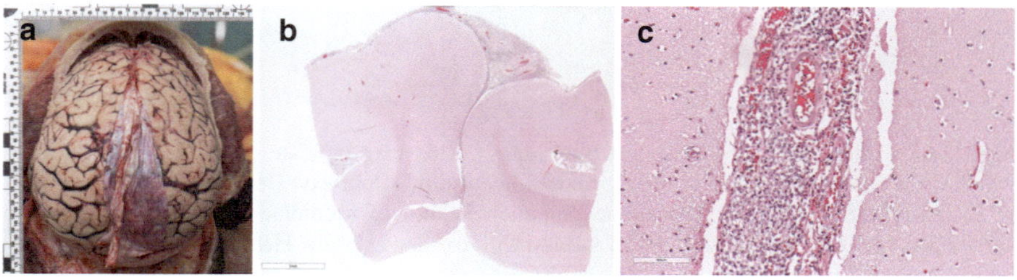

Fig. 12.11 Meningitis can be challenging to detect, especially in a younger person and in the absence of purulent exudate. Histological examination can be helpful. (**a**) Top of the brain with calvarium removed and scalp reflected. Purulent exudate is not observed. (**b**) Photomicrophraghs of the frontal cortex, H&E, low power. (**c**) Photomicrophraghs of the frontal cortex, H&E, higher power, showing an acute meningitis

Ancillary Investigations

Depending on the jurisdiction, there is a wide variety of ancillary investigations that may have not been sought. This may require additional histological and toxicological sampling (Fig. 12.12).

Table 12.11 The evidence that may be collected in the internal examination

• Weight & examine individual organs
• Injuries
• Natural disease
• Congenital anomalies
• Medical/surgical interventions

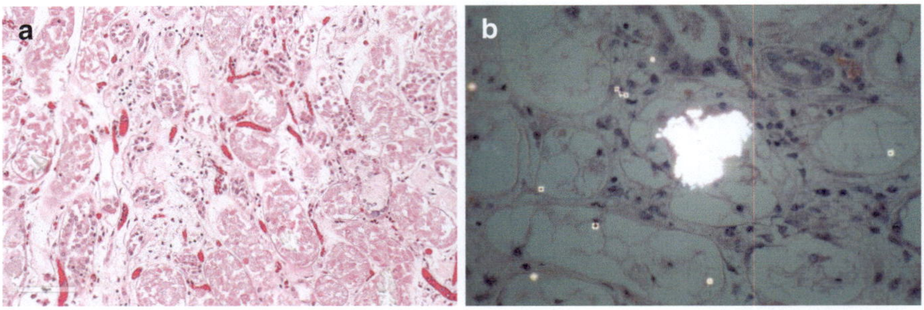

Fig. 12.12 Calcium oxalate crystal in the kidneys. This may indicate ethylene glycol toxicity, which is not usually tested for on routine toxicology testing. (Courtesy: Dr. M. Shkrum Department of Pathology and Laboratory Medicine, Schulich School of Medicine and Dentistry, Western University). (**a**) Microscopic section of kidney with oxalate crystals, H&E. (**b**) Birefringent oxalate crystals. H&E and polarised

Conditions that Should Not Be Invoked as a Cause of Death

There are a variety of observations at autopsy that should not invoke a cause of death. These include mechanisms of death (i.e., pulmonary edema), which can be observed at autopsy but are not etiologically specific and can arise in a variety of consequences. In addition, to funerary artifacts, resuscitation-related artifacts (Fig. 12.13) and tissue donation for transplantation (Fig. 12.14, Table 12.12).

Autopsy findings that require additional findings to support a cause of death include sickle red blood cells and potential aspiration of gastric contents. In individuals with sickle cell disease or trait, the red blood cells sickle antemortem and postmortem (Fig. 12.16). Red blood cells sickle postmortem due to the anoxic and acidotic environment. However, in the right context, where the sickled red blood cells can be ascertained to occur in life, the histological finding of sickled red blood cells may support a cause of death. Similarly, the presence of gastric contents in the airway may or may not serve as a cause of death. Gastric contents in the airway may be found in the airways at autopsy (Fig. 12.17). The gastric contents can be displaced during resuscitation-related chest compressions, during postmortem handling of the body and increased abdominal pressure during decomposition. However, if there is a history of internal airway obstruction ("choking") or evidence of an inflammatory reaction in the lungs on histology, this would support that the gastric contents were present in the airways in life.

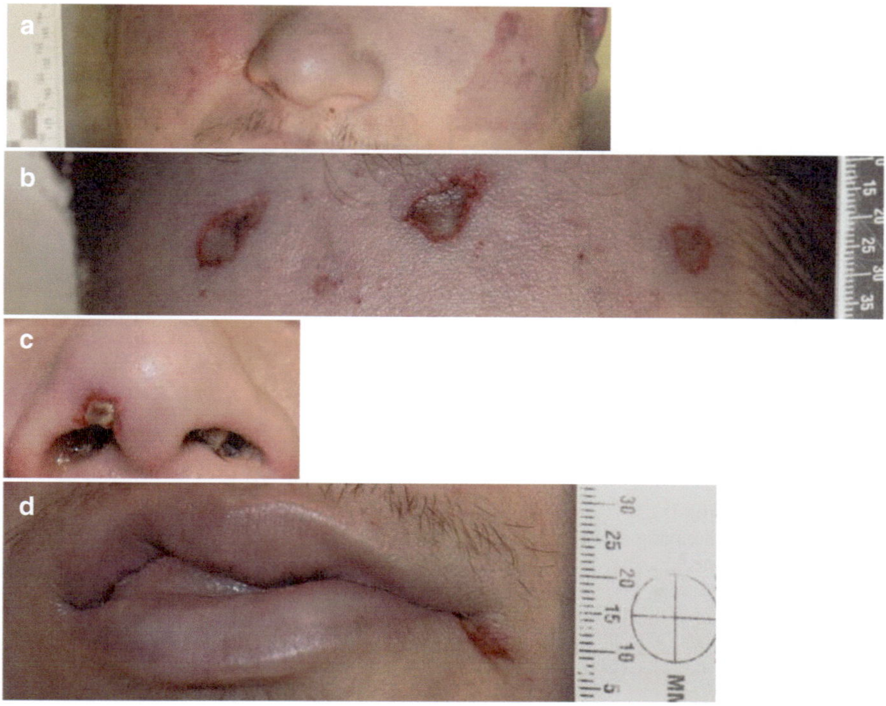

Fig. 12.13 Therapeutic and resuscitation-related artifacts. (**a**) Lividity of the cheeks due to blood pooling under the oral endotracheal tube (breathing tube) strap. (**b**) Pressure injuries due to metal electrodes for the assessment of an electroencephalogram that measures the electrical activity of the brain. (**c**) Pressure injury due to nasogastric tube placement for the purpose of feeding and administering medications. (**d**) Pressure injury due to oral endotracheal tube placement

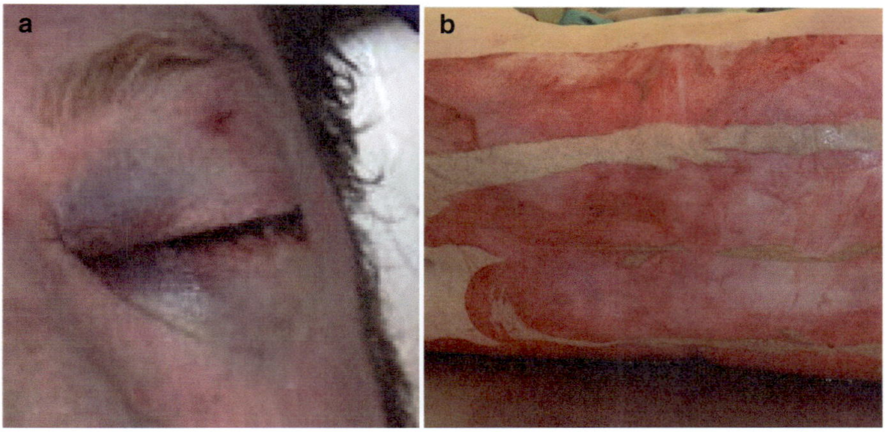

Fig. 12.14 Tissue donation artifacts. (**a**) Periorbital bruising and abrasion due to postmortem removal of the eye for corneal donation. Elevating the head, application of pressure and packing the site can minimize this artifact. In addition, newer techniques and training that results in removing just the cornea *in situ* can minimise this artifact. (**b**) Postmortem skin donation of the back that can be used in individuals that have been critically injured by burns

Table 12.12 Autopsy findings that do not invoke a cause of death

• Interpreting epicardial fat in the anterior right ventricle as arrhythmogenic right ventricular cardiomyopathy
• Lividity of the myocardium
• Minute foci of chronic inflammation of the heart is not myocarditis
• Sleep apnea (unless cor pulmonale present)
• Gastromalacia
• Undertaker's fracture (postmortem fracture usually of the lower cervical vertebrae) (Fig. 12.15)
• Basal skull fracture in the wrong context (may be a postmortem artifact)

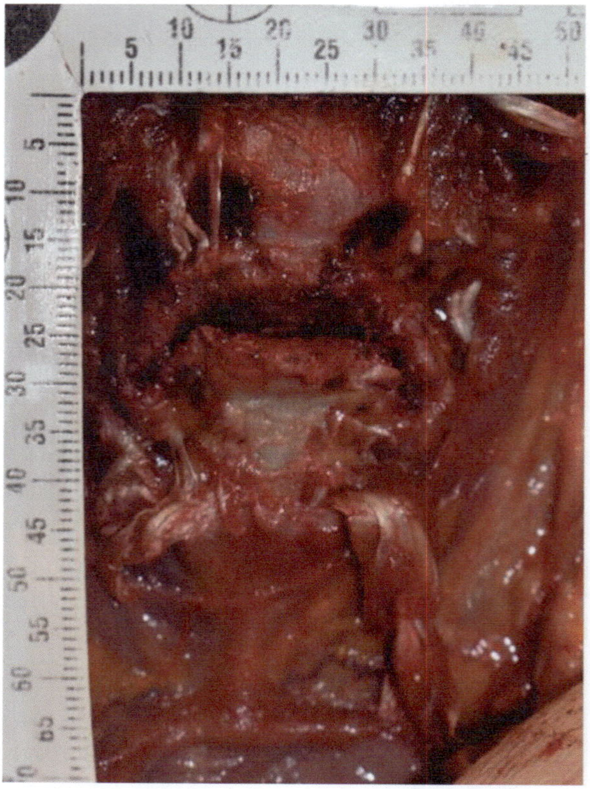

Fig. 12.15 Postmortem fracture of the lower cervical vertebrae (also referred to as an undertaker's fracture). Is thought to arise in breaking rigor mortis of the neck, which causes subluxation of the cervical spine

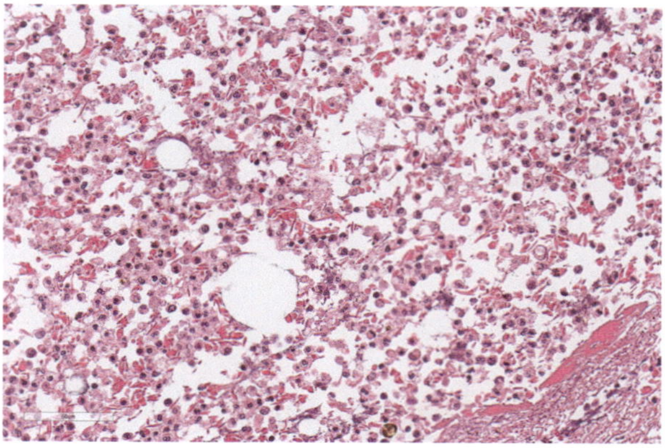

Fig. 12.16 Sickled red blood cells can occur antemortem and postmortem in individuals with sickle cell disease and trait. On its own is not a cause of death

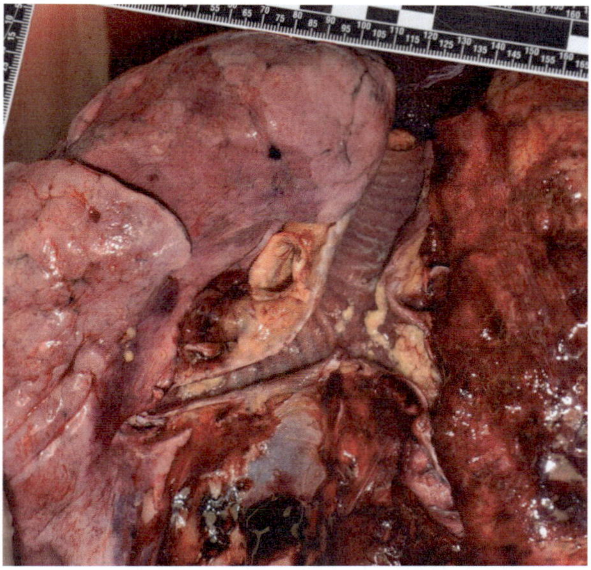

Fig. 12.17 Postmortem shifting of stomach contents into the airway following handling of the body. A readily explainable cause of death was present

Appropriate to Call the Cause of Death Undetermined (Negative Medicolegal Autopsy)

It is appropriate to call a negative medicolegal autopsy when the following conditions are considered:

1. A complete autopsy was performed. This is when all the anticipated questions are answered by the autopsy. The ability to anticipate later questions in part depends on past experiences and training.
2. Threshold for calling a case negative is case dependent. The ancillary investigations required in a recently dead person are greater than skeletal remains.

Summary

A small percentage of correctly conducted autopsies, with appropriate ancillary investigations, will not yield a cause of death. This will vary with the pattern of work and the experience of the pathologist.

References

1. Biswas H, et al. Autopsy rate at forensic medicine department of Dhaka Medical College. Dinajpur Med Col J. 2008;1(1):21–3.
2. Knights and Knight B. The obscure autopsy. Forensic Sci Int. 1980;16:237–40.
3. Pervez A, et al. Critical appraisal of autopsy work. APMC. 2016;10(4):194–202.
4. Sanchez O, et al. Natural and undetermined sudden death: value of postmortem genetic investigation. PLoS One. 2016;11(12):e0167358. https://doi.org/10.1371/journal.pone.0167358.
5. Lawler W. The negative coroner's necropsy: a personal approach and consideration of difficulties. J Clin Pathol. 1990;43:977–80.
6. Nordum I, et al. Unexplained and explained natural deaths among persons above 1 year of age in a series of medico-legal autopsies. Forensci Sci Int. 1998;93:89–98.
7. Modi K, et al. The study of negative autopsy among the post mortem cases referred from medical officers to forensic medicine department, Ahmedabad, India. Int J Med Toxicol Forensic Med. 2017;7(2):138–43.
8. Khan MY, et al. Frequency of negative autopsy and their demographic evaluation at Khyber medical college, Peshwar. JPMI. 2007;21(2):132–5.
9. Adelson L. No anatomic cause of death. Conn State Med J. 1954;18:732.
10. Wright RK, Wetli CV. A guide to the forensic autopsy-conceptual aspects. Pathol Annu. 1981;16:273–88.
11. Brinkmann B. Harmonisation of medico-legal autopsy rules. Int J Legal Med. 1999;113:1–14.
12. Sandler G. Costs of unnecessary tests. Br Med J. 1979;2:21–4.
13. Peterson MC, et al. Contributions of the history, physical examination, and laboratory investigation in making medical diagnoses. West J Med. 1992;156(2):163–5.
14. Roshan M, Rao AP. A study on relative contributions of the history, physical examination and investigations in making medical diagnosis. J Assoc Physicians India. 2000;48(8):771–5.
15. Hampton JR, et al. Relative contributions of history-taking, physical examination, and laboratory investigation to diagnosis and management of medical outpatients. Br Med J. 1975;2(5969):486–9.
16. Miall LS, Davies H. An analysis of paediatric diagnostic decision-making: how should students be taught? Med Educ. 1992;26(4):317–20.
17. Gruppen LD, Woolliscroft JO, Wolf FM. The contribution of different components of the clinical encounter in generating and eliminating diagnostic hypotheses. Res Med Educ. 1988;27:242–7.
18. Wagemakers HP, et al. Diagnostic value of history-taking and physical examination for assessing meniscal tears of the knee in general practice. Clin J Sport Med. 2008;18(1):24–30.
19. Vroomen PC, et al. Diagnostic value of history and physical examination in patients suspected of lumbosacral nerve root compression. J Neurol Neurosurg Psychiatry. 2002;72(5):630–4.

Part III
Medicolegal Death Investigations of Special Populations

Chapter 13
Pediatrics

Rebekah Jacques

Pediatric (childhood) mortality has a powerful public presence. The vast majority (85%) of pediatric deaths occur in the first 5 years of life [1]. There are various causes of death that fall under all manners of death; however, an unknown cause of death (i.e. undetermined) is more common in infants than other ages of children.

The pediatric population does not simply represent small adults. The pediatric population represents a heterogenous group of anatomic, developmental, and physiologic range of differences. Pediatric pathology and deaths encompass a wide spectrum of findings that are more common or unique to this population. This is reflected in a different range of cause of death, included a higher incidence of undetermined causes among infants. The pediatric and perinatal post-mortem examination represents the unique challenges associated with this population. Depending on the context that the baby is born, the pathologist needs to examine the placenta (if available) in addition to the decedent's body determine the fetal age, if the baby was born dead (i.e., Stillborn) or alive, identification, and possible causes of death.

Despite awareness of child abuse beginning in the 1960s in many countries, pediatric forensic pathology is a subset of cases within forensic pathology that can generate its own acadmic literature and experiential learning, and is not considered a separate medical subspecialty.

R. Jacques (✉)
London Health Sciences Centre, University Hospital, London, ON, Canada
e-mail: rebekah.jacques@lhsc.on.ca

R. Jacques (ed.), *Forensic Pathology*,
https://doi.org/10.1007/978-3-031-42038-2_13

Perinatal Postmortem Examination

Stillbirth

The term stillbirth has a variety of different definitions but is broadly understood as a viable fetus (depending on jurisdiction this can include a variable gestational age cutoff 20 weeks and even 28 weeks) [2] that did not breathe, have a heartbeat, pulsation of the umbilical cord, or unmistakable movement of voluntary muscle after being completely expelled from the pregnant person. Heartbeats are distinguished from transient cardiac contractions, and respiration is distinguished from fleeting respiratory gasps or efforts [3]. These findings require a reliable history to determine. Prior to 20 weeks, the expelled or extracted fetus or embryo (i.e. gestational age before 8 weeks gestation) are often considered miscarriages (spontaneous abortion) and usually have no medico-legal significance. This description can have challenges in the death investigation system. The majority of stillbirths die in utero followed by the early stages of parturition. Stillbirth is a common complication and the incidence can be highly variable depending on the gestational age and nation [4]. A retained fetus that has died in utero will have developed maceration over time but sometimes this can be challenging to differentiate from putrefactive decompositional changes.

Not all medicolegal death investigation systems interpret their role as including the investigation of stillbirths because legally there was no life and thus no death [5]. However, when there is doubt about the status of a livebirth versus a stillbirth, the pathologist can become involved to make the determination. The scenarios can be highly variable and include clandestine circumstances, discarded fetuses, a non-natural component to the pregnant person that temporally was followed by a stillbirth, concealed pregnancy concerns of care, and unattended delivery. The pathologist can function in determining the identity, live birth versus stillbirth, and cause of death.

Determination of Live Birth

The determination between and live birth Determining that the potentially viable fetus was born alive (i.e. had signs of life) and had a separate existence is challenging in the absence of a reliable history. Separate existence indicates that the baby was completely extracted or expelled from the parental passages, even if still attached to the placenta. This has been traditionally determined by considering the following:

1. Absence of maceration
2. Maturity estimation
3. Extra-uterine contents in the gastrointestinal tract
4. Hydorstatic test
5. Inflammatory reaction at the stump of the umbilical cord
6. Absence of non-viable congenital defects (i.e. anencephaly)

Maceration

Maceration is in utero decompositional changes of a fetus (Fig. 13.1). The latin etymology of maceration is macerare, which means "to soften." The presence of maceration changes indicates that the fetus died in utero and therefore there was no

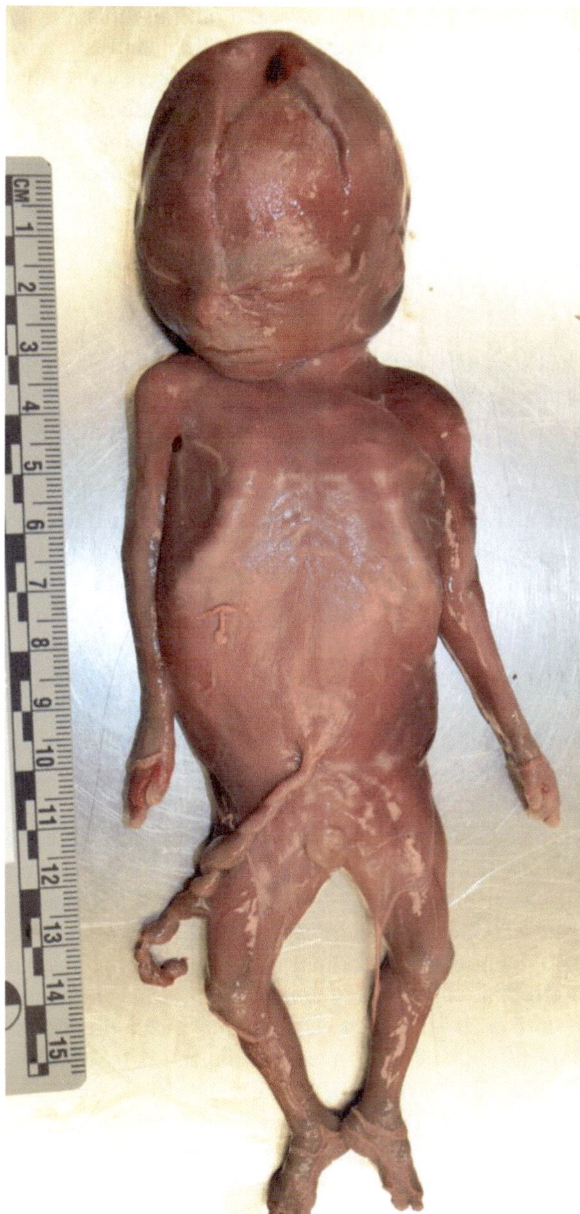

Fig. 13.1 Stillborn with evidence of maceration (e.g. skin slippage and moulding of skull bones). The hypercoiled umbilical cord may explain the intrauterine fetal demise

livebirth that occurred. The absence of maceration is not helpful in differentiating liveborn from stillborn but its presence does.

One of the earliest changes of maceration includes skin slippage and dark discoloration of the umbilical cord may appear if there is prolonged retention. In live births, the umbilical cord has a yellow appearance but this can also be observed in stillbirths. Macroscopically, maceration changes start 6 hours after in utero retention in the form of skin slippage, pink discoloration and eventually skull plate hypermobility [6]. After 2 weeks of retention, the fetus may appear mummified (e.g. fetus papyraceous) [6]. However, maceration can be accelerated with intrauterine infection [2]. Maceration differs from putrefactive decomposition as the former tend to have pink appearance rather than green associated with putrefaction but in practice this assessment can be challenging. In addition, decomposition can develop in all fetuses regardless if liveborn or stillborn and decomposition can obscure maceration.

Maturity Estimation

The estimation of the age of maturity of a fetus has medical and legal relevant issues as this has implications on whether the fetus was too immature to survive (i.e., viable) outside of the uterus. The gestational age cutoff of viability will depend on local laws and the medical intervention standards available. In a very premature fetus survival is not possible or unlikely if delivered without immediate medical attention. Methods to determine gestation age estimation can include using findings of the placenta and the fetus, such as foot length, gross brain development, microscopic lung development, and skeletal age based on ossification center and lengths of long bones [7, 8]. The body weight and external measurements, such as crown to rump, crown to foot, head circumference, and foot length should be compared to appropriate standardized measurements, that considers syndromes. The same is repeated for organ weights. In addition, thoracic circumference at the level of the nipples, and abdominal circumference at the level of the umbilicus can be compared to ultrasound estimations. The reliability of the accuracy is dependent on decomposition, maceration, intrauterine growth restriction, and if there is prolonged hospital stays. In general, the foot length is the most reliable external measurement to assess fetal age [2]. Macroscopic and microscopic of the internal organs and tissues, in addition to the placenta, can also give indication of gestational age. Neuropathological examination of the brain can determine gestational age based on the macroscopic assessment of gyral formation and microscopic evaluation of neuronal migration, differentiation, and myelination [2]. Macroscopically, earlier gestation shows smooth external surface. Histological evaluation of the lungs is classified into four main developmental stages: glandular (5–16 weeks), canalicular (16–24 weeks), saccular (24–35 weeks), alveolar (35 weeks onwards) [2]. Essentially, the older gestational age is associated with increased branching and complexity of the airways. Radiological estimation can be performed on the routine skeletal survey that is often performed in circumstances where maturity estimation is required. Human variation would result in a range of observations that would overlap with different gestational ages. In addition, postmortem changes may hinder determination of gestational age. For example, maceration may increase body length but foot length is thought to remain quite accurate.

Presence of Extra-Uterine in the Gastrointestinal Tracts

The presence of food, such as curdled milk or other extra-uterine elements, in the gastrointestinal tract is interpreted that not only was the fetus born alive but was also fed.

Inflammatory Response at the Stump of the Umbilical Cord

Time estimation using histopathology has similar limitations as determining time interval between injury and death. In stillbirths, the umbilical cord is described as red at the stump [9, 10] but can also be yellow if there is not a prolonged in utero retention.

Microscopic examination of the umbilical cord as a means to determine that the newborn was liveborn is controversial. The presence of acute inflammatory cells at the infant side of a previously transected umbilical cord and absence of acute inflammatory cells on the placental side of a non-retained placenta indicates a live birth. Inflammatory changes of the umbilical cord can be identified as polymorphonuclear leukocyte infiltrates [2]. An immunohistological study found that that the presence of mast cell tryptase, CD68 (a histiocytic stain) and alpha-1-antichymotrypsin showed a statistically significant different expression in stillborn and liveborn. Liveborn umbilical tissue has an increased level of mast cell tryptase expression [11]. The inflammatory changes would have to be differentiated from other inflammatory processes such as funisitis that commonly is associated with chorioamnionitis. Chorioamnionitis is associated with stillbirth.

"Hydrostatic Test"

The "hydrostatic test" or "floatation test" is a controversial test as well that has been used to demonstrate that there was evidence of breathing in the newborn (Fig. 13.2). In general, lungs in a stillborn exhibit primary atelectasis and are dark red, non-expanded with a rubbery consistency. In aerated lungs, the appearance is pink, expanded and spongy. The test is variable described as taking sections of lungs or the entire thoracic pluck of organs (i.e. heart, mediastinum, and neck structure with attached lungs) in water and observes if the lung tissue floats. The floating lung tissue indicates aeration and the inference is that the newborn was able to breath. Limitations to this assessment and interpretation are the decompositional changes (microscopic or macroscopic) can result in floatation of lung tissues in a stillbirth

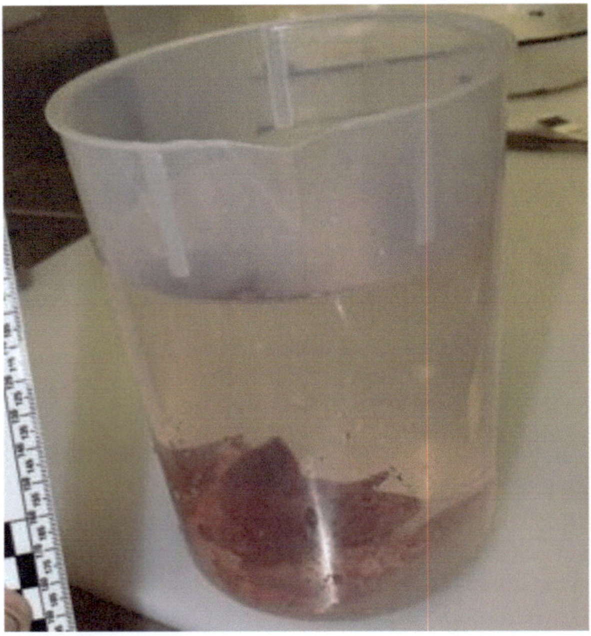

Fig. 13.2 The 'hydrostatic' test where the thoracic pluck is placed in water to test for floatation. If the organs sink, as shown here, this may indicate that the fetus was a stillbirth and was not breathing and aerating the lungs. The test is controversial and has false negatives and false positives to consider

due to the production of decompositional gases. In addition, resuscitation efforts can artificially introduce air into the lungs, resulting in floatation of the lungs in a stillbirth. Further, pneumonia or diffuse alveolar damage in a live birth would fail the hydrostatic test. Histological evaluation of lungs, in congenitally normally lungs, for expanded alveoli is of no use because they have been observed as expanded in stillbirths [12]. The value of the hydrostatic test is limited to newborns that have maximally respired lungs without decomposition or evidence of resuscitation. The interpretation of this finding cannot independently determine post-natal survival and must be interpreted using the constellation of findings.

The absence of lung aeration is not the equivalent to the presence of a beating heart. A beating heart may be present in the absence of breathing due to poor tone or other circumstances.

Non-Viable Congenital or Placental Anomalies

There are multiple congenital anomalies that would not be viable. These can include malformation, disruptions, deformations, and syndromes. Anencephaly, arthrogryposis, severe hydrops, severe spina bifida, gastroschisis, type 2 osteogenesis imperfecta or amniotic deformity adhesions, and mutilation of the head, umbilical cord, or other vital areas of the body are examples of a congenital anomaly that are non-viable (Figs. 13.3, 13.4, 13.5). Assessment of the placenta may also indicate no-viability such as a large retroplacental hematoma and chorioamnionitis.

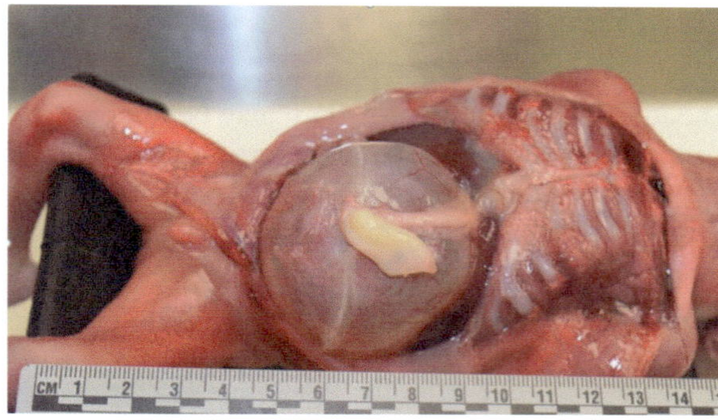

Fig. 13.3 The presence of an omphalocele would indicate that the newborn would not have lived long following delivery without immediate medical intervention

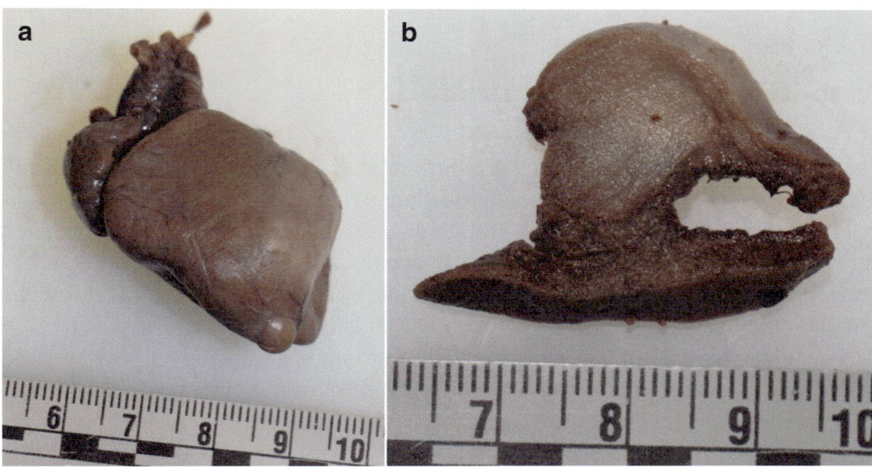

Fig. 13.4 Congenital cardiac rhabdomyoma (heart tumor). This tumor would have not been compatible with separate existence following delivery. (**a**) Anterior (front) view of the heart showing a mass extending from apex that a histological examination confirmed was a rhabdomyoma. (**b**) Cross-section of the same heart at the level of the right and left ventricle showing a pale mass that was a rhabdomyoma

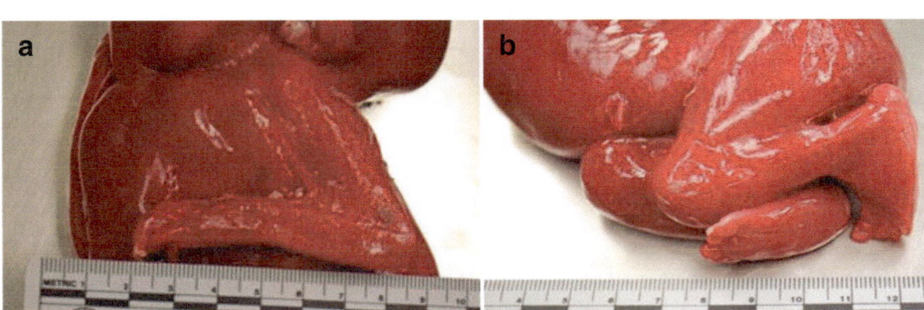

Fig. 13.5 Arthropryposis multiplex with ptergia (web of skin) would be incompatible with separate existence outside of the uterus. (**a**) ptergia of the left arm. (**b**) ptergia of the legs

Identification

The identification of the newborn may be in question. The identification of a stillbirth starts at the scene and investigation by law enforcement. This can include the bags, blankets, and other items that the body was wrapped in. The apparent ethnicity of the baby can also guide identification. The appearance of the umbilical cord (i.e., presence of a cord clamp) and clean cut, rather than an irregular cut end, can also indicate that the birth was attended by healthcare professionals and that the birth was recorded in a local hospital or clinic. Positive identification will require collecting a DNA sample from the baby for profiling but a successful identification can only occur if a presumptive parent can be identified and legal venues are available for obtaining a DNA sample in the absence of volunteering a biological sample.

Birth-Related Injuries and Death

There are a variety of traumas that are birth related that can occur in both assisted and non-assisted deliveries. These injuries largely fall into scalp injuries, intracranial bleeding of multiple types (i.e., subdural, subarachnoid, intraparenchymal, and intraventricular) and fractures of the skull, clavicle, ribs, upper and lower extremities. Operative vaginal deliveries include the use of a vacuum extractor and forceps to assist in the vaginal delivery of a fetus. The vacuum extractor can also be used in caesarean delivery. Scalp injuries are relatively common during the birthing process. Scalp injuries can include cutaneous (skin) abrasions and bruises typically in vaginally assisted delivery (Fig. 13.6). In addition, vacuum-assisted deliveries can cause

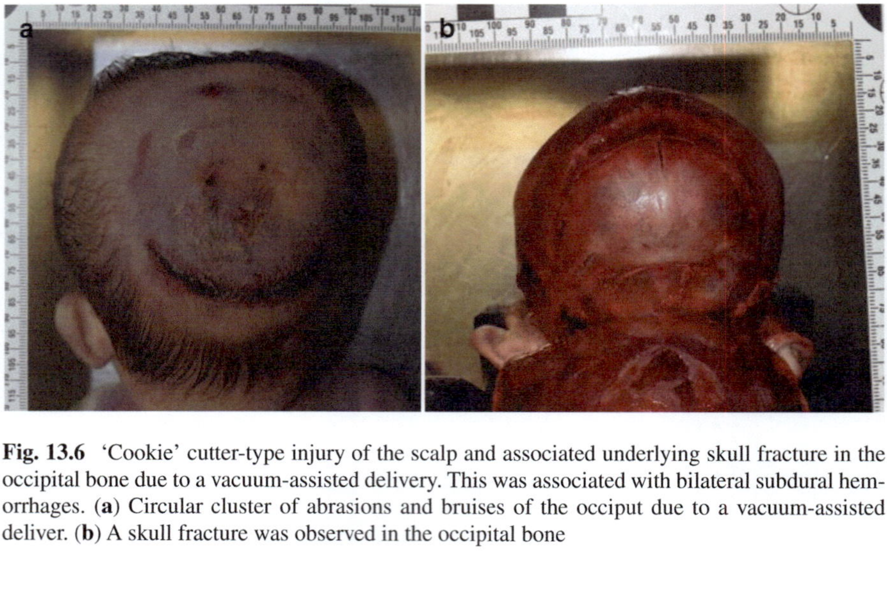

Fig. 13.6 'Cookie' cutter-type injury of the scalp and associated underlying skull fracture in the occipital bone due to a vacuum-assisted delivery. This was associated with bilateral subdural hemorrhages. (**a**) Circular cluster of abrasions and bruises of the occiput due to a vacuum-assisted deliver. (**b**) A skull fracture was observed in the occipital bone

what is referred to as 'cookie-cutter' injuries to the fetal scalp [13]. There are various scalp hemorrhages that have different names depending on location of bleeding but are usually non-fatal. For example, Subgaleal hematoma is bleeding into the subaponeurotic layer of the fetal scalp due to lacerated emissary veins that connect the scalp veins to the dural sinuses. The bleeding is not confined to a single bone. This space can hold as much as 260 mL of blood and can lead to hypovolemic shock [14]. A cephalhematoma is a localized area of subperiosteal bleeding that is limited by sutures resulting in well-defined edges. A caput succedaneum (scalp edema) is a non-hemorrhaguc injury that can result in diffuse edema that overlies more than one skull bone resulting in ill-defined edges. This arises from molding of the head causing overriding of the parietal bones during vaginal delivery. An internal examination can facilitiate differentiating birth-related scalp injuries. Fractures from both vaginal and Caesarean deliveries are rare. Rarely, skull fractures can occur during deliveries and commonly involve the clavicule (collar bone). Clavicle fractures occur as a result of the anterior shoulder of the fetus being compressed against the maternal symphysis pubis or obstetric maneuvers to minimize the chest circumference in shoulder dystocia [15]. Rarely, the rib fractures can occur in association with clavicle fractures [16]. If these are unrecognized at the time of delivery, this can lead to challenges at the postmortem examination. In general, birth-associated fractures will show radiographic evidence of healing (i.e., subperiosteal new bone formation and callous formation) 10 days after delivery (Fig 13.7) [17]. Humerus (upper arm bone) fractures can also arise during delivery in the setting of shoulder dystocia and can arise in both vaginal and caesarean section with cephalic presentation [15]. Femur fractures have been reported in difficult vaginal breech delivery and malpositions during caesarean deliveries that is related to the extraction methods used [15]. In addition, the classical metaphyseal lesions, that have been considered highly specific for abuse, can occur in uncomplicated and challenging caesarean sections [18]. Obtaining the delivery records can help inform the significance of injuries.

Subdural and retinal hemorrhage may also be complications related to birth. Nearly half of neonates have asymptomatic subdural hemorrhages [2]. The incidence of retinal hemorrhages is comparable and can be quite extensive and persists for 2 months after delivery [2]. The incidence of retinal hemorrhages is indicated to be due to raised intracranial pressures, in addition to hypoxia and hypercapnia [2].

Placenta

The macroscopic and microscopic examination of the placenta, if available, is a fundamental part of the perinatal postmortem examination. The placenta can be used for a variety of purposes including establishing a cause of death and age estimation of the fetus.

Intrauterine infections are a common cause of stillbirth and early neonatal deaths. Infections are most commonly due to ascending infection but can also be acquired from vascular dissemination that passes through the placenta. Acute

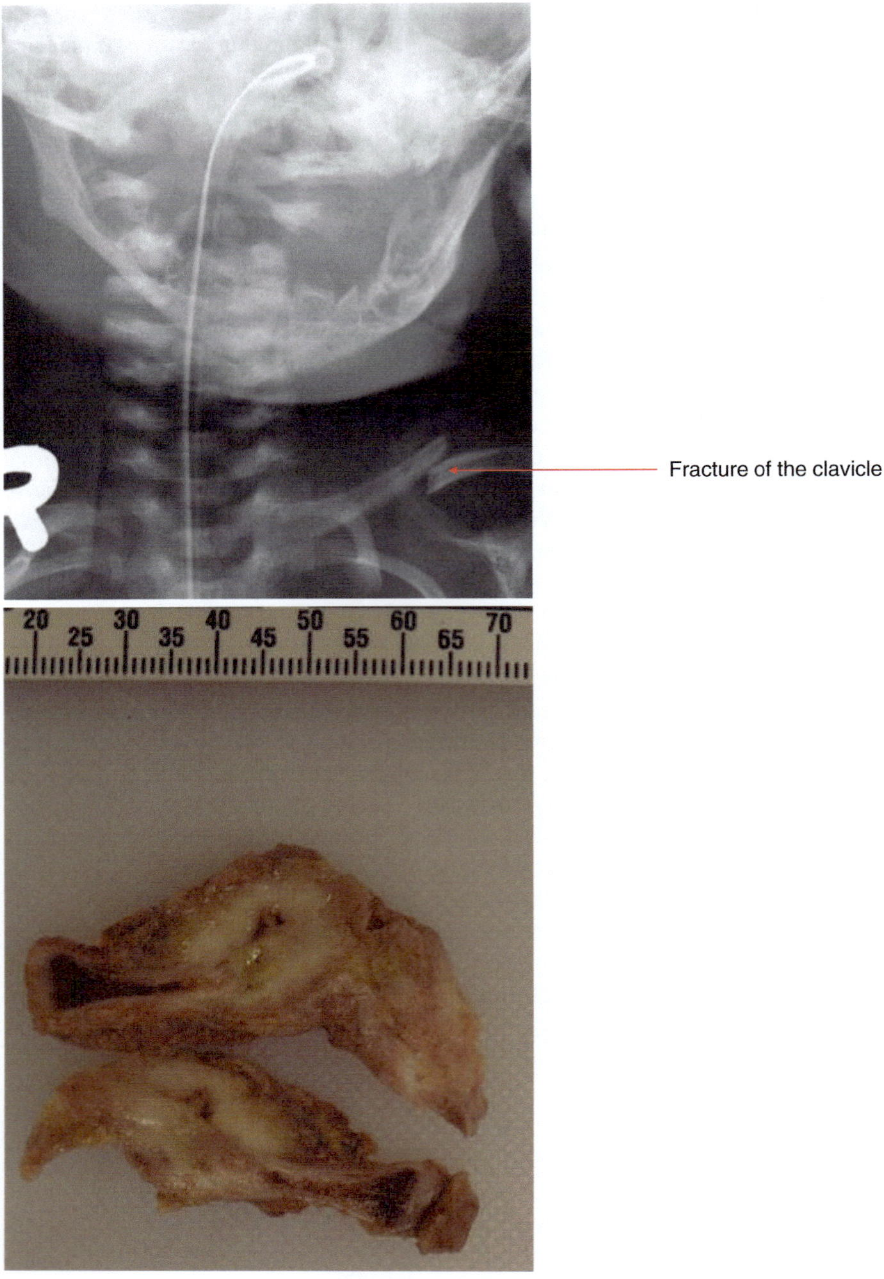

Fig. 13.7 Healing clavicle (collar bone) fracture that was related to birth-related injury. (**a**) Radiograph of the left clavicle does not visualise the cartilage phase of healing bones. (**b**) Macroscopic examination of the clavicle showing a cartilagnous callus (healing fracture)

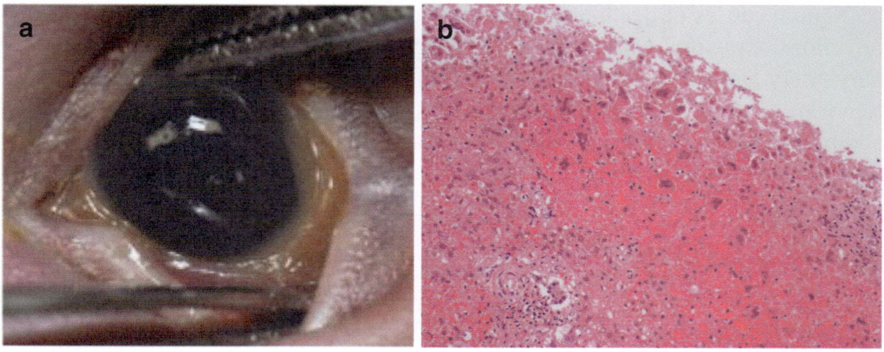

Fig. 13.8 Liver failure due to congenital herpes simplex infection involving the liver. (**a**) Scleral icterus (yellowing of the eye sclera). (**b**) Herpes virus was detected in the liver, H&E, 20×

chorioamnionitis can be associated with congenital pneumonia commonly due to bacterial organisms, TORCH infections and more recently Zika and Covid-19 viruses. TORCH infections are organisms that are caused by Toxoplasma gondii, rubella cytomegalovirus, syphilis, and herpes simplex virus (Fig. 13.8).

Deaths in Infancy

Deaths in infancy are those deaths that occur in the pediatric population during the first year of life. The majority of deaths in this population are unknown. In recent years there has been a shift from ascribing unknown causes of death in infants from "sudden infant syndrome" to undetermined. The term "sudden infant death syndrome" (SIDS) is used to describe an infant death where a full investigation of the scene, medical records, complete external and internal examinations, multiple ancillary investigations including histology, microbiological cultures, radiological examination, and toxicology testing, fail to identify a definite cause of death. Proffering a SIDS opinion as a cause of death implied that the manner of death was natural. However, collectively, these deaths are thought to represent a variety of underlying natural diseases, unrecognized asphyxial deaths, such as suffocation, or even hyperthermia from overheating. Many deaths of unknown cause involve an infant that was found dead in their crib, the so-called crib deaths. It has been shown that infants are more likely to die in their sleep if in the prone position (i.e. lying on their stomachs). The exact reason for prone sleeping as being a risk factor for infant death is unknown. Consequently, it is recommended that infants are placed in the supine position (i.e. lying on their backs) when put to bed in their cribs. In addition, to the position of the infant, there is growing interest in the sleeping environment of infants as a possible risk factor for death that include abundant bedding, bedsharing with others, cigarette smoke in the residence.

Natural causes of death among infants that can be identified at autopsy include infections, structural cardiac anomalies, including some types of congenital coronary artery anomalies, in addition to pediatric malignancy (cancer) such as Wilms' tumor of the kidney, hepatoblastoma of the liver, and retinoblastoma of the eye in addition leukemias of the blood, brain cancers, and bone cancers.

Sudden Infant Deaths

The certification of sudden unexpected deaths in infancy is an ongoing issue due to the lack of standardized classification of deaths in this age-group. Causes of death may be heterogenous in this group and can range from natural disease that is not ascertainable at autopsy and associated ancillary investigations to mechanical asphyxia.

Sudden infant death (SUID) also referred to as sudden death in infants (SUDI) applies to the death of an infant (less than 1 year old) in which the investigation, autopsy, medical history review, and appropriate laboratory testing do not identify a specific cause of death. This can include injuries of unknown significance and an "unsafe" sleep environment [19, 20]. The spectrum of findings for an "unsafe" sleeping environment is wide and includes prone sleeping position, type and quantity of bedding, others sleeping with the infant. The safest sleeping environment is an infant sleeping on their back, alone, in a crib. A single baby blanket is also considered safe. Sudden infant death syndrome (SIDS) falls under the classification of SUID/SUDI [19–21]. SIDS is the sudden death of an infant under 1 year of age that remains unexplained after a thorough case investigation, including performance of a complete autopsy, examination of the death scene, and review of the clinical history [22]. Risk factors for SIDS include:

- Low birth weight
- Premature
- Age: Most unexplained deaths in infants occur between 2 and 7 months [9, 23, 24]
- Sex: There are slightly more male infants. But this is not observed in Indigenous cultures in Australia, Alaska, United States, and New Zealand [24–38]
- Multiple gestation: Infants that were the product of multiple gestations often are also premature and of a lower birth rate
- Seasonal variance: In temperate zones, there is a higher incidence in the cooler months and may relate to increase circulating viruses
- Social determinants: The social economic status is known to affects mortality and morbidity in general but also includes infants

The autopsy findings are non-specific and often include petechial hemorrhages of the visceral pleura, epicardium, and thymus. Extensive histological sampling of organs and tissues, in addition to metabolic, vitreous biochemistry, toxicology, metabolic studies, radiographs, bacterial, and viral culture are non-contributory. Over time, there has been a wide variety of explanations. The current theory to explain sudden infant syndrome is the triple risk model that involves the intersection of the following risks [39]:

1. Vulnerable infant
2. Critical developmental period in homeostatic control
3. Exogenous stressors

Child Maltreatment

There are various definitions of child abuse but in general child maltreatment is an act, or failure to act, that results in death, serious physical, or emotional harm, sexual abuse or exploitation, or imminent risk of serious harm that involves a child. Pathologists, like other physicians, have an ethical and legal obligation to identify and report child abuse. During a pediatric autopsy, the pathologist needs to cognizant of abuse but also to think broadly and objectively about differential diagnoses that mimic abuse. At autopsy, a pathologist may see four types of abuse: physical, sexual, and neglect.

The approach is using the 5 steps of the autopsy. In the history phase of the autopsy, is considering if the history plausible to the autopsy findings; that the injuries align with the child's motor skills and milestones that are appropriated for the child's stage of development. The external examination in physical abuse may be unremarkable or shows multiple cutaneous bruises or other blunt force injuries and sometimes burns.

Although child abuse can be similar to homicides observed in adults, such as sharp force injuries, strangulation, and firearm injuries, blunt force injuries are more common in the pediatric cohort followed by burning and suffocation [40, 41, 44–46] Most pediatric homicides occur in children under the age of 3 years old [23]. Anatomically, the most common areas of fatal injuries involve the head followed by the abdomen [24, 47]. In the case of fatal child abuse, there is a legal component of exclusive opportunity. Indicating that there are a limited number of individuals that would have access to the child when the fatal injuries occurred. As the child will be in the care of a parent or another guardian in which the inference of fatal injuries is that the adult caregiver was responsible for these injuries if the timing of injuries intimately connected with the exclusive opportunity of that caregiver party?

For the pathologist, it may not always be clear if the injuries are accidental or non-accidental in nature based on the autopsy findings alone. Using causes of death that indicate that the cause of death in non-accidental in nature has pejorative and judgmental effect. For example, the term "shaken baby syndrome" is not diagnosis per se but a conclusion about why someone died. Shaken baby syndrome is an "event" rather than a diagnosis and the finding of abuse is a legal—not a medical—conclusion. It is preferable to use a more neutral description and leave legal issues around motive, etc. to others in the legal system. Although there are various patterns that may be concerning for child abuse, each case must be measured on its own merits and considers all of the relevant investigational information. Findings that may be concerning for child abuse include:

- Delay in seeking treatment for injuries and medical conditions
- Injuries that are not congruent with the provided history
- Injuries that are improbable or impossible with milestones
- Multiple severe injuries of various stages of healing

It is important for death investigation systems to recognize fatal child abuse to prevent the recurrence in other children but it is also equally important to not falsely accuse and convict parents or guardians where the injuries were accidental.

Child Abuse and Neglect

The determination of fatal child abuse and neglect is a challenge for the pathologist. Proffering opinions about injuries that are concerning for child abuse are not done in isolation. Instead they rely on a comprehensive death investigation. The pathological findings are interpreted in a holistic way that involves scene information, health history of the child, relevant ancillary investigations and where relevant special dissections and consultations are performed. Using a systemic, evidenced-based approach in collaboration with the death investigation team can lead to an accurate determination of the cause and manner of death.

The postmortem examination should be recorded such that the pertinent positive and negative findings are recorded in the written and visual record such that a peer review can be completed.

Malnourishment

Malnourishment can be due to natural causes or can be an indicator of abuse. Natural causes to consider include structural anomalies of the oral cavity and along the gastrointestinal tract, malignancy, malabsorption diseases such as celiac disease, cystic fibrosis, diabetes, and congenital heart disease. Starvation is a type of malnourishment, which can be a deliberate act or an indicator of neglect by the caregiver. It can also be a manifestation of extreme poverty without adequate social supports. For example, prolonged breastfeeding without adequate supplementation or overdilution of formula can lead to failure to thrive can be the result inaccessible formula. Malnutrition can also be related to low-protein diets or diets that are overly restrictive. Infants and children are vulnerable to starvation because of their inability to independently obtain food. Malnourished infants and children are vulnerable to acquiring infections. The mechanisms of death can include arrhythmia, hypoglycemia, and ketoacidosis. Previous episodes of malnourishment but also disease may be observed as growth arrest lines in the long bones (Fig. 13.9).

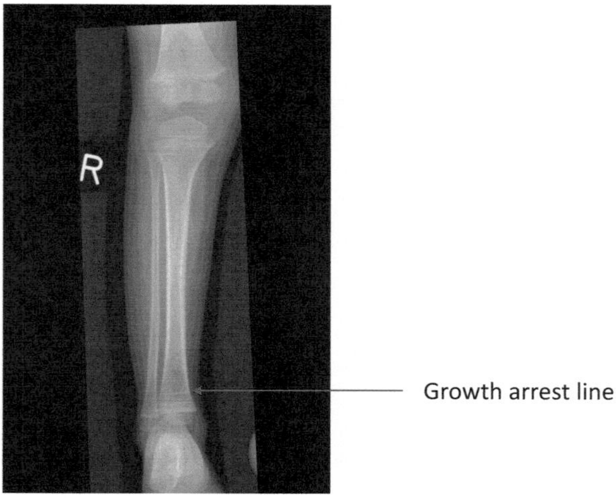

Fig. 13.9 Radiograph showing growth arrest lines that is readily apparent as traverse lines of the three long bones (femur, tibia and fibula) of the right leg. These sclerotic (white) lines indicate increased bone density at the position of the growth plate at the time of stress during bone development. Stress that can cause growth arrest lines include periods of disease and malnutrition

Autopsy findings that may indicate malnourishment include:

1. Decreased body weight which results in prominence of bones of the face, ribs, and pelvis
2. Signs of dehydration: sunken eyes, sunken fontanelles, desiccated tissues, hypernatremia, on vitreous biochemistry
3. Skin may have a wrinkled appearance due to dehydration and loss of subcutaneous adipose (fat) tissue
4. Thin brittle hair
5. Dental caries
6. Loss of adipose tissue
7. Muscle atrophy
8. Decreased visceral organ weights
9. Atrophy/involution of the thymus
10. Hepatic steatosis (Fatty liver)
11. Stomach and bowels are empty; however, desiccated stool may be present

There are a number of classification systems that can be used to classify the degree of malnutrition. The Gomez classification examines the body weight and length for age [48], the Waterlow classification determines stunted growth and wasting also based on body length and weight [49] and the Welcome's classification assess weight but also the presence of edema [25]. Malnutrition can also be divided into kwashiorkor, where the protein malnourishment accompanies edema, and marasmus, where the protein malnourishment is without edema.

Spectrum of Injuries

At autopsy, the spectrum of injuries can be highly variable depending on the type of trauma inflicted on the infant or child. Given that blunt force injuries are the most common mode of trauma, the recognition of this type of fatal injury may range from being obvious externally or the complete absence of any external injuries despite massive fatal internal injuries [26].

Injuries to the Skin

Bruising to the skin is one of the more common injuries observed in child abuse [50]. Concerning injuries to the skin include:

1. **Patterned injuries:** The patterned surface or the features of the implement that impacted the body can leave a patterned injury on the skin. These include rods, shoes, human and animal bites, etc. Bite marks are characterized by two opposing arcs of bruises or abrasions. Seeking an opinion from a dentist with training in forensics can be helpful in the determination of patterned injuries thought to be due to human bite marks. Collection of a DNA swab for any bite mark may ascertain the source of the patterned injury.
2. **Injuries at different time intervals:** Determination of time interval between bruising and death is suggested to be based on different colors of bruises. The different colors of bruises, red, blue, purple, brown, green, and yellow suggest different stages of healing and therefore the result of separate traumatic results. Based on colour, yellow bruises are the only bruises that have shown certainty on timing based on macroscopic evaluation (See Antemortem injuries in the Blunt Trauma chapter). Histological evaluation of a bruise can determine the age by assessing for hemorrhage, inflammation, and other signs of healing. It is good practice to sample for histology the periphery with adjacent normal skin because this is where the most advanced inflammatory response often lies.
3. **Distribution of injuries:** The distribution of bruises, abrasions (scrapes), and lacerations (tears) should correlate with the history provided. A history of a fall would include that the protuberant areas of the body could be bruised including the bony prominence of the forehead, tip of nose, posterior elbow, knees, and shins. Blunt force trauma around the eyes, in the absence of a basal skull fracture of the anterior cranial fossa or other explanation, ears, lips, oral mucosa, neck, backs of hands, thighs, buttocks, genitals, and soles of feet are concerning for child abuse [50].

Burns

Like other injuries, burns can be a result of child abuse or accidental that are often classified as contact burns and scalding. Contact burns are the result of a hot object against the skin [51]. The injury will be well demarcated and can be patterned. Contact burns suggestive of a cigarette burn have a discoid appearance of a few millimeters. Scalding is a burn from a hot liquid. Immersion into bathtub with hot water can show symmetrical burns of the buttocks and lower extremities often with sparing in the flexed area of the body such as the groin as flexing the lower extremities is a natural defense response when scalded. Unilateral scalding can occur when a hand or foot is forced into hot water. Mimickers of burns include dermatitis, impetigo, and epidermolysis bullosa [27].

Osseus (Skeletal) Injuries

At autopsy, the skull, hyoid bone, vertebral bodies, chest, and pelvic cavities are routinely directly examined. The remainder of the skeletal system is not routinely directly examined. Consequently, it is standard practice to perform a radiological skeletal survey prior to the internal examination to determine for the presence of recent and healing fractures, in addition to the presence of congenital anomalies and diseases. This allows radiological examination of the skeletal system, and allows for a focused macroscopic and microscopic examination of osseus injuries that would otherwise would not be directly examined.

The skeletal system in the pediatric population differs from adults in terms changing anatomic structure due to evolving maturation and development [52]. These include higher elasticity, thicker periosteum, thinner bone, and the presence of growth plates. These can result in different osseous injuries that are not observed in skeletally mature individuals, such as classic metaphyseal lesions and green stick fractures.

If there has been a hospital admission, a bone radionuclide scintiscan or bone scan may be performed that was the advantage of detecting early fractures but may be confused with growth plates [28].

Radiological studies play a role in identifying recent or healing injuries. Skeletal injury is present in about a third of abused children, often in children under the age of 2 years [29]. Things to consider in determining the nature of skeletal injuries include the context, past medical history, location, quantity, and spectrum of healing. Fractures that are concerning, but not diagnostic, for child abuse include multiple fractures of various ages, classic metaphyseal fractures, spiral fractures, and posterior rib fractures. The mechanism of injury of the classic metaphyseal fracture is the most concerning because the mechanism of injury is due to traction or torsion of the growth plate of a long bone. Some consider that this fracture in young children as diagnostic for child abuse as it usually does not arise accidentally.

Microscopically, there is disruption of the trans-metaphyseal in the sub-physeal area [30]. Spiral fracture is a diaphyseal fracture that is more frequently observed than classic metaphyseal fractures [31]. The mechanism of injury is due to the twisting of a limb. This can arise accidentally from a fall; however, in non-ambulatory (non-walking) children, this fracture is concerning for abuse. Rib fractures can be accidental, from cardiopulmonary resuscitation chest compressions, intrinsic bone diseases, or abuse. A systematic literature review of autopsy and clinical studies found that the cardiovascular (CPR) and thoracic injury rate following standard CPR ranged from 32 to 45% [32]. It rose to 58–75% with active compression-decompression (ACD) devices, and up to 100% when standard CPR was followed by ACD-CPR. Major injuries occurred in up to 3% and 7% of CPR-treated pediatric and adult patients, respectively. Hoke et al. found no difference in the adverse effects from CPR administered by lay and trained individuals. The incidence of rib fractures based on autopsy data was 12.9–96.6% following conventional CPR [33]. Sternal fractures ranged from 1.3 to 31% [33]. Bilateral fracture of the second to seventh ribs along the mid-clavicular line is a common pattern [34]. Costochondral junction separation is less frequent [32]. Clavicle and vertebral fractures are rare [32]. The sternum is typically fractured at the level of the fourth ribs [32, 33]. Rib fractures tend to be left-sided [33], but fracture distribution can vary due to hand placement. The average number of fractures ranges usually from six to eight [33]. The risk of fractures and CPR-related injuries increases in older individuals and during long CPR [35]. CPR in infants and children seldom results in fractures [36–38]. In a review of four autopsy studies of CPR in children (0–240 mo. of age), rib fractures were found in 0 to 2.1%. [33]. Posterior rib fractures have been observed in infants when two-handed CPR has been applied [53, 54]. Birth-related posterior rib fractures are rare and are associated with macrosomia and shoulder dystocia [16, 44].

The detection of rib fractures can be subtle in infants, especially those that are fresh, linear, and non-displaced. Consideration of oblique radiological views of the ribcage can facilitate the detection of rib fractures that are not always visible on lateral (sides) and anteroposterior (front to back) views of the chest. During the internal examination, stripping the parietal pleura will facilitate visualizing the fracture because the pleural surface overlying the fracture may be intact and obscure the fracture. Although resuscitation-related rib fractures are uncommon, these are typically parasternal, anterior, and/or anterolateral [36].

Head Injuries

Head injuries result in the most common traumatic cause of death in children. Head injuries that exhibit an impact site in the form of a scalp injury and/or skull fracture that are also associated with bleeding of the subdural space, retina and with hypoxic-ischemic encephalopathy are more readily explainable. However, the pattern or “triad” of subdural hemorrhage (SDH), retinal hemorrhages (RHs), and encephalopathy [hypoxic-ischemic encephalopathy (HIE), cerebral edema] has been ascribed to infants who present in cardio-respiratory arrest and are thought to have been shaken. This collection of findings is sometimes referred to a Shaken Baby Syndrome (SBS) and is a controversial area in medicine. A brief summary of some issues follows.

Early authors linked subdural hemorrhage with certain extracranial injuries (e.g., long bone fracture) and considered that any infant with these findings who died suddenly was a victim of "the battered-child syndrome" [45, 46]. Guthkelch proposed that cases of SDH from proved or suspected assault that had no external evidence of direct head impact could have been shaken [55]. Due to the relatively large head and weak neck muscles, an infant's brain was vulnerable to acceleration/deceleration from repetitively jerking the body in an anterior-posterior direction while holding the child at the chest and/or limbs. Guthkelch wrote that all cases of infantile SDH were "best assumed to be traumatic unless proved otherwise." In 1972, Caffey added that long bony traction injuries ("metaphyseal avulsions") could occur in whiplash-shaken infants and that bilateral SDHs and intraocular hemorrhages in the absence of external head and neck trauma could be explained by whiplash [56, 57].

Biomechanical studies were divided on whether shaking alone or shaking with head impact ("shaken impact syndrome") was necessary to generate the forces resulting in the triad [58–60]. The American Academy of Pediatrics (AAP) Committee on Child Abuse and Neglect wrote that a combination of shaking and blunt impact, as well as shaking could cause neurologic injury [61]. The AAP recommended "abusive head trauma" (AHT) as a "less mechanistic term", but this term was criticized because it still had an etiological implication [61, 62]. Evidence of head impact (e.g., scalp injury, skull fracture) or other trauma indicative of forcible chest compression (finger impressions, rib fractures) were considered signs that an infant could have been shaken [63, 64]. The National Association of Medical Examiners Ad Hoc Committee on SBS wrote that the lack of physical signs of head trauma was explained by impact occurring on a broad or padded surface [65]. Hyperextension of the cervical spine resulting in neck injuries from violent shaking could damage the underlying respiratory control centers in the brainstem leading to apnea and cardio-respiratory arrest [66].

Geddes et al. proposed a "unified hypothesis" that severe hypoxia, brain swelling, and increased intracranial pressure from any cause of apnea [e.g., Apparent Life-threatening Event = ALTE or Brief Resolved Unexplained Event = BRUE] could lead to leakage of blood from oxygen-deprived intracranial veins and cerebral blood vessels. This could explain not only the presence of intradural (IDH) and thin-film subdural hemorrhage but also cerebral edema in apparent SBS cases [67–70]. Interference of blood flow from the eyes by cerebral edema could account for peri-optic nerve sheath and retinal hemorrhages. Postmortem studies of fetuses, infants, and children up to 3 years old found a statistically significant association between SDH and HIE [71]. IDH and SDH were more common in infants under 1 month corrected age, but rarely these hemorrhages were found in the absence of trauma in children aged 1 month to 3 years. Geddes et al. suggested that for "triad only" cases, a descriptive non-etiological diagnosis—"infantile encephalopathy with subdural and retinal bleeding"—be used. The Geddes hypothesis predicts that RH and SDH occur after brain swelling in contrast to the SBS hypothesis that bleeding occurs at the time of the traumatic incident [70]. Time may elapse following an infant's collapse and subsequent resuscitation before there is expert assessment of the retina and Computed tomography scan of the brain to assess the meninges [70].

Lynoe et al. in a systematic SBS medical literature review of the diagnostic accuracy of the "triad"(SDH, RHs, encephalopathy) observed in infants up to 12 months of age concluded that there was insufficient scientific evidence to assess the diagnostic accuracy of the "triad" in the identification of trauma arising from shaking [72]. The authors wrote that the main reason the scientific evidence linking the "triad" with traumatic shaking was of "low quality" was due to circular or self-fulfilling medical reasoning. If the triad was present, and no other acceptable explanations were provided by a caregiver, then physicians concluded that the infant had been shaken. A caregiver's credibility was considered suspect when an initial statement about the denial of shaking was followed by an admission to it in response to the infant's distress (dyspnea or apnea, loss of consciousness) [62].

In response to Lynoe et al., a consensus statement was published stating that the diagnosis of an inflicted head injury is reliable provided an appropriate multidisciplinary workup has been carried out even in those triad cases lacking scalp and/or skull trauma [73, 74]. The American Academy of Pediatrics had specified a range of clinical specialties involved on the diagnostic team [75], but forensic pathologists were not mentioned.

Abdominal Injuries

Following head injuries, abdominal injuries are the second most common cause of traumatic death [76]. Anatomically, the abdominal wall in children is more vulnerable to trauma of the abdominal organs because the muscles of the abdominal wall are thinner, the omentum is thinner and the liver and spleen have less protection from the overlying ribs. Blunt force trauma is a common mechanism of injury and can cause crushing, shearing, and barotrauma to the viscus and solid organs. The solid organs can be crushed against the vertebral bones, thorax, and pelvic bones. The intestines can lacerate due to the sudden increase in intraluminal pressure [76]. Shearing forces can cause lacerations of the mesentery, and viscus [76]. The liver and small bowel are the most commonly injured.

Thoracic Injuries

Fatal thoracic injuries are rare but can result in cardiac lacerations (Fig. 13.10), pneumothorax, chylothorax, pulmonary contusions, and lacerations. Intrathoracic injuries are usually associated with rib fractures [77].

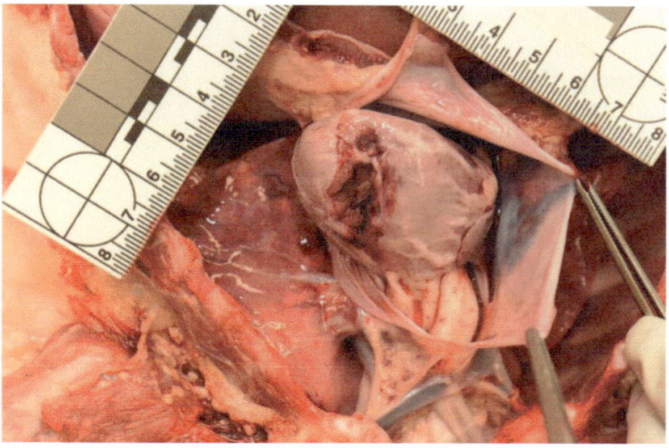

Fig. 13.10 Lacerations of an infant heart due to blunt impact trauma to the chest. There were no external injuries

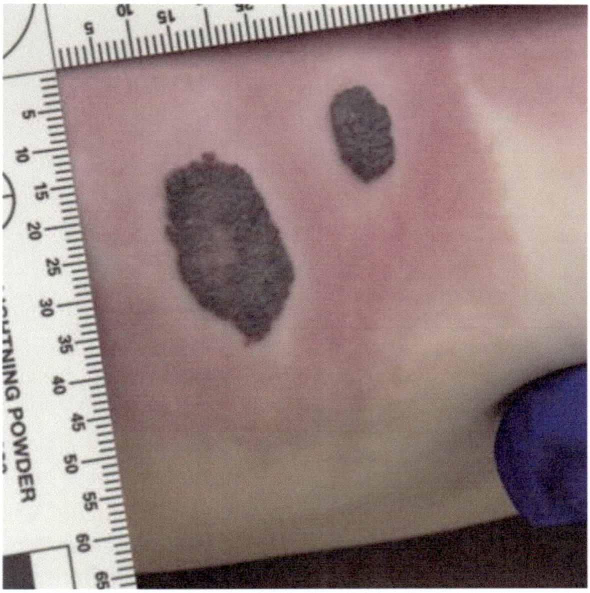

Fig. 13.11 Cutaneous lesions can be mistaken as bruise. Shown are two hemangiomas of the back

Mimickers of Child Abuse

The literature is filled with examples of medical mimics of child abuse (Figs. 13.11, 13.12, 13.13, 13.14). Differentiating these medical conditions from abuse requires an awareness of uncommon diseases, common diseases with uncommon presentations, willingness to consider alternative diagnoses, recognition of biases that can affect medical decision-making and incorporating an objective and rational approach in evaluating the medical evidence.

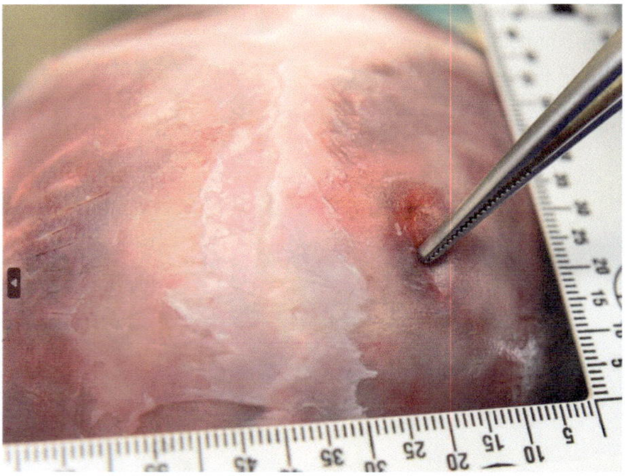

Fig. 13.12 Craniotabes of the infant skull is a focal area of softening of the skull, typically of the parietal bone and can be bilaterally. This finding is often related to prematurity

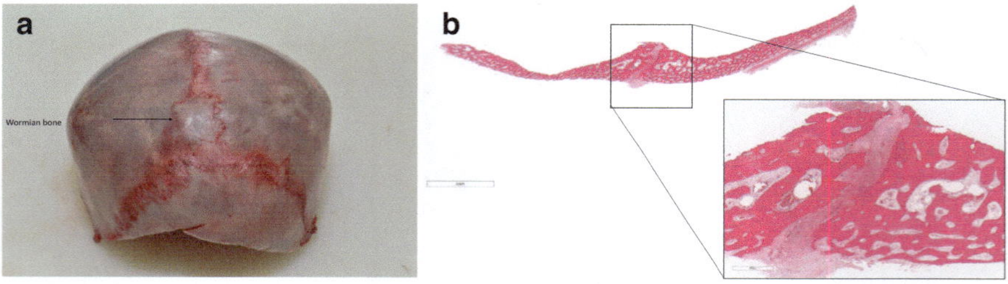

Fig. 13.13 A Wormian bone adjacent to the occipital bone of the skull that can be mistaken as a skull fracture at autopsy and by radiography. Histology can facilitate differentiating between the two. (**a**) Macrocopic view. (**b**) Microscopic view of suture, H&E. Inset is higher power image of the suture

Cutaneous mimics of abuse include coagulation disorders, connective tissue diseases, and inflammatory responses. Coagulation disorders can cause more extensive bleeding, which may result in more and larger bruises than children without a coagulation disorder. Coagulation disorders can be heritable or acquired. The heritable coagulation disorders that can undergo genetic testing postmortem include hemophilia A and B. A family history of bleeding disorders can direct investigations. There are other coagulation studies that can be performed but requires antemortem samples. If there is a hospital admission blood sample, often a coagulation panel and history is obtained. Acquired coagulation disorders include aplastic anemia, liver disease, and infections. These can be assessed by microscopic examination of the bone marrow and liver. Routine samples of blood and lung in addition to a nasopharyngeal swab can be sent for microbiological studies such as bacterial cultures and viral PCR (polymerase chain reaction) studies.

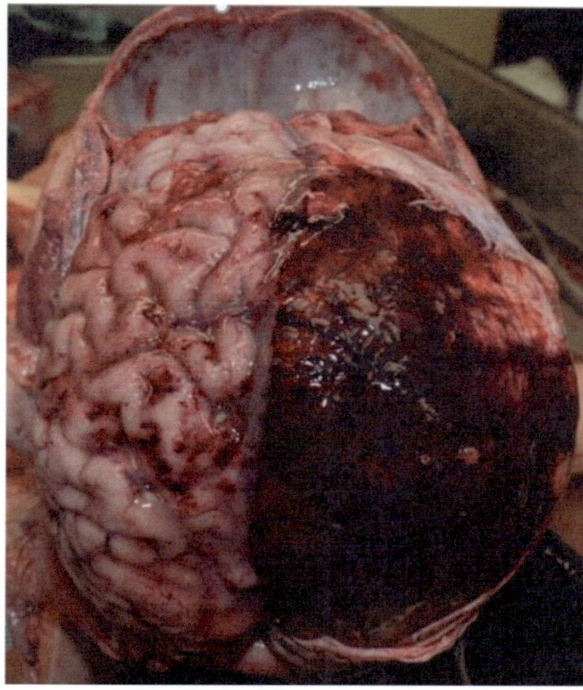

Fig. 13.14 Subdural hemorrhage due to infection in a young child

Connective tissue disorders can manifest as bruising and other skin injuries. Heritable connective tissue disorders such as Ehlers-Danlos syndrome (EDS) has a spectrum of manifestations that are subclassified into different types that is characterized by joint hypermobility, hyperextensibility and fragility of the skin, internal organs, and blood vessels. EDS is rarely diagnosed in infants but is usually confused with abuse in young school-aged children [78]. Rarely EDS can present with fractures that has been described as a mixed EDS and Osteogenesis phenotype [79]. Acquired vitamin C (ascorbic acid) deficiency can also lead to skin fragility, including bruising and and gingival (gum) disease [80].

Diseases that make bones vulnerable to fractures are those that affect collagen and bone mineralization, skeletal dysplasias, inborn errors of metabolism, prematurity, infection, and neoplasia. Many of these diseases are inheritable and can be distinguished from abuse based on history, radiographic findings, histology, and other investigations [81]. Histological examination of the ossification center can detect anomalies (i.e., rib with the costochondral junction) related to rickets, osteogenesis imperfecta, osteomalacia, and scurvy. The proximal femur functions as a preferable location to identify dysplasias in younger infants because of the broader surface area and ossification center (Fig. 13.15).

Fractures of the metaphysis, posterior ribs, scapula, and spinous process are concerning for abuse.

Fig. 13.15 To look for change of dysplasia the proximal femur has a broader ossification and is better to assess

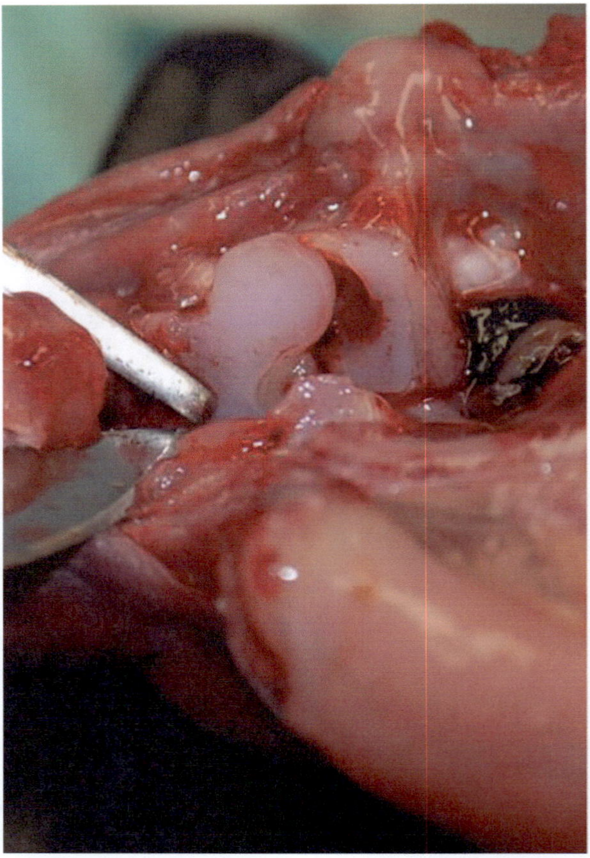

Osteogenesis Imperfecta

Osteogenesis imperfecta (OI) is one of the most common inherited diseases that predisposes to fractures. OI is caused by a genetic mutation that is responsible for collagen production. The severity and manifestation of OI are variable and can include blue sclera, multiple fractures from minor trauma (Fig. 13.16), and dentinogenesis imperfecta. Given this variability and that fractures in OI can arise in areas of the body that are suspicious for abuse, OI is commonly misinterpreted as abuse [82]. Especially in individuals whose phenotype shows the classic stigmata of OI.

Caffey Disease

Caffey disease is a rare inflammatory disorder of the bone and soft tissue that is due to a genetic mutation in one of the collagen genes that arises in the first months of life. Radiographs may be cortical thickening and new marked subperiosteal bone

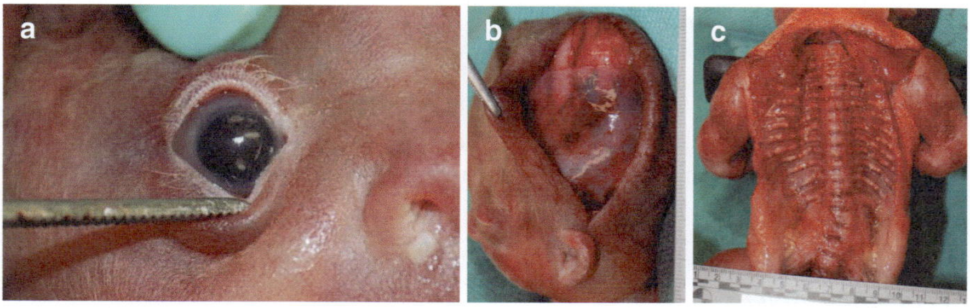

Fig. 13.16 External and internal features of osteogenis imperfecta. (**a**) Blue sclera. (**b**) Skull is not ossified. (**c**) Innumerable rib fractures and shortened upper limbs due to multiple fractures

formation that typically involves the ascending ramus and angle of the mandible (jaw) but can also include the clavicle, scapula, skull, ilium, and diaphysis of the long bones [83].

Osteopathy of Prematurity

Osteopathy of prematurity is a metabolic bone disease of premature infants that arises due to sub-optimal bone matrix development. Premature infants, typically under 32 weeks gestation, and with low birth weights are at risk of developing fracture-associated osteopathy [84]. In addition, chronic lung disease, chronic parental nutrition, diuretic treatment and liver disease [84]. Fractures typically involve the diaphyseal long bones and anywhere along the rib arc and can be multiple.

Rickets

Rickets is a metabolic bone disease that results in the failure of bone mineralization in new bone [85]. The radiographic and histological features can make the determination rickets. Histologically, rickets show marked architectural disorganization of the endochondral ossification of the costochondral junctions and growth plates of long bones [86]. Vitamin D deficiency is a common cause of rickets and the levels be tested in postmortem blood. Rickets are not associated with a higher risk of fractures in particular bone types.

Hyper IgE Syndrome

Hyper IgE syndrome is a rare primary immunodeficiency disease due to a mutation that impairs cytokine signaling [87]. At autopsy, atopic dermatitis, staphylococcal abscesses, and pneumonia in addition to fractures of the long bones and ribs [88].

Metabolic Diseases

Inherited metabolic diseases are due to inherited mutations in the enzymes or cofactors needed to metabolize protein, carbohydrates, or fats. These mutations impact the metabolic pathways typically due to absent, deficient, or insufficient enzymatic activity. At autopsy, features that are suggestive of a metabolic disease include a range of dysmorphic features such as microcephaly (small head), micrognathia (small chin), anteverted nares (nostrils), hepatomegaly, cardiomegaly, hepatosteatosis among others. However, dysmorphic features can be subtle and not always appreciated with fetuses or small infants. Some countries perform a screening test for metabolic diseases at the time of delivery for all neonates. Similarly, some death investigation jurisdictions submit blood and bile samples for metabolic testing in infant deaths with no explained cause of death at autopsy. A few drops of whole blood and bile onto filter paper (i.e., a Guthrie card) is the most convenient method of collection.

Toxicology

Toxicological deaths in younger pediatric populations are rare in countries' that improved medicine safety such as child-resistant closures. Toxicological investigations in the pediatric population pose a number of challenges. In the younger pediatric population, the blood volume is much smaller, there are multiple competing investigations that require a blood sample, and limited scientific data on the impacts of substances on children. Consequently, a smaller sample of blood is available for toxicological analysis. Further, many substances such as carbon monoxide, ethanol, and methanol are very toxic to the younger pediatric population due to their small size and naïve drug status [89]. This population is also physiologically vulnerable to medicines such as Reye's syndrome due to the administration of aspirin, especially in the setting of a viral infection. In addition, are the confounding effects of substances and drugs passing in utero and breast milk. The effects of in utero exposure of maternal opioids can lead to neonatal abstinence syndrome.

Summary

Pediatric deaths often bring intense public interest. The patterns of injury and disease are unique to this cohort as they have evolving maturities and physiologies. Both the triad cases and sudden unexpected deaths remain the most problematic in forensic pathology as these deaths largely remained unexplained. Further research and reflection are required to arrive at the truth of why these young children die.

References

1. World Health Organization. Trends and Levels in Child Mortality. United Nations Children's Fund; 2019.
2. Cohen MC, Scheimberg I. Forensic aspects of perinatal deaths. Acad Forensic Pathol. 2018;8(3):452–91.
3. Incerpi MH, et al. Stillbirth evaluation: what tests are needed? Am J Obstet Gynecol. 1998;178:1121–5.
4. Anonymous. Management of stillbirth: obstetric consensus. Obstet Gynecol. 2020;135(3):e110–32.
5. Hanzlick R, Parrrish RG. The role of medical examiners and coroners in public health and surveillance and epidemiologic research. Annu Rev Public Health. 1996;17:383–409.
6. Generst DR, et al. Estimating the time of death in stillborn fetuses: I histological evaluation of fetal organs: an autopsy study of 150 stillborns. Obstet Gynecol. 1992;80:575–84.
7. Conway DL, et al. An algorithm for the estimation of gestational age at the time of fetal death. Pediatr Perinatal Epidemiol. 2013;27(2):145–57.
8. Van der Harten, et al. The prenatal development of the normal human skeleton: a combined ultrasonographic and postmortem radiographic study. Pediatr Radiol. 1990:52–6.
9. Genest DR, Singer DB. Estimating the time of death in stillborn foetuses: III. External fetal examination: a study of 86 stillborns. Obster Gynecol. 1992;80(4):593–600.
10. Baergen RN. Umbilical cord pathology. Surg Pathol Clin. 2017;6(1):61–85.
11. Neri M, et al. Stillborn or liveborn? Comparing umbilical cord immunohistochemical expression of vitality markers (typtase, alpha(1)-antichymotrypsin and CD68) by quantitative analysis and confocal laser scanning microscopy. Pathol Res Pract. 2009;205(8):534–41.
12. Kuroda S, et al. Medicolegal studies in the fetus and infant with special reference to the histological characteristics of the lungs of liveborn and stillborn infants. Tohoku J Exp Med. 1965;85:40–54.
13. Unzila AA, Norwitz ER. Vacuum-assisted vaginal delivery. Rev Obstet Gynecol. 2009;2(1):5–17.
14. Davis DJ. Neonatal subgaleal haemorrhage: diagnosis and management. CMAJ. 2001;164(10):1452–3.
15. Högberg U, et al. Difficult birth is the main contributor to birth-related fracture and accidents to other neonatal fractures. Acta Paediatr. 2020;109:2040–8.
16. van Rijn RR, et al. Birth-related mid-posterior rib fractures in neonates: a report of three cases (and a possible fourth case) and a review of the literature. Pediatr Radiol. 2009;39:30–4.
17. Walters MM, et al. Healing patterns of clavicular birth injuries as a guide to fracture dating in cases of possible infant abuse. Pediatr Radiol. 2014;44:1224–9.
18. Lee GS, et al. Classic metaphyseal lesion of distal tibia following footling breech delivery. Pediatr Radiol. 2019;49(13):1840–2.
19. Corey TS, et al. NAME Ad Hoc Committee on Sudden Unexplained Infant Death. A functional approach to sudden unexplained infant deaths. Am J Forensic Med Pathol. 2007;28:271–7.

20. Shapiro-Mendoza CK, et al. Classification system for the sudden unexpected infant death case registry and its application. Pediatrics. 2014;134:e210–1.
21. Krous HF, et al. Sudden infant death syndrome and unclassified sudden infant deaths: a definitional and diagnostic approach. Pediatrics. 2014;134:e210–9.
22. Willinger M, et al. Defining the sudden infant death syndrome (SIDS): deliberations of an expert panel convened by the National Institute of Child Health and Human Development. Pediatr Pathol. 1991;11:677–84.
23. Vanezis P. Interpreting bruises at microscopy. J Clin Pathol. 2001;54:348–55.
24. Pinneri K, Matshes E. Recommendations for the autopsy of an infant who has died suddenly and unexpectedly. Acad Forensic Pathol. 2017;7:171–81.
25. Bhattacharyy AK. Protein-energy malnutrition (Kwashiorkor-Marasmus syndrome): terminology, classification, and evolution. World Rev Nutr Diet. 1986;47:80–133.
26. Klotzbatch H, et al. Postmortem diagnosis and age estimation of infants' fractures. Int J Leg Med. 2003;117:82–9.
27. Patel B, Butterfield R. Common skin and bleeding disorders that can potentially masquerade as child abuse. Am J Med Genet C Semin Med Genet. 2015;169:328–36.
28. Conway JJ, et al. The role of bone scintigraphy in detecting child abuse. Semin Nucl Med. 1993;23:321–33.
29. Merten DF, et al. The abused child: a radiological reappraisal. Radiology. 1983;146:370–81.
30. Walker A, et al. Are there hallmarks of child abuse? I. Osseus injuries. Acad Forensic Pathol. 2016;6(4):568–90.
31. Leonidas JC. Skeletal trauma in child abuse syndrome. Pediatr Ann. 1983;12:875–81.
32. Miller AC, et al. A systematic review and pooled analysis of CPR-associated cardiovascular and thoracic injuries. Resuscitation. 2014;85(6):724–31.
33. Hoke RS, Chamberlain D. Skeletal chest injuries secondary to cardiopulmonary resuscitation. Resuscitation. 2004;63(3):327–38.
34. Yang KM, Lynch M, O'Donnell C. "Buckle" rib fracture: an artifact following cardiopulmonary resuscitation detected on postmortem CT. Leg Med (Tokyo). 2011;13(5):233–9.
35. Ram P, et al. Breaking your heart—a review on CPR-related injuries. Am J Emerg Med. 2018;36(5):838–42.
36. Maguire S, Mann M, John N, Ellaway B, Sibert JR, Kemp AM, Welsh Child Protection Systematic Review Group. Does cardiopulmonary resuscitation cause rib fractures in children? A systematic review. Child Abuse Negl. 2006;30(7):739–51.
37. Weber MA, Risdon RA, Offiah AC, Malone M, Sebire NJ. Rib fractures identified at postmortem examination in sudden unexpected deaths in infancy (SUDI). Forensic Sci Int. 2009;189(1–3):75–81.
38. Matshes EW, Lew EO. Two-handed cardiopulmonary resuscitation can cause rib fractures in infants. Am J Forensic Med Pathol. 2010;31(4):303–7.
39. Guntheroth WG, Spiers PS. The triple risk hypothesis in sudden infant death syndrome. Pediatrics. 2022;110(5):e64. https://doi.org/10.1542/peds.110.5.e64.
40. Tieder JS, et al. Clinical practice guideline: brief resolved unexplained events (formerly apparent life-threatening events) and evaluation of lower-risk infants: executive summary. Pediatrics. 2016;137(5):e20160591.
41. Byard RW. Unexpected infant death: lessons from Sally Clark case. Med J Aust. 2004;181:52–4.
42. Green FC. Child abuse and neglect: a priority problem for the private physician. Pediatr Clin North Am. 1975;22:329–39.
43. Pollanen MS, et al. Fatal child abuse-maltreatment syndrome. A retrospective study in Ontario, Canada. 1990–1992. Forensic Sci Int. 2002;126:101–4.
44. Lonergan GJ, Baker AM, Morey MK, Boos SC. From the archives of the AFIP. Child abuse: radiologic-pathologic correlation. Radiographics. 2003;23(4):811–45.
45. Caffey J. Multiple fractures in the long bones of infants suffering from chronic subdural hematoma. Am J Roentgenol Radium Ther. 1946;56(2):163–73.

46. Kempe CH, Silverman FN, Steele BF, et al. The battered-child syndrome. JAMA. 1962;181(1):17–24.
47. Akbarnia B, et al. Manifestations of the battered-child syndrome. J Bone Joint Surg Am. 1974;56:1159–66.
48. Gomez F, et al. Malnutrition in infancy and childhood, with special reference to Kwashiorkor. Adv Pediatr. 1955;7:131–69.
49. Madea B, et al. Forensic aspects of starvation. Forensic Sci Med Pathol. 2016;12:276–98.
50. Maguire, et al. Are there patterns of bruising in childhood which are diagnostic or suggestive of abuse. A systematic review. Arch Dis Child. 2005;90:182–6.
51. Tsokos M. Diagnostic criteria for cutaneous injuries in child abuse: classification, findings and interpretation. Forensic Sci Med Pathol. 2015;11:235–42.
52. Ross AH, Juraez CA. Skeletal and radiological manifestations of child abuse: Implications for study in past populations. Clin Anat NYN. 2016;29:844–53.
53. Duval JV, Andrew TA. Two thumb method of infant CPR: Is there an increased risk for posterior rib fractures? Paper presented at National Association of Medical Examiners 41st Annual Meeting, Savannah, Georgia; 2007.
54. Clouse JR, Lantz PE. Posterior rib fractures in infants associated with cardiopulmonary resuscitation. Paper presented at American Academy of Forensic Sciences Annual Meeting, Washington, DC; 2008.
55. Guthkelch AN. Infantile subdural haematoma and its relationship to whiplash injuries. 2. British Med J. 1971:430–1.
56. Caffey J. On the theory and practice of shaking infants. Its potential residual effects of permanent brain damage and mental retardation. Am J Dis Child. 1972;124(2):161–9.
57. Caffey J. The whiplash shaken infant syndrome: manual shaking by the extremities with whiplash-induced intracranial and intraocular bleedings, linked with residual permanent brain damage and mental retardation. Pediatrics. 1974;54(4):396–403.
58. Duhaime AC, Gennarelli TA, Thibault LE, Bruce DA, Margulies SS, Wiser R. The shaken baby syndrome. A clinical, pathological, and biomechanical study. J Neurosurg. 1987;66(3):409–15.
59. Bruce DA, Zimmerman RA. Shaken impact syndrome. Pediatr Ann. 1989;18(8):482–94.
60. Cory CZ, Jones BM. Can shaking alone cause fatal brain injury? A biomechanical assessment of the Duhaime shaken baby syndrome model. Med Sci Law. 2003;43(4):317–33.
61. Christian CW, Block R, Committee on Child Abuse and Neglect, American Academy of Pediatrics. Abusive head trauma in infants and children. Pediatrics. 2009;123(5):1409–11.
62. Elinder G, Eriksson A, Hallberg B, Lynøe N, Sundgren PM, Rosén M, Engström I, Erlandsson BE. Traumatic shaking: the role of the triad in medical investigations of suspected traumatic shaking. Acta Paediatr. 2018;107(Suppl 472):3–23.
63. Nelson EL, Melton LJ 3rd, Annegers JF, Laws ER, Offord KP. Incidence of skull fractures in Olmsted County, Minnesota. Neurosurgery. 1984;15(3):318–24.
64. Gurdial ES, Gurdjian ES. Acute head injury: a review. Surg Annu. 1980;12:223–41.
65. Gurdjian ES. Impact head injury: Mechanistic, clinical and preventive correlations. Springfield, IL: Charles C. Thomas; 1975.
66. Matschke J, Büttner A, Bergmann M, et al. Encephalopathy and death in infants with abusive head trauma is due to hypoxic-ischemic injury following local brain trauma to vital brainstem centers. Int J Leg Med. 2015;129(1):105–14.
67. Geddes JF, Whitwell HL. Inflicted head injury in infants. Forensic Sci Int. 2004;146(2–3):83–8.
68. Geddes JF, Tasker RC, Hackshaw AK, et al. Dural haemorrhage in non-traumatic infant deaths: does it explain the bleeding in 'shaken baby syndrome'? [published correction appears in Neuropathol Appl Neurobiol. 2003;29(3):322]. Neuropathol Appl Neurobiol. 2003;29(1):14–22.
69. Lynøe N, Eriksson A. Is there a common denominator for brief resolved unexplained events, sudden infant death syndrome, and alleged shaken baby syndrome? Med Hypotheses. 2020; https://doi.org/10.1016/j.mehy.2020.10993.

70. Acres MJ, Morris JA. The pathogenesis of retinal and subdural haemorrhage in non-accidental head injury in infancy: assessment using Bradford Hill criteria. Med Hypotheses. 2014;82(1):1–5.
71. Scheimberg I, Cohen MC, Zapata Vazquez RE, et al. Nontraumatic intradural and subdural hemorrhage and hypoxic ischemic encephalopathy in fetuses, infants, and children up to three years of age: analysis of two audits of 636 cases from two referral centers in the United Kingdom. Pediatr Dev Pathol. 2013;16(3):149–59.
72. Lynoe N. et al. Insifficnent eveidence for 'shaken baby syndrome' - a systematic review. Acta Peadiatr. 2017;106(7):1021–7.
73. Choudhary AK, Servaes S, Slovis TL, et al. Consensus statement on abusive head trauma in infants and young children. Pediatr Radiol. 2018;48(8):1048–65.
74. Choudhary, et al. 2019 Endorsements of consensus statement on abusive head injury. Pediatr Radiol. 2019;49:421.
75. American Academy of Pediatrics Committee on Child Abuse and Neglect. Shaken baby syndrome: inflicted cerebral trauma. Pediatrics. 1993;92(6):872–5.
76. Huntimer CM, et al. Can falls on stairs result in small intestine perforations? Pediatrics. 2000;106:301–5.
77. Maguire SA, et al. A systematic review of abusive visceral injuries in childhood—their range and recognition. Child Abuse Negl. 2013;37:430–45.
78. Owen SM, Durst RD. Ehlers-Danlos syndrome simulating child abuse. Arch Dermatol. 1984;120:97–101.
79. Shur N, Carey JC. Genetic differentials of child abuse: is your case rare or real? Am J Med Genet C Semin Med Genet. 2015;169:281–8.
80. Agrawal A, et al. Scurvy in pediatric age group: a disease often forgotten? J Clin Orthop Truama. 2015;6:101–7.
81. Bronicki LM, et al. Beyond osteogenesis imperfecta: causes of fractures during infancy and childhood. Am J Med Genet C Semin Med Genet. 2015;169:314–27.
82. Oandya NK, et al. Unexplained fractures: child abuse or bone disease? A systematic review. Clin Orthop. 2011;469:805–12.
83. Ved N, Haller JO. Periosteal reaction with normal-appearing underlying bone: a child abuse mimicker. Emerg Radiol. 2002;9:278–82.
84. Wei C, et al. Fractures in a tertiary neonatal intensive care unit in Wales. Acta Paediatr. 2012;101:587–90.
85. Elder CJ, Bishp NJ. Rickets. Lancet. 2014;383:1665–76.
86. Kepron C, Pollanen MS. Rickets or abuse? A histologic comparison of rickets and child abuse-related fractures. Forensic Sci Med Pathol. 2015;11:78–87.
87. Minegishi Y. Hyoer-IgE syndrome. Curr Opin Immunol. 2009;21:487–92.
88. Freeman AF, Holland SM. Clinical manifestations, etiology, and pathogenesis of the hyper IgE syndromes. Pediatr Res. 2009;65:32R–7R.
89. Morley SR, et al. Drug and alcohol-related deaths in paediatric institutions in the United Kingdom. Am J Forensic Med Pathol. 2012;330:390–4.

Chapter 14
Maternal Deaths

Joseph A. Prahlow and Theodore T. Brown

Introduction

Pregnancy is considered a normal biologic process for the purpose of reproduction. Associated with the hormonal changes that accompany pregnancy, there are a variety of physiologic and anatomic changes which occur in a female's body. Some of these changes can increase the risk for morbidity and mortality. Depending on the general health and lifestyle, and the particulars of a given pregnancy, the "normal" physiologic and anatomic changes associated with pregnancy may or may not be tolerated well during pregnancy. Classic physiologic changes associated with pregnancy include increased blood volume, heart rate, and cardiac output, as well as ventricular dilatation, decreased vascular resistance (systemic and pulmonary), relative anemia, resistance to insulin, and increased measurable levels of several coagulation factors [1, 2]. Normal anatomic changes include weight gain, abdominal distension, increased uterine size (Figs. 14.1 and 14.2), and placental development.

Per the World Health Organization (WHO), maternal mortality is "the annual number of female deaths from any cause related to or aggravated by pregnancy or its management (excluding accidental or incidental causes) during pregnancy and childbirth or within 42 days of termination of pregnancy, irrespective of the duration and site of the pregnancy." [3] Furthermore, "a late maternal death is the death of a woman from direct or indirect obstetric causes, more than 42 days but less than one year after termination of pregnancy." [3] In 2017, there were approximately 295,000 maternal deaths worldwide [4]. The majority (approximately 86%) of maternal deaths occurred in Sub-Saharan Africa and Southern Asia where resources,

J. A. Prahlow (✉)
SSM Health and Saint Louis University School of Medicine, St. Louis, MO, USA

T. T. Brown
Department of Public Safety, Arkansas State Crime Laboratory, Little Rock, AR, USA

R. Jacques (ed.), *Forensic Pathology*,
https://doi.org/10.1007/978-3-031-42038-2_14

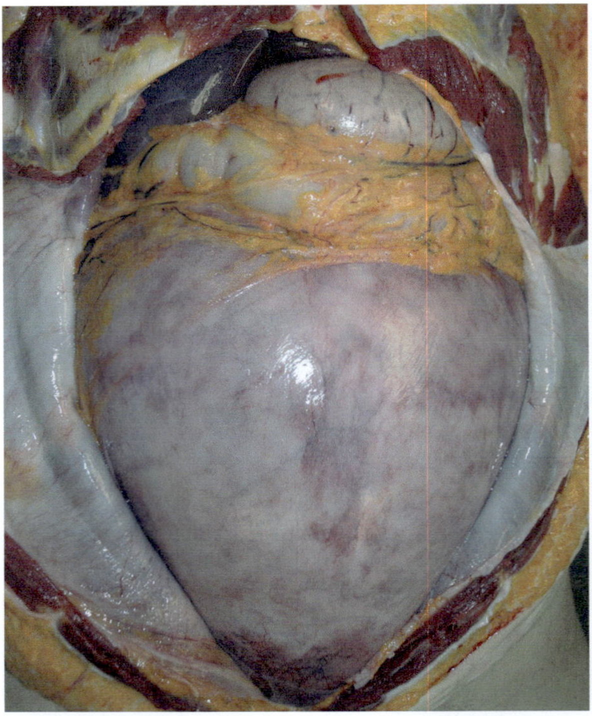

Fig. 14.1 Full-term gravid uterus in situ at autopsy from a decedent who died from non-pregnancy related causes

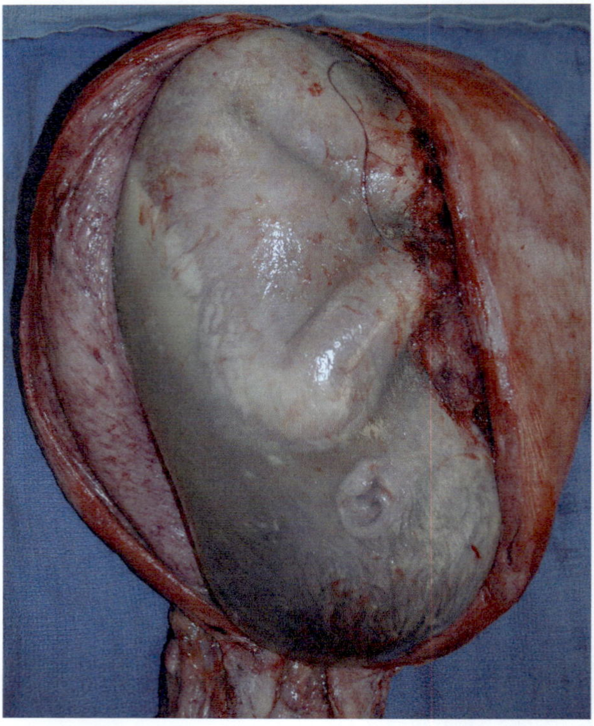

Fig. 14.2 The same uterus as shown in Fig. 14.1, after removal at autopsy, showing the fetus within an intact amniotic sac

including lack of quality health services, are low [4]. It is worth noting that certain "pregnancy-related deaths" may occur beyond the one-year time limit that encompasses the "maternal death" definition as described above.

The most common mechanisms of maternal mortality, comprising nearly 75% of maternal deaths, include significant bleeding, infections, preeclampsia and eclampsia, delivery-related complications, and unsafe abortions [5]. In an effort to decrease maternal mortality, WHO is collaborating with stakeholders worldwide toward "addressing inequalities in access to and quality of reproductive, maternal, and newborn health care services; ensuring universal health coverage for comprehensive reproductive, maternal, and newborn health care; addressing all causes of maternal mortality, reproductive and maternal morbidities, and related disabilities; strengthening health systems to collect high quality data in order to respond to the needs and priorities of women and girls; and ensuring accountability in order to improve quality and equity." [4]

Forensic pathologists are in a strong position to ensure that a thorough medicolegal death investigation and autopsy are completed on all maternal and late maternal deaths to best understand the circumstances and causes of deaths. The completion of a thorough medicolegal death investigation and autopsy are critical to learn from and prevent future maternal deaths. Many medical examiner and coroner offices are active contributors of community and statewide maternal mortality review committees that bring together multiple stakeholders that share the common goal of improving maternal morbidity and mortality.

Prior to the autopsy, a review of all available clinical history of the decedent should be obtained and reviewed, to include medical records prior to pregnancy, obstetric history, ultrasound reports, and procedural records [6]. In addition, strong consideration should be given to complete postmortem imaging (X-ray or CT) as soon as possible if an air embolism is in the differential diagnosis [6]. At autopsy, besides a complete external and internal examination of the mother, when available, the placenta and fetus should also be carefully examined, both grossly and microscopically. If the placenta is not with the mother, a request for a pathologic examination by a surgical pathologist should be made and a report of the findings should be obtained.

The literature reports several ways to categorize and evaluate the deaths of pregnant or postpartum women. For example, deaths are sometimes divided into direct maternal deaths, indirect maternal deaths, and incidental maternal deaths. Direct maternal deaths result from complications of the pregnant state, indirect maternal deaths result from diseases that were worsened or developed due to the pregnant state, and incidental maternal deaths are unrelated to the pregnant state (including accidental and intentional traumatic deaths). Worldwide, direct maternal deaths are most common, while in the United States, indirect maternal deaths are most common [7, 8]. Maternal deaths can also be divided by the stage of pregnancy (first trimester, second trimester, third trimester, during labor or birth, and postpartum). Within this overview, pregnant and postpartum deaths are classified by pathologic conditions and whether they are unique to pregnancy, associated with pregnancy, or exacerbated by pregnancy, with the caveat that there may be some overlap.

Maternal Deaths Unique to Pregnancy

Hemorrhagic Conditions (Ruptured Ectopic Pregnancy, Placenta Previa, Placenta Abruption, Uterine Rupture, Postpartum Hemorrhage)

Ectopic pregnancy occurs when a fertilized egg implants outside of the uterus, most commonly within the fallopian tube [9]. Reported risk factors for ectopic pregnancy include prior fallopian tube disease or surgical intervention, previous ectopic pregnancy, intrauterine devices, smoking cigarettes, and in utero diethylstilbestrol exposure [9]. Rupture can occur spontaneously and result in death due to massive intraperitoneal hemorrhage. At autopsy, documentation of the rupture site along with blood within the peritoneal cavity can confirm the diagnosis of a ruptured ectopic pregnancy (Figs. 14.3, 14.4, 14.5). Microscopic confirmation of the pregnancy should be performed (Fig. 14.6).

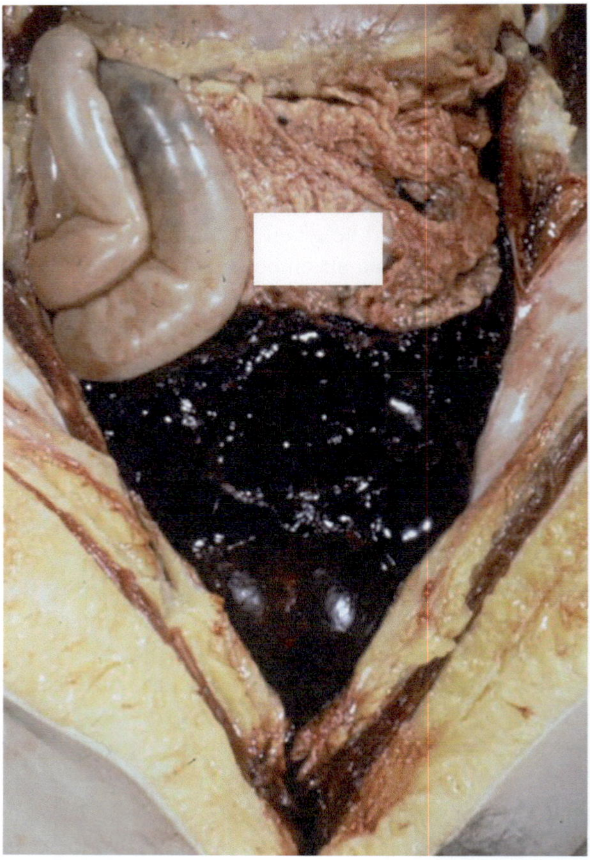

Fig. 14.3 Hemoperitoneum related to a ruptured ectopic pregnancy

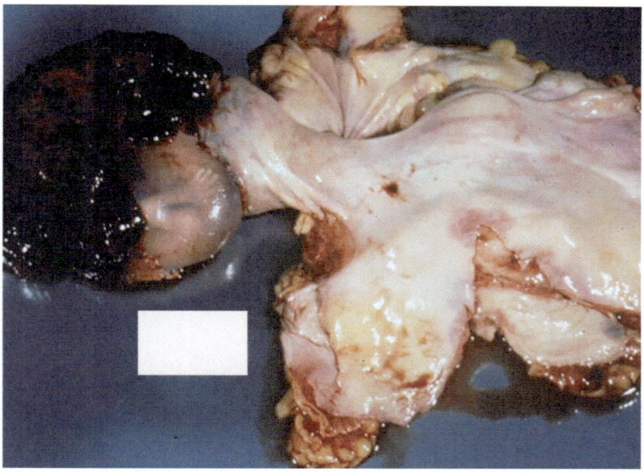

Fig. 14.4 The uterus, tubes, and ovaries from the case depicted in Fig. 14.3, with hemorrhagic ectopic pregnancy (note the visible fetal extremity)

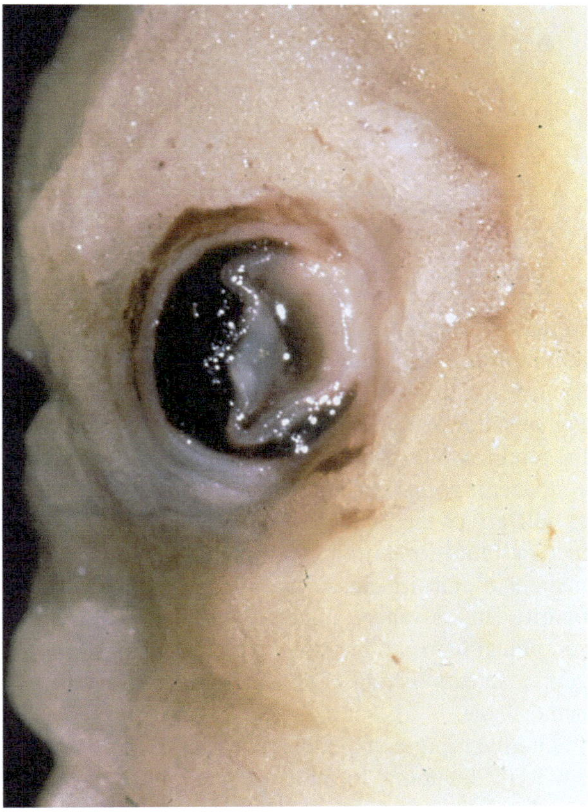

Fig. 14.5 Another ectopic pregnancy, with hemorrhage involving a fallopian tube

Placenta previa occurs when the placenta implants in the uterine lining such that the placenta nearly or completely covers the cervical opening. This finding can be demonstrated at autopsy by careful examination of the uterus and placenta together.

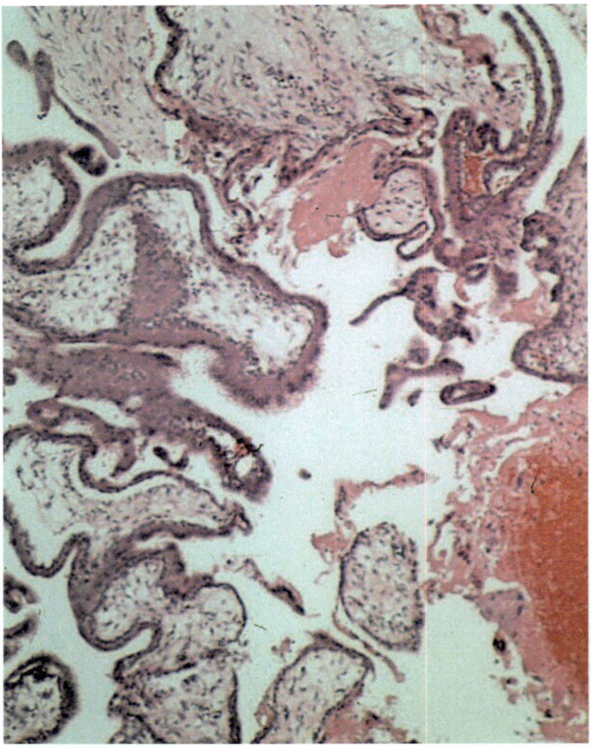

Fig. 14.6 Microscopic examination of a hemorrhagic, dilated fallopian tube reveals the presence of chorionic villi, indicative of an ectopic pregnancy

Reported risk factors for placenta previa include previous placenta previa, prior uterine procedures, uterine trauma, drugs use, multiparity, and advanced maternal age (greater than 35 years) [10, 11]. Placenta previa may present as recurrent bleeding episodes and may lead to placenta accreta (growth of the placenta deep within the uterine wall), postpartum hemorrhage, and rare maternal death [10, 11].

Placenta abruption occurs when the placenta detaches from the uterine wall prior to delivery of the infant (Figs. 14.7 and 14.8). Risk factors for placenta abruption include blunt force traumatic injury to the abdominal/pelvic region and nontraumatic etiologies, such as drug use, underlying natural disease (hypertension), multiparity, and advanced maternal age [11, 12]. Placenta abruption may present as abdominal pain and bleeding in the last trimester of pregnancy. Treatment is emergent cesarean section [11, 12]. Maternal death can occur as a result of severe hemorrhage.

Uterine rupture, which may be traumatic (commonly at the fundus of the uterus due to the anatomic location) or nontraumatic, occurs when the uterine wall completely ruptures and results in a full-thickness tear of the uterine wall with resultant hemorrhage into the peritoneal cavity [13, 14]. Nontraumatic uterine rupture may be spontaneous (Figs. 14.9 and 14.10), and risk factors include previous uterine rupture, prior uterine surgery (especially cesarean section), oxytocin or prostaglandin use, placenta abruption, malposition of the fetus, and underlying connective

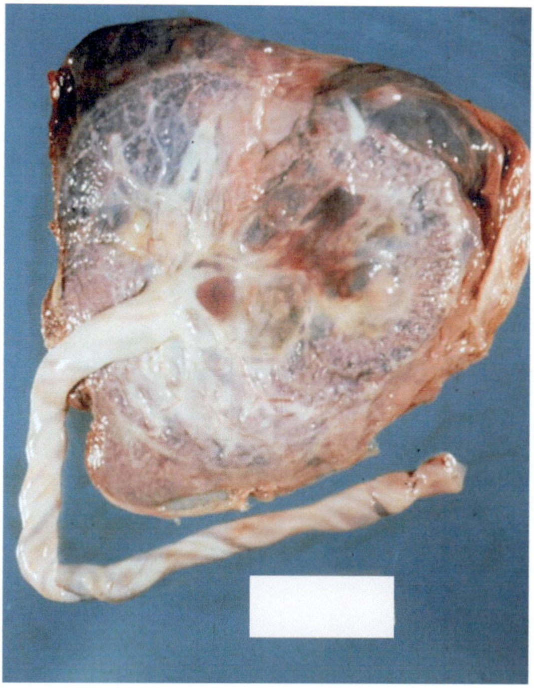

Fig. 14.7 Fetal surface of an abrupted placenta that resulted in maternal death related to severe hemorrhage

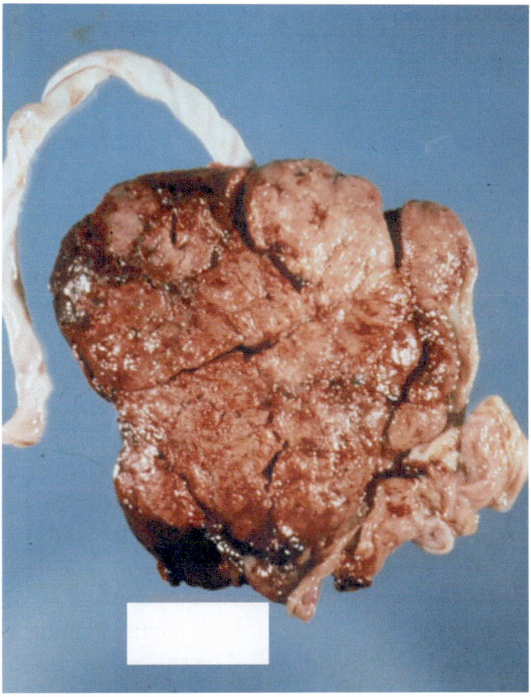

Fig. 14.8 The maternal surface of the abrupted placenta shown in Fig. 14.7

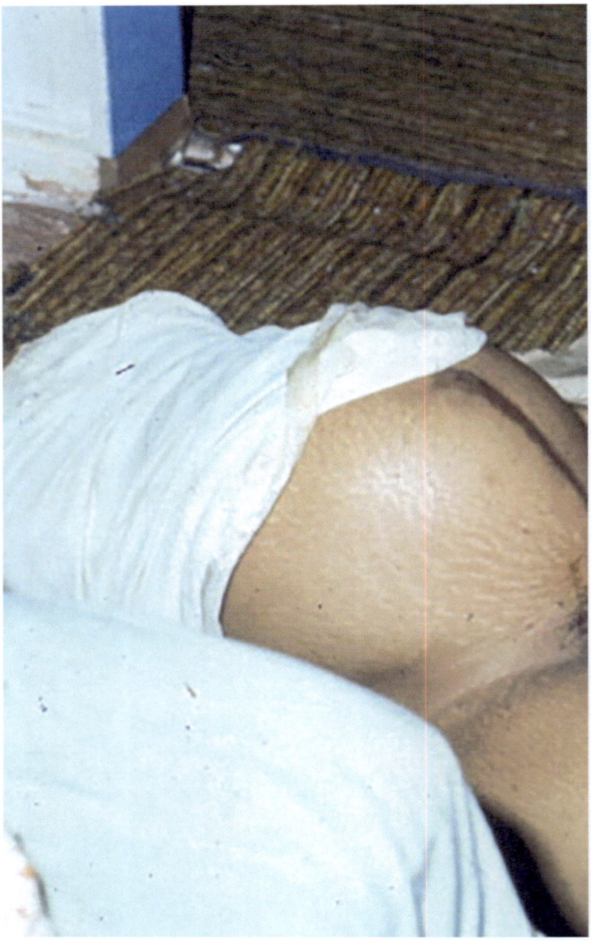

Fig. 14.9 Scene photograph of a woman in the late second/early third trimester of pregnancy, in which she was found dead at home

tissue disorders [13, 15]. Traumatic uterine rupture occurs when an external force contributes to the rupture. This can involve accidental blunt or other forms of trauma, but it can also involve various obstetrical interventions, including externally applied pressure and instrumentation. Uterine rupture often occurs during labor and necessitates emergent surgical treatment [13, 14]. In cases of uterine rupture, pathologists should consider the possibility that the woman has a predisposing underlying connective tissue disorder, such as Ehlers-Danlos syndrome.

Postpartum hemorrhage, which is described as more than one half of a liter of bleeding within the first 24 h after birth, can occur due to multiple etiologies and includes soft tissue (puerperal) hematoma, retained placenta, uterine inversion, and uterine atony [16, 17]. There are paravaginal, paracervical, and parametrial puerperal hematomas [16, 17]. Risk factors include tears during childbirth, episiotomy, and other instrumentation. Depending on the location, puerperal hematomas can

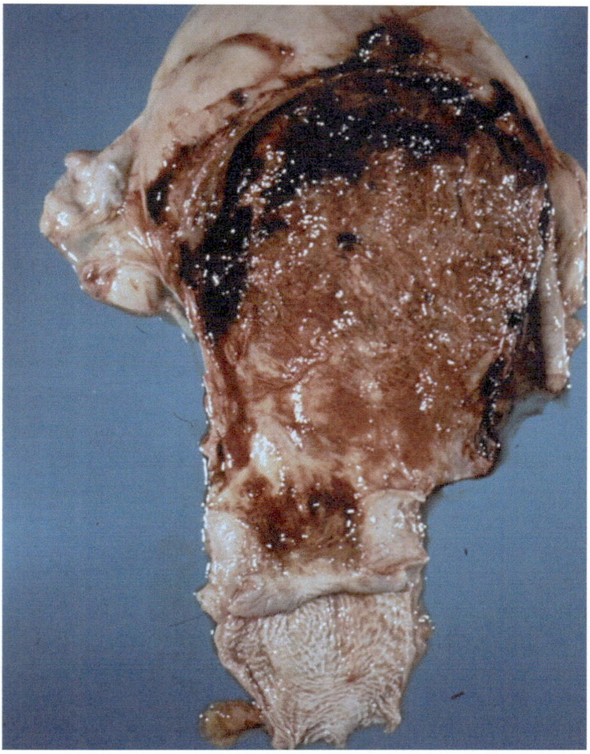

Fig. 14.10 At autopsy in the case shown in Fig. 14.9, a hemoperitoneum was discovered and was related to the spontaneous uterine rupture shown

appear as enlarging soft tissues masses. Retained placenta can occur in many clinical settings, to include placenta accreta, increta, and percreta [16, 17]. Risk factors include previous retained placenta and uterine surgery. Uterine inversion occurs when the uterus prolapses following birth and uterine atony occurs when the muscular tone of the uterus is diminished or non-existent [16–18]. While not as common in incidence or in causing maternal death, these etiologies of postpartum hemorrhage can be life-threatening.

It is important that the autopsy includes a full examination of not only the mother, but also, if applicable, the placenta and fetus. If the placenta is not available for examination, requesting the hospital pathology placental report should be considered.

Pregnancy-induced Hypertension (Preeclampsia and Eclampsia)

Per the International Society for the Study of Hypertension in Pregnancy, preeclampsia is "de novo hypertension developing after 20 weeks of gestation combined with proteinuria (>300 mg/day), other maternal organ dysfunction, such as renal insufficiency, liver involvement, neurologic or hematological complications, uteroplacental dysfunction, or fetal growth restriction." [19] Eclampsia is a progression of preeclampsia to include neurologic disorders that include hyperreflexia, seizures, decreased level of consciousness, or coma [20–22]. Risk factors include first pregnancy, advanced maternal age, family history, and underlying natural diseases to include obesity and diabetes mellitus [19, 23]. Death can result, which is most commonly due to intracerebral hemorrhage [24]. Microscopic changes of preeclampsia of the uterus include vascular fibrinoid necrosis associated with lipid-laden macrophages and mononuclear cell inflammation [25]. Additional microscopic changes include edematous changes of the endothelial cells and occlusion of the glomerular capillaries, "flame" hemorrhages of the heart, and adrenal gland necrosis and hemorrhage [26]. HELLP syndrome is an associated disorder occurring in some women with preeclampsia. It is defined by the presence of *H*emolysis, *E*levated *L*iver enzymes, and *L*ow *P*latelets, and it carries with it a significant risk of death [6]. Obtaining all available medical records, especially prenatal records, to review with the autopsy findings will best position the pathologist to opine on the cause of death.

Pregnancy-Specific Embolic Disorders (Amniotic Fluid Embolism and Trophoblastic Tissue Embolism)

Amniotic fluid embolism occurs when amniotic fluid enters the maternal venous circulation by a tear in the placental membranes and uterus, cervix, or vagina, resulting in sudden hemodynamic and circulatory compromise [27–32]. While obstruction of the pulmonary microvasculature system may occur, it is more likely that the circulatory collapse is related to the response of the amniotic fluid in the vasculature that induces the complement system or an anaphylactoid reaction [33, 34]. Risk factors include uterine hypercontractility, cesarean section, assisted births, advanced maternal age, placental or uterine pathology, and maternal diabetes mellitus [6]. At autopsy, a tear in the uterus, cervix, or vagina should be sought-out, while nonspecific findings, which may include pulmonary edema and a dilated heart, are more commonly noted [27–32]. Microscopic identification of findings consistent with amniotic fluid material, which may include squamous cells from fetal skin, lanugo hair from the fetus, and mucous within the maternal pulmonary circulation is critical for the confirmation of amniotic fluid embolism (Fig. 14.11). Multiple representative sections of all lobes of the right and left lungs should be examined microscopically. Additional stains, such as cytokeratin, modified Attwood stain, and mucin stains, can help demonstrate the amniotic fluid under the microscope (Fig. 14.12) [6, 24].

Trophoblastic tissue embolism occurs when trophoblastic tissue (chorionic villi, syncytiotrophoblast, and cytotrophoblast) enters the maternal circulation and embolizes typically during a pregnancy-related procedure [35]. The reported occurrence is rare and requires microscopic confirmation of trophoblastic tissue within the maternal pulmonary vasculature [35].

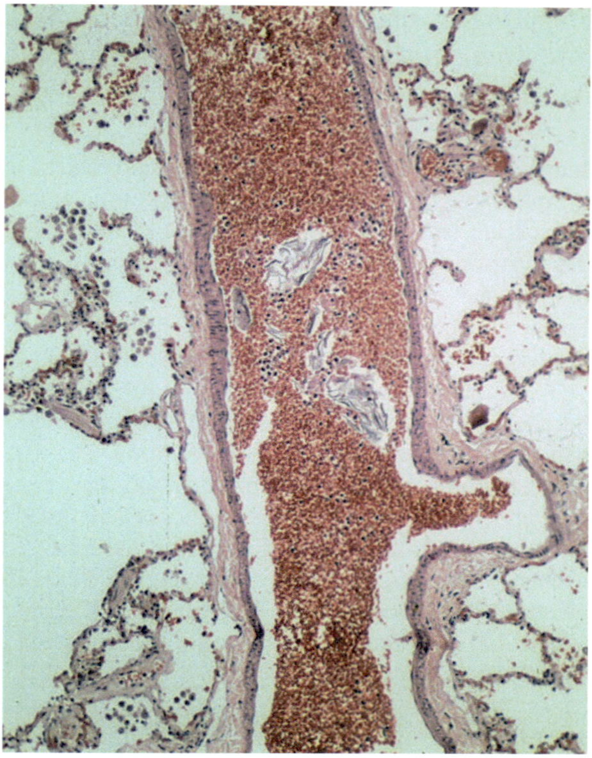

Fig. 14.11 Microscopic image of the maternal lung at autopsy, from a woman who died from amniotic fluid embolism. Note the fetal squamous cells and other amniotic “debris” within the blood vessel

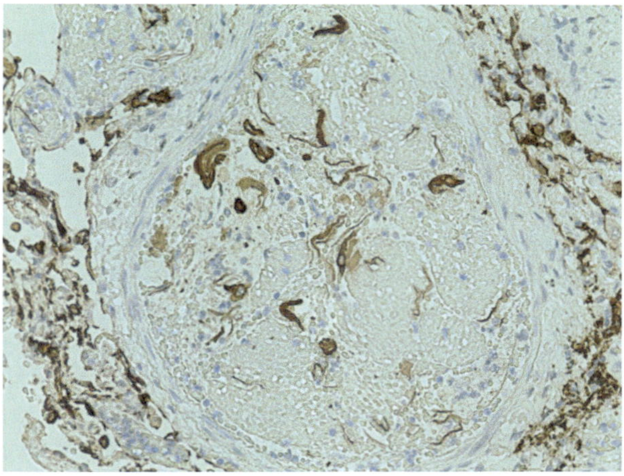

Fig. 14.12 A high-power photomicrograph of the pulmonary microvasculature from a case of amniotic fluid embolism, stained with a cytokeratin immunoperoxidase stain, which highlights fetal cells within the maternal microcirculation

Hepatic Disorders (Intrahepatic Cholestasis of Pregnancy and Acute Fatty Liver of Pregnancy; and HELLP Syndrome—As Above)

Intrahepatic cholestasis of pregnancy is cholestasis, which manifests with clinical symptoms that may include pruritis, dark discoloration of the urine, and jaundice, that occurs late in pregnancy [36]. Risk factors may include family history, and genetic variants that are believed to increase the risk of an abnormal hepatic response to hormones, such as estrogen, during pregnancy [36]. Microscopically, there may be hepatic cholestasis with intracellular bile and canalicular plugs [36]. Maternal death is rare, but adverse fetal outcomes, which include stillbirth, are increased [36].

Acute fatty liver of pregnancy has a higher maternal fatality rate compared to intrahepatic cholestasis of pregnancy and can present clinically with abdominal pain, vomiting, jaundice, and renal failure [37]. Risk factors include primiparity, especially primiparous women with a multi-fetus gestation or male fetus [36]. The etiology of acute fatty liver of pregnancy is believed to be related to a mitochondrial fatty acid beta-oxidation dysfunction in the fetus, which can result in maternal hepatic failure [36]. At autopsy, the maternal liver is characterized by microvesicular steatosis, ballooning of the hepatocytes, and periportal inflammation [24].

HELLP Syndrome—Please refer to discussion above (Pregnancy-induced hypertension).

Maternal Deaths Associated with Pregnancy

Pregnancy-associated Cardiac Disorders (Peripartum Cardiomyopathy, Peripartum Myocarditis, and Pregnancy-associated Spontaneous Coronary Artery Dissection)

Peripartum cardiomyopathy, which is characterized by heart failure that manifests during the peripartum period (third trimester to five months postpartum), most commonly occurs postpartum, but can present late during pregnancy [38, 39]. Importantly, for a diagnosis of peripartum cardiomyopathy to be made, there can be no other explanation of heart failure. The etiology of peripartum cardiomyopathy is likely multifactorial and includes inflammatory and hemodynamic-related changes [40–42]. Risk factors include advanced maternal age, multiparity, and previous peripartum cardiomyopathy [38, 39]. At autopsy, the heart is dilated (Fig. 14.13) and does not have any other pathologic reason to be dilated. The lungs may have

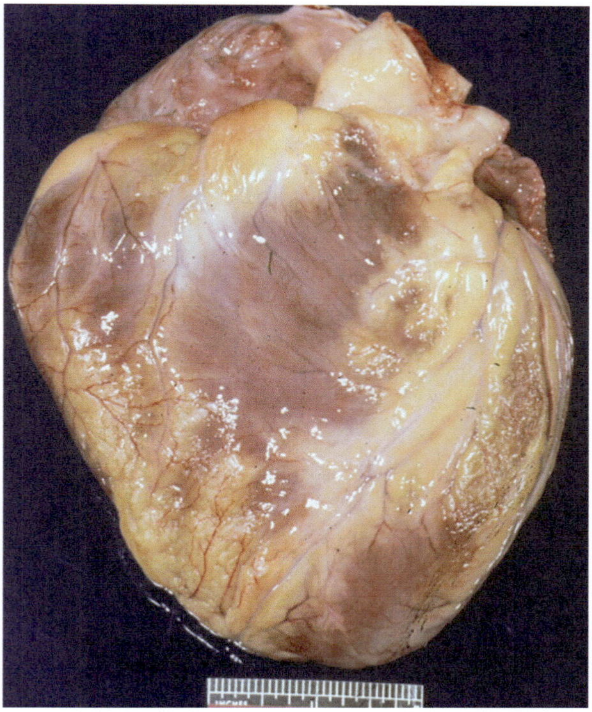

Fig. 14.13 Enlarged and dilated heart in a woman who died from peripartum cardiomyopathy

excess congestion and edema. Microscopically, the heart may have findings that include myocardial hypertrophy and interstitial fibrosis [39]. A woman may survive many years following the onset of a pregnancy-related dilated cardiomyopathy, yet succumb to the disorder. As such, this would be an example of a situation where the death might still be considered a pregnancy-related death, even though it falls outside of the timeframe established by the WHO to be considered a "late maternal death."

Peripartum myocarditis can also present with heart failure and is likely related to a viral infection or other immunologic disorders [43]. Like peripartum cardiomyopathy, a dilated heart can be identified at autopsy. Microscopically, peripartum myocarditis is associated with myocarditis (lymphohistiocytic inflammation) [43].

Pregnancy-associated spontaneous coronary artery dissection most frequently occurs in the last trimester of pregnancy or presents postmortem in individuals who often do not have underlying coronary artery disease [44, 45]. When the diagnosis of a pregnancy-associated spontaneous coronary artery dissection is made or confirmed at autopsy, histological sampling of the dissected coronary artery may exhibit periadventitial eosinophils, although their presence is not well understood [46]. The disorder is characterized by arterial dissection involving a coronary artery (Figs. 14.14 and 14.15).

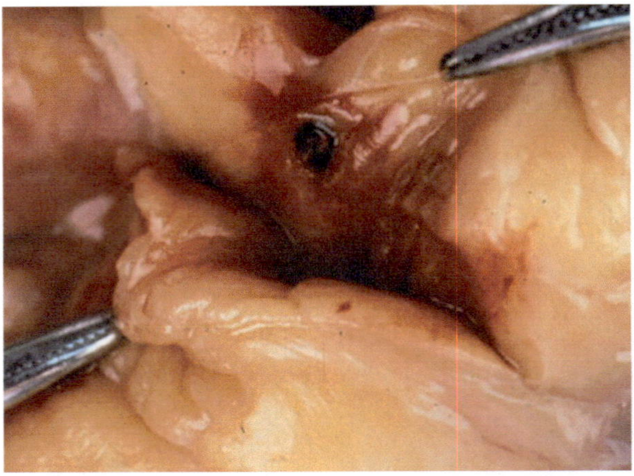

Fig. 14.14 A coronary artery dissection present in a woman who collapsed and died late in pregnancy

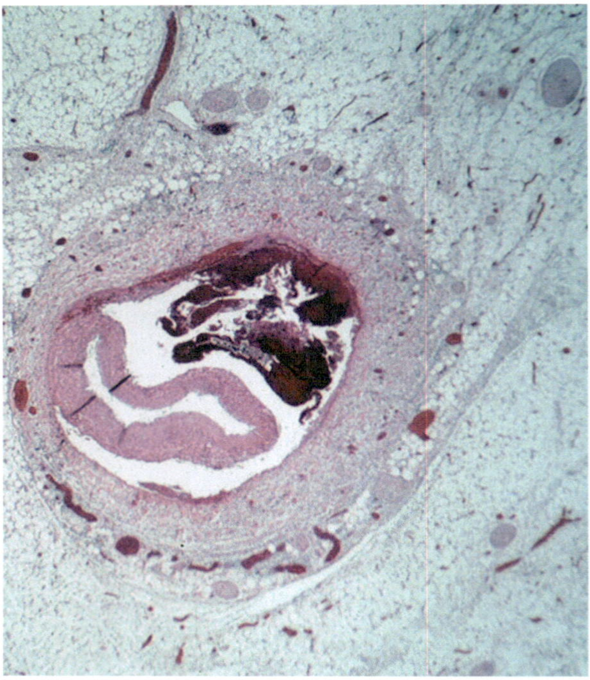

Fig. 14.15 The microscopic appearance of the coronary artery dissection depicted in Fig. 14.14

Embolic Disorders (Pulmonary Thromboembolism and Air Embolism)

The risk for the development of a pulmonary thromboembolism increases during pregnancy and persists up to approximately 2 months after birth due to a variety of factors, which include the hypercoagulable state of pregnancy itself, trauma associated with birth, and venous stasis associated with decreased mobility [6]. Other risk factors, similar to non-pregnant individuals, include obesity and genetic mutations that increase one's risk of a hypercoagulable state. Sources of pulmonary thromboembolism can be deep venous thrombosis of the lower extremities and within the veins of the pelvic region. Clinical manifestations of a pulmonary thromboembolism include sudden shortness of breath. At autopsy, an occlusive, adherent thrombus obstructing the pulmonary arterial system is diagnostic of a pulmonary thromboembolism (Figs. 14.16 and 14.17). If discovered, the source of the thromboembolism should be identified (deep leg veins or pelvic veins). Postmortem genetic testing for hypercoagulable states is possible and can provide additional valuable information for surviving family members.

An air embolism occurs when air enters and collects in the venous system, travels to the heart, and causes obstruction [31]. Air can enter the venous circulatory system of the female genitalia by multiple mechanisms and includes sexual activity, hygienic activity, and surgical intervention [31]. Clinical symptoms of an air embolism may include sudden shortness of breath [31]. Prior to the autopsy, radiographic images of the chest should be obtained as soon as possible following death to look for collections of air pockets within the right side of the heart (Fig. 14.18). A postmortem CT scan, if available, provides an excellent method for identifying an air embolism [6]. An autopsy approach to help ascertain the presence of an air embolism involves

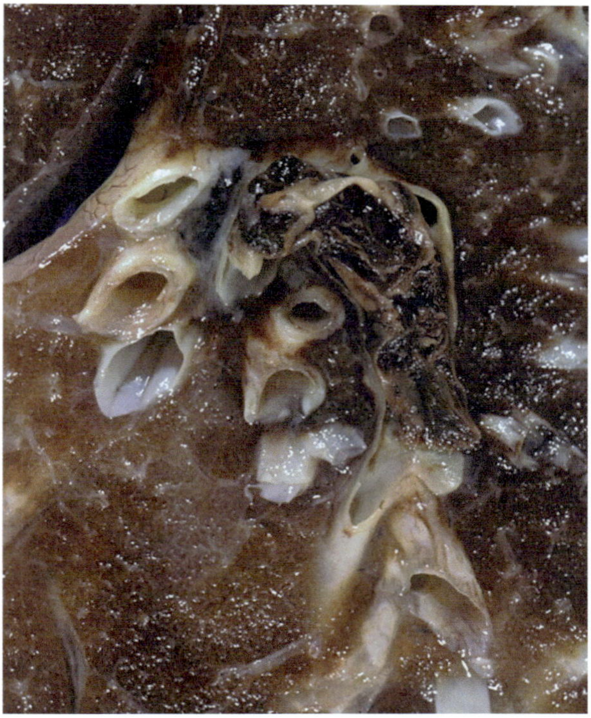

Fig. 14.16 Pulmonary thromboembolism seen at autopsy in a young pregnant woman who suddenly collapsed and died

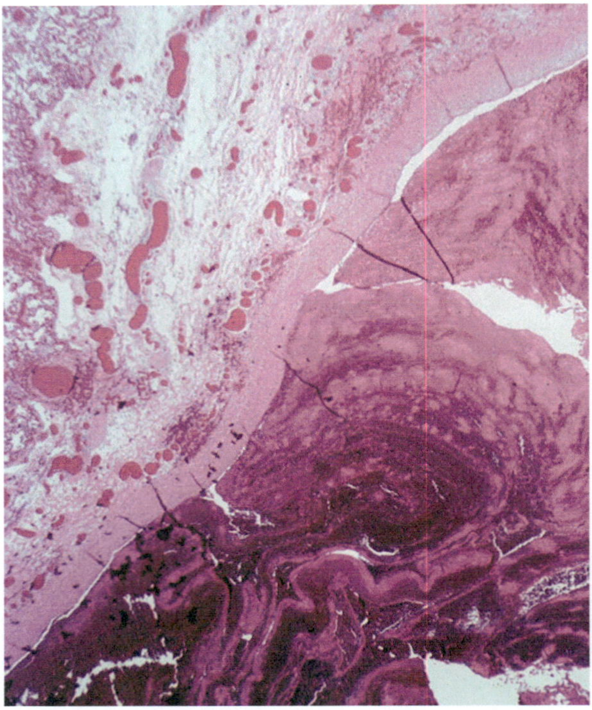

Fig. 14.17 Microscopic appearance of the pulmonary thromboembolism shown in Fig. 14.16

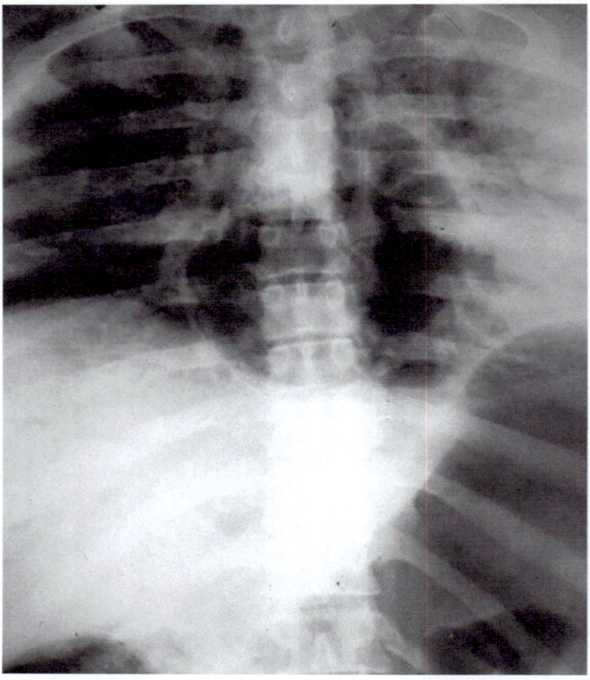

Fig. 14.18 A postmortem chest radiograph from a young pregnant woman who died during sexual activity. Note the large radiolucent (dark) area of air within the right side of the heart

filling the pericardial sac with water, creating a small defect on the submerged right side of the heart, and watching for the presence of air bubbles [47].

Thrombotic Microangiopathies of Pregnancy (Thrombotic Thrombocytopenia Purpura and Hemolytic Uremic Syndrome; Disseminated Intravascular Coagulation)

Thrombotic thrombocytopenia purpura (TTP) and hemolytic uremic syndrome (HUS) are primary thrombotic microangiopathies that lead to microthrombi within the vasculature. TTP has the classic clinical features that include fever, neurologic changes, renal dysfunction, microangiopathic hemolytic anemia, and thrombocytopenic purpura due to the widespread involvement of multiple organs affected by microthrombi [48–50]. HUS is more limited and has the classic clinical features that include microangiopathic hemolytic anemia, thrombocytopenia, and acute renal failure [48, 50]. At autopsy, petechial hemorrhages may be noted grossly in multiple organs (Fig. 14.19), and microthrombi are evident microscopically (Fig. 14.20). The kidney is most significantly affected in HUS due to renal microthrombi. Pregnancy-related deaths can occur as a result of either of these conditions.

It should also be noted that disseminated intravascular coagulation (DIC) may occur in the setting of pregnancy, from a variety of underlying conditions. For example, women experiencing pre-eclampsia/eclampsia may develop DIC. The morphologic/histologic features of DIC can be identical to other thrombotic microangiopathies.

Endocrine Disorders (Gestational Diabetes Mellitus; Pituitary Insufficiency)

Gestational diabetes mellitus is the diagnosis of abnormal glucose metabolism due to the inability to produce sufficient insulin during pregnancy [51]. Gestational diabetes may be clinically recognized by maternal intolerance to carbohydrates and can increase maternal risk of infection and heart disease [51]. Gestational diabetes mellitus also increases the risk of fetal macrosomia, and the overall morbidity and mortality of the fetus increase [51]. Maternal deaths may be secondary to complications associated with large fetus size, such as difficult labor and subsequent uterine injury.

Pituitary insufficiency most commonly manifests in one of two ways: lymphocytic hypophysitis (autoimmune disorder characterized by chronic inflammation of the pituitary gland during the peripartum period) and pituitary gland infarction (also known as Sheehan syndrome in the postpartum setting) [52]. If an excess amount of blood is lost by the mother during or after delivery, ischemic necrosis of the pituitary gland can result, which can appear gray-red at autopsy [53].

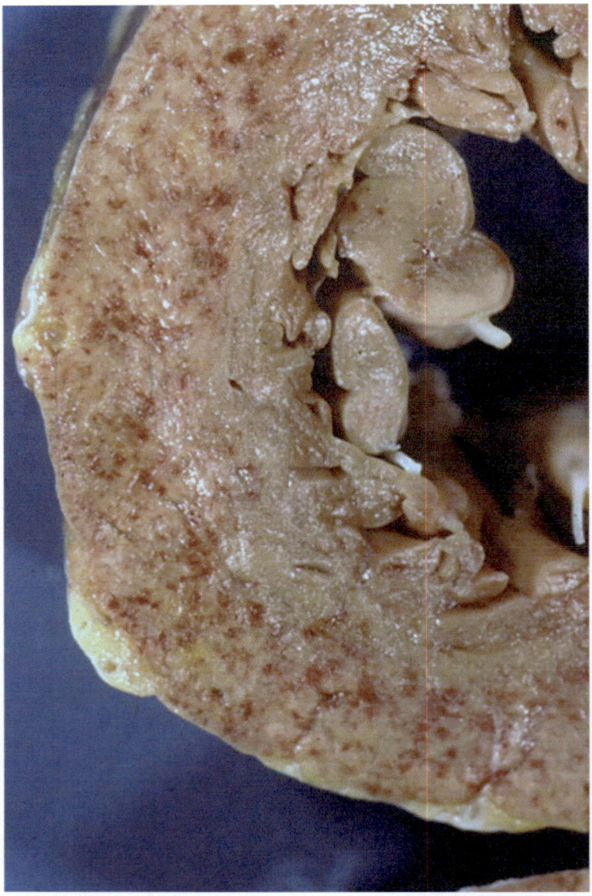

Fig. 14.19 Gross image of a cross section of a heart from a pregnant woman who died from TTP

Infectious Diseases

Infectious diseases, most commonly involving gram-negative anaerobes, gram-positive aerobes, and gram-positive anaerobes, contribute to maternal morbidity and mortality [54]. Types of infections include Group A beta-hemolytic *Streptococcus* (toxic shock syndrome), endometritis, and uterine gas gangrene (*Clostridium perfringens*) [26]. If an infectious disease is in the differential diagnosis of a maternal death, aerobic and anaerobic blood cultures should be obtained, as well as cultures of any potential infection source. In addition, the placenta and umbilical cord should be microscopically evaluated for evidence of infection [26].

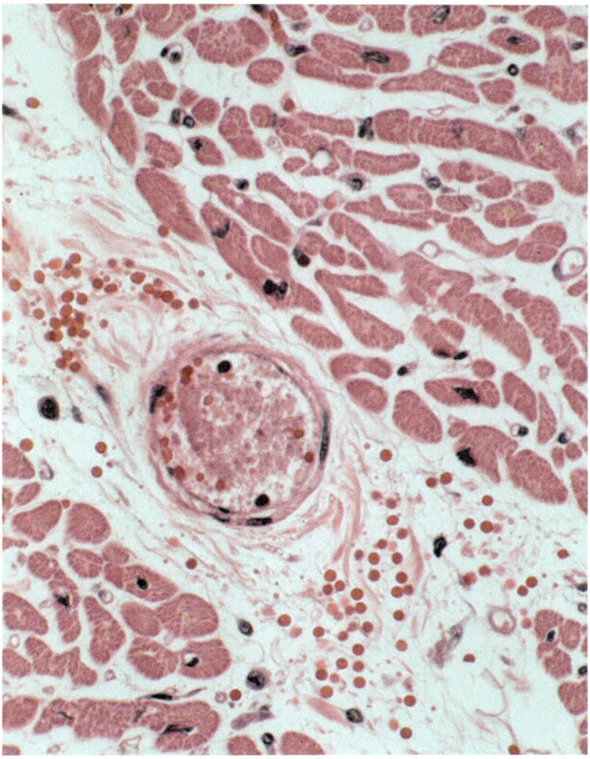

Fig. 14.20 Microscopic image from the same TTP case as shown in Fig. 14.19, showing a microthrombus

Gestational Trophoblastic Disease

Gestational trophoblastic disease occurs when there is abnormal neoplastic placental tissue trophoblastic proliferation that produces human chorionic gonadotropin (hCG). Types of malignant forms of gestational trophoblastic disease include the invasive mole, choriocarcinoma, placental site trophoblastic tumor, and epithelioid trophoblastic tumor [55, 56]. If widespread, malignant gestational trophoblastic disease can be lethal [55, 56].

Maternal Deaths Exacerbated by Pregnancy

Cardiac Diseases (Congenital Heart Disease, Acquired Valvular Disease, Hypertensive Cardiovascular Disease, Atherosclerotic Cardiovascular Disease, Arrhythmogenic Heart Disease)

Known or unknown underlying cardiac diseases, including congenital heart disease, acquired valvular disease, hypertensive cardiovascular disease, atherosclerotic cardiovascular disease, and arrhythmogenic cardiac disease, can be worsened during pregnancy [57]. Careful examination of the heart, with consideration of a cardiac pathology consultation, may be warranted.

Pulmonary Diseases (Primary Pulmonary Hypertension and Asthmatic Bronchitis)

Primary pulmonary hypertension is defined as high blood pressure in the lungs. The mortality rate of this condition increases when associated with pregnancy [58]. Autopsy findings may include firm pulmonary arteries on cut surface of the lungs. Histologic findings of primary pulmonary hypertension include thickening of the pulmonary arterial vasculature, proliferation of endothelial and smooth muscle cells, and possible thrombosis [59].

Asthma may be exacerbated during pregnancy, especially when asthma is not controlled well prior to pregnancy [60]. At autopsy, hyperexpanded lungs, mucus within the airways, and thickened bronchial walls may be observed with asthmatic bronchitis (Fig. 14.21). Microscopic changes of asthmatic bronchitis include mucus within the airway, increased bronchial submucosal inflammation with eosinophils, bronchial basement membrane thickening, and peribronchial smooth muscle cell hypertrophy (Fig. 14.22).

Fig. 14.21 Grossly hyperinflated lungs in an asthmatic death

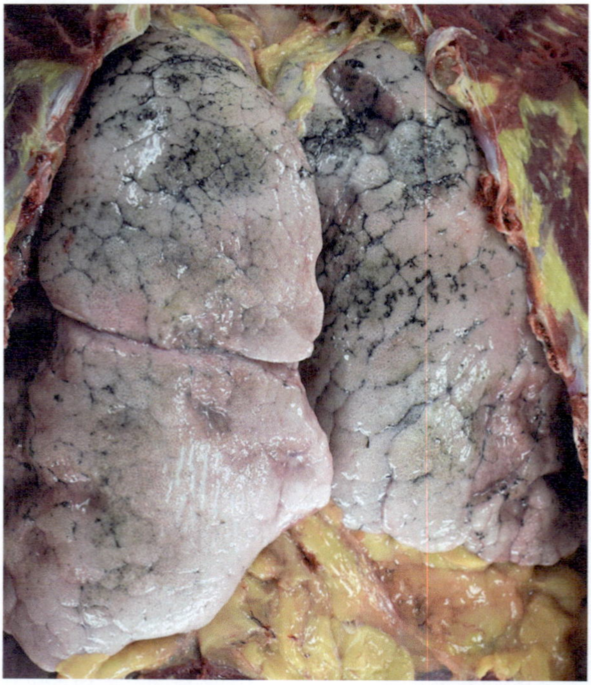

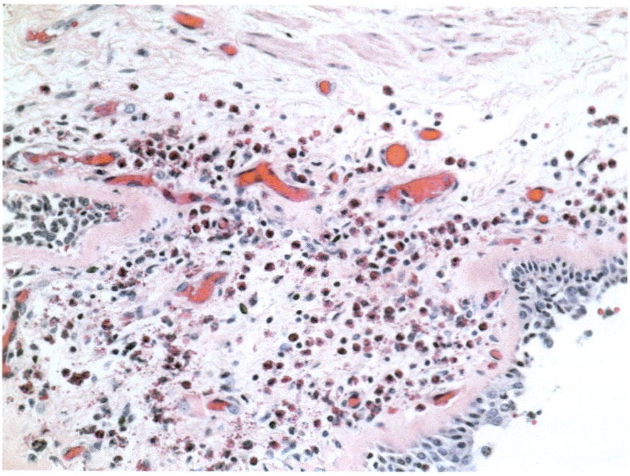

Fig. 14.22 Microscopic image of bronchial mucosa in a death due to acute and chronic asthmatic bronchitis

Hematologic Diseases

Anemia, thrombocytopenia, bleeding disorders, thrombosis, and thrombophilia may impact pregnancy in part due to physiologic changes that can affect hematologic indices [61]. Anemia is the most common hematologic disorder encountered during pregnancy [61]. During pregnancy, there is an increase in plasma volume relative to red blood cell mass that results in decreased hemoglobin concentration [61, 62]. Furthermore, an increase in daily iron intake during pregnancy can prevent iron deficiency anemia given the increased demand on bone marrow during pregnancy [63]. Significant complications can arise from individuals with sickle cell disease, a hypochromic microcytic anemia, and include eclampsia, stillbirths, spontaneous abortions, and low birth weight that require early and aggressive treatments should they arise [64–67].

Thrombocytopenia may occur in up to approximately 10% of pregnancies, often secondary to increased blood volume, platelet activation, and increase platelet clearance [68]. The most common thrombocytopenia encountered during pregnancy is gestational thrombocytopenia, most of which are not associated with poor outcomes [61]. Thrombocytopenia is also seen in the setting of immune thrombocytopenia, preeclampsia, HELLP syndrome, and neonatal alloimmune thrombocytopenia [61].

Bleeding disorders, both inherited and acquired, can lead to complications during pregnancy, especially during the postpartum period, to include immediately after delivery [61]. Of note, individuals with Von Willebrand disease are at a significant increased bleeding risk in the postpartum setting if von Willebrand factory activity levels are less than 50 IU/dL [69]. However, significant postpartum bleeding is more oftentimes associated with delivery complications versus an inherited coagulopathy [61]. Severe postpartum hemorrhage in this setting may be due to hemodilution, disseminated intravascular coagulation, acute fatty liver of pregnancy, placenta accrete, HELLP syndrome, and amniotic fluid embolism [61].

Venous thromboembolism is associated with significant maternal morbidity and mortality due to the combination of a hypercoagulable state due to alterations of coagulation factors, acquired resistance to activated protein C, decreased free protein S, and altered fibrinolysis, stasis due to decreased lower extremity blood flow, and endothelial damage during delivery [61]. For individuals with an inherited thrombophilias, such as factor V Leiden and prothrombin 20210A mutation, special preventative care is essential to reduce the risk of developing a venous thromboembolism [61].

At autopsy, pulmonary thromboembolism is typically readily evident on gross examination of the lungs. Residual deep venous thrombosis may be evident within the deep veins of the legs or in uterine/pelvic veins. Consideration should be given to collecting a DNA sample for genetic hypercoagulability testing if an inherited coagulopathy is considered based on the autopsy findings and not previously diagnosed.

Neurologic Disorders

While rare, neurologic disorders, especially stroke and cerebral venous thrombosis, have an increased frequency during pregnancy and postpartum [70]. Neurologic disorders account for approximately 20 percent of maternal deaths [71]. Due to the physiologic and hemodynamic alterations during pregnancy, both ischemic and hemorrhagic strokes carry a significant risk of maternal morbidity and mortality [72]. Hemorrhagic strokes carry a higher mortality rate versus ischemic and are most commonly associated with preeclampsia/eclampsia, arteriovenous malformations, and cerebral artery aneurysm rupture [73]. Individuals with known arteriovenous malformations and cerebral artery aneurysms often elect to deliver by cesarean section due to the possible rupture risk associated with the physiologic stress of labor and vaginal delivery [70]. Cerebral venous and sinus thrombosis, a subtype of stroke which may result in either ischemic and/or hemorrhagic neurologic consequences, most commonly involve the superior sagittal and transverse sinuses [70]. Clinically, they may present with headache, papilledema, and seizures [70]. Seizures during pregnancy can be caused by multiple etiologies and include cerebrovascular conditions like cerebral venous thrombosis, hypertension, structural abnormalities, infections, drugs, metabolic abnormalities, and epilepsy [74]. The authors are aware of a pregnancy-induced seizure disorder being the cause of death in a woman many years following the initial onset of seizures, which was considered to be pregnancy-related. This represents another example of a pregnancy-related death occurring beyond the official WHO definition of a "late maternal death." If a neurologic disorder is suspected at autopsy, consideration to fix the brain in formalin prior to examination and to obtain a neuropathologist consultation is recommended for optimal evaluation.

Unnatural Maternal Deaths

Unnatural deaths, which occur when a pregnant woman dies from an accident, suicide, or homicide, were reported at an average rate of 4.9 per 100,000 live births [75]. In one study of unnatural pregnancy deaths in a large metropolitan city in the United States, accidental deaths most commonly involved motor vehicle accidents, suicide deaths most commonly involved drug overdoses, and homicide deaths most commonly involved gunshot wounds [76]. Obtaining DNA specimens from both the mother and fetus, for example, a blood spot card, should be considered should paternity questions arise [6].

Complications of Anesthesia

Anesthesia poses a risk for complications in pregnant women in part because of maternal physiologic changes and other potential factors, including obesity and increased maternal age [77]. Central neuraxial blockade complications may include post-dural puncture headache, spinal cord injury, epidural abscess, epidural hematoma, and cardiovascular reactions to include hypotension, bradycardia, and cardiac arrest [77]. Non-central blockage regional anesthetic complications include adverse outcomes of general anesthesia to include lack of appropriate airway control, pulmonary aspiration, and drug toxicity [77]. If death occurs in this setting, special attention to the histologic evaluation of the brain, lungs, and spinal cord should be considered.

Death Certification

The appropriate completion of the death certificate is essential for vital statistics and public health reporting. During the course of the medicolegal investigation of a female of reproductive age, efforts to obtain medical records and complete interviews with individuals who knew the decedent best will allow the certifier to best report the decedent's pregnancy status within the past year on the death certificate. When determining the cause of death in a pregnant female or a female who was pregnant within up to 1 year prior to death, the certifier should consider whether pregnancy caused or contributed to death. Pregnancy-associated direct cause of death or contributing factor statements that should be considered on the death certificate include: "abortion, amniotic, antepartum, birth, delivery or delivered, ectopic, gestational age, labor, miscarriage or miscarried, obstetric, peripartum or postpartum, placenta or placental, pregnancy or pregnant, pregnancy termination, prenatal, trimester, uterine." [78] Furthermore, a pregnancy checkbox is included on the death certificate to document the pregnancy status of all females, which should be completed. Accurate completion of the entirety of the death certificate will allow for the most appropriate *International Statistical Classification of Diseases and Related Health Problems, 10th Revision* (ICD-1) assignment [78].

Conclusion

Maternal deaths can be unique to pregnancy, associated with pregnancy, or exacerbated by pregnancy. A full medicolegal death investigation into all maternal deaths, to include obtaining all available medical records, interviewing appropriate individuals who can provide information to the circumstances of death, and completion of a full autopsy with ancillary studies will position the certifier to best opine on the cause and manner of death. The information gained from this process can then be succinctly reported on the death certificate which can help ensure accurate reporting of maternal mortality statistics, provide a clearer picture for future research endeavors as it relates to maternal health, and allow stakeholders to work together to learn from and prevent future maternal deaths.

References

1. Crapo R. Normal cardiopulmonary physiology during pregnancy. Clinical obstetrics and gynecology. 1996;39(1):3–16. http://ovidsp.ovid.com/ovidweb.cgi?T=JS&NEWS=n&CSC=Y&PAGE=fulltext&D=ovft&AN=00003081-199603000-00004. https://doi.org/10.1097/00003081-199603000-00004.
2. Greer IA. Thrombosis in pregnancy: Maternal and fetal issues. The Lancet (British edition). 1999;353(9160):1258–65. https://doi.org/10.1016/S0140-6736(98)10265-9.
3. Maternal deaths. https://www.who.int/data/gho/indicator-metadata-registry/imr-details/4622. Accessed 17 Aug 2022.
4. Maternal mortality. https://www.who.int/news-room/fact-sheets/detail/maternal-mortality. Updated 2019. Accessed 17 Aug 2022.
5. Say L, Chou D, Gemmill A, et al. Global causes of maternal death: A WHO systematic analysis. The Lancet Global Health. 2014;2(6):e323–33. https://www.clinicalkey.es/playcontent/1-s2.0-S2214109X1470227X. https://doi.org/10.1016/S2214-109X(14)70227-X.
6. Garland J, Little D. Maternal death and its investigation. Acad Forensic Pathol. 2018;8(4):894–911. https://doi.org/10.1177/1925362118821485.
7. Hay SI, Naghavi M, Pinho C, et al. Global, regional, and national levels of maternal mortality, 1990–2015: a systematic analysis for the global burden of disease study 2015. Lancet. 2016;388(10053):1775–812. https://www.clinicalkey.es/playcontent/1-s2.0-S0140673616314702. https://doi.org/10.1016/S0140-6736(16)31470-2.
8. Pregnancy Mortality Surveillance System. https://www.cdc.gov/reproductivehealth/maternal-mortality/pregnancy-mortality-surveillance-system.htm. Updated 2022. Accessed 17 Aug 2022.
9. Pisarska M, Carson S. Incidence and risk factors for ectopic pregnancy. Clinical obstetrics and gynecology. 1999;42(1):2–8. http://ovidsp.ovid.com/ovidweb.cgi?T=JS&NEW

S=n&CSC=Y&PAGE=fulltext&D=ovft&AN=00003081-199903000-00004. https://doi.org/10.1097/00003081-199903000-00004.
10. Lavery JP. Placenta previa. Clin Obstet Gynecol. 1990;33:414–21.
11. Baron F, Hill W. Placenta previa, placenta abruptio. Clinical obstetrics and gynecology. 1998;41(3):527–32. http://ovidsp.ovid.com/ovidweb.cgi?T=JS&NEWS=n&CSC=Y&PAGE=fulltext&D=ovft&AN=00003081-199809000-00008. https://doi.org/10.1097/00003081-199809000-00008.
12. Lowe TWCF. Placental abruption. Clin Obstet Gynecol. 1990;33:406–13.
13. Phelan JP. Uterine rupture. Clin Obstet Gynecol. 1990;33:432–7.
14. Miller DA, Goodwin TM, Gherman RB, Paul RH. Intrapartum rupture of the unscarred uterus. Obstetrics and gynecology (New York. 1953). 1997;89(5):671–3. https://doi.org/10.1016/S0029-7844(97)00073-2.
15. Pepin M, Schwarze U, Superti-Furga A, Byers PH. Clinical and genetic features of Ehlers Danlos syndrome type IV, the vascular type. The New England Journal of Medicine. 2000;342(10):673–80. http://content.nejm.org/cgi/content/abstract/342/10/673. https://doi.org/10.1056/NEJM200003093421001.
16. Zahn C, Yeomans E. Postpartum hemorrhage: placenta accreta, uterine inversion, and puerperal hematomas. Clinical obstetrics and gynecology. 1990;33(3):422–31. http://ovidsp.ovid.com/ovidweb.cgi?T=JS&NEWS=n&CSC=Y&PAGE=fulltext&D=ovft&AN=00003081-199009000-00006. https://doi.org/10.1097/00003081-199009000-00006.
17. Druelinger L. Postpartum emergencies. Emerg Med Clinic North Am. 1994;12:219–37.
18. Hostetler DR, Bosworth MF. Uterine inversion: a life-threatening obstetric emergency. Journal of the American Board of Family Medicine. 2000;13(2):120–3. http://www.jabfm.org/cgi/content/abstract/13/2/120. https://doi.org/10.3122/15572625-13-2-120.
19. Mol BWJ, Roberts CT, Thangaratinam S, Magee LA, de Groot CJM, Hofmeyr GJ. Preeclampsia. Lancet. 2016;387(10022):999–1011.
20. Hernandez CCF. Eclampsia. Clin Obstet Gynecol. 1990;33:460–6.
21. Zamorski MA, Green LA. Preeclampsia and hypertensive disorders of pregnancy. American family physician. 1996;53(5):1595–610. https://www.ncbi.nlm.nih.gov/pubmed/8623688
22. Witlin D, Andrea G, Sibai M, Baha M. HYPERTENSION IN PREGNANCY: Current concepts of preeclampsia. Annual review of medicine. 1997;48(1):115–27. https://doi.org/10.1146/annurev.med.48.1.115.
23. Fillipi V, Chou D, Ronsmans C, et al. Chapter 3, levels and causes of maternal mortality and morbidity. In: Reproductive, maternal, newborn, and child health: Disease control priorities, third edition (volume 2). Washington: International Bank for Reconstruction and Development/The World Bank, pp. 51–70.
24. Dolinak D, Matshes E, Lew EO. Forensic pathology. Burlington: Elsevier Science & Technology; 2005. https://ebookcentral.proquest.com/lib/[SITE_ID]/detail.action?docID=286692
25. Rushton DI, Dawson IM. The maternal autopsy. J Clin Pathol. 1982;35(9):909–21.
26. Schandl CA. Maternal autopsy. In: Autopsy performance and reporting, 2nd ed. Northfield (IL): College of American Pathologists, pp. 135–49; 2003.
27. Chatelain S, Quirk J. Amniotic and thromboembolism. Clinical obstetrics and gynecology. 1990;33(3):473–81. http://ovidsp.ovid.com/ovidweb.cgi?T=JS&NEWS=n&CSC=Y&PAGE=fulltext&D=ovft&AN=00003081-199009000-00013. https://doi.org/10.1097/00003081-199009000-00013.
28. Clark S. New concepts of amniotic fluid embolism: a review. Obstetrical & gynecological survey. 1990;45(6):360–8. http://ovidsp.ovid.com/ovidweb.cgi?T=JS&NEWS=n&CSC=Y&PAGE=fulltext&D=ovft&AN=00006254-199006000-00003. https://doi.org/10.1097/00006254-199006000-00003.
29. Prahlow JALP. Amniotic fluid embolism with paradoxical embolization. Am Soc Clin Pathol Check Sample. 1993;35:1–4.

30. Lau G. Amniotic fluid embolism as a cause of sudden maternal death. Medicine, science, and the law. 1994;34(3):213–20. https://journals.sagepub.com/doi/full/10.1177/0025802494034003005. https://doi.org/10.1177/002580249403400305.
31. Dudney TM, Elliott CG. Pulmonary embolism from amniotic fluid, fat, and air. Progress in cardiovascular diseases. 1994;36(6):447–74. https://doi.org/10.1016/S0033-0620(94)80053-7.
32. Martin RW. Amniotic fluid embolism. Clin Obstet Gynecol. 1996;39:101–6.
33. Hikiji W, Tamura N, Shigeta A, Kanayama N, Fukunaga T. Fatal amniotic fluid embolism with typical pathohistological, histochemical and clinical features. Forensic Sci Int. 2013;226(1-3):16.
34. Jecmenica D, Baralic I, Alempijevic D, Pavlekic S, Kiurski M, Terzic M. Amniotic fluid embolism-apropos two consecutive cases. J Forensic Sci. 2011;56(Suppl 1):247. https://doi.org/10.1111/j.1556-4029.2010.01588.x.
35. Cohle S, Petty C. Sudden death caused by embolization of trophoblast from hydatidiform mole. Journal of forensic sciences. 1985;30(4):1279–83.
36. Schorr-Lesnick B, Lebovics E, Dworkin B, Rosenthal WS. Liver diseases unique to pregnancy. The American journal of gastroenterology. 1991;86(6):659–70. https://www.ncbi.nlm.nih.gov/pubmed/2038986
37. Papafragkakis H, Singhal S, Anand S. Acute fatty liver of pregnancy. South Med J. 2013;106(10):588–93.
38. Forssell G, Laska J, Olofsson C, Olsson M, Mogensen L. Peripartum cardiomyopathy—three cases. Journal of internal medicine. 1994;235(5):493–6. https://onlinelibrary.wiley.com/doi/abs/10.1111/j.1365-2796.1994.tb01109.x. https://doi.org/10.1111/j.1365-2796.1994.tb01109.x.
39. Lampert MB. Peripartum cardiomyopathy. Am Heart J. 1995;130:860–70.
40. Okeke TC, Ezenyeaku CCT, Ikeako LC. Peripartum cardiomyopathy. Ann Med Health Sci. 2013;3(3):313–9.
41. Ramaraj R, Sorrell VL. Peripartum cardiomyopathy: causes, diagnosis, and treatment. Cleveland Clinic journal of medicine. 2009;76(5):289-296. http://www.ccjm.org/content/76/5/289.abstract. doi: https://doi.org/10.3949/ccjm.76a.08004.
42. Johnson-Coyle L, Jensen L, Sobey A. Peripartum cardiomyopathy review and practice guidelines. American journal of critical care. 2012;21(2):89–98. https://www.ncbi.nlm.nih.gov/pubmed/22381985. https://doi.org/10.4037/ajcc2012163.
43. Melvin KR, Richardson PJ, Olsen EGJ, Daly K, Jackson G. Peripartum cardiomyopathy due to myocarditis. The New England journal of medicine. 1982;307(12):731–4. https://doi.org/10.1056/NEJM198209163071207.
44. D'Ovidio C, Sablone S, Carnevale A. Spontaneous coronary artery dissection: case report and literature review. J Forensic Sci. 2015;60(3):801–6.
45. Tweet MS, Hayes SN, Codsi E, Gulati R, Rose CH, Best PJM. Spontaneous coronary artery dissection associated with pregnancy. J Am Coll Cardiol. 2017;70(4):426–35.
46. Appleby CE, Barolet A, Ing D, et al. Contemporary management of pregnancy-related coronary artery dissection: a single-centre experience and literature review. Experimental and clinical cardiology. 2009;14(1):e8–e16. https://www.ncbi.nlm.nih.gov/pubmed/19492033
47. Prahlow JABJ. Pregnancy-related maternal deaths. Am J Forensic Pathol. 2004;25:220–36.
48. Kemp WL, Barnard JJ, Prahlow JA. Death due to thrombotic thrombocytopenic purpura in pregnancy: Case report with review of thrombotic microangiopathies of pregnancy. The American journal of forensic medicine and pathology. 1999;20(2):189–98. https://www.ncbi.nlm.nih.gov/pubmed/10414663. https://doi.org/10.1097/00000433-199906000-00017.
49. May HV, Harbert GM, Thornton WN. Thrombotic thrombocytopenic purpura associated with pregnancy. American journal of obstetrics and gynecology. 1976;126(4):452–8. https://doi.org/10.1016/0002-9378(76)90638-4.
50. Miller J, Pastorek J. Thrombotic thrombocytopenic purpura and hemolytic uremic syndrome in pregnancy. Clinical obstetrics and gynecology. 1991;34(1):64–71. http://ovidsp.ovid.com/ovidweb.cgi?T=JS&NEWS=n&CSC=Y&PAGE=fulltext&D=ovft&AN=00003081-199103000-00010. https://doi.org/10.1097/00003081-199103000-00010.

51. Boden G. Fuel metabolism in pregnancy and in gestational diabetes mellitus. Obstetrics and gynecology clinics of North America. 1996;23(1):1–10. https://doi.org/10.1016/S0889-8545(05)70241-2.
52. Molitch ME. Pituitary diseases in pregnancy. Seminars in perinatology. 1998;22(6):457–70. https://doi.org/10.1016/S0146-0005(98)80026-8.
53. Kovacs K. Sheehan syndrome. The Lancet (British edition). 2003;361(9356):520–2. https://doi.org/10.1016/S0140-6736(03)12490-7.
54. Pearlman M, Faro S. Obstetric septic shock: A pathophysiologic basis for management. Clinical obstetrics and gynecology. 1990;33(3):482–92. http://ovidsp.ovid.com/ovidweb.cgi?T=JS&NEWS=n&CSC=Y&PAGE=fulltext&D=ovft&AN=00003081-199009000-00014. https://doi.org/10.1097/00003081-199009000-00014.
55. Lewis JL. Diagnosis and management of gestational trophoblastic disease. Cancer. 1993;71(S4):1639–47. https://onlinelibrary.wiley.com/doi/abs/10.1002/cncr.2820710430. https://doi.org/10.1002/cncr.2820710430.
56. Berkowitz RSGD. Gestational trophoblastic disease. Cancer. 1995;76:2079–85.
57. Clark SL. Cardiac disease in pregnancy. Crit Care Obstet. 1991;18:237–56.
58. Kiss H, Egarter C, Asseryanis E, Putz D, Kneussl M. Primary pulmonary hypertension in pregnancy: a case report. American journal of obstetrics and gynecology. 1995;172(3):1052–4. https://www.ncbi.nlm.nih.gov/pubmed/7892851
59. Ghamra ZW, Dweik RA. Primary pulmonary hypertension: an overview of epidemiology and pathogenesis. Cleveland Clinic journal of medicine. 2003;70(Suppl 1):S2. http://www.ccjm.org/content/70/Suppl_1/S2.abstract. https://doi.org/10.3949/ccjm.70.Suppl_1.S2.
60. Abbott J. Medical illness during pregnancy. Emergency medicine clinics of North America. 1994;12(1):115–28. https://www.ncbi.nlm.nih.gov/pubmed/8306928. https://doi.org/10.1016/S0733-8627(20)30454-5.
61. Townsley DM. Hematologic complications of pregnancy. Semin Hematol. 2013;50(3):222–31. https://doi.org/10.1053/j.seminhematol.2013.06.004.
62. Sifakis SPG. Anemia in pregnancy. Ann N Y Acad Sci. 2000;900:125–36.
63. Trumbo P, Yates AA, Schlicker S, Poos M. Dietary reference intakes: vitamin A, vitamin K, arsenic, boron, chromium, copper, iodine, iron, manganese, molybdenum, nickel, silicon, vanadium, and zinc. Journal of the American Dietetic Association. 2001;101(3):294–301. https://doi.org/10.1016/S0002-8223(01)00078-5.
64. Smith JA, Espeland M, Bellevue R, Bonds D, Brown AK, Koshy M. Pregnancy in sickle cell disease: experience of the cooperative study of sickle cell disease. Obstetrics and gynecology (New York. 1953). 1996;87(2):199–204. https://doi.org/10.1016/0029-7844(95)00367-3.
65. Serjeant GR, Loy LL, Crowther M, Hambleton IR, Thame M. Outcome of pregnancy in homozygous sickle cell disease. Obstetrics and gynecology (New York. 1953). 2004;103(6):1278–85. https://www.ncbi.nlm.nih.gov/pubmed/15172865. https://doi.org/10.1097/01.AOG.0000127433.23611.54.
66. Sun PM, Wilburn W, Raynor BD, Jamieson D. Sickle cell disease in pregnancy: Twenty years of experience at Grady memorial hospital, Atlanta, Georgia. American journal of obstetrics and gynecology. 2001;184(6):1127–30. https://doi.org/10.1067/mob.2001.115477.
67. Villers MS, Jamison MG, Castro D, James LM, Andra H. Morbidity associated with sickle cell disease in pregnancy. American journal of obstetrics and gynecology. 2008;199(2):125.e1–5. https://www.clinicalkey.es/playcontent/1-s2.0-S0002937808004079. https://doi.org/10.1016/j.ajog.2008.04.016.
68. Burrows RF, Kelton JG. Incidentally detected thrombocytopenia in healthy mothers and their infants. The New England Journal of Medicine. 1988;319(3):142–5. http://content.nejm.org/cgi/content/abstract/319/3/142. https://doi.org/10.1056/NEJM198807213190304.
69. James AH, Jamison MG. Bleeding events and other complications during pregnancy and childbirth in women with von Willebrand disease. Journal of thrombosis and haemostasis. 2007;5(6):1165–9. https://onlinelibrary.wiley.com/doi/abs/10.1111/j.1538-7836.2007.02563.x. https://doi.org/10.1111/j.1538-7836.2007.02563.x.
70. Hosley CM, McCullough LD. Acute neurological issues in pregnancy and the peripartum. Neurohospitalist. 2011;1(2):104–16.

71. Berg CJ, Chang J, Callaghan WM, Whitehead SJ. Pregnancy-related mortality in the united states, 1991–1997. Obstetrics and gynecology (New York. 1953). 2003;101(2):289–96. https://doi.org/10.1016/S0029-7844(02)02587-5.
72. Feske S. Stroke in pregnancy. Semin Neurol. 2007;27(5):442–52.
73. Fewel ME, Thompson J, Gregory B, Hoff JT. Spontaneous intracerebral hemorrhage: a review. Neurosurgical focus. 2003;15(4):1. https://www.ncbi.nlm.nih.gov/pubmed/15344894. https://doi.org/10.3171/foc.2003.15.4.0.
74. Kaplan PW. Neurologic aspects of eclampsia. Neurologic clinics. 2004;22(4):841–61. https://doi.org/10.1016/j.ncl.2004.07.005.
75. Palladino C, Singh V, Campbell J, Flynn H, Gold K. Homicide and suicide during the perinatal period: Findings from the national violent death reporting system. Obstetrics and gynecology (New York. 1953). 2011;118(5):1056–63. http://ovidsp.ovid.com/ovidweb.cgi?T=JS&NEWS=n&CSC=Y&PAGE=fulltext&D=ovft&AN=00006250-201111000-00013. https://doi.org/10.1097/AOG.0b013e31823294da.
76. Mahesan Paul AB, Simms L, Paul AE, et al. Unnatural pregnancy deaths in las vegas: a descriptive study. Journal of forensic and legal medicine. 2016;44:79–83. https://www.clinicalkey.es/playcontent/1-s2.0-S1752928X16301123. https://doi.org/10.1016/j.jflm.2016.08.018.
77. Jadon A. Complications of regional and general anaesthesia in obstetric practice. Indian J Anaesth. 2010;54(5):415–20.
78. A reference guide for certification of deaths associated with pregnancy on death certificates. National Center for Health Statistics; 2022.

Chapter 15
The Pathology of Elder Abuse and Neglect

Rebekah Jacques and Qi Zhang

Despite early reports concerning elder maltreatment [1–3], advancement in understanding this ubiquitous public health and human rights issues remains limited [4]. Research into elder maltreatment is estimated to lag a couple of decades behind child abuse [5, 6]; despite the rate of elder abuse being roughly equivalent to child abuse [6–8]. Segments of the population that are dependent on others for care are vulnerable to abuse and neglect. This has been recognized in infants and children, which has resulted in the development of social and medicolegal adjustments to detect and investigate deaths among the pediatric population. Similarly, older adults can become reliant on others for care and subsequently vulnerable to maltreatment because of the high prevalence of age-related changes, diseases, and associated complex polypharmacy that can result in physical and cognitive decline. However, unlike the pediatric population, the criteria of detecting elder maltreatment have not been established. In addition, elder maltreatment is considered more difficult to detect than child abuse because of the social isolation of some older adults may result in an increase in the risk of maltreatment and the ability of identifying that maltreatment [9]. This social isolation is generally not the case with the pediatric population that do not live alone and often interact with non-family members through school participation [9]. The abuse of older people is slowly emerging as a public health and criminal justice concern. As a cohort, older people have a unique pathophysiology due to age-related changes and diseases. Both age-related diseases and maltreatment place this cohort at risk of death [10].

A recurring theme in elder maltreatment publications is the challenge of defining elder abuse and maltreatment. Definitions of elder abuse vary [11, 12], and this challenges the ability to assess the scope of the problem, comparing incidence, and prevalence rates [13–16]. The most commonly used definition was developed by Action on Elder Abuse in the United Kingdom and adopted by the International

R. Jacques (✉) · Q. Zhang
London, ON, Canada
e-mail: rebekah.jacques@lhsc.on.ca

R. Jacques (ed.), *Forensic Pathology*,
https://doi.org/10.1007/978-3-031-42038-2_15

Network for the Prevention of Elder Abuse (IPNEA) and World Health Organization is "a single, or repeated act, or lack of appropriate action, occurring within any relationship where there is an expectation of trust, which causes harm or distress to an older person" [17]. This definition highlights many issues to consider including any act(s) of omission or commision and the relational aspect of elder maltreatment. The expectation of trust includes certain relationships that can be kin relationships, social relationships and healthcare worker or related aides. Maltreatment of older people is often classified into the following, non-mutually exclusive, categories: physical, psychological, sexual, neglect, and/or financial exploitation. Further, this can be identified as domestic elder abuse, institutional elder maltreatment, and self-neglect (Fig. 15.1). The forms of abuse that are often observed by forensic pathologists are physical abuse, neglect, and sexual abuse. Self-neglect and neglect may look the same at autopsy but the latter has no criminal implications.

Consideration of elder maltreatment as a distinct forensic entity is important because ignorance around fatal complications of this entity has resulted in wrong classification of manner of death [18] and could result in lost opportunity for criminal justice. Conversely, age-related changes and diseases can also be a mimicker of inflicted harm and could lead to miscarriage of justice. The role of ageism and stigmatization of older people as a possible obstacle that has adversely affected professional recognition of elder abuse has yet to be properly investigated [1]. In addition, many older people have an underlying natural disease that serve as an explanation for death can lead to these deaths being less thoroughly investigated deaths [6, 7]. This chapter focuses on abuse of older individuals, either in their homes or in other institutional settings. It does not cover causally obvious forms of elder homicides, such as sharp force and firearm-related death.

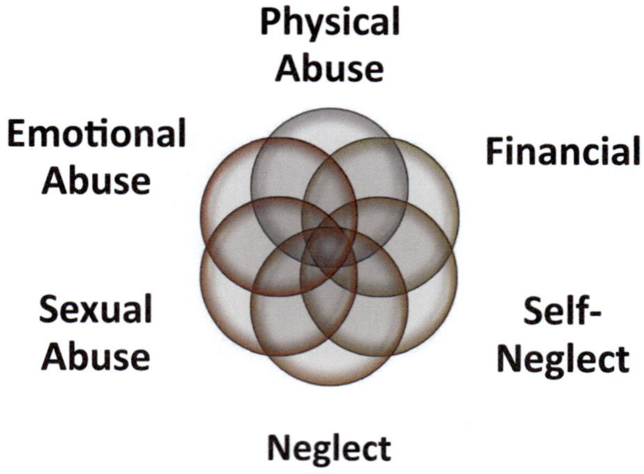

Fig. 15.1 Common types of elder abuse and neglect. Evidence of neglect, physical and sexual abuse may be present at autopsy for the forensic pathologist to assess but others forms of elder maltreatment such as emotional and financial abuse are better evaluated by other non-medical evidence. Self-neglect can appear similar to neglect at autopsy but requires historical and circumstantial information to differentiate. This is important as self-neglect as it does not become a criminal matter. Self-neglect is included here for completion

Aging Population

Older age is generally considered as the time when individuals demonstrate a decline that impairs their ability to physically, physiologically, and cognitively function in society. When "older age" begins is not precisely defined, with the published age cut-off ranging from 55 to 65 years [16, 19–22]. Understanding that using an age cut-off is arbitrary as a large percentage of these people lack age-related changes and diseases. In addition, age-related changes and diseases do not immediately appear at a given age.

Concern over the mistreatment of older adults has been heightened by the realization that the coming decades, in both developed and developing countries, there is expected to be a dramatic increase in this demographic. The proportion of the global population that was 65 years or older in the world in 1990 was 1% or 15 million and 6% or 342 million in 1992 [23]. This is predicted to increase by approximately 22% of the population by 2020 [23]. The fastest growing segment is the "oldest old"—individuals that are older than 85 years. This group is more susceptible to cognitive impairment, chronic and disabling disease and therefore at risk of being more dependent [24–26] and requiring institutional living [27], which is emerging as a risk factor for elder maltreatment.

Elder Abuse as a Problem

Maltreatment of the elderly is a global problem that affects millions of older adults worldwide. This demographic is projected to have a greater prevalence of chronic diseases, disabilities, and cognitive decline [28]. The combination of a growing number of older adults with the accompanying prevalence of diseases that are dependent on relatively fewer familial, financial, and societal resources may lead to the rise of elder maltreatment cases and associated deaths (Fig. 15.2).

Elder abuse is associated with significant morbidity and premature mortality [29–33]. In a long-term study that compared the percentage of surviving elderly, the cohort members with confirmed mistreatment had poorer survival rates (9%) than either those for self-neglect (17%) or other non-mistreated cohort members (40%) [34]. Despite the growing evidence of prevalence of elder maltreatment with its associated mortality, the rate of autopsies decline with increasing age after the ages of 15–24 years [35]. In the United States, the autopsy rate for the 15–24 years was 60.3, however, between 55 and 64 years of age was 11, 4.2 of 65–74-year-old and 2 of 75 to 84 and less than 1 over the age of 85 years [35]. This inverse relationship between age and autopsy rate indicates that the older the decedent the less likely they are to receive an autopsy [23, 35–37]. In addition, there is a further decrease in rate of autopsies when the death of an older person occurrs in an institution [23, 36, 37]. Many elderly death certificates are completed without a complete medicolegal death investigation and without an examination by a physician or autopsy [38].

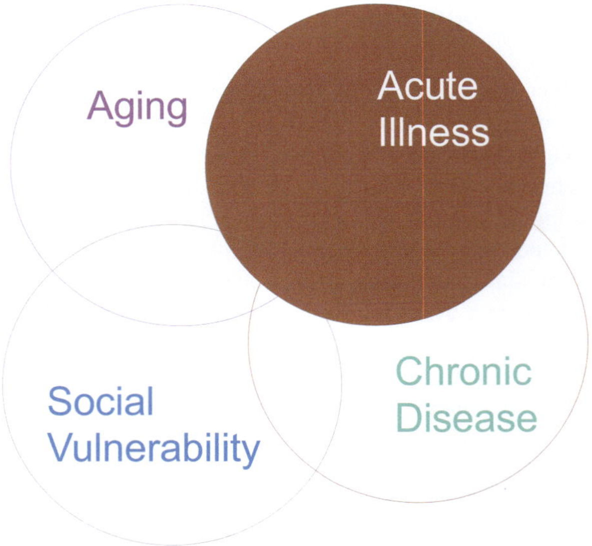

Fig. 15.2 The overlapping of physical and social vulnerabilities make the cohort of older adults vulnerable to abuse but the high incidence of chronic disease make detection of sudden and unexpected deaths a challenge to determine whether the death investigation system ought to investigate their deaths

Part of the reason of a decline in medicolegal autopsy rate of deaths among older adults is that the death may not clearly fall within the relevant statues that typically investigate sudden and unexpected deaths. The challenge is to determine what constitutes sudden and unexpected deaths among the elderly with chronic diseases. In general, it is reasonable expectation that most deaths among the elderly, especially with chronic disease, are the result of natural processes. As a result, these deaths may not be reported to the death investigator. In addition, deaths in institutions, such as nursing homes, would need to be reported by nursing home staff or surviving family members. Self-reporting by institutional staff represents a conflict of interest and may permit the failed detection of serial killer health workers [39].

Recognizing the signs of elder abuse and neglect is the first step to reach a correct diagnosis. As a result, it is important for forensic pathologists and other death investigators to identify markers of abuse and neglect among older adults. The forensic pathologist and their application of the discovery and documentation of the autopsy remain the final opportunity to detect of elder maltreatment. Education of forensic pathologists regarding this entity is a critical component of knowledge and skill development and this chapter will provide a foundation upon which to build knowledge.

Physiology of Aging

The healthcare problems of the elderly are often more complex than those of other age groups. The number of diseases and their associated medications are often multiple and can result in functional disabilities, physiological and metabolic changes that make this cohort unable to provide self-care but also maltreatment.

Further, age-related diseases and changes may resemble abuse. The forensic pathologist is tasked with the responsibility to different causes of death by abuse and neglect from findings related to senescence.

Normal aging is characterized by loss in every body system, which fosters dependency and manifestations of maltreatment.

Examples include:

- **Dehydration:** Older adults are at risk of dehydration due to water metabolism and due to altered thirst sensation, renal metabolism, and high prevalence of medications that are diuretics [40]
- **Hyperthermia and hypothermia:** Among this cohort, there is a decreased temperature perception and impaired temperature regulation therefore making this cohort at risk to hypo- and hyperthermia [23]
- **Sarcopenia:** Sarcopenia is the involuntary reduction in skeletal muscle tissue and strength with age that leads to a functional decline and subsequent loss of independence [41]. Sarcopenia can begin as early as the fourth decade of life and decline in a linear fashion with up to half of skeletal mass being lost by the eighth decade [41]. The etiology of sarcopenia is multifactorial and includes decline in physical activity, altered endocrine function, chronic diseases, inflammation, insulin resistance, and nutritional deficiencies [41]. This results in an elderly body habitus and limits the applicability of using body mass index (BMI) as an underweight indicator and therefore malnourished. Muscles are a reserve of proteins and energy that can be used in periods of acute illness and starvation.
- **Other findings:** An unsteady gait due to decreased proprioception and the effects of certain medications may result in orthostatic hypotension and result in falls and their related injuries. Older adults are prone to abrasions and lacerations because of age-related loss of skin thickness, elasticity, and tensile strength [42, 43]. Bruising and purpura are common in older people as their skin is more easily bruised secondary to vascular fragility. Senile purpura, steroid use-steroid purpura, and photoaging are commonly observed in older adults (Fig. 15.3). Purpura indicates that there is hemorrhage under the skin but is a non-specific term. Purpura can arise in minor injuries due to the fragile nature of the skin and may persist long after the injury. Senile purpura are red-purple areas that are typically on the flexor surfaces of the upper hands. Bateman purpura are restricted to areas of chronic sun damage, and similarly steroid purpura are limited to areas of steroid application [44].

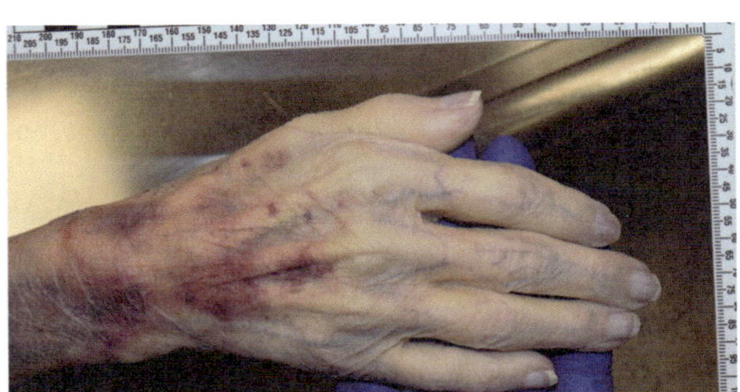

Fig. 15.3 Age-related changes can be mistaken as injuries. In older adults, senile pupura of the back of the hands and forearms is common and does not denote trauma

Age-related Diseases

Approximately, 80% of the population over 65 years have at least one chronic condition and 50% have two chronic conditions [45]. Older adults often have multiple chronic illnesses that make them dependent and require the use of more medications. In addition, natural diseases can mask or resemble abuse and neglect. The distinction between normal aging and disease is an essential foundation to the recognition of possible cases of elder abuse. In addition, distinguishing diseases caused by abuse or neglect from naturally occurring conditions is complex. The common age-related diseases that make this cohort vulnerable to fatal maltreatment and mimickers of abuse and neglect include age-related bone diseases, dementia, and acquired disease resulting in coagulation.

Age-related bone diseases such as osteoporosis, renal osteodystrophy, and osteomalacia are risk factors for fractures as they can occur with minimal provocation of force. In the setting of osteoporosis, the vertebral bodies and the hip are common sites for fractures. Other pathological factors include those of malignancy, which can occur at any site, thereby may require histopathological evaluation.

Dementia is not a normal part of aging. It is a disease in which older age is a risk factor for the development of dementia. In addition, dementia is a risk factor for elder maltreatment as this disease impairs cognitive domains including attention, information processing, and praxis. This impaired executive function makes individuals with dementia at risk of being violent and sexually disinhibited [46]. The diagnosis of dementia is clinicopathological diagnosis and includes evidence of memory loss plus the loss of function in at least one other cognitive domain including language, judgment, and visuospatial ability. The most common types of dementia include Alzheimer's diseases, Lewy body dementia, Parkinson's disease, frontotemporal dementia, and vascular dementia. Neurodegenerative disorders and normal age-related changes result in atrophy of the brain. This puts tension on the bridging veins between the brain and dura. As a result, minor falls can result in a massive subdural hemorrhage. Further, intracerebral hemorrhage may be associated with hypertension, congophilic amyloid angiopathy due to Alzheimer's disease, anticoagulation, and trauma.

Subdural hemorrhage can occur "spontaneously" or after 'minimally appreciated' head trauma in the elderly with mild cognitive impairment and individuals treated with anticoagulation. Bleeding in the subdural space is commonly due to the laceration of "bridging veins" between the brain and the dura. These veins become increasingly vulnerable to lacerations as a consequence of "physiological" brain atrophy or neurodegenerative disorders. The dura remains tightly adherent to the inner table of the calvarium, while the distance between the dura and brain increases, thereby placing tension onto the bridging veins.

If available, neuropathology consultation is recommended for brain examination for suspected neurodegenerative disorders. Detailed neuropathological examination and complete staging of certain neurodegenerative disorder are beyond the scope of this chapter. Here we recommend a concise protocol to examine and sample the brain regions needed for diagnosis of common neurodegenerative disorders.

- After the standard brain removal (with or without spinal cord), document fresh brain weight
- Reflect the dura and document any chronic/acute hemorrhage, exudate or other anomaly
- Perform an external examination of the whole brain, document the arrangement of circle of Willis for any vascular malformation, presence/absence and degree of atherosclerosis of the major branches, cerebral atrophy and distribution, and other lesions (infarcts, contusions, brain swelling/herniation, hemorrhages)
- If possible, the whole brain should be fixed in formalin for 2 weeks and further examined by a neuropathologist. If the brain has to be sectioned freshly, serial coronal sections of the cerebral hemispheres, parasagittal sections of the cerebellum, and horizontal sections of the brainstem are recommended (Fig. 15.3)
- Examine the brain slices for atrophy, including cerebral white matter atrophy and discoloration, ventricular enlargement, hippocampal atrophy, discoloration of substantia nigra or locus coeruleus, cerebellar atrophy (vermis, hemisphere, and dentate). Examine for any old infarct or intraparenchymal hemorrhage, particularly in the deep gray matter (basal ganglia and thalamus)
- The following sections are recommended for microscopic examination: motor and somatosensory cortex, mid frontal gyrus, superior temporal gyrus, inferior parietal lobule, occipital lobe with calcarine, anterior and posterior cingulate, amygdala, hippocampus at the level of lateral geniculate nuclei, basal ganglia, mamillary bodies, thalamus at the level of subthalamic nuclei, centrum semiovale, midbrain, pons, medulla, cerebellar vermis, and cerebellar hemisphere with dentate (Fig. 15.4).

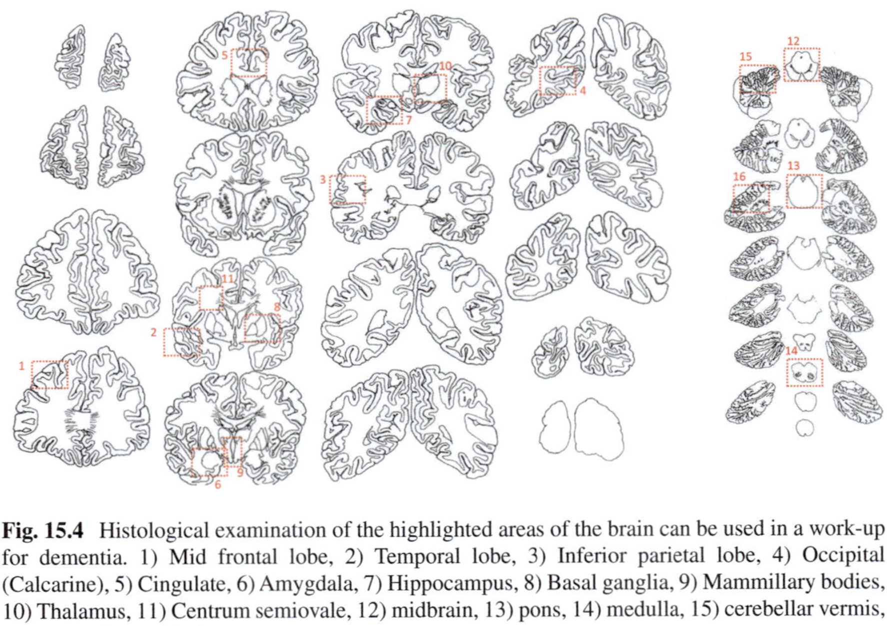

Fig. 15.4 Histological examination of the highlighted areas of the brain can be used in a work-up for dementia. 1) Mid frontal lobe, 2) Temporal lobe, 3) Inferior parietal lobe, 4) Occipital (Calcarine), 5) Cingulate, 6) Amygdala, 7) Hippocampus, 8) Basal ganglia, 9) Mammillary bodies, 10) Thalamus, 11) Centrum semiovale, 12) midbrain, 13) pons, 14) medulla, 15) cerebellar vermis, 16) cerebellum with dentate

- Special stains (including hematoxylin/eosin/Luxol fast blue and Bielschowsky sliver stain) and immunohistochemistry with antibodies to phosphorylated tau, beta-amyloid, alpha-synuclein, and TDP-43 are commonly performed and summarized in Table 15.1.

Despite the different clinical presentations, neurodegenerative diseases share several common histological features: (1) neuronal loss, associated gliosis, and microglia activation in the affected regions; (2) abnormal accumulation of specific proteins, either intracellularly (i.e., neurofibrillary tangles or various inclusion bodies) or extracellularly (i.e., amyloid plaques); (3) these changes are region specific, closely correlated with the clinical features. In the dementing diseases, the degenerative changes are primarily located in the cerebral cortex. Here we will briefly discuss the three most common neurodegenerative diseases related to cerebral cortex and dementia.

Alzheimer disease (AD) is the most common degenerative disease, characterized by presence of neurofibrillary tangles, amyloid plaques, and neuritic plaques. Macroscopically, features of cortical atrophy, such as narrowed cerebral gyri and widened sulci, are more prominent in the medial temporal region, corresponding to the amygdala, hippocampus, and parahippocampal gyri. The frontal and parietal lobes are also involved, but the occipital lobes are usually spared. On the cross-sections, cortical atrophy with dilated ventricles, particularly the temporal horns on the lateral ventricles, is evident. Pigment loss is more evident in the locus coeruleus than the substantia nigra. Microscopically, plaques and tangles are readily identifiable with special stains and immunohistochemistry. Amyloid plaques are highlighted with beta-amyloid immunohistochemistry. Depending on the disease

Table 15.1 Summary of the brain regions, special stains, and immunohistochemistry recommended for suspected neurodegenerative workup

	Brain region	H/E/LFB	p-Tau	Beta-amyloid	α-Syn	TDP-43
1	Mid frontal lobe	x	x	x	x	x
2	Temporal lobe	x	x		x	
3	Inferior parietal lobe	x				
4	Occipital (calcarine)	x	x			
5	Cingulate	x			x	
6	Amygdala	x	x		x	x
7	Hippocampus (LGN)	x	x	x	x	x
8	Basal ganglia	x		x		
9	Mammillary bodies	x				
10	Thalamus	x				
11	Centrum semiovale	x				
12	Midbrain	x		x	x	
13	Pons (locus coeruleus)	x			x	
14	Medulla	x				x
15	Cerebellar vermis	x				
16	Cerebellar hemisphere	x		x		

severity, the amyloid pathology is present in the neocortex at the earlier stage, and progresses to the hippocampus, basal ganglia, thalamus, midbrain, pons, and cerebellum (*Thal* stage). Neurofibrillary tangles, on the other hand, follow a different sequence. The tangles and dystrophic neurites can be detected using Bielschowsky silver stain or immunohistochemistry with antibodies to phosphorylated tau. The neurofibrillary tangles and dystrophic neurites are first detected in the transentorhinal and entorhinal cortex, followed by the hippocampal CA1 sector, the remainder of the hippocampus, and lastly spread to the association neocortex and the primary motor/sensory cortex (*Braak* and *Braak* stage). The degree of cognitive decline is correlated with both amyloid and tau pathology. Amyloid angiopathy, with accumulation of beta-amyloid in the blood vessel wall, is commonly seen in patients with Alzheimer's disease. Cerebral amyloid angiopathy (CAA) is a risk factor for lobar intracerebral hemorrhage.

Lewy body disease (LBD) is another common type of dementia. Clinically, patients usually present as cognition fluctuation with early hallucinations (more commonly cited as well-formed visual hallucination). The brain atrophy is not as severe as seen in AD. The depigmentation is commonly identified in substantia nigra and locus coeruleus. Histologically, LBD is characterized by the presence of neuronal intracytoplasmic round eosinophilic inclusions (Lewy bodies) at different brain regions. Lewy bodies can be highlighted with immunohistochemistry with antibody to alpha-synuclein. Again, depending on the disease severity and clinical progression, the Lewy bodies can be found in the brainstem, limbic structures, and neocortex.

Frontotemporal lobar degenerations (FTLD) are a heterogeneous group, characterized by degenerative changes of the frontal and temporal lobes. Clinically the patient can present with behavioral disturbance, primary aphasia, and memory loss. A classic gross feature of FTLD brain is the severe frontal temporal lobe atrophy and the relative sparing of the occipital lobes, giving a "knife edge" appearance (Fig. 15.5). Microscopically, the involved frontotemporal neocortex often have vacuolated neuropil due to massive neuronal loss and gliosis. Depends on the underlying pathology, the neuronal inclusions can be highlighted by immunohistochemistry with antibodies to phosphorylated tau, TDP-43, p62, or FUS (fused in sarcoma).

Concomitant proteinopathies are not uncommon in neurodegenerative diseases. Patients with mixed pathologies of tau, beta-amyloid, alpha-synuclein, and TDP-43 have more severe cognitive decline.

Bruising is common in older people, and it cannot be used as a definitive indicator of abuse. There are mimickers of physical abuse of the skin. Physical changes that are associated with aging as previously mentioned, as well as increased susceptibility to injuries must be considered in cases of fatal abuse. Acquired bleeding disorders, such as liver disease and warfarin therapy, are common. Other cutaneous mimics of elder abuses include burn injuries that have a glove/stocking distribution maybe a glove/footwear contact dermatitis [44]. Photodermatitis, photosensitive dermatitis, paraneoplastic syndromes, and the side effects of drugs can be mistaken for vitamin B3 deficiency, pellagra (e.g., Casal necklace) [44].

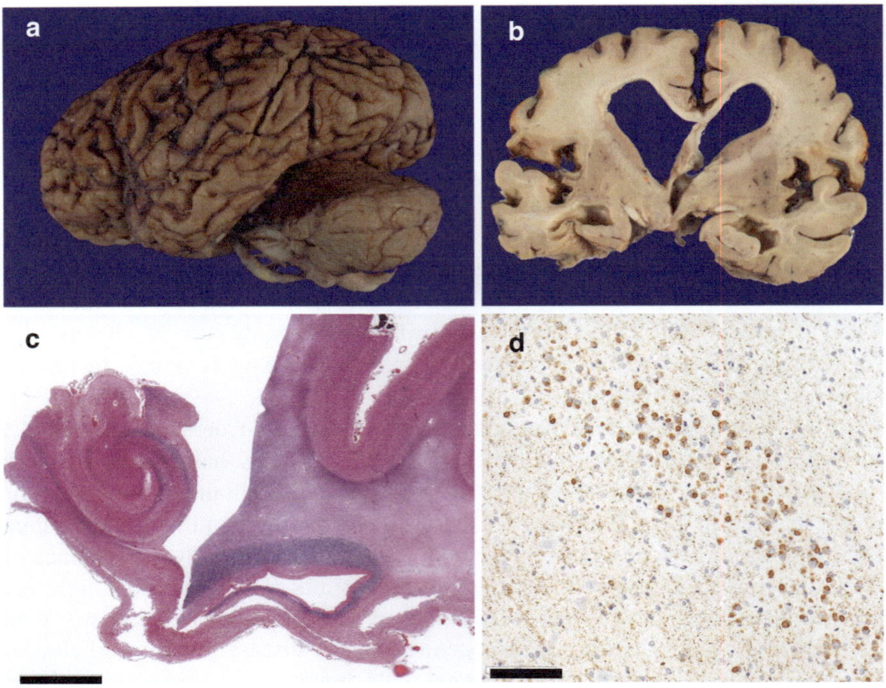

Fig. 15.5 The brain of a 68 year old male with frontotemporal lobar degeneration. There is severe cerebral atrophy at the frontal and temporal lobes, but sparing the parietal and occipital lobes (**a**). The cortical ribbon is thin, the ventricles are dilated. Severe atrophy is at the mesial temporal lobe (**b** and **c**). Immunohistochemistry with pTau shows abundant neuronal inclusions as "Pick bodies". Scale bar: 3 mm in **c**, 100 μm in **d**

Neglect vs Self-neglect

The failure of meeting the needs of Instrumental Activities of Daily Living (IADL) and Activities of Daily Living (ADL) results in neglect and self-neglect. ADLs include fundamental skills that are needed to manage basic physical needs of personal care including personal hygiene, toileting, eating, taking medications, dressing, and ambulating. IADL are more complex activities that permit independent community living based on a higher level of cognitive abilities and include cleaning and maintaining one's home, preparing meals, managing finances and medications. At autopsy, neglect and self-neglect can appear the same. Self-neglect has been defined as the behavior of an older adult that threatens their own health and safety [9]. This definition does not address the issue of cognitive impairment or competence. While neglect implies that a caregiver has not met the needs of the older adult. Neglect by others, or by oneself, may appear the same at autopsy and include pressure injuries, malnutrition, dehydration, and poor hygiene (Fig. 15.6). The two need to be differentiated because self-neglect generally does not have criminal

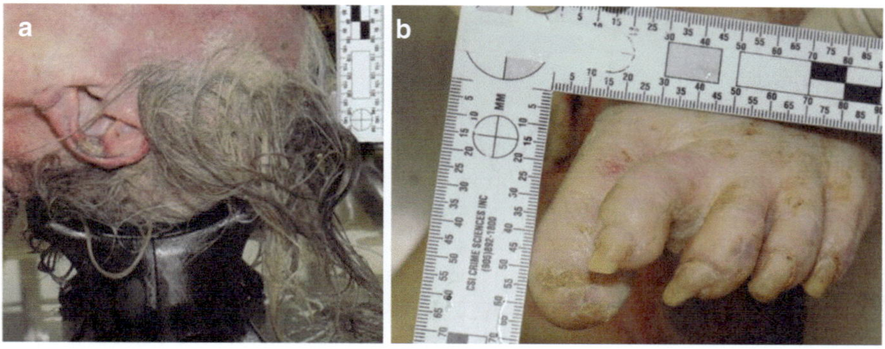

Fig. 15.6 Neglect and self-neglect can present as poor hygiene. (a) Hair sebum due to unwashed hair and pressure injury of the ear. (b) Long toenails and unwashed skin

justice implications. The difference is determined through the history, scene, circumstances, and the police investigation.

Self-neglect, or Diogenes syndrome, named after a fourth century controversial Greek philosopher who believed in the virtue of poverty is characterized by social withdrawal, poor personal hygiene extreme squalor, and lack of concern about one's living conditions [47]. Diogenes syndrome is also referred to as senile squalor, senile breakdown, and social withdrawal in the elderly [48–50]. The incidence of self-neglect is estimated to be 1 in every 2000 individuals over the age of 60 years [49]. The scene is often in a state of marked disrepair, broken windows, peeling paint, piles of garbage, odor of rotting food, urine and feces, unflushed toilets and may have evidence of hoarding. The decedent may be in filthy and advanced decomposition because of social isolation, and there may be signs suggestive of hypothermia or hyperthermia [47, 51]. Usually self-neglect occurs among individuals who live alone; however, there are cases of married couples and siblings that show the same features, this is termed Diogenes à deux [48, 52–54].

Signs and Symptoms of Neglect and Self-Neglect:

- Malnutrition
- Dehydration
- Pressure injuries
- Poor personal hygiene: sebum, lice, scabies, soiled clothes, poor oral care
- Contractures
- Filthy living conditions: soiled bedding, animal/insect infestations
- Lack of prescribed medications present in toxicology tests
- Unattended or untreated health problems
- Hazardous or unsafe living conditions: improper electricity, appropriate plumbing, heat and access to clean water
- Inadequate clothing
- Lack of necessary medical aids: eyeglasses, hearing aids, and dentures

Features:

Malnutrition

Malnutrition is a common and serious problem among older adults [55]; however, it is commonly unrecognized by health workers [56, 57]. The reported prevalence of malnutrition among older adults ranges from 10 to 85% [58–60]. This wide variance is due to differences in the study methods employed, the setting the study occurred and how malnutrition was defined [61]. Herein, malnutrition will refer to the insufficient dietary intake to meet the energy or protein requirements [62]. There is no single feature that has emerged as optimal in defining malnutrition in the elderly. Diagnosing malnutrition among older adults can be a challenge [61]. This can be due to lack of adequate food intake of the essential nutrients or by inadequate intake in the face of illness such as infections or pressure injuries, or medical treatment, wherein nutrients cannot be ingested, absorbed, or metabolized adequately at the rate of utilization when external losses are excessive [63].

Risk factors for developing malnutrition include poor dentition and poorly fitting dentures [64], age-related loss of smell and taste, disease states, and medication [65]. Medications can result in malnutrition because they can reduce food intake due to the side effects of anorexia, nausea, and vomiting. Reduced oral intake can be due to inadequate finances, edentia, poor-fitting dentures and food insecurity, or the deliberate withholding of food by caregivers. In addition, poor appetite is common with older adults, this has been referred to as the anorexia of aging [66]. All cause of reduced oral intake have the same effect.

Findings at autopsy include:

- External findings: pronounced rib cage, pelvic, and vertebral bones
- Internal findings: loss of fat stores (e.g., absent subcutaneous and visceral fat tissue, thin omentum/mesentery, atrophy of muscles and internal organs, absent stomach contents, lack of stool in the bowel

Malnutrition increases susceptibility to infection, delayed wound healing, reduced rate of drug metabolism, and impaired physical and cognitive function [59]. In turn, infection increase demand on energy requirements and can result in a vicious cycle of clinical deterioration that can lead to death as infection can lead to increased caloric and protein requirements, thus making the malnutrition worse, which, again, predisposes to pressure injuries and infection.

Medical Causes

(a) Chronic disease conditions that make eating difficult (e.g., paralysis due to stroke)
(b) Increase caloric or protein requirements due to infection or the healing wounds
(c) Medications that impair the desire to eat (e.g., psychotropic drugs)

Dehydration

The elderly are prone to dehydration due to age-related alterations in control of fluid hemostasis. Explanations of dehydration include illness (e.g., fever and infection) and medication (e.g., diuretics). Other explanations include decreased fluid intake. Assessing for dehydration is based on external findings such as sunken globes and dry organ surfaces on cut section, desiccated stool, empty urinary bladder, dry mucous and serosal membranes. The diagnosis can be confirmed with a "dehydration pattern" using vitreous biochemistry [67, 68]. The postmortem vitreous fluid will show an elevation of sodium, chloride, creatinine, and urea levels [69]. Using skin turgor in the elderly is not useful given that loss of elasticity is a common finding in older persons.

Pressure Injuries

Pressure injuries, are also known as decubitus ulcers, pressure sores, ischemic ulcers, and bed sores, are areas of tissue necrosis and ulceration that form when blood flow is reduced to the soft tissues due to sustained pressure (Fig. 15.7). When pressure on soft tissue closes capillary blood flow, this results in oxygen deprivation to the tissue area and accumulation of metabolic end products. Pressure injures commonly occur in areas overlying bony prominences. The distribution of pressure injuries indicates the sustained positions an individual had in life (Fig. 15.8). For example, in supine individuals pressure injuries commonly occur in the sacrum, coccyx, hips, and heels. Pressure injuries are a serious medical problem because skin is a part of the innate immune system and breaches to the skin in the form of pressure injuries can lead to death through sepsis or bacteremia due to the colonization of pressure injuries with microorganisms can lead to infectious complications such as osteomyelitis,

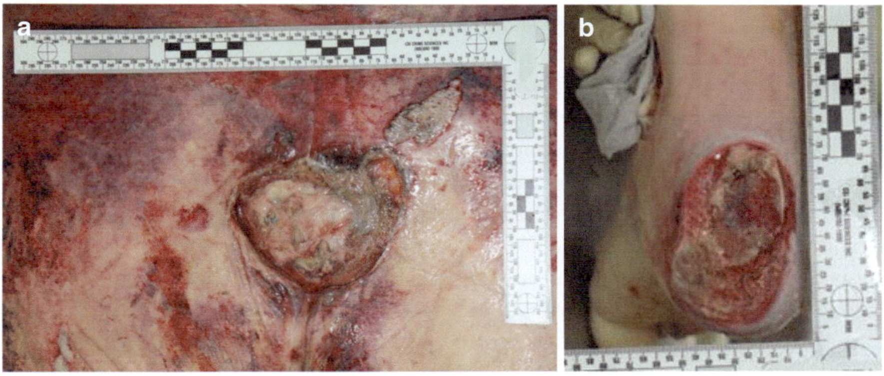

Fig. 15.7 High grade pressure injuries. (**a**) Pressure injury of the sacrum. The fat is exposed in the right upper hand coroner of the pressure injury and the pelvic bone is exposed at the base of the pressure injury. (**b**) Pressure injury of the heel showing the exposed calcaneous bone

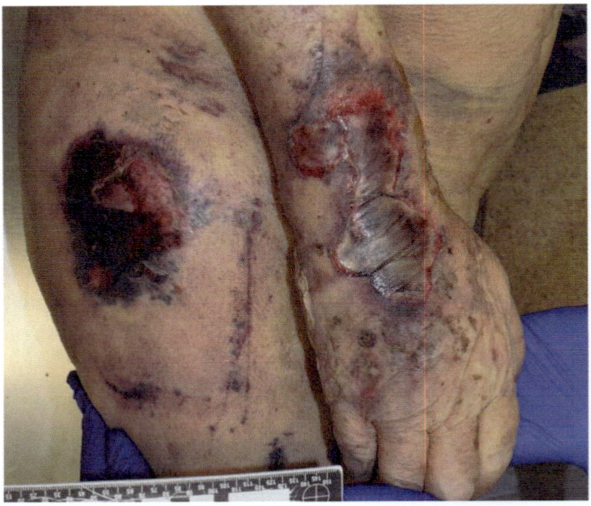

Fig. 15.8 The distribution of pressure injuries can indicate a prolonged position of the body in life. The hip and the wrist were in contact with the floor as demonstrated by the location of these pressure injuries and scene findings

bacteremia, and septicemia. Septicemia related to pressure injuries is associated with a mortality rate of up to 50 to 55% [70, 71]. Unfortunately, the prevalence of pressure injuries is commonly encountered in geriatric patients that are institutionalized in retirement homes, nursing homes, and hospitals [72–74]. Pressure injuries constitute a preventable and usually treatable, yet potentially fatal condition in the elder [75].

A study of pressure injuries among older adults found that pressure injurieswere more frequently discovered among seniors that died in retirement homes or nursing homes than in any other category of the place of death, such as a private home or hospital. The overall prevalence of pressure injuries among older adults ranges from 1.3 to 11.2% [72, 76, 77]. This may be due to risk factors of the populations within these domicilies rather than difference in care standards. Among long-term care home residents, there is a significant correlation between the prevalence of pressure injuries with advance age and certain diseases, such as trauma, dementia, neurological diseases, apoplexy, and marasmus [72] Various disease states in which individuals are immobile, including dementia, and incontinence and malnutrition augment skin breakdown. The resultant pressure injury in both appearance and extent inevitable raise questions about the quality of health care, neglect, and mistreatment. A fallacy is that complications of pressure injuries as an inevitable sequelae of "normal disease process" are a natural death. However, pressure injuries can be successfully prevented, or minimised, by early risk assessment scores, modifications of risk factors, consistent monitoring, and utilization of prophylactic measures [72]. Pressure injuries can result in death usually do to bacteremia that arose from an infected pressure injury that has gained access to the blood stream. Deaths that arise from complications of pressure injuries may be due to any manner of death; however, those that arise in the setting of neglect and/or abuse, the manner of death maybe erroneously certified as natural death.

The skin serves many functions including protection, body temperature regulation, and sweat excretion. The most superficial layer of skin, is an avascular epidermis with rete pegs that protrude into the deeper fibro-elastic dermis that contain blood vessels. The deepest layer is the subcutis, which is a loose connective tissue deep to the dermis that is composed predominantly of fat cells with little vascularity. This layer is compressible but lacks significant tensile strength and is therefore vulnerable to shear forces that may compromise its blood supply by angular stretching of the vessels [78]. Depending on the location of the body, deep to subcutis is muscle and soft tissues. Muscles are vascular and tolerate compression poorly but is actively resistant to tension. The amount of muscle overlying bony or cartilaginous prominences are variable. The periosteum and perichondrium are the deepest soft tissues overlying bone and cartilage, respectively. Pressure on any bony prominence is transmitted from the surface of the skin to the underlying bone, compressing all intervening layers. The elasticity of these tissues results in the force being distributed maximally over the bony prominence and diminishing progressively to the periphery. A pressure gradient exists from the surface to the bone with each succeeding layer [78]. The mean blood pressure of normal, healthy skin capillaries varies from 12 to 70 mmHg [78]. Pressure that exceeds this will be sufficient to obstruct and compromise blood flow will result in localized ischemia and eventually cell death. This is observed as a pressure injury. This is compounded by the maceration effects of urine, stool, and sweat and their associated bacterial populations.

Risk Factors for the formation of pressure injuries:

(a) Decrease sensory/motor function
(b) Altered consciousness
(c) Pressure over bony prominences
(d) Malnutrition: Muscle atrophy and reduction in subcutaneous fat make the pressure more significant. Allows for padding when it is a normal amount of fat
(e) Shearing forces: Sliding of one tissue layer over another with stretching and angulation of blood vessels, which results in injury and thrombosis. Friction and perspiration cause fixation of the skin and superficial fascia to the sheets/clothing, while deep fascia slides down. This is aggravated by loose skin commonly seen in the elderly because of aging, loss of subcutaneous tissue, and dehydration
(f) Moisture (fecal/urinary incontinence): Reduces skin resistance to other factors
(g) Dementia
(h) Obesity: Adipose tissue is poorly vascularized and the underlying tissue becomes more susceptible to ischemia
(i) Immobilized paraplegic patients
(j) Trauma
(k) Inappropriate use of restraints

There are a number of clinical pressure injury classification systems [78–82]. The pressure injury classification used here will incorporate common macroscopic descriptions and the histopathological description often not used in antemortem circumstances. Each stage describes the severity but also predicts significant mortality [78].

Stage I: Reactive hyperemia (reddening of the skin) of an irregular, ill-defined area of soft tissue swelling over a bony prominence. The redness is caused by a sudden increase in blood flow to the area compressed after relief from the pressure of compression. This lesion can occur within two hours. This type of pressure ulcer is difficult to assess postmortem, often due to the obscuring impact of lividity. Histologically, there is an acute inflammatory response involving all soft tissues and edema. There is no ulceration.

Stage 2: Blister to ulceration of the skin. The ulcer can be full thickness of the skin but does not penetrate into the subcutaneous fat. The ulcer edges are more distinct with early fibrosis and pigmentation changes that blend into a broad indistinct area of erythema. Histologically, the section shows an ulcer that penetrates through the full thickness of the dermis to the junction with the subcutaneous fat. The underlying dermis shows fibrotic infiltrate and a mixed acute and chronic inflammation involving the superficial and deeper. In addition, there may be edema and thrombosed blood vessels.

Stage 3: Full thickness ulcers extending through the skin and subcutaneous fat up to the fascia. There is usually undermining of the skin. The base of the ulcer is usually necrotic, foul-smelling, and infected. Histological evaluation shows an intense mixed acute and chronic inflammatory infiltrate. Myocytes may be edematous and lose fibrillar detail. The ulcer margins are thickened due to epidermal reaction. The subcutaneous fat is obliterated with necrosis.

Stage 4: Full thickness ulcer that extends to the muscle, bone, cartilage, and joint(s). This stage is at risk of the following complications: osteomyelitis and septic arthritis with subluxation and dislocation. Postmortem radiological imaging can be used to examine for bone involvement with osteomyelitis and loss of bone substance; however, if there is underlying osteoporosis or osteoarthritis, this can limit radiological assessment. To confirm osteomyelitis, examination of the bone histologically can confirm the presence of absence of osteomyelitis.

Closed pressure injuries: This is a special pressure injury that is caused by the same pathologic process but externally appears to be a small benign-appearing cutaneous ulcer that has extensive pathology internally and extend along the deep fascial planes. These commonly occur over bony prominence of the pelvis. Microscopically, there is a narrow, but deep ulcer lined by thickened epidermis.

The evaluation of pressure injuries can include photodocumenting the ulcer with a scale, macroscopic descriptions including stage, tissues involved, evidence of treatment, quantity, location, size, presence of granulation or necrotic tissue, re-epithelialization, nature of the exudate, if present, presence of osteomyelitis, microbiological studies of the pressure injury and a blood sample, and histopathological evaluation. Currently, the imaging studies of pressure injuries are used in the clinical context, especially if there are concerns for osteomyelitis, and but not on postmortem cases [83]. Radiological imaging techniques may not sufficiently discriminatate between soft tissue infections alone and accompanying bone infections [84–87] because current radiological imaging techniques are sometimes insufficient to differentiate between infectious and pressure-induced osseous changes, that include reactive bone formation [86]. Histopathological studies of pressure injuries were based on clinicopathological features [86–88]. There are few postmortem studies examining the implications for pressure injuries [89] and few studies that examine the histopathological appearance of pressure injuries [90, 91]. The advantage of postmortem studies, compared to clinicopathological studies, is that postmortem tissues permit a more precise assessment of extent of bone involvement [92], other osseous pathologies and purulent exudate in the soft tissues.

The casual relationship of a pressure injury as the etiology of fatal infectious complication has to be clearly demonstrated based on the forensic evidence. The microbiological cultures have to be differentiated from postmortem contamination and overgrowth. The microbiological investigations of the ulcer and blood are important because this will identify the focus of the bacteremia. The histological evaluation of the ulcer identifies the focus of septicemia, documents the inflammatory tissue changes, and demonstrates the necrosis of the ulcer. Together, microbiological and histological investigations can identify a pressure injury as the place of entry of bacteremia and the focus of septicemia, which is the evidentiary casual link between the pressure injuries, bacteremia, and death. Bacteremia or sepsis as a consequence of pressure ulcer formation may be regarded as an unnatural cause of death when the possibility of neglectful care leads to the formation of the pressure injury. Other findings need to be taken into account to determine the manner of death.

Poor Hygiene

Poor hygiene can manifest through soiled clothing, unwashed hair, and unwashed skin that results in the accumulation of sebum, unkempt fingernails, and toe nails that may grow through clothing. In addition, assessment for lice and scabies is warranted.

Contractures

Contractures is an abnormal, usually permanent, condition characterized by flexion and fixation of a limb at a joint. Contractures leave the joint in a non-functional position that is resistant to bending or extension. This can occur in prolonged periods of bed rest, including bed rest in intact neuromuscular systems and functionally normal individuals. The muscle becomes weak, atrophic, change shape and shorten with disuse. Eventually, there is replacement with fibrous connective tissue, progressing to fibrosis and fatty metaplasia.

Theses can be prevented by passive range-of-motion exercises. Development of contractures may indicate inadequate appropriate joint exercises.

Physical Abuse

Physical abuse is a broad classification of elder maltreatment that is the result of the infliction of mechanical injury [93]. Physical abuse accounts for up to 14% of elder maltreatment and results in death more frequently than younger adults [23]. Physical abuse markers include abrasions/lacerations, bruises, traumatic alopecia, fractures, evidence of restraints, evidence of trauma, patterned injuries, and burns/scalds. This also includes unexplained injuries, injuries that are incongruent with the explanation and delay in seeking and receiving treatment. Injuries to the eyes, mouth, and posterior torso need to be explained. Concerning blunt force injuries include bruises or abrasions of different ages, bruises and abrasions in certain parts of the body including of the inner thighs, palms, ears, neck, mastoid regions, and axilla [23].

Findings suggestive of physical abuse:

- The explanation of injuries is in congruent with injuries
- Injuries located with areas that are not typical of terminal collapse
- Patterned injuries
- Injuries in different stages of healing
- Delay between injury and seeking treatment

Restraints

The use of physical and chemical restraints ranges from 8.5 to 18.5% with reported increased use the older the patient [94]. Physical restraints can be mechanical devices, materials, or equipment that restrict individuals freedom of movement or normal access to their bodies. Individuals in restraints are at risk of ligature strangulation, traumatic or positional asphyxia.

In the context of using restraints, these include authorized and inappropriate use of restraints. Restraints can be used to control an institutionalized older adult if they have a tendency to be violent or wander. Restraints can be divided into chemical and physical restraints. Physical restraints are the use of an object to limit an individuals' freedom of movement [95]. These can include a geriatric chair with a table, belts tied to a chair or a bed with bedrails, tipping chairs, blankets, sheets, vets, wrists and elbow restraints, and manipulation of furniture [95, 96]. The use of physical restraints in the elderly is common in hospitals and nursing homes, with the prevalence being up to 2/3s of the elderly patients [96]. The prevalence of restraints in home care is unknown [96]. Use of restraints requires an explanation as restraints can have negative physical impacts for the elderly and can result in death. The physical impacts include increase risk of falls, loss of muscle mass, joint contractures, and traumatic asphyxia [96, 97]. Physical restraints appear to be used most frequently to prevent falls and fall-related injuries, ironically have also been associated with falls and an increase of death [96]. Clinical documentation including medical indication, duration and method of restraint, and photograph of the decedent in situ (or reenactment of the positioning of the decedent by a witness) needs to be conveyed to the forensic pathologist. If the decedent has been removed, a description of the decedent relative to the restraint will be necessary. Autopsy features supportive of restraint-associated asphyxia include a possible ligature mark of neck or torso, demarcation above the restraint the congestion, petechiae of the conjunctivae; with possible involvement of the oral mucosa and face. An apparent ligature mark on the skin may not be obvious with soft broad ligatures. Chemical restraints can include medications that impact consciousness.

Bruises

Bruises are a common blunt force injury within the geriatric community and on their own can be difficult to distinguish what is accidental and what is inflicted [98]. In addition, vitamin C and K deficiencies or liver disease may result in coagulopathies that can make individuals prone to bruising.

The dating of bruises by macroscopic attributes of color is inexact and forensically unreliable because of the individual variation in response to injury. This is particularly true of the elderly that have systemic age-related changes that delay healing. Timing of the injuries may require histological examination [99]. The microscopic dating of injuries is scientifically based on an understanding of the dynamic process of cutaneous would healing and has significant limitations [100, 101]. Histopathological assessment allows the forensic pathologist to make general conclusions by considering the timing of the stages of healing. Cutaneous wound healing is an orchestra of biological phenomena that consists of three sequential, overlapping phases: inflammation, proliferation, and maturation. Forensic pathologists are often asked to give their opinion on the age of wounds, and the interpretation may have significant medicolegal consequences. However, biological variability introduces a wide margin of uncertainty. Changes will vary depending on the size of wound, nature of wound, age, nutrition and health of the person, and local factors. Limitations at all stages are subject to multifactorial conditions that overlap in time and are dependent on constitutional factors that limit healing, such as diabetes mellitus, which is commonly the geriatric population.

Multiple bruises that are at different stages may be a sign of maltreatment or alcohol dependence. In fatal cases without internal injury and there is extensive external soft tissue bleeding, attempts to quantitate the injuries should be measured and corroborated indicators of hypovolemic shock such as decrease in intravascular blood volume, decrease/absence of lividity, and/or subendocardial hemorrhages of the left ventricle [102, 103].

Injuries due to terminal collapses with individuals with deteriorating medical conditions may suggest an assault [104] but their distribution focused on the prominent areas of the face can help distinguish between the two.

Fractures

The medicolegal meaning of fractures in the elderly differs compared to infants and children. While in the pediatric population, the manner of death follows very closely from the nature of the injuries, this is not so with the elderly. For example, fractures of long bones and posterior ribs almost always should be investigated further in

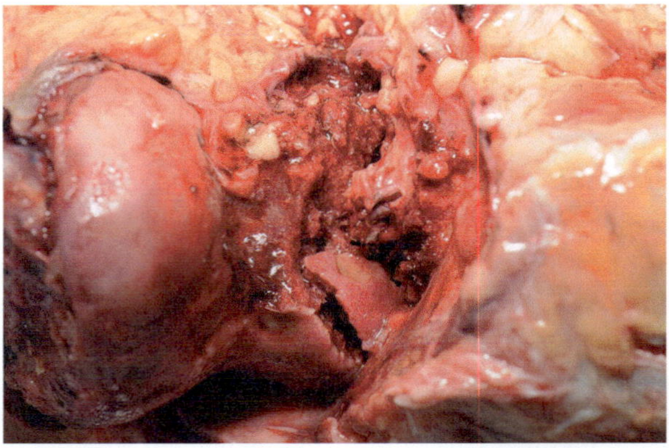

Fig. 15.9 Fracture of the distal femur in an elderly person that was bed bound. No medical attention was sought by caregivers

non-ambulatory infants. A fracture of the hip or a fracture of the vertebrae may not be. Fractures that raise suspicion of abuse include fractures of the mid and lower face, including avulsed teeth [105] and spiral fractures [106].

Fractures as an indication of physical abuse can also pose a serious dilemma. The occurrence of so-called spontaneous fractures of the long bones in older nursing home patients can be misleading as an indicator of abuse [107, 108]. Fractures that occur with or without the degree of trauma that is typically required to cause a bone break can occur in the vertebrae and pelvis and rarely long bones [107–110]. Fractures of the vertebrae often occur in the setting of osteoporosis or osteopenia. However, fractures of long (limb) bones, such as the humerus, ulna, femur, tibia, and fibula, are not typically seen in individuals with osteoporosis but can occur in the setting of prolonged periods of being bed bound (Fig. 15.9). Turning or transfers in individuals with prolonged bed rest are referred to as long bone insufficiency fractures [111]. Recognition that they are a complication of prolonged bed rest, as a form of disuse atrophy, may lessen accusations of abuse or neglect. Torque forces in the context of bones with decrease mass and quality can result in long bone fractures [108]. However, these long bone insufficiency fractures of the humerus are less frequent as there is less torque of the upper limbs on transfer [108].

Burns

Injuries that are concerning for elder maltreatment include [112–115]

Signs and Symptoms of Elder Maltreatment:

- Inadequate supervision of an adult who is seriously mentally impaired at the time of injury.
- Delay in seeking treatment of a burn injury.
- An injury that is not consistent with the story described or conflicting reports of injury.
- Scalds with clear-cut immersion lines and with no splash marks.

- Scalds that involve the anterior or posterior half of an extremity and/or the buttocks and genitals, or a flexion pattern.
- The nature of the fire indicates the decedent did not have the physical and/or cognitive capacity to perform.
- Inadequate supervision of an individual who is physically and cognitively impaired.
- Delay in seeking treatment of a burn injury.

Burns can be mistaken as pressure injuries, Stevens–Johnson syndrome, and Staphylococcal infection.

Traumatic Alopecia

Hair pulling, traumatic alopecia, is a possible sign of elder maltreatment [116]. Normal patterned hair loss typically occurring at the vertex or frontotemporal regions (e.g. frontal fibrosing alopecia) is common but diffuse hair loss can also occur in men and can be observed in elderly women. Hair loss in atypical areas may represent traumatic alopecia.

Sexual Abuse

Sexual abuse is the least reported form of elder maltreatment and is reported to represent less than 1% of abuse [117–119]. Further, elder sexual abuse is perhaps the most understudied and least well-understood form of elder abuse [120–123]. Sexual abuse can occur in the home and in institutionalized residences. Disabled elders who are unable to independently bathe and toilet are particularly vulnerable [124]. Like other forms of abuse, elder sexual abuse can cause physical harm [125, 126]. Sexual abuse includes genital injuries, human bite marks, imprint injuries such as fingermarks, bruising on the thighs, buttocks, breasts, and anogenital injuries. A normal aging process in among woman is the level of estrogen decreases and makes them prone to anogenital injuries due to increased vaginal dryness, thinning of genital tissues and tissue friability. When sexual abuse is suspected, DNA samples are taken for further analysis. In the setting of injuries, the injuries ought to be documented with photo and consider histological sampling. Concerns for sexually transmitted disease require microbiological or virological sampling.

Bite marks are a patterned form of blunt force injury and are curvilinear bruises and abrasions and sometimes lacerations. These require proper evaluation and documentation by a forensic dentition and a DNA sample obtained.

Vaginal bleeding is suspicious, as are certain patterns of bruising to the abdomen and pelvis. Bite marks on breasts and genitalia. Elderly who are incapable of rendering consent due to cognitive deficiencies are vulnerable to sexual abuse [127].

Signs and Symptoms of Sexual Abuse:

- Bruises around the breasts or anogenital areas
- Unexplained venereal disease or genital infections
- Unexplained vaginal or anal bleeding

Considerations of mimics of anogenital injury include lichen sclerosus.

Ancillary Investigations: Toxicological & Radiological Investigations

The role of toxicology may help asses for the presence of improper medication(s), over- and under-medication. Medications that are designated for elderly patients may be misappropriated by formal and informal caregivers for personal use, street sale or with-held for other non-medically indicated reasons. Over-medicating is the administration of an excessive amount of medicines that are not according to instructions. It can be used as a means of behavioral modification can cause central nervous system depression and respiratory depression that can lead to pulmonary thromboembolism and pneumonia and ultimately death. Under-medicating is the refusal or limiting to administered medicine. The absence of medications can be due to multiple causes including non-compliance and withholding of medications.

With multiple chronic illness among older adults, as a cohort they are prone to take multiple medications. Older patients utilize prescription and non-prescription medications, and the improper use of these medications can lead to cognitive impairment and even death. Polymedicine is the use of multiple medications for the treatment of multiple comorbid conditions [128]. Toxicological studies in addition to medical records and an understanding of pharmacokinetics are helpful. Due to the high prevalence of medical conditions, older people take approximately three times as many prescription medications compared to younger patients [128]. Utilizing multiple medications increases the risk of adverse drug events. A long-term care home study found that the rate of adverse drug events is double in patients taking nine or more medications compared to those taking less [129]. In addition, polypharmacy is the use of more medications than are medically necessary [130]. This includes duplicative similar medications, drug-to-drug interactions, and insufficient attention to pharmacokinetic and pharmacodynamic principles, medications that are not indicated, not effective or constitus a therapeutic duplication [128, 131]. Polypharmacy occurs among nearly half of elderly individuals [131]. Approximately, 40% of hospitalized elderly and 35% of outpatients experience an adverse drug event. Among long-term care homes, drug classes that are associated with adverse drug reactions include anticoagulants, non-steroidal anti-inflammatory drugs, cardiovascular medications, diuretics, antibiotics, anticonvulsants, benzodiazepine, and hypoglycemic medications [131]. In addition, polypharmacy may result in an increased risk of *in vitro* synthesis of concerning substances. For example, the metabolite specific for heroin use is 6-monoacetymorphine (6-MAM). The detection of 6-MAM without a history of heroin use may lead to the erroneous determination of elder maltreatment if the formation of 6-MAM in gastric contents containing both morphine and aspirin is not considered [132].

Given that many elderly will have chronic natural diseases that can be observed at autopsy. The majority of older adults at autopsy will often exhibit a chronic, potential cause of death, often of cardiovascular origin such coronary artery atherosclerosis. Attributing death to an anatomical cause, in the absence of appropriate toxicological analysis may result in misclassification of the cause and manner of death [133]. Given the prevalence of multiple comorbidities and associated possible polypharmacy highlights the importance of detecting and quantifying prescription and non-prescription medication levels in toxicology testing.

Polypharmacy can also be used as a form of restraints in older adults. Chemical restraints are drugs administered for the purposes of discipline or conveniences and not required for the treatment of a resident's medical condition [94]. Common medications used for chemical restraint include haloperidol, lorazepam, loxapine, clonazepam, diazepam, acetaminophen with codeine and diphenhydramine [134]. In a Finnish study that examined elderly patients in long-term hospital cares, 53% of patients had 3 or more psychotropics regularly and irregularly, respectively. The use of psychotropic drugs was used to control the behavior of patients and the lack of documentation of the effects implicated that psychotropics were used as a chemical restraint [94]. Utilization of psychotropic medications and other drugs, such as opioids, serotonergic, and anticholinergic drugs can cause side effects, such as extrapyramidal symptoms that may mimic symptoms of agitation [94]. In addition, the concomitant use of many of these medications can induce behavioral problems, such as smearing with feces and urine [94]. Further, administration of psychotropics is considered inappropriate to manage the side effects of these medications [94].

Scene

As society and individuals deal with this rapidly growing cohort of older adults within the general population, this change will result in greater pressures for families and residential institutions the inevitable task of establishing long-term care arrangements for seniors. Providing care for chronically diseased and disabled seniors, without appropriate systemic and individual planning will inevitable increase the incidence of neglect.

Death Scene Examination

The domicile that elder abuse and neglect can occur can be broadly divided into domestic elder abuse and institutional abuse. Domestic settings include residential homes and retirement homes. Institutional settings can include a wide-range of settings including hospitals, adult day care facilities, geriatric units, group homes, long-term care facilities, which include nursing homes and homes for the aged. Circumstantial and scene findings require careful investigation to evaluate elder maltreatment.

Institutional Deaths

The prevalence of maltreatment is reported to be higher among older adults requiring care, especially those residing in long-term care facilities. In an American survey, 24.3% of elderly relatives reported at least one incident of physical abuse by nursing home staff in the last year [135]. In rural China, more than 1/3 of elderly people reported elder abuse, with caregiver neglect being one of the most common type of abuse [136]. Dementia also appears to be an independent risk factor for elder abuse [137–139]. Patients with dementia that exhibit disruptive behavior are particularly at risk of physical abuse [140]. In addition, disabilities [141, 142] and chronic health problems [143] contribute to increase dependence on caregivers and thus risk of elder maltreatment.

The role of institutionalized homes for seniors will have a greater role in society as the population has an extended life expectancy resulting in an increasing number of geriatric patients in their final years requiring advanced care. The percentage of older individuals that live in long-term care homes ranges from 4 to 7% in developed and developing countries [144, 145]. Among those aged 65–69 years this was about 1% and for seniors aged 85 and over was 29.6% [145]. The standard of care provided in institutions for older adults is under increasing scrutiny by the government and the community. Long-term care homes are a type of residential care facility that provide permanent and short-term 24-hour nursing care and are predominantly composed of the elderly population. Reasons for admission to a nursing home are variable and include declining health, limited/no support from caregivers, and increased dependence [29].

The majority of nursing home residents are elderly and reside in institutions because of increase dependence due to negative changes financially and/or health. As the worldwide population ages, this will be reflected as an increasing numbers of long-term care home residents. All manners of death in nursing homes are possible and all forms of elder maltreatment are possible in institutional deaths. However, most are attributed to natural causes. Deaths in long-term care homes are, for the most part, natural and usually do not fall under the jurisdiction of the local death investigation system. Unless, there is concerned for (1) resident on resident violence, (2) drug overdose due to either (i) drug mix-up, (ii) does mix-up, (iii) allegations/confessions of long term care home staff giving medications to cause death, (iv) euthanasia, (3) asphyxia due to (i) bedrails, (ii) restraints, (iii) falls, (iv) running water, including hot water and (4) neglect.

Ibrahim and colleagues conducted a descriptive epidemiological analysis of premature of nursing home residents in Australia that has documented an increased incidence of premature and potentially preventable deaths of nursing home residents [29]. Most of the non-natural deaths were related to falls, choking, and suicides. In addition, the majority of nursing home deaths were not investigated because of the high prevalence of disease among residents. However, part of the lack of investigation may be due to concealment of non-natural deaths [146].

Prevalence of institutional maltreatment is challenging without incorporating postmortem data. In Arkansas, all deaths in nursing homes are investigated by the medical death investigation system which show that nursing home records can contain misleading data or omit important data and antemortem surveys by government oversight do not identify all serious deficiencies, such as preventable weight loss and pressure injuries [147].

Another challenge to identifying deaths that require death investigation oversight, is when there is a delay between the injury and death as the older person may linger in hospital subsequently dying from complications from the injury but also because of the fickleness of memory, among other things, their death goes unrecognized as related to the injury. Consequently, the death may not enter the death investigation system. Resident on resident violence is often physical, verbal, and sexual abuse that occurs between long-term home care residents. Elderly homicide victims are more likely to suffer a lingering death than younger victims [148]. This delay has the risk of doubting the causal link between injury and death and amnesia about why the individual was brought to hospital.

Drug Overdose

Most drug overdose deaths in the care of trained professionals are inadvertent; however, there are rare cases of intentional administration of medications. Long-term care home residents can be given either too much medication or the wrong medication. When deaths due occur from medication mix-up, the death may be missed as drug-related and misattributed to natural causes. Often, when these cases do not fall within the jurisdiction of the death investigation, the onus lays with employees of the long-term care homes. In addition, advances in policy, regulation, and technology are means to reduce medication errors.

Serial Killers/Homicides

Serial homicides are relatively rare and as such can present with many significant challenges due to this rarity to link a series of homicides to a single accused [149]. Identification of serial homicides is challenging because of its rarity, limited understanding of the subpopulation of serial killers, limited physical evidence, absence of personal relationship between offender and decedent, and inadequate communication between different law enforcements and judicial jurisdictions [149]. Although, there is lack of consensus on a definition, serial killers and serial homicides are defined as 2 or more deaths by homicide over a period of time and over temporal separation between the events committed by the same offender(s) in a civilian context [150, 151]. The civilian context is included to exclude military actions and political assassinations by terrorists groups. The death investigation and postmortem findings of two or more decedents may share characteristic or forensic evidence (i.e., DNA of the offender(s) suggesting the possibility that their deaths were committed by the same offender(s)). Serial homicides is differentiated from mass murders, which is defined as four or more murders that occur in a single event with no distinctive time lapses between the deaths or spree-killing, which is at least two deaths without an emotional cooling off period [152]. Forensic psychology research on serial killers is fraught with challenges; however, a common feature appears some degree of sexual behavior in relation to some or all of their murders but not all are sexually motivated [153]. This element of sexual behavior is not usually described among healthcare serial killers. The causes of death, disposal of bodies, and characteristics of the decedent in serial murders are variable between and within those who kill serially [153]. Features that a single autopsy may indicate serial homicides include dismemberment, cleaning of the genital areas, anogenital injuries, burning, administration of drugs, placement of items in the orifices and display the decedents bodies in a gruesome and offensive ways but these are uncommon features in single homicide-related offences [153, 154]. The autopsy is a tool that must be used in concert with other death investigative methods to ascertain serial homicides.

Healthcare serial killer, also referred to as caregiver associated serial killings (CASKs) [155], is a poorly understood but increasingly identified issue; however, the scale of deaths can be greater, in part because of the privileged position and access to medicines and trusting patients. Healthcare workers are in positions that allow for prolonged periods undetected. Further, the causes of deaths are typically donot result in physical injuries; there are no signs of struggle or wounds present [156]. The deaths typically attract little attention because the patients may be vulnerable, terminally ill, unable to communicate because of their young age or too ill [156]. However, many patients that die from CASK are ambulatory and have intact cognitive capacity [155]. Examples of CASK include Dr. Harold Shipman, a 54-year-old general practitioner who was found guilty of the death of 15 patients with a lethal injection of heroin may have murdered 260 to 450 patients in total [156] and Dr. Michael Swango who reportedly killed 60 patients across several American states and Africa [156]. Registered nurses have also confessed to killing multiple patients over multiple hospitals and long-term care homes [155]. Suspicions may be aroused when there is a cluster of cardiopulmonary arrests and deaths that occur in a particular population [155]. The common methods used include injection of insulin, potassium chloride, epinephrine, paralyzing agents (i.e., succinylcholine or Pavulon), opiates, and cardiac medications (i.e., digoxin or lidocaine) and air embolus, drowning, oral medications, tampering with equipment, and suffocation [155]. Many of these methods are difficult to determine postmortem. For example, a fatal administration of potassium chloride unreliable to detect in autopsy samples as potassium levels normally increases in the postmortem period. A retrospective analysis of the hospital samples taken at the time of arrest and analysis of syringes with traces of concentrated potassium chloride and the decedent's DNA can be considered. Similarly, hypoglycemia due to exogenous insulin administration is challenging to determine in the postmortem context [157, 158]. The magnitude of patient deaths due to healthcare serial killers demands systemic changes that track adverse patient events associated with the presence of a specific healthcare worker (physician, nurse, and allied healthcare worker), quality assurance and changes in control of all medicines beyond opioids.

Manner of Death

Recognizing elder maltreatment requires a multidisciplinary death investigation that can include law enforcement, pathologists, paramedics, institutions, and other physicians, while incorporating scene and circumstantial findings. There is a tendency to write off the death of an older adult as inevitable. It is argued that because of a patient's conditions (e.g., bedridden, incontinence, inability to perform ADL), then it is expected that they will become malnourished, develop contractures and pressure injuries. With proper nursing care, pressure injuries would be prevented or minimised, the elderly would have access to nutritious meals, even if bedridden.

Among German nursing homes, the prevalence of pressure injuries is up to 25% and is dependent on the individual risk profiles of the individual [73]. In cases of septicemia and bacteremia, for the causality to pressure injury the micro-organism in the blood most correlate with the bacteria in the pressure injury and the exclusion of other infectious foci. Pressure injuries are an example of a disease that if occurs in the setting of elder maltreatment a manner of homicide can be considered.

The increased frequency of multiple comorbidities and frailty that is among older adults make death investigation a challenge as it is difficult to discriminate between disease progression from non-natural causes of death, including complications of care and remote trauma.

Fatal elder abuse is characterized by the following criteria:

- An act of commission and/or omission toward an older person
- Demonstrable physical harm to the older person
- Causal link between caretaker behavior and harm to the older person
- Determination that the abuse and/or neglect is sufficiently severe related to the cause of death

Summary

Seniors often have numerous underlying medical problems, and functional dependencies and are assumed to be more vulnerable to stressors causing death. Thus, when a senior dies their death is rarely carefully scrutinized, if at all, regardless of risk factors or indications of possible abuse or neglect. In addition, old age often brings medical conditions and physiological attributes that may mimic or mask the markers of elder abuse and neglect, further complicating the analysis and detection. Consequently, the current state of medical science and forensic science in abuse and neglect among older adults is about where child abuse was in 1970s, when medical disciplines began to look at whether or not there were diagnostic injuries in child abuse and neglect [5].

There is increasing global awareness that some older people die as a result of maltreatment. Further, elder maltreatment can coexist with other conditions that make determination of fatal elder maltreatment a challenge for the forensic pathologist. In addition, cases of elder maltreatment are a challenge to ascertain due to a lack of guidelines, paucity of instruction and awareness, and many cases of elder maltreatment may be passing as accidents or natural deaths.

Death investigators have an important role in identifying fatal elder maltreatment. These are reportable deaths, and death investigators have a role of informing relevant stakeholders of features of elder maltreatment. To capture fatal elder maltreatment may require expanding what are reportable deaths. This may include removal of the requirement to not report all natural causes of death in institutions. This change may increase documentation of deaths that are misclassified as natural cause deaths because of diagnostic minimization of the significance of illnesses or contributing injury-related factors. The multiple comorbidities and fragility that often accompanies the elderly cohort make it difficult to demarcate disease progression from sudden and unexpected causes of death, including complications of care and non-recent trauma.

References

1. Butler RN. Ageism: another form of bigotry. Gerontologist. 1969;9(4):243–6.
2. Brostoff P, et al. The public interest: report No.6 "Beating up" on the elderly: police, social work, crime. Aging Human Dev. 1972;3(4):319–22.
3. Burston GR. Granny-battering (letter). BMJ. 1975;3:592.
4. Dong et al. Elder self-neglect and abuse and mortality risk in a community dwelling. JAMA 2009;302(5):517-526.
5. Steigel L. Recommendations for the elder abuse, health, and justice fields about medical forensic issues related to elder abuse and neglect: special report. J Elder Abuse Neglect. 2006;18(1):41–80.
6. National research council. Elder mistreatment: abuse, neglect and exploitation in an aging America. Washington, DC: National Academic Press; 2003.
7. Dyer CB, Connolly MT, McFeeley P. The clinical and medical forensics of elder abuse and neglect. In: National Research Council (US) Panel to Review Risk and Prevalence of Elder Abuse and Neglect
8. Jones JS. Elder abuse and neglect: responding to a national problem. Ann Emerg Med. 1994;23:845–8.
9. The National elder abuse incidence study. The National Center on Elder Abuse, 1998
10. Lachs M, Pillemer KA. Elder abuse. N Engl Med. 2015;373:1947–56.
11. Callahan JJ elder abuse: some questions for policymakers. Gerontologist 1988; 28(4), 453-458.
12. Pedrick-Cornell C, Gelles RJ. Elder abuse: the status of current knowledge. Family Relations. 1982;3:457–65.
13. Salend E, et al. Elder abuse reporting: limitations of statues. Gerontologist. 1984;24(1):61–9.
14. Cooper C, Selwood A, Livingstone G. The prevalence of elder abuse and neglect: a systematic review. Age Ageing. 2008;37:151–60.
15. Into the light: national survey on the mistreatment of older Canadians, 2015. National Initiative for the Care of the Elderly. pp. 1–136

16. AMA Council on Scientific Affairs: elder abuse and neglect. JAMA. 1987;257:966–71.
17. What is elder abuse? Action on Elder Abuse Bulletin, 1995, 11 (May-June) and adopted by the International Network for the Prevention of Elder Abuse (IPNEA) and World Health Organization is "a single, or repeated act, or lack of appropriate action, occurring within any relationship where there is an expectation of trust, which causes harm or distress to an older person" (World Health Organization (WHO). The Toronto declaration on the global prevention of elder abuse/Geneva: WHO; 2002.
18. Collins KA, Presnell SE. Elder neglect and the pathophysiology of aging. Am J Forensic Med Pathol. 2007;28:157–62.
19. Dumont-Smith C. Aboriginal elder abuse in Canada. Aboriginal Healing Foundation; 2010.
20. Brennan S. Victimization of older Canadians; 2009.
21. Juristat article. Stats Canada; 2012:85-002-X.
22. Shields L, Hunsaker D, Hunsaker J. Abuse and neglect: A ten-year review of mortality and morbidity in our elders in a large metropolitan area. J Forensic Sci. 2004;49(1):122–7.
23. Collins KA, Presnell SE. Elder homicide. Am J Forensic Med Pathol. 2006;27:183–7.
24. Schiamberg LB, Barboza GG, Oehmke J, Zhang Z, Griffore RJ, Weatherill RP, et al. Elder abuse in nursing homes: an ecological perspective. J Elder Abuse Negl. 2011;23(2):190–211.
25. McDonald L, Beaulieu M, Harbison J, Hirst S, Lowenstein A, Podnieks E, et al. Institutional abuse of older adults: what we know, what we need to know. J Elder Abuse Negl. 2012;24(2):138–60.
26. Buzgová R, Ivanová K. Elder abuse and mistreatment in residential settings. Nurs Ethics. 2009;16(1):110–26.
27. Frazão SL, et al. Physical abuse against elderly persons in institutional settings. J Forensic Legal Med. 2015;36:54–60.
28. Centers for disease control and prevention. Trends in aging—United States and wordlwide. MMWR. 2003;52:101–6. http://www.cdc.gov/mmwr/PDF/wk/mm5206.pdf
29. Ibrahim JE, et al. Premature deaths of nursing home residents: an epidemiological analysis. MJA. 2017;206(10)
30. Wolf R. Elder abuse and neglect causes and consequences. J Geriatric Psychiatry. 1997;30(1):153–74.
31. Dong X, et al. Association of cognitive function and risk of elder abuse in a community-dwelling population. Dement Geriatr Cogn Discord. 2009;302(5):517–26.
32. Laumann EO, et al. Elder mistreatment in the United States: prevalence estimates from a nationally representative study. J Gerontol B Psychol Sci Soc Sci. 2008;63(4):S248–54.
33. Dong X, et al. Elder self-neglect and abuse and mortality risk in a community dwelling population. JAMA. 2009;302(5):517–26.
34. Lachs MS, et al. The mortality of elder mistreatment. JAMA. 1998;280:428–32.
35. Hoyert DL. The changing profile of autopsied deaths in the United States, 1979–2007. NCHS data brief. 2011;(67):1–8.
36. Gruszecki AC, et al. Investigation of elderly deaths in nursing homes by the medical examiner over a year. Am J Forensic Med Pathol. 2004;25(3):209–12.
37. CDC and Prevention. Characteristics of elderly nursing home current residents and discharges. Adv Data. 2000;312:1–15.
38. Isaac CV, et al. An investigative tool for detecting elder abuse. Acad Forensic Pathol. 2014;4(4):524–31.
39. Esmail A. Physician as serial killer—the shipman case. NEJM. 2005;352:18.
40. Ayus JC, Arieff AI. Abnormalities of water metabolism in the elderly. Sem Nephrol. 1996;16:277–88.
41. Walston JD. Sarcopenia in older adults. Curr Opin Rheumatol. 2012;24(6):623–7.
42. Giles TE, Williams AR. The post-mortem incidence of senile ecchymoses. Am J Forensic Med Pathol. 1994;115:208–10.
43. Malone M, et al. The epidemiology of skin tears in the institutionalised elderly. J Am Geriatrics Soc. 1991;39:591–5.

44. Danesh BS, Chang ALS. The role of the dermatologist in detecting elder abuse and neglect. J Am Acad Dermatol. 2015;73:285–93.
45. National Center for Chronic Disease Prevention and Health Promotion, CDC. Chronic disease notes and reports: special focus. Healthy Aging. 1999;12:3.
46. Cipriani G, et al. Violent and criminal manifestations in dementia patients. Geriatr Gerontol Int. 2016;16:541–9.
47. Byard RW, Tsokos M. Forensic Issues in cases of diogenes syndrome. Am J Forensic Med Pathol. 2007;28:177–81.
48. Macmillan D, Shaw P. Senile breakdown in standards of personal and environmental cleanliness. BMJ. 1966;ii:1032–7.
49. Cooney C, Humid W. Review: diogenes syndrome: age. Aging. 1995;24:451–3.
50. Clark ANG, et al. Diogenes syndrome: a clinical study of gross neglect in old age. Lancet. 1975;i:366–8.
51. Self-neglect by older adults. Health Canada; 1999
52. Cole AJ, et al. A case of self neglect in a married couple: "Dogenes" à deux? Int J Geriatr Psychiatry. 1992;7:839–41.
53. Esposito D, et al. Diogenes syndrome in a pair of siblings. Can J Psychiatry. 2003;48:571–2.
54. Spear J, et al. Diogenes' syndrome and folie à deux in a married couple. Psychiatr Case Rep. 1997;2:53–7.
55. Seiler WO, Stahelin HB. Malnutrition in the elderly. New York: Springer; 1999.
56. Mowe M, Bohmer T. The prevalence of undiagnosed protein-calorie undernutrition in a population of hospitalized elderly patients. J Am Geriatr Soc. 1991;39:1089–92.
57. Kelly IE, et al. Still hungry in hospital: identifying malnutrition in acute hospital admissions. Q J Med. 2000;93:93–8.
58. Mion LC, et al. Nutritional assessment of the elderly in the ambulatory care setting. Nurse Practitioner Forum. 1994;5:46–51.
59. Sullivan DH. The role of nutrition in increased morbidity and mortality. Clin Geriatr Med. 1995;11:661–74.
60. Thomas DR. Causes of protein-energy malnutrition. In: Seiler WO, Stahelin HB, editors. Malnutrition in the elderly. New York: Springer; 1999. p. 59–68.
61. Chen CC, et al. A concept analysis of malnutrition in the elderly. J Adv Nurs. 2001;36(1):131–42.
62. Roy BV. The role of malnutrition in the failure to thrive syndrome. In: Watson RR, editor. Handbook of nutrition in the aged. Boca Raton, FL: CRC Press; 1994. p. 303–8.
63. Braunwald E, Isselbacher KL, Petersdorf RG, Wilson JD, Martin JB, Fauci AS, editors. Rudman D. Protein and energy undernutrition. In Harrison's Principles of Internal Medicine. McGraw-Hill, New York, 1987. Pp 393-397
64. Saunders MJ. Nutrition and oral health in the elderly. Dental Clin North Am. 1997;41:681–98.
65. Schiffman S. Taste and smell losses in normal aging and disease. J Am Med Assoc. 1997;278:1357–62.
66. Morley JE. Anorexia of aging: physiologic and pathologic. Am J Clin Nutr. 1997;66:760–73.
67. Coe JI. Postmortem chemistries on human vitreous humor. Am J Clin Pathol. 1969;51:741–0.
68. Coe JI. Some further thoughts and observations on post-mortem chemistries. Forensic Sci Gazette. 1973;4:2–5.
69. Coe JL. Postmortem chemistry update. Am J Forensic Med Pathol. 1993;14:91–117.
70. Bryan CS, et al. Bacteremia associated with decubitus ulcers. Arch Intern Med. 1983;143:2093–5.
71. Galpin JE, et al. Sepsis associated with decubitus ulcers. Am J Med. 1976;61:346–50.
72. Tsokos M, et al. Pressure sores: epidemiology, medicolegal implications and forensic argumentation concerning causality. In J Legal Med. 2000;113:283–7.
73. Heinemann A, et al. Medicolegal aspects of pressure sores. Legal Med. 2003;5:S263–6.
74. Galpein JE, et al. Sepsis associated with pressure ulcers. Am J Med. 1976;61:346–50.
75. Rothchild JM, et al. Preventable medical injuries in older patients. Arch Int Med. 2000;160:2717–28.

76. Barbenel JC, Jordan MM, Nicol SM, Clark MO. Incidence of pressure-sores in the greater Glasgow health board area. Lancet. 1977;2:548–50.
77. Barrois B, Allaert FA, Colin D. A survey of pressure sore prevalence in hospitals in the greater Paris region. J Wound Care. 1995;4:234–23.
78. Shea JD. Pressure sores: classification and management. Clin Orthop Relat Res. 1975;12:89–100.
79. Reid J, Morrison M. Classification of pressure sore severity. Nurs Times. 1994;90(20):46–50.
80. Hitch S. NHS Executive Nursing Directorate—strategy for major clinical guidelines-prevention and management of pressure sores, a literature review. J Tissue Viability. 1995;5(1):3–24.
81. Agency for health Care and Research. Pressure ulcers in adults: prediction and prevention. Rockville, MD: AHCPR; 1992.
82. EPUAP. Guidelines on the treatment of pressure ulcers. EPUAP Rev. 1999;2:31–3.
83. Alok K, et al. Magnetic resonance imaging for diagnosing foot osteomyelitis: a meta-analysis. Arch Intern Med. 2007;167:125–32.
84. Borgstrom PS, et al. Radiography of pressure ulcers. Acta Radiol. 1988;29(Fasc 5):581–4.
85. Lewis, et al. The diagnosis of osteomyelitis in patients with pressure sores. Plast Reconstr Surg. 1988;81:229–32.
86. Darouchie RO, et al. Osteomyelitis associated with bed sores. Arch Intern Med. 1983;143:683–8.
87. Sugarman B. Pressure sores and underlying bone infection. Arch Intern. 1987;147:553–5.
88. Sugarman B, et al. Osteomyelitis associated with pressure ulcers. Ach Intern Med. 1983;143:683–8.
89. Heinemann A, et al. Medico-legal aspects of pressure sores. Legal Med. 2003;5:S263–6.
90. Tsokos M, et al. Pressure sores: epidemiology, medico-legal implications and forensic argumentation concerning causality. Int J Legal Med. 2000;113:283–7.
91. Turk EE, et al. Autopsy-based assessment of extent and type of osteomyelitis in advanced-grade sacral decubitus ulcers: a histopathologic study. Arch Pathol Lab Med. 2003;127:1599–602.
92. Turk EE, et al. Autopsy-based assessment of extent and type of osteomyelitis in advanced-grade sacral decubitus ulcers: A histopathological study. Arch Pathol Lab Med. 2003;127:1599–602.
93. Wyandt MA. A review of elder abuse literature: An age old problem brought to light. California J Health Promotion. 2004;2(3):40–52.
94. Nurminen J, et al. The use of chemical restraints for older long-term hospital patients: a case report from Finland. J Elder Abuse Neglect. 2009;21:890104.
95. Hantikainen V. Physical restraint: a descriptive study in Swiss nursing homes. Nurs Ethics. 1998;5:330–46.
96. Hamers JPH, Huizing AR. Why do we use physical restraints in the elderly. Z Gerontol Geriat. 2005;38:19–25.
97. Karger B, et al. Fatalities related to medical restraint devices-asphyxia is a common finding. Forensic Sci Int. 2008;178(2-3):178–84.
98. Wiglesworth A, Austin R, Corona M, Schneider D, Liao S, Gibbs L, Mosqueda L. Bruising as a marker of physical elder abuse. J Am Geriatr Soc. 2009;57(7):1191–6.
99. Langlois NEI, Gresham GA. The ageing of bruises: a review and study of the colour changes with time. Forensic Sci Int. 1991;50:227–38.
100. Singer AJ, Clark RAF. Cutaneous wound healing. N Engl J Med. 1999;341:738–46.
101. Robertson I, Hodge PR. Histopathology of healing abrasions. Forensic Sci. 1972;1:17–25.
102. Cluroe AD. Superficial soft-tissue injury. Am J Forensic Med Pathol. 1995;16:142–6.
103. Cebelin MS, Hirsch CS. Human stress cardiomyopathy. Myocardial lesions in victims of homicidal assaults without internal injuries. Hum Pathol. 1980;11:123–32.
104. Hamilton JR, et al. Fatal hemorrhages from simple lacerations of the scalp. Forensic Sci Med Pathol. 2005;4:267–72.
105. Fenton SJ, et al. Orofacial considerations for pediatric adult, and elderly victims of abuse. Emerg Med Clin North Am. 2000;18:601–17.

106. Schor JD. Geriatric assessment in the diagnosis and treatment of elder abuse. N J Med. 1995;92:108–10.
107. Kane RS, Goodwin JS. Spontaneous fractures of the long bones in nursing home patients. Am J Med. 1991;90:263–6.
108. Chen GI, Garcia MB. Spontaneous fractures in nursing homes. Proc UCLA Healthcare. 2014;18:1–2.
109. Rodondi A, Chevalley T, Rizzoli R. Prevalence of vertebral fracture in oldest old nursing home residents. Osteoporos Int. 2012;23(11):2601–6.
110. Benzinger P, Becker C, Kerse N, Bleibler F, Büchele G, Icks A, Rapp K. Pelvic fracture rates in community-living people with and without disability and in residents of nursing homes. J Am Med Dir Assoc. 2013;14(9):673–8.
111. Martin-Hunyadi C, Heitz D, Kaltenbach G, Pfitzenmeyer P, Mourey F, Vogel T, Niederberger B, Kiesmann M, Berthel M, Kuntzmann F. Spontaneous insufficiency fractures of long bones: a prospective epidemiological survey in nursing home subjects. Arch Gerontol Geriatr. 2000;31(3):207–14.
112. Bowden ML. The elderly, disabled and handicapped adult burned through abuse and neglect. Burns Incl Therm Int. 1988;14(6):447–50.
113. Greenbaum AR, et al. Burn injuries inflicted on children or the elderly: a framework for clinical assessment. Plast Reconstr Surg. 2006;118(2):46e–58e.
114. Krob MJ, et al. Burned-and-battered adults. J Burn Care Rehabil. 1986;7:529.
115. Purdue GF, Hunt JL. Adult assault as a mechanism of burn injury. Arch Surg. 1990;125:268–9.
116. Gray-Vickrey P. Recognising elder abuse. Nursing. 1999;29:52–3.
117. AMA Council on Scientific Affairs. Elder abuse and neglect. JAMA. 1987;257:966–71.
118. AMA White paper on elderly health: report of the Council on Scientific Affairs. Arch Intern Med. 1990;150:2459–72.
119. Swagerty DL Jr, et al. Elder mistreatment. Am Fam Physician. 1999;59:2804–8.
120. Ramsey-Klawsnik H. Elder abuse: preliminary findings. J Elder Abuse Neglect. 1991;3(3):73–90.
121. Burgress A, et al. Sexual abuse of nursing home residents. J Psychosoc Nurs. 2000;38(6):10–8.
122. Holt M. Elder sexual abuse in Britain: preliminary findings. J Elder Abuse Neglect. 1993;5(2):63–71.
123. Teaster P, et al., et al. Sexual abuse of older adults: Preliminary findings of cases in Virginia. J Elder Abuse Neglect. 2000;12(3/4):1–16.
124. Ramsey-Kawsnik H. Elder sexual abuse within the family. J Elder Abuse Neglect. 2003;15(1):43–58.
125. Ramsey-Klawsnik H. Dynamics of sexual assault/abuse against people with disabilities and the elderly. In Wisconsin Coalition Against Sexual Assault. Widening the circle: Sexual assault/abuse and people with disabilities and the elderly. Madison WI, author 1998
126. Ramsey-Klawsnik H. Assessing physical and sexual abuse in health care settings. In: Baumhover LA, Beall SC, editors. Abuse, neglect, and exploitation of older persons. Baltimore: Health Professions Press.
127. Pillemer K, Finkelhor D. The prevalence of elder abuse: a random sample survey. Gerontologist. 1988;28:51–7.
128. Monane M, et al. Optimal medication use in elders: key to successful aging. Successful aging. West J Med. 1997;167:233–7.
129. Nguyen JK, et al. Polypharmacy as a risk factor for adverse drug reactions in geriatric nursing home residents. Am J Geriatric Pharmacother. 2006;4:36–41.
130. Tija, et al. Studies to reduce unnecessary medications use in frail older adults: a systematic review. Drugs Aging. 2013;30:285–307.
131. Maher RL, et al. Clinical consequences of polypharmacy in elderly. Expert Opin Drug Saf. 2014;13(1) https://doi.org/10.1517/14740338.2013.827660.
132. Naso-Kaspar CK. In vitro formation of acetylmorphine from morphine and aspirin in postmortem gastric contents and deionised water. J Anal Toxicol. 2013;37:500–6.

133. Yang E, et al. 5-year retrospective review of diltiazem associated deaths. Research and reviews. J Hosp Clin Pharm. 2017;3(3):1–4.
134. Kow JZ, Hogan DB. Use of physical and chemical restraints in medical teaching units. CMAJ. 2000;162(3):339–40.
135. Sciamberg LB, Oehmke J, Zhang Z, Barboza GE, Griffore RJ, Von Heydrich L, et al. Physical abuse of older adults in nursing homes: a random sample survey of adults with an elderly family member in a nursing home. J Elder Abuse Neglect. 2012;24:65–83.
136. Wu L, Chen H, Hu Y, Xiang H, Yu X, Zhang T, et al. Prevalence and associated factors of elder mistreatment in a rural community in People's Republic of China: a cross-sectional study. PLoS One. 2012;7(3):e33857.
137. Cooper C, Selwood A, Blanchard M, Walker Z, Blizzard R, Livingston G. Abuse of people with dementia by family carers: representative cross sectional survey. BMJ. 2009;338:b155.
138. Dyer CB, Pavlik VN, Murphy KP, Hyman DJ. The high prevalence depression and dementia in elder abuse or neglect. J Am Geriatr Soc. 2000;48:205–8.
139. Hansberry MR, Chen E, Gorbien MJ. Dementia and elder abuse. Clin Geriatr Med. 2005;21:315–32.
140. McDonald L, Collins A. Abuse and neglect of older adults: a discussion paper. Family Violence Prevention Unit. Health Canada; 2000. p. 1–82.
141. Ansello EF, O'Neill P. Abuse, neglect, and exploitation: consideration in aging with lifelong disabilities. J Elder Abuse Neglect. 2010;22:105–30.
142. Laumann EO, Leitsch SA, Waite LJ. Elder mistreatment in the United States: prevalence estimates from a nationally representative study. J Gerontol Ser B Psychol Sci Soc Sci. 2088;63:S248–54.
143. Lowenstein A, Eisikovits Z, Band-Winterstein T, Enosh G. Is elder abuse and neglect a social phenomenon? Data from the First National Prevalence Survey in Israel. J Elder Abuse Neglect. 2009;21:253–77.
144. Kane RL, Kane RA. Long-term care in six countries: implications for the United States. Washington, DC: United States Department of Health, Education and Welfare; 1976.
145. Statistics Canada. Living arrangements of seniors. Census in brief; 2011.
146. Corey TS, et al. Unnatural deaths in nursing homes. J Forensic Sci. 1992;37(1):222–2227.
147. GAO. Nursing home deaths: Arkansas coroner referrals confirm weakness in state and federal oversight of quality of care. Report to Congressional Requesters, pp. 1–74; 2004.
148. Block CR. Homicide against or by the elderly in Chicago 1965-2000. Homicide Studies. 2013;17(2):154–83.
149. Campobass CP, et al. A serial killer of elderly women: analysis of multi-victim homicide investigation. For Sci Int. 2009;185:e7–11.
150. Sturup J. Comparing serial homicides to single homicides: a study of prevalence, offender and offence characteristics in Sweden. J Investig Psychol Offender Profil. 2018:1–15.
151. Wilson W, Hilton T. Modus operandi of female serial killers. Pschol Reports. 1998;82:495–8.
152. Marono AJ, et al. A behaviour sequence analysis of serial killers; livers: from childhood abuse to methods of murder. Psychiatr Psychol Law. 2020;27(1):126–37.
153. Beasley JO. Serial murder in America: case studies of seven offenders. Behav Sci Law. 2004;22:395–414.
154. Promish DJ, Lester D. Classifying serial killers. For Sci Int. 1999;105:155–9.
155. Yorker BC, et al. Serial murder by healthcare professionals. J Forensic Sci. 2006;51(6) https://doi.org/10.1111/j.1556-4029.2006.00273.x.
156. Kaplan R. The clinicide phenomenon: an exploration of medical murder. Austr Psychiatry. 2007;15(4):299–304.
157. Marks V, Teale JD. Hypoglycemia: factitious and felonious. Endocrinol Metab Clin Nort h Am. 1999;28(3):579–601.
158. Pounder DJ, Jones GR. Postmortem drug redistribution—a toxicological nightmare. Forensci Sci Int. 1990;45(3):253–63.

Index

A
Abdominal injuries, in children, 358
Accidental sharp force injuries, 246
Accountability for Reasonableness (A4R), 68
Activities of Daily Living (ADL), 406
Acute fatty liver of pregnancy, 380
Acute intraparenchymal hemorrhages, 155
Acute ischemic injury, 135
Adipocere formation (saponification), 14
Age of maturity of baby, 342
Age-related diseases
  bone disease, 402
  dementia, 402
  neurodegenerative disorders, 402, 404
    Alzheimer's disease, 404, 405
    frontotemporal lobar degenerations, 405
    Lewy body disease, 405
  subdural hemorrhage, 402
Aging, physiology of, 400, 401
Air embolism, 383
Algor mortis, 13
Alzheimer's disease, 404, 405
Ammunition, 287, 291
  See also Firearms
Amniotic fluid embolism, 378
Anal transition zone, 277
Anatomical Gift Act of 1968, 72
Anatomy of the courtroom, 105–107
Anemia, 389
Anesthesia, complications of, 391
Anogenital anatomy, 270
Anogenital injury
  causation, 270
  consensual and non-consensual sexual activity, 269
  prevalence, 269
Antemortem injury, 193
Anterior neck structure, forensic anatomy of, 257, 259
Aortopathy, 131
Arrhythmic death, 134–137
Asphyxia
  chemical, 249–251
  mechanical, 252
  positional, 256
  signs of, 249
  traumatic, 256
Asphyxial death, 137–139
Asphyxiating gas, 252
Assaults
  cause of death
    commotio cordis, 221–222
    commotio medullaris, 222
    homicide by heart attack, 221
    oculocardiac reflex, 221
  craniocerebral trauma, 218
  head trauma, 217, 218
  TBSAH, 220–221
Assistant Crown Attorney, 98
Asthmatic bronchitis, 388
Atlanto-occipital (AO) junction, 213
Autoerotic asphxyia, 261
Autolysis, 14
Autopsy, 15–17, 319
  report, 24
  See also Negative medicolegal autopsy

R. Jacques (ed.), *Forensic Pathology*, https://doi.org/10.1007/978-3-031-42038-2

B
Behcet's arteritis, 132
Benzodiazepines, 174
Bereavement, 36
Biochemical and metabolic death, 140
Bioethical theories, 68
Bioethics, 53, 55, 57–59, 68, 83, 89
Biological female anatomy
  vagina, 272
  vulva, 270–272
Birdshot, 288
Birth related injuries, 346
  fractures, 347
  scalp injuries, 346
  subdural and retinal haemorrhage, 347
  subgaleal hematoma, 347
Bleeding death, 143, 144
Bleeding disorders, 389
Blunt impact trauma, neck, 267
Blunt trauma
  acute injuries
    external, 191
    internal, 192
  assaults
    cause of death, 221
    craniocerebral trauma, 218
    head trauma, 217, 218
    TBSAH, 220–221
  CPR, 223, 224
  descent from heights, 222
  external examination, 189
    antemortem injury, 193–194
    degree and direction of force, 195
    patterned injuries, 196–198
    perimortem, 193
    postmortem, 193
  falls from standing height, 214–215
  fat embolism syndrome, 225–226
  injury interpretation, 190
  MVCs
    cervical spine, 212–214
    chest trauma (*see* Chest trauma)
    craniocerebral trauma, 208–212
    injury patterns, 198
    lower extremity injuries, pedestrians, 198–200
  past medical history, 191
  radiographic findings, 190
  scene visitation or review, 191
  skin wounds, 189
Bone diseases, age-related, 402
Bristol inquiry, 58, 75, 76, 78
Bruising, in elderly population, 401, 415
Buckshot, 288
Burns and fire-related deaths
  artifacts, 310
  body surface area, 308
  chemical burns, 311
  contact burns, 311
  depth of burn, 309–310
  in elderly population, 416, 417
  scald, 311

C
Caffey disease, 362
Canadian Inquiry, 58
Carbon monoxide, 250, 251
Carboxyhemoglobin, 250
Cardiac diseases, 387
Cardiomyopathies syndrome, 136
Cardiopulmonary resuscitation (CPR), 223, 224
Cartridge cases, 289, 291
Case history, 83
Cause of death, 8
Cellular death, 12
Central neuraxial blockade complications, 391
Cerebral amyloid angiopathy (CAA), 155
Chemical asphyxia, 249
  carbon monoxide, 250, 251
  cyanide, 251
  hydrogen sulfide, 251
Chest trauma
  chest wall fractures, 202–203
  first-generation air bags, 201
  hemoperitoneum, 203
  hemorrhagic shock, 206
  hemothorax, 203
  pelvis, 207–208
  pneumothorax, 201
  retroperitoneal hemorrhage, 205–206
  thoracolumbar spine, 206
Child abuse, 351, 352
  abdominal injuries, 358
  burns, 355
  head injuries, 356–358
  medical mimics, 359–364
  and neglect, 352
  osseus (skeletal) injuries, 355, 356
  skin injuries, 354
  thoracic injuries, 358
Chop wounds, 243
Chronic alcoholics, 214
Clavicle fractures, 347
Clinical, academic/hospital autopsy, 17

Close range
of gunshot wounds, 296
of shotgun wounds, 299
Closed pressure injury, 412
Coagulation disorders, 360
Cocaine, 173
Code of ethics, 54, 58, 69–70
Collagen vascular disease, 140
Colorectal zone, 277
Commotio cordis, 221–222
Commotio medullaris, 222
Communitarian ethics, 66, 67
Conducted electrical weapon (CEW), 316
Connective tissue disorders, 361
Consciousness criterion, 71
Consequentialist ethics, 63, 64
Conservation of momentum, 187
Contact range
of gunshot wounds, 296
of shotgun wounds, 299
Contractures, 413
Coronary artery anomaly, 133
Coroner system, 5
COVID-19, 138
Courtroom testimony
anatomy of the courtroom, 105–107
criminal versus civil cases, 97–99
doctors as witnesses, 100–103
notification of court appearance, 105
oral evidence, 119–121
oral testimony, 111–114, 116
steps of the examination, 116, 118, 119
structure of the court system, 96
testimony, preparation of, 107–110
trial and adversarial system, 99
Craniocerebral trauma
brain retention, 208
cerebral edema and herniation, 211–212
DAI and DVI, 209
HIE, 209–211
scalp wound, 208
skull fracture, 208
Cricoid cartilage, 259
Criminal justice system, 16
Criminal vs. civil cases, 97–99
Crown attorney, 98
Crown counsel, 98
Cyanide, 251

D

Day of Expert Testimony (Oral Evidence), 109, 110
Death, cause of, 322
additional autopsy findings, 332
continuum of evidence, 322
definitely fatal acute or perimortem pathological findings, 322, 324
non-definitive/non-specific pathological findings, 325
potentially fatal acute/perimortem pathological findings, 324
potentially fatal chronic pathological findings, 324
undetermined/negative medicolegal autopsy, 326
Death certificate, 6, 391
Death, in elderly population, manner of, 423
Death investigation, 11, 12, 55, 57–61, 63–69, 73–78, 83, 86–90, 319
autopsy, 15–17, 24
bioethics, 54–59, 61, 67, 90
duties, 55, 56
ethical paradigms and institutional relationships, 56
non-traditional physician–patient relationship, 57
pathology ethics, 57, 58
procedural trust, role of, 56
public inquiries, 58
cause of death, 8
continental system, 6
coroner system, 5
death certificate, 6
experience of loss, 34–36, 38, 39, 41, 43–47
forensic pathology, 18–20
histology, 21, 22
identification, 7
manner of death, 10
mechanism of death, 11
medical examiner, 6
photography, 25, 27
quality assurance and peer review, 29, 30
social determinants of health, 31, 32, 34
Death scene examination, 419
drug overdose deaths, 421
institutional abuse/deaths, 420, 421
Deaths in infancy, 349, 350
Decomposition, 13
Defence pathologist, 103, 104
Defensive injuries, 245, 246
Dehydration, in elderly population, 401
Dementia, 402
Deontology ethics, 63
Diatom studies, 255

Diffuse axonal injury (DAI), 209
Diffuse vascular injury (DVI), 209
Diogenes syndrome, *see* Self-neglect
Direct examination, 117
Direct maternal death, 371
Disseminated intravascular coagulation (DIC), 385
Distant range, of shotgun wounds, 299
DNA analysis, 279
Doctors as witnesses, 100–103
Drowning, 253–255
Drug interactions, 176–177
Drug overdose deaths, 421
Drug-related deaths
  analytical testing, 170
  autopsy finding, 163
  history, 163
  interpretation of results
    alcohol concentration, 177–178
    benzodiazepines, 174
    cocaine, 173
    drug interactions, 176–177
    drug tolerance, 174, 175
    ethanol concentrations, 173
    GHB concentrations, 174
    hospital vs. forensic alcohol testing, 178
    pharmacogenomics, 175
    postmortem alcohol interpretation, 177–179
    postmortem redistribution, 172
    stability, 172–174
    subdural or epidural hematomas analysis, 179
    tetrahydrocannabinol (THC), 174
    trauma and blood transfusion effect, 179
  opioid crisis, 180
  sample collection
    blood, 167
    gastric contents, 168
    liver, 168
    urine, 167
    vitreous fluid, 168
  sample submission, 169
  scene, 163
Drug tolerance, 174, 175
"Duret" hemorrhages, 211

E
Eclampsia, 378
Ectopic pregnancy, 372, 373
Ehlers-Danlos syndrome (EDS), 361
Elder abuse
  prevalence, 399
  problem, 399, 400
  signs, 400
Elder maltreatment, 397, 399, 400
  See also Physical abuse
Electrocution, 313–316
Endocrine death, 139, 140
Entrance vs. exit gunshot wounds, 292, 294
Environmental injuries
  burns and fire-related deaths
    artifacts, 310
    body surface area, 308
    chemical burns, 311
    contact burns, 311
    depth of burn, 309–310
    scald, 311
  electrocution, 313–316
  handheld conducted electrical weapon, 316
  mechanism of death, 309, 312–313
  mechanism of injury, 312
  temperature-related deaths, 303–305
Ethical dilemma, 54, 55, 59–63, 66, 67, 70, 83, 89
Ethical frameworks, 67–68
Ethical theory, 61–67, 89
  communitarian ethics, 66, 67
  consequentialist, 63, 64
  deontology, 63
  principilism, 64
  virtue ethics, 61–63
Ethics, 53–54, 63–64, 66–68, 80–82
Examination in chief, 117
Exhumation, 31, 32
Expert witness, 55, 59, 70, 80–82, 101
External male genitalia
  anus, 277, 279
  penis, 275
  perineum, 276
  scrotum, 276
External neck compression, blunt impact trauma, 267
External neck injuries, 264, 265
Extrinsic factors of injury
  conservation of momentum, 187
  first law of motion, 187
  second law, 187
  third law, 187

F
Fact witness, 100

Families, benefits for, 16
Family Indigenous Liaison Units (FILU), 48
Family Liaison Units, 48
Fatal elder abuse characterisation, 423
Fat embolism syndrome, 225–226
Female genital cutting, 274, 275
Female genital mutilation, 274, 275
Firearms
  anatomy and function, 283, 285
  classification, 285
  cylinder and muzzle gap, 300
  injuries, 292, 294
  kinetic energy and wounding, 291
First-generation air bags, 201
Flame burns, 311
Flash burns, 311
Floatation test, 343, 344
Forensic pathologists
  action, 84, 85
  consequences, 85
  context, 87
  moral agent, 84
Forensic pathology, 18–20
Fractures, 266, 267
Fractures in elderly population, 415, 416
Frontotemporal lobar degenerations (FTLD), 405

G

Gamma-Hydroxybutyric Acid (GHB), 174
Gauge, 285
Genetic criterion, 71
Gestational diabetes mellitus, 385
Gestational trophoblastic disease, 387
Gettler chloride test, 255
Gomez classification, 353
Goudge inquiry, 58
Government-sponsored medicolegal death investigation, 3
Graze gunshot wound, 300
Grief and mourning, 36
Gunshot residue (GSR), 291
Gunshot wounds
  entrance *vs.* exit, 292, 294
  entry, pathological range, 294–298
  graze, 300

H

Handguns, 285
Handheld conducted electrical weapon, 316
Hangings, 260–262
Head injuries, in children, 356–358
Healthcare and legal systems, 55, 87
HELLP syndrome, 378
Hematologic diseases, 389, 390
Hemolytic uremic syndrome (HUS), 385
Hemoperitoneum, 203
Hemorrhages, 266
Hemorrhagic shock, 206
Hemothorax, 203
Hepatic disorders, 380
Homicides, 11
Hot-tubbing, 122
Humanitarian forensic action, 34
Hydrogen sulfide, 251
Hydrostatic test, 343, 344
Hyoid bone, 258
Hyopthermia, in elderly population, 401
Hyper IgE syndrome, 364
Hyperthermia, 305, 401
Hypothermia, 303–305
Hypoxic ischemic encephalopathy (HIE), 209–211

I

Immunological/inflammatory death, 140, 141
Incidental maternal death, 371
Incised-stab wounds, 243
Incised wounds, 237, 241–243
Indeterminate/distance range, of gunshot wounds, 298
Indeterminate range, of shotgun wounds, 299
Indigenous communities, 88
Indirect maternal death, 371
Infarct involving the insular cortex, 156
Infectious death, 138–139
Infectious diseases, 386
Injured female anatomy, tissue management of, 274
Injury classification, 187–188
Instrumental Activities of Daily Living (IADL), 406
Intermediate range, of gunshot wounds, 297
Intermediate wounds, 300
Internal airway obstruction, 256
Internal neck injuries, 265, 267
Intracranial hemorrhages, 154
Intrahepatic cholestasis of pregnancy, 380
Intraparenchymal hemorrhages, 154
Intraventricular tumors, 156

J
Judicial colloquia, 122

L
Larynx (voice box), 258
Latrogenic-induced death, 145, 146
Lesions involving medulla, 156
Lewy body disease (LBD), 405
Ligature strangulation, 262, 263, 265
Liquid chromatography–tandem mass spectrometry (LC–MS-MS), 170
Livor mortis, 12

M
Maceration, 14, 341, 342
Malnourishment, in children, 352, 353
Manner of death, 10
Manual strangulation, 262, 264
Markula Center for Applied ethics, 68
Maternal death
 associated with pregnancy
  embolic disorders, 382, 385
  endocrine disorders, 385
  gestational trophoblastic disease, 387
  infectious diseases, 386
  pregnancy-associated cardiac disorders, 380, 381
  thrombotic microangiopathies of pregnancy, 385
 direct, 371
 exacerbated by pregnancy
  cardiac diseases, 387
  hematologic diseases, 389, 390
  neurologic disorders, 390
  pulmonary diseases, 388
 incidental, 371
 indirect, 371
 unique to pregnancy, 372
  ectopic pregnancy, 372
  hepatic disorders, 380
  placenta abruption, 374
  placenta previa, 373, 374
  postpartum hemorrhage, 376
  pregnancy-induced hypertension, 377
  pregnancy-specific embolic disorders, 378
  uterine rupture, 374
 unnatural, 391
Maternal mortality, 369, 371
Mechanical asphyxia, 252
 asphyxiating gases, 252
 drowning, 253–255
 environmental/entrapment, 252
 internal airway obstruction, 256
 plastic bag asphyxia, 252
 smothering (external airway obstruction), 252, 253
Mechanism of death, 11, 259
Medication-induced death, 145
Medicine and public health, 16
Medicolegal autopsy, 58, 68, 73, 75, 76, 89
Medicolegal/forensic autopsy, 17
Metabolic diseases, 364
Morality, 53, 54, 69
Morals, 53–54
Moral status, 70–72, 74
Motor vehicle collisions (MVCs)
 cervical spine, 212–214
 chest trauma (*see* Chest trauma)
 craniocerebral trauma, 208–212
 injury patterns, 198
 lower extremity injuries, pedestrians, 198–200
Multiple gunshot wounds, 300
Mummification decomposition, 14
Murdered Indigenous Women (MMIW) Inquiry, 75

N
Natural death
 arrhythmic death, 134–137
 asphyxial death, 137–139
 biochemical and metabolic death, 140
 bleeding death, 143, 144
 endocrine death, 139, 140
 Iatrogenic-induced death, 145, 146
 immunological/inflammatory death, 140, 141
 infectious death, 138–139
 medication-induced death, 145
 neoplastic deaths, 144
 obstructive death, 139
 occlusive thrombotic and infarction death, 142, 143
Neck compression, 257
 hanging, 260–262
 strangulation, 264, 265
Neck injuries
 external, 264, 265
 internal, 265, 267
Negative medicolegal autopsy
 case type, 321
 decedent characteristics, 321

incidence, 319, 320
pathologists experience, 320
recommended conditions, 335
reexamination approach, 328
ancillary investigations, 331
external examination, 330
history and circumstances, 328–330
internal examination, 330
Neglect, 406
contractures, 413
dehydration, 409
malnutrition, 408
poor hygiene, 413
pressure injuries, 409–413
Neoplastic deaths, 144
Neurological determination of death, 12
Neurologic disorders, 390
Nitrobenzodiazepines, 174
NOK Clinic Meeting/Post Autopsy Family Conference, 47
Non-central blockage regional anesthetic complications, 391
Non-malignant gastric ulceration, 133
Nonspecific interstitial pneumonitis (NSIP) disease, 141
Nontraumatic uterine rupture, 374
Notification of court appearance, 105
Novel psychoactive substances (NPS), 170

O

Oath taking, 116
Obstructive death, 139
Occlusive thrombotic and infarction death, 142, 143
Oculocardiac reflex, 221
Oral evidence, 119–121
Oral testimony, 111–114
Organ and tissue donation for transplantation, 77–78
Organ retention, 57, 58, 67, 78, 79, 81, 85, 86
Osseus (skeletal) injuries, 355, 356
Osteogenesis imperfect (OI), 362
Osteopathy of prematurity, 363
Over-medication, 418

P

Parkinson's disease (PD), 156
Pathologist experience, in medicolegal autopsy, 320
Patterned skin injuries, 354
Pediatric forensic pathology, 339
Pediatric pathology and deaths, 339
Perianal skin, 278
Perinatal postmortem examination
placenta, 347, 349
separate existence determination, 340
extra-uterine elements in gastrointestinal tract, 343
hydrostatic test, 343, 344
inflammatory response, 343
maceration, 342
maturity estimation, 342, 343
non-viable congenital/placental anomalies, 344
stillbirth, 340
Peripartum cardiomyopathy, 380
Peripartum myocarditis, 381
Petechial haemorrhages, 263, 264
Photography, 25, 27
Physical abuse, 413
bruises, 415
burns, 416, 417 (*see also* Elder abuse)
fractures, 415, 416
restraints, 414, 415
sexual abuse, 417, 418
traumatic alopecia, 417
Physical restraints, 414
Pituitary insufficiency, 385
Placenta abruption, 374
Placenta, examination of, 347, 349
Placenta previa, 373, 374
Plastic bag asphyxia, 252
Polycystic adult kidneys, 133
Polymedicine, 418
Polypharmacy, 418, 419
Positional asphyxia, 256
Postmortem changes, 12
Postmortem examination, 128–130
Postmortem redistribution, 172
Postpartum hemorrhage, 376
Practice of morality, 53
Preeclampsia, 377
Pregnancy, 369
Pregnancy-associated cardiac disorders, 380, 381
Pregnancy-associated spontaneous coronary artery dissection, 381
Pregnancy-induced hypertension, 377
Pregnancy-specific embolic disorders, 378
Pressure ulcers, in elderly population, 409–411
Pre-testimonial meeting, 108
Primary arrhythmia syndromes, 136
Primary methemoglobinemia, 251
Primary pulmonary hypertension, 388

Principilism, 62, 64–66
Prinsloo-Gordon artefact, 266
Professional ethics, 54, 65, 82
Professionalism, 54
Psychotropic medications, 419
Public condemnation, 83
Pulmonary blastomycosis, 132
Pulmonary thromboembolism, 382, 383
Purpura, in elderly population, 401
Putrefaction, 14

Q
Quadrupole time-of-flight mass spectrometry (QTOF-MS), 170

R
Radiological investigations, in elderly population, 418, 419
Radiology, 22
Reasonable doubt, 98, 102, 118
Research, in forensic pathology, 88, 89
Restraints, 414, 415
Retroperitoneal hemorrhage, 205–206
Rickets, 363
Rifles, 285
Right atrial cardiac myxoma, 132
Rigor Mortis, 13
Risk of attornment, 102
Rotational force (torque), 187

S
Sacroiliac joint widening, 207
Sarcopenia, 401
SARS-CoV-2 infection, 138
Scalp injuries, 346
Scientific investigations, 88
Scientific uncertainty, 121
Scientific Working Groups for Medicolegal Death Investigation (SWGMDI), 35
Secondary methemoglobinemia, 251
Self-neglect, 406
  contractures, 413
  dehydration, 409
  malnutrition, 408
  poor hygiene, 413
  pressure injuries, 409–413
Serial killers/ homicides, 421–423
Sexual abuse, in elderly population, 417, 418
Sharp force injuries
  accident, suicide, or homicide, 244, 246
  ancillary investigations, 244
  chop wounds, 243
  decomposed and embalmed bodies, 247
  defensive injuries, 245, 246
  history and scene findings, 233–237
  incised wounds, 241–243
  mechanism of death, 246, 247
  morphology, 237–248
  stab wounds
    corners/angles, 237
    edges of, 237
    features of, 240
    knives, 241
Shored exit wound, 292
Shotgun shells, 287, 289
Shotgun slug, 289
Shotgun wounds
  entry, pathological range in, 298–300
  injury related to wadding, 300
Siderophages, 215
6-Monoacetymorphine (6-MAM), 418
Skin injuries, 354
Skull fractures, 347
Smothering (external airway obstruction), 252, 253
Social criterion, 71
Social determinants of health, 31
Social recognition, 54
Somatic death, 12
Spinal cord injury can occur in adults and children without radiological evidence (SCIWORA), 214
Squamous zone, 277
Stab wounds
  edges of, 237
  features of, 240
  knives, 241
Stillbirth, identification, 346
Strangulation, 262, 264, 265
Strontium, 255
Structure of the court system, 96
Structured Learning In Clinical Ethics (S.L.I.C.E.), 68
Subarachnoid hemorrhages (SAH), 154
Subdural and retinal haemorrhage, 347
Subdural hemorrhage (SDH), 215, 402
Subgaleal hematoma, 347
Sudden death, central nervous system (CNS) disorders
  intracranial hemorrhages, 154
  MSA patients, 156
  SUDEP
    causes, 146

general autopsy findings and toxicology, 148
molecular pathology, 152–153
neuropathology, 148–152
Sudden infant death syndrome (SIDS), 349, 350
Sudden unexpected death in epilepsy (SUDEP), 146
causes, 146
general autopsy findings and toxicology, 148
molecular pathology, 152–153
neuropathology, 148–152
Suspected laryngohyoid injuries, tissue management of, 267

T

Taphonomy, 14
Temperature-related deaths, 303–305
Testimony, preparation of, 107–110
Tetrahydrocannabinol (THC), 174
Theory of morality, 53
Thomas A. Swift's Electric Rifle (TASER), 316
Thoracic injuries, in children, 358
Thoracolumbar spine, 206
Thrombocytopenia, 389
Thrombophilias, 390
Thrombotic thrombocytopenia purpura (TTP), 385
Tissues, 186
TORCH infections, 349
Toxicological deaths, in younger pediatric populations, 364
Toxicological investigations, in elderly population, 418, 419
Transparent and accountable process, 80
Traumatic alopecia, 417
Traumatic asphyxia, 256
Traumatic Basal Subarachnoid Hemorrhage (TBSAH), 220–221
Traumatic uterine rupture, 376
Trier of fact, 107
Trier of law, 107
Triticerous cartilage, 259, 268
Trophoblastic tissue embolism, 378
Truth Telling, 47

U

Under-medication, 418
Unnatural maternal death, 391
Urine alcohol concentration (UAC), 177
Uterine rupture, 374
Utilitarianism, 64

V

Vagina, 272
Venous bleeding, 208
Venous thromboembolism, 390
Virtue ethics, 61–63
Virtue theory, 61
Vitreous biochemistry, 21
Voir dire, 101, 113
Vulva, 270–272

W

Waterlow classification, 353
Witness, 104
World Health Organization, 75
Wounds, 185
bullet/firearm injuries, 291 (*see also* Gunshot wounds; Shotgun wounds)
intermediate, 300

Z

Zone of coagulation, 312
Zone of hyperemia, 312
Zone of stasis, 312

MIX
Papier aus verantwortungsvollen Quellen
Paper from responsible sources
FSC® C105338

If you have any concerns about our products,
you can contact us on
ProductSafety@springernature.com

In case Publisher is established outside the EU,
the EU authorized representative is:
Springer Nature Customer Service Center GmbH
Europaplatz 3, 69115 Heidelberg, Germany

Printed by Libri Plureos GmbH
in Hamburg, Germany